Stuttering

Stuttering

Its Nature, Diagnosis, and Treatment

Edward G. Conture

Vanderbilt University

Allyn and Bacon

Boston • London • Toronto • Sydney • Tokyo • Singapore

Executive Editor: Stephen D. Dragin
Editorial Assistant: Barbara Strickland
Senior Editorial-Production Administrator: Joe Sweeney
Editorial-Production Service: Walsh & Associates, Inc.
Composition Buyer: Linda Cox
Manufacturing Buyer: Chris Mason
Cover Administrator: Brian Gogolin

Copyright 2001 by Allyn & Bacon
A Pearson Education Company
160 Gould Street
Needham Heights, MA 02494

www.abacon.com

Library of Congress Cataloging-in-Publication Data

Conture, Edward G.
    Stuttering : its nature, diagnosis, and treatment / Edward G. Conture
        p. cm
    Includes bibliographical references and index.
    ISBN 0-205-31924-6
    1. Stuttering.   I. Title
RC424.C575   2000
616.85'54 — dc21   00-040594

Printed in the United States of America

10   9   8   7   6   5   4   3   2   1   04   03   02   01   00

To People Who Stutter and the People Who Care About Them

CONTENTS

Preface   xvii

Acknowledgments   xix

1 Introduction   1

What Is the Purpose of This Book?   1

Not a Cookbook   2

Learning from Rather Than Hiding Our Mistakes   3

Relative Versus Absolute Descriptions of "Stuttering" and "Stutterer"   3

What Is Stuttering?   4

Stuttering Versus People Who Stutter   4

The Role of Listener Judgments   7

Speakers Differ; So Do Listeners   7

How Do We Measure Stuttering?   8

Frequency of Disfluency as a Means of Differentiating   9

Type of Speech Disfluency as a Means of Differentiating   10

Physical Effort, Tension, and Avoidance Associated with Stuttering: The "Effortless-Avoidance" Continuum   12

Norms to Establish Whether a Person Stutters   13

The One Constant About Stuttering Is Change   14

What Nonspeech Behaviors Are Associated with Stuttering?   15

What Are Some Basic Generalizations About Stuttering?   15

Some Relatively Safe Generalizations About Stuttering   17

Cures Are for Hams and Other Edibles   22

What Are the Characteristics of People Who Stutter?   23

Why Do People Stutter (Subtitled, What Causes Stuttering)?   26

Lay Opinion About Cause   26

Professional Opinions About Cause   26

Theories of Stuttering   27

Temporal Misalignment: One Essential Aspect of Many Modern-Day Theories of Stuttering   38

The Assembly Line: An Analogy for Mismatches Within the Person Who Stutters   40

Mismatches Between People Who Stutter and Their Environments   45

Nature Interacting with Nurture: One Source of Mismatches   46

**General Orientation Toward the Treatment of Stuttering
and People Who Stutter   48**
**How to Talk About Stuttering When Speaking with Clients
and/or Families   50**
An Example Is in Order   50
Recognizing Differences in People and Behavior   51
Sometimes Cub Scouts Are More Important Than Speech-
Language Therapy   52
What Is the Point?   53
Tolerating Differences in People and Behavior   53
Intolerance for Individual Differences in the Ability to Communicate   53
Individuals Stutter but They Are Still Individuals   54
We Typically Don't See What We Typically See   54
Enthusiasm for Changing People and Behavior   55
The Common Cold and Stuttering   55
Rationales Versus Recipes   56
Certainty in an Uncertain World   57
Summary   57

2   Assessment and Evaluation   59

Some Basic Beliefs That Guide Our Assessment Procedures   60
Gaining Perspective on the Client's Unique Circumstances   60
Examining the Examiner   60
Facilities   61
Equipment   62
Audio Recordings   62
Video Recordings   63
Informed Consent or the Client's Right-to-Know   64
Components of the Stuttering Evaluation   64
The Intake Form   65
The Interview Procedure: Areas and Types of Inquiry   66
Assessing Communicative and Related Behaviors   78
Fluency   78
(In)formal Tests of Stuttering   91
Expressive/Receptive Language (Syntax)   96
Expressive/Receptive Language (Vocabulary)   97
Voice   99
Hearing   102
Reading   103
Academic Abilities and Status   104
Attention Deficit Hyperactivity Disorders (ADHD)   105

Tourette's Syndrome   107

Neuromotor Speech and Nonspeech Behavior   108

Word Finding   110

Psychosocial Adjustment   111

Temperament   115

Who Is and Who Is Not Referred for Therapy   118

General   120

Those at Moderate Risk for Continuing Stuttering   120

Those at Low to No Risk   121

Children   122

Parents and Relatives of Children   122

Older Clients: Those Who Need Therapy   123

Older Clients: Those for Whom Treatment Is Uncertain   124

Those Who Appear to Stutter in Their Heads Not Their Mouths   124

Older Clients: Those Who Have Problems Other Than Stuttering   125

Some Parting Thoughts   125

Summary   126

3   Remediation: Children Who Stutter   129

Stuttering Is a Disorder of Childhood   129

The Clinician   129

Six Characteristics of Successful Clinicians   130

Problem-Specific Empathy   131

Clinician/Client Reluctance to Deal with Childhood Stuttering   133

Knowing Literature Pertinent to Children Who Stutter   134

Remediating Children May Mean Involvement with Their Parents   135

Talking to Parents About the Cause of Stuttering   136

Parents Generally Want to Do the Right Thing   138

Therapy   138

When to Start, How Long, and How Often   138

Suggested Guidelines   139

Three Issues All Clinicians Encounter   140

Saying the "S" Word   141

Talking to the Child About Talking in General and the Child's
    Talking in Specific   141

The Child's Age in Relation to the Type of Therapy Prescribed   143

Direct Versus Indirect Approaches   143

Age Grouping for Therapy   144

Four Categories of Children Who Receive Services   145

**Young Children with No Communicative Problems Whose
Parents Are Reasonably to Quite Concerned   145**

Parents' Concerns   147

Counseling the Parents and Keeping in Touch   150

Reevaluation of the Child and Keeping in Touch with the Parents   153

Children with Some Stuttering Whose Parents Are Unconcerned   153

Who Knows Who Will Become Fluent and Who Will Continue
to Stutter?   154

Concomitant Speech and/or Language Problems Exhibited by
Children Who Stutter Somewhat   155

Using a Concomitant Problem to Get Therapy Going   156

Dealing with Delays in Language in a Child Who Stutters   157

Dealing with Articulation/Phonological Concerns in a Child
Who Stutters Somewhat   158

The Child Who Begins to Stutter AFTER Therapy for
Articulation Problems   160

The Young Child Who Stutters and Exhibits Speech Sound Problems   161

Young People Who Stutter Who Are Almost or
Completely Unintelligible   161

Dealing with Voice Problems in Children Who Stutter   162

Dealing with Other Problems in Children Who Stutter   163

Modifying the Stuttering of Children Who Exhibit Some Stuttering
but Whose Parents Are Minimally or Completely Unconcerned   166

The Parent/Child Fluency Group   167

**Children with Some Stutterings Whose Parents
Are Also Concerned   177**

Getting Therapy Started   177

Introducing the Concept of Hard and Easy Speech   178

Nature of Communicative Interaction Between Clinician and Client   180

The Child's Communicative Interaction ("Pragmatic" or
Usage) Abilities   181

Parents' Reading to Their Children   183

Deciding When a More Direct Approach Is Warranted   185

**Children with Some to a Great Deal of Stuttering Whose Parents
Are Reasonably to Somewhat Concerned   187**

Try Not to Bug the Children Just Like Their Parents Do   188

Helping the Child Accept a More Active Role in the
Changing of Stuttering   188

Helping Parents Understand That Many Aspects of Speaking
Are out of Sight and Therefore out of Mind   189

Helping Parents Understand What It Feels Like to Stutter   190

The Garden Hose Analogy   193

Helping the Child See, Hear, and Feel Stuttering   205

Helping the Child Understand "Forward Movement" in Speech
(Changing Arresting and Releasing Gestures)   207

Cursive Writing as an Analogy to "Forward Movement" in Speech   208
Trying Not to Turn off Child and Parents to Speech Therapy   210
Referrals to Other Professionals   212
Concluding Remarks   214
Segue into the Land of Teens Who Stutter   215
Summary   215

4   Remediation: Older Children and Teenagers Who Stutter   217

Older Children Are Not Just Older, They Are Different as Well   217
Paralysis Through Analysis   218
**Understanding the Parents of the Older Child and Teenager
Who Stutter   219**
How Older Children Differ in General from Younger Children   220
**How Stuttering Problems of Older Children Who Stutter
Differ from Those of Young People Who Stutter   222**
The Age of the Client Is a Guide Not an Imperative   223
Variations Among Older Children and Teenagers Who Stutter   223
Older Children with Minimal or Little Awareness of Stuttering   224
Awareness of Stuttering: What It Is, What It Means, and How to
Deal with It Therapeutically   224
Matter-of-Fact, Objective Approach Helps Counteract
Negative Aspects of Awareness   226
"Everybody Makes Mistakes" as Another Means for Counteracting
the Negative Aspects of Awareness   227
Use of "Awareness" as a Positive Influence on Changing Behavior   228
Desensitization   228
Beginning to "Desensitize" the Young Client   229
Introducing "Barbs" or Fluency Inhibitors   230
Inattentive Listeners: A Potent but Difficult to Discern
Fluency Disrupter   231
Evaluating Successfulness of Desensitization Approach   232
Encouraging the Child to (Non)verbally Interact with Peers   233
The Gradual Process of Learning or Learning About Learning   233
**Older Children with Definite (Cognitive/Emotional)
Awareness of Stuttering   235**
Motivation   236
Identification   237
Modification   240
Teenagers with Definite Awareness of Stuttering   254
Twelve- to Fourteen-Year-Old People Who Stutter: Turning
the Corner into Adolescence   254
Teenagers' Interest in and Cooperation with Therapy   255

Using Other People to Assist with the Teenager's Therapy Program   256

Differences Between Young Teenagers and the Younger
Child Who Stutters   257

Some "Demographics" Re: Teenagers Who Stutter   257

Planning Therapy: Factors to Consider   260

When to Begin and When Not to Begin Therapy   263

Objectively Changing Speech Behavior   264

Motivating Client to Make Speech Changes   270

Practice and/or Carryover of Change   271

Assessing Changes in Speech Outside of Therapy   273

Related Concerns: Academics, Social Life, and Employment   274

Some Parting Thoughts   279

Clinician as Guide Not Curer   279

Objective Awareness Before Speech Objectively Changes   279

Sometimes Some Kinda Help Is the Kinda Help People Who Stutter
Can Do Without   280

Summary   280

5   Remediation: Adults Who Stutter   283

The General Lay of the Land   283

The Past Many Times Influences the Present   283

Habitual Inappropriate Behavior May Feel More "Normal" Than
Novel, Appropriate Behavior (Subtitle: Better to Deal with a
Known Devil Than an Unknown Angel)   283

Levels of Emotionality   284

Cautious Optimism Is Not the Same as Pessimism   285

Problem Dictates Procedure   285

Late Onset   285

Similarities to Other Problems   286

Referrals from Employers   286

A(Affect), B(Behavior), C's(Cognition) of Stuttering   287

Group Therapy for Adults Who Stutter   289

Adult Fluency Groups   289

Client Reluctance to Participate in Group Therapy   289

Logistics of Group Therapy   290

Composition of Group Members   290

Group Therapy by Itself   291

The SLP as Group Leader   291

Mechanics of Versus Feelings About Speech   291

Individual Therapy for Adults Who Stutter: Starting Up   292

First Impressions   292

How Many Times per Week?   294

Trial Therapy   294
Individual Therapy for Adults Who Stutter: Identification Phase   295
Identifying and Physically Feeling (In)appropriate Behavior   295
"Devices" Used with Identification   296
Adults' Reactions to Identification   296
Amount of Time Spent on Identification per Session   297
Three Early Signs of Improvement   297
Continuing with Identification   298
Off-Line Identification   299
Bridge Between Off-Line and On-Line Identification   301
On-Line Identification   301
Further Reactions to Identification   303
Bridging Between Identification and Modification   304
Spontaneous Modification   305
If Identification Fails to Develop   305
Individual Therapy for Adults Who Stutter: Modification Phase   306
Movement Between Rather Than Movement Within Sounds   306
The Problem Relates to the Nature of Speaker's Speech Behavior
    Not the Nature of Speech Sounds Spoken   307
Where and What to Begin Modifying   307
After and Then During the Instance of Stuttering   309
When the Client Fails to Change   311
When the Client Produces Real Change   312
Within-Therapy Carryover   313
Changing Speech in Conversation   315
Homework or Further Work Outside Therapy   316
Some Client Reactions to Change   317
Knowing When to Dismiss   318
Maintenance/Follow-up Therapy   320
Some Parting Thoughts   322
"This Is What We Think Needs to Be Considered"   322
It's the Therapist, Not Merely the Technique   322
Avoid Being Overly Certain About the Uncertain   323
Summary   323

6 Conclusions   327

Basic Assumptions About Stuttering   327
Evaluation Precedes Remediation   329
Do as I Say Not as I Do: An Example   329
Identification   331
The Importance of Physically Feeling Behavior That Interferes
    with Speech-Language Production   331

The Clinician's Ability to Identify   332

Helping the Client Identify Stutterings Should Not Take the Place
of Helping the Client Learn to Modify Stutterings   333

Doing It "to" Clients Versus Having Them Do It "for" Themselves   333

Modification   334

Behavior Modification   334

How to Behave Before All the Data Are In   335

Being Able to Modify Stuttering Behavior (in the Present) Does Not
Mean We Know What Stuttering Behaviors Need Modifying
(for Future Success)   335

Different Behaviors, Different Etiologies: Different Therapies?   336

Some of the Things We Do Know About STUTTERED
Speech Production   337

Starting with "Simple" and Working Toward "Complex" Behavior   338

Spoken Versus Orthographic Behavior   338

Psyche, Soma, and Their Interaction   339

Transfer   340

SLPs Modify Stuttering but Can People Who Stutter Maintain
the Modification?   340

Carryover Problems Are Not the Exclusive Domain of Stuttering   341

The Need for Pre- Versus Post-Therapy Research   342

Future Directions: General Considerations   344

Change, the One Constant   344

Drowning in a Sea of Information   345

Allowing Information to Cloud Our Judgment   345

Data Are Not Always Reflected in Discussion   346

Science Advances by Small Increments in Knowledge as Much as It
Does by Quantal Leaps   346

It Is Replication by Independent Researchers Not Size of Sample
That Counts in the Long Run   347

Future Directions: Opportunities   348

Children   348

Subgroups   350

Attention Deficit Hyperactivity Disorder (ADHD)   351

Temperament   352

Linguistic Activities and Behavior (e.g., Syntactic, Semantic,
and Phonological Encoding)   354

Concomitant Speech and Language Problems of People Who Stutter   356

Cortical Activity and Structure of People Who Stutter   357

Motor Activity and Behavior (e.g., Temporal Coordination of
Tongue and Jaw Movements During Speech)   360

Transitions   364

Treatment Efficacy   367

Naturalness, Suitability, and Utility of Speech   371

Self-Help Organizations   373

Some Parting Thoughts   375

The Future Is a Carte Blanche We Write on with Hope   375

Two Trains Running in Parallel   375

Nature INTERACTING with Nurture   376

Explicating a Common Thread Gives the Lay Public Something to
Hold onto   376

What Can Be Changed, What Can't, and the Ability to Recognize
the Difference   377

Hammers Versus Swiss Army Pocketknives   378

**Appendix A   Interview Questions for the Parent(s) of
a Disfluent Child   379**

**Appendix B   Note to a Beginning Speech–
Language Pathologist   383**

**Appendix C   An Example of a Diagnostic Report for a
Child Who Stutters   391**

Appendix D   Twelve Minus One Report-Writing Concerns   397

**Appendix E   Ten Common Mistakes Observed During
a Diagnostic   401**

**Appendix F   Children Who Stutter: Suggestions for
the Classroom Teacher   405**

References   407

Author Index   429

Subject Index   437

PREFACE

Hindsight, it is said, is twenty-twenty. After studying and working in the area of stuttering for nearly thirty years, I now believe I may better understand what I don't understand as well as know what I don't know. Looking back to the first edition of this book (published in 1982), I can more clearly see my own growth as well as that of our field. Would that such growth were smooth and linear; however, like most human endeavors, the field's understanding of stuttering as well as my own has lurched from periods of knowledge stagnation to periods of knowledge growth. And, as I suggested in the preface to a previous edition, it would be ". . . nice to see the treatment and understanding of stuttering rapidly advance through a quantum leap in knowledge based on a once-in-a-lifetime discovery, (but) the plain truth is that most disciplines advance through the systematic, albeit slow, accretion of relatively small bits of information" (Conture, 1990b, vii).

With this edition we offer, for the readers' consideration, a window through which they might be able to glimpse, no matter how murky the view, some appreciation for the author's understanding of stuttering. It probably goes without saying that such understanding has been based on countless academic, clinical, and research experiences with stuttering. Certainly, no corner on the market of understanding will be claimed; neither will the reader be spared the author's honest opinions, regardless of their relative (un)popularity. While one should neither disagree merely to disagree or be disagreeable when disagreeing, there is also no apparent reason, after reason has been employed, to fail to share one's opinion. That said, it has been our goal throughout the book, whenever possible, to make the abstract reasonably concrete by using readable but appropriately scholarly expression. Hopefully, we have been relatively successful in achieving this goal.

In many places, the text purposely has one foot in the real world and the other in the best-of-all-possible worlds. Such an approach will, undoubtedly, challenge the thinkers as well as the doers in this field—that is, it will challenge those who study stuttering when all possible variables are controlled and those who treat stuttering when few variables are possible to control. This should not be construed as a John Lennon plea to "come together . . . ," but it is to strongly suggest that without science our practice lacks much of its motivation and without practice, our science is similarly unmotivated. Attempting to have the thinkers consider the great unwashed problems of practice and to have the doers ponder the theoretical questions that must be answered if practice is to ever grow is a large part of what this book is all about. In essence, the book attempts to strike a balance between the formality required by the world of empirical science and the informality necessitated by the realities of the world of clinical services.

This essentially clinically oriented book is intended for advanced undergraduate and graduate-level students as well as beginning clinicians in speech–language pathology who are assessing, evaluating, treating, and trying to further their understanding of stuttering. As with previous editions, the author also believes that more experienced clinicians will find that the book covers various issues that they may want to know more about or review in light of current experience or information. Throughout, we have tried to consider people who stutter as humans first and people who stutter second. Many, many insights into the problem of stuttering are lost, by both researchers and clinicians alike, when the person who stutters is viewed solely through the lens of stuttering. Placing the part of the person called "stuttering" into the whole of the person who stutters called "the person" is the challenge we assumed in writing this text, a challenge the reader will hopefully believe we met.

ACKNOWLEDGMENTS

An old song contains a line something like "you never, ever walk alone . . ." Surely, the same is true of writing a book. You never write alone. When I put fingers to keyboard, or editing pencil to rough draft, I convey what I know and believe through what I have been taught by and learned from teachers, students, colleagues, friends, family, and life. While I want to leave no room for doubt that I accept full responsibility for the text and attribute all mistakes it may contain to myself, I nonetheless owe a great deal to others. In the past, I have acknowledged my instructors at Emerson College and Northwestern University, in particular my mentor, Dr. Dean E. Williams, at the University of Iowa (whom I owe a debt I can never repay). I also acknowledged doctoral students through about 1990. Since that time, in the 1990s, there have been other, equally excellent doctoral students, first at Syracuse and now Vanderbilt Universities—J. Anderson, K. Logan, K. Melnick, M. Pellowski, and J. S. Yaruss—who have been tremendous sources of assistance, inspiration, and information. Teachers influence students and students, in turn, influence teachers; perhaps, like a dance, teachers sometimes lead and sometimes follow the student. And as I've said in this space before, thank you all, my present and former doctoral students and ". . . may you be as fortunate as I and have students as good as you" (Conture, 1990, p. viii).

There are several people I'd like to acknowledge in terms of manuscript preparation: Kathy Rhody, for her incredibly good cheer, patience, and support through countless drafts and corrections; Judy Warren for her assistance with the many pieces of minutiae attendant in such a project; and Tamara Altman for her assistance with the development and illustration of figures. Special thanks to Patricia Kenyon for her love and support throughout and her valuable assistance proofing prose and developing rough drafts of several illustrations. I would also like to acknowledge the assistance of my Vanderbilt University colleagues Christine Adkins, Jennifer Ask, and Jodi Roos for their models of clinical excellence from which I have learned a great deal about the superlative blending of technical/professional and interpersonal skills. I am particularly indebted to my many European/Dutch colleagues, especially Dr. Herman Kolk, but also Drs. Wouter Hulstijn, Herman Peters, Pascal van Lieshout, from whom I learned so much about research, science, and theory during a year's sabbatical leave at the Nijmegen Institute for Cognition and Information, University of Nijmegen, Nijmegen, The Netherlands. We were also fortunate to have the administrative support and encouragement of colleagues in Vanderbilt University's Department of Hearing and Speech Sciences as well as NIH/NIDCD research grant (DC00523) to Vanderbilt University. I am also very appreciative of Kathy Whittier, of Walsh & Associates, Inc., for her incredible attention to detail, insights, and support during the long editorial journey into night of making rough draft become final book. Above all, I would like to thank Steve Dragin, Publisher and Executive Editor, Allyn & Bacon, for his assistance, patience, and support during a project that was, to say the least, a long time coming, interrupted by a sabbatical leave to Europe and a move to another university.

Finally, I would like to acknowledge you, the reader, for you are reason such books are written in the first place. Through many a quandary in writing regarding matters great and small, it was helpful to know that someone, in the end—perhaps with less than a great deal of experience with and knowledge about stuttering—must read my words. Your "presence" was definitely of benefit to me, and as I said before in this space, "may my influence on you be as positive as I felt yours was on me" (Conture, 1990b, p. ix).

1

Introduction

. . . a riddle wrapped in a mystery inside an enigma . . .
—Churchill, 1939

What Is the Purpose of This Book?

It has been said that if one's only tool is a hammer, then everything looks like a nail. For example, if all we understand is physiology, then the only aspects of stuttering we may be willing to examine is the *soma* (i.e., the physiological). Conversely, if all we understand is psychology, then the only aspects of stuttering we may be willing to examine is the *psyche* (i.e., the psychological). Human beings, however, reside at neither the somatic nor psychic poles. Instead, most people generally inhabit the large in-between temperate zones where elements of physiology and psychology jointly reside, interact, and, at times, collide.

Of course, it would be nice if we solely consisted of a psyche or a soma. Then our lives, or at least the lives of people like me, who try to write about people, would be so much simpler! Common sense, however, which is not all that common, tells us that most humans are composed of a complex mixture of soma and psyche. So, wading into this melange of physiological and psychological events, the present writer dares venture—a feat that you can either chalk up to courage or stupidity!

Venturing forth, this writer enters a place where ambiguity, uncertainty, and lack of complete understanding reign. For *ambiguity* comprises the sum and substance, the *sine qua non*, if you will, of much of our everyday "reality." Indeed, stuttering comprises one part of the ambiguous whole that we term "reality." Thus, the part we call "stuttering" is probably going to be at least as ambiguous as the whole we call "reality." And it is reality, I think, that readers of these pages would probably prefer this writer to focus on as he tries to discuss what stuttering is and how we might best diagnose and treat it. Indeed, rigor may be the name, but ridiculous is the game for those with zero tolerance for ambiguity and expectations of invariance when dealing with highly variable events such as human behavior.

Therefore, it is the purpose of this book to discuss the evaluation and treatment of stuttering. I will do this by sharing with the reader approaches to the evaluation and treatment of stuttering that I have found useful as well as the rationale and/or reason for their use and use-fulness. To accomplish these goals I will need to cover four interrelated areas (i.e., research, theory, diagnosis, and therapy), but not necessarily in equal amounts. Why do I need to cover some research and theory in a book whose primary emphasis is on *clinical* assessment and treatment of people who stutter? Certainly, I will not to stray too far from this primary empha-sis, but I will need to cover some relevant research and theory. Such coverage is necessitated by the fact that in many instances, this research and theory strongly influence what we do when we assess and treat stuttering in children, teenagers, and adults. Our clinical practice can-not and should not develop devoid of scientific backing (see Curlee & Yairi, 1997, Ingham & Riley, 1998, for similar discussion). Instead, as much as possible, what we do clinically should be grounded in, enhanced, and motivated by information resulting from objective research.

Further, as the reader of this book will see, some topics that are covered have been thoroughly studied and are quite well understood. Conversely, the reader will also see that other topics are less well understood, still controversial in nature, and often less than thor-oughly studied. More than anything, the present writer hopes to imbue you, the reader, with some of the same curiosity about and interest in stuttering that he has had for over thirty years. Indeed, as I hope to make clear, stuttering touches upon just about every facet of the human condition imaginable: academic, communicative, emotional, neurological, psycho-logical, physiological, social, and vocational (see Blood & Conture, 1998). Because stut-tering involves many aspects of the human condition, those who study and treat stuttering have an opportunity to develop their understanding beyond that of a solitary speech and language disorder. Students of this problem have the opportunity to increase the breadth and depth of their understanding of many aspects of the human condition.

Not a Cookbook

Beginning with the first edition of this book (1982), I have never intended this to be a "how-to" book. Instead, the writer intends this to be a "most things that need to be considered" book. The book presents concepts, ideas, notions, procedures, and strategies that the author has found and/or believes to be pertinent to consider in the evaluation and management of stuttering. This book was not written to teach readers how to serve their clients' fast fluency at the drive-through therapy window. Popping the contents of this book in the readers' con-ceptual microwaves will not make instant experts among its readers. Nor will readers sim-ply heat and serve the contents of this book to their clients and hope to achieve immediate success in the management of stuttering. Instead, we will try to provide both the stu-dent–clinician as well as practicing speech-language pathologist (SLP) with meaningful insights into and information about some of the more central, relevant aspects that need to be considered when assessing and treating children, teenagers, and adults who stutter.

But before we journey to the center of this chapter, it seems appropriate to recognize that stuttering is a multidimensional problem that has defied a variety of unidimensional explanations. It would certainly be nice to say, for example, that we will tell our readers what causes stuttering. Yes, that would be comforting, reassuring, and a minimally ambigu-ous thing to say. However, to suggest that we know, in any absolute or certain fashion, what causes stuttering would be intellectually, ethically, and professionally dishonest. The truth of the matter is that no one knows what causes stuttering. Yes, we have some excellent guesstimations of what may or may not cause stuttering; but these statements remain, at least at present, statements of probability rather than certainty.

Learning from Rather Than Hiding Our Mistakes

Unfortunately, the hype surrounding certain therapies has contributed to feelings of inadequacy by SLPs who are less successful than the famous Dr. X, even though, in reality, the famous Dr. X also has clinical failures when treating people who stutter. Instead, what is needed for this field to grow and mature is to stop ignoring or downplaying our clinical failures. Rather, we need to realize that systematic study of our failures can lead to powerful new insights into the problem. For example, such study may help us identify, prior to beginning a therapy regimen, those clients most apt to take longer to recover or those most likely to relapse. Such information, in the beginning of therapy, should help us make the necessary adjustments in our timelines and expectations. To paraphrase a popular song, our mistakes are one of the few things we can truly call our own. If we can't learn from our mistakes, who can?

The reader should be just as clear, however, that none of the foregoing cautionary notes suggests that we know little or nothing about stuttering and/or its treatment. Or that we have little knowledge of what stuttering is, or what it sounds, acts, looks like, and so forth. Quite the contrary, we know a great deal about stuttering, based on years of research and clinical experience. For example, we know a considerable amount about when stuttering occurs, what it sounds and looks like, under what conditions it will increase and decrease, and some of the better ways to assess and treat it. Do we know everything we need to or should know about these issues? No, of course not, but a large number of solid facts will be covered in considerable detail within this text.

But, as mentioned above, much of what passes for reality can be ambiguous. Thus, stuttering, as part of that reality, can also be ambiguous. So right at the outset, this writer would like to suggest that as educated professionals (whether of the inservice [clinicians] or preservice [student] variety), we need to develop and maintain a high tolerance for ambiguity. If we couple a tolerance for ambiguity together with a dedication to a lifetime of learning, we increase our chances for keeping up with the future whose one constancy will be change.

Relative Versus Absolute Descriptions of "Stuttering" and "Stutterer"

It is difficult, if not impossible, as we will shortly discuss, to develop *absolute* definitions of what is and what is not a stuttering as well as who is and who is not a person who stutters (Bloodstein, 1995). We can, however, develop *relative* definitions of what is stuttering and who is a person who stutters. Relative definitions that capture the essentials of this problem (e.g., Wingate, 1964). We use the word *apt* on purpose to highlight the fact that this definition involves a statement of probability rather than one of certainty (e.g., it is a statement of certainty that the sun will come up tomorrow but a statement of probability that a particular horse will win the Kentucky Derby). For example, comics who attempt to imitate people who stutter as part of their act are *apt* or *most likely* to produce repetitions of parts of words, for example, sounds or syllables, rather than repetitions of one or more words, for example, a phrase. Once again, the phrase *most likely* denotes an event that is relatively (probably) rather than absolutely (certainly) likely to occur.

In recent years, considerable energy has seemingly been spent trying to develop a zero-tolerance-for-error definition of stuttering or events surrounding stuttering. Such efforts, no matter how well intended, are apparently driven by a notion that definitions of stuttering, unlike definitions of all other perceptually identified events (e.g., hoarseness of voice, identification of phonological processes) must contain, in essence, NO error to be of any value in either laboratory or clinical settings. Instead, what would be welcome, in this writer's opinion, would be a clear documentation of the average amount or percentage (and range) of error associated with various reasonably objective definitions of stuttering (after being tested out on a large number of subjects by a fairly large number of clinicians across a wide variety of speaking situations). Clinicians and researchers alike could then take such inherent error into consideration when using X, Y, or Z definitions to measure stuttering for various research and clinical purposes.

For example, suppose we knew that by defining stuttering as sound/syllable repetition and/or sound prolongations we could account for about 90 percent of all listener judgments of stuttering (i.e., a 10% error term). In other words, the definition misses, on average, about 10 percent of those behaviors people judge to be stuttered. Thus, when we read that a particular therapy, using this definition, resulted in a 25 percent decrease of stuttering (pre- versus posttreatment), we'd know that was considerably beyond the 10 percent difference we'd expected merely by employing this definition. Of course, we'd also know that more than a small percentage of the 25 percent was due merely to the way we defined stuttering and had nothing to do with the treatment. But we put the cart before the horse. Before we can argue about which definition is more or less error prone, we probably need to know something about what stuttering typically sounds and looks like, what we need to consider when measuring stuttering, what nonspeech behaviors are typically associated with stuttering, how we might characterize people who stutter, and so forth.

What Is Stuttering?

To describe stuttering, perhaps it is best to first look at how we might describe other problems, for example, alcohol abuse. It is clear that alcohol and the person with an alcohol addiction are related but two distinct entities. The first, alcohol, the substance, can be measured or quantified in terms of amount and percentage per volume. The second, the person with an addiction to alcohol, cannot be adequately described by merely measuring the amount and percentage of alcohol he or she consumes. Indeed, to thoroughly understand the nature and severity of the person's alcohol addiction, we'd want to know much more than the mere amount of alcohol consumed. However, some of the other things we would want to know about, for example, the person's ability to function on the job, are much more difficult to quantify or objectively measure than the mere amount and percentage of alcohol consumed.

Stuttering Versus People Who Stutter

As with our description of alcohol and the person with an alcohol problem, so it is when we describe "stuttering" and the "person who stutters." The first term, "stuttering," relates to a *behavior* and can be measured in terms of frequency, duration, severity, associated nonspeech behaviors (e.g., eyeblinks), and the like. The second term, "stutterer" or "person who stutters" (PWS), relates to a *person*, someone who interacts with the world and his or her problem in a multitude of ways. Thus, due to these multitudinous interactions, the person cannot be as easily measured. For purposes of our present discussion, we will focus on stuttering, the behavior, and related relatively measurable aspects, for example, speaking rate. However, we hasten to point out that if we add up all these measurable behaviors they do not equal a "stutterer," any more than adding up the amount and percentage of alcohol consumed would completely describe a person's alcohol addiction and/or its role and influence in his or her life. Yes, people who stutter *do* exhibit stuttering, but to fully understand and treat these individuals we must know more than just the stuttering part of their communicative, psychological, physiological, social, etc. whole. Indeed, later on we will discuss some of those things that go beyond, well beyond, the audible and visual aspects of stuttering (i.e., the impairment or behavior described as stuttering), for example, limitations in the ability to communicate and/or disadvantages resulting from stuttering (for further, relevant discussion regarding the impairment, disability, and handicap of stuttering see Curlee, 1993; Prins, 1991, 1999; Yaruss, 1998a, 1999c).

Returning to the focus of this section ("what is stuttering"?), this writer has stated elsewhere (Conture, 1990b; Conture, 1996) that while no universally accepted definition of stuttering exists, certain observations can reasonably be made:

> Speech, like many other human behaviors, is occasionally produced by speakers with hesitations, interruptions, prolongations, and repetitions. These disruptions in . . . ongoing speech are termed *disfluency* and the frequency, duration, type, severity, and so forth of these speech disfluencies vary greatly from person to person and from speaking situation to speaking situation. Some of these speech disfluencies, particularly those which involve within-word disruptions (such as sound or syllable repetitions), are most apt to be classified or judged by listeners as *stuttering*. (Conture, 1990a, p. 2)

Table 1.1 shows those types of disfluency most and least likely to be judged as stuttering. Of course, as we have pointed out elsewhere (Conture, 1996), different types of speech disruptions, for example, between-word pauses, can and are perceived as stuttering, particularly in adults. I will, however, for the purpose of this text describe or define *stuttering* or *stuttered* speech as *typically* involving: (1) sound or syllable repetitions; (2) sound prolongations; (3) monosyllabic whole-word repetition; or (4) within-word pause. These types of speech disfluency are oftentimes referred to as *within-word* disfluencies. Again, we are dealing with the *probability*, not *certainty*, of being judged as stuttering—for example, a sound/syllable repetition has a much higher probability than a phrase repetition of being judged as an instance of stuttering. Yairi and his colleagues (e.g., Yairi, Ambrose, & Niermann, 1993) have used the term *stuttering-like disfluencies* to describe some of these same types of disfluencies (i.e., part-word repetition, single-syllable word repetitions, and disrhythmic phonation) that we consider to be *stuttering*. (Although it is not technically correct to consider monosyllabic whole-word repetitions as "within-word," they are sufficiently close in structure to sounds and syllables [e.g., often involving one-sound or syllable words like "I" or "he"] and are so often stuttered, especially by young children, that they can be, for all practical purposes, considered "within-word").

It should be pointed out, however, that all within-word speech disfluencies are not always consistently perceived or judged as stuttering. For example, mothers of children

TABLE 1.1   Examples of Various Types of Speech Disfluency That Are Likely to Be Judged by Listeners as "Stuttered" or "Normal"

Most Likely to Be Judged:

Disfluency Type	Stuttered	Not Stuttered/ Normal	Examples
Sound/syllable repetitions			"He is run-ruh-running." "It is abou-about time." "See the ba-ba-baby." "You t-t-take it."
Sound prolongation	X		"Mmmmmmore cake please." "T-(silence while person holds articulatory posture for "t")-oday is Monday."
Broken word	X		"I was g-(pause)-oing." Distinguishing broken words from sound prolongations is not always possible or easy.
Monosyllabic whole-word repetitions[1]	X	X	"I-I-I can't do that." "He-he-he is a big boy."
Multisyllabic whole-word repetitions		X	"She really-really is here."
Phrase repetition		X	"I was – I was there."
Interjection		X	I will, uhm, you know, be late."
Revision		X	"She is – she was here."

[1]Monosyllabic whole-word repetitions are sometimes judged stuttered and other times as nonstuttered. This judgment seems to be dependent on associated physical tension, rate of repetition, and other as yet unknown factors. For the present discussion, monosyllabic whole-word repetitions will be considered to be within-word or stuttered disfluencies. Note that sometimes "between-word" disfluencies can also be judged as stuttered (see text).

Note: Not all listeners, under all conditions, for all speakers, will *always* arrive at these judgments. For example, it is sometimes possible that some listeners may judge a sound/syllable repetition as "normal" or a phrase repetition as "stuttered." While these possibilities can and do happen, on occasion, they are generally not as likely as those listed in this table. Whether talking about the rule or the exception to the rule regarding judgments of instances of stuttering, however, we are making statements of probability rather than statements of certainty.

who do and do not stutter *infrequently* (15 to 30% of the time) judge sound prolongations of relatively brief duration (i.e., less than 300 msec) to be stuttered. In other words, very brief sound prolongations (a within-word disfluency) are not always judged as stuttering; thus, we cannot categorically assume that all kinds and duration of within-word disfluencies will be judged as "stuttered." Conversely, these same mothers *very frequently* (i.e., 83% or more of the time) judge sound or syllable repetitions of any duration as stuttered (Zebrowski & Conture, 1989); thus, some within-word disfluencies (i.e., sound/syllable repetitions) are almost always judged as stuttered.

It should also be pointed out that stuttering or stuttered speech can also be perceived as occurring in the intervals *between* words (e.g., Cordes & Ingham, 1995; Curlee, 1981; Mac-

Donald & Martin, 1973), such disruptions sometimes being referred to as *between-word* disfluency. For example, stuttering is sometimes judged to occur on effortful-sounding or appearing disfluency perceived between words, such as hesitations, tense pauses, or blocks. (A "block" is typically exemplified by the person's speech production mechanism *ceasing* to move forward to the next sound position. During a "block," the person's speech mechanism appears stuck, fixed, or "frozen" in position—for example, the speaker's lower jaw may be dropped and the tongue may be lying on the floor of the mouth for longer than the period needed to produce the intended sound, syllable, or word.) Recently (e.g., Cordes, Ingham, Frank, & Ingham, 1992), it has been suggested that the presence/absence of stuttering is more reliably judged within a given time-interval or epoch of time during speech (e.g., every one second), rather than on specific sounds, syllables, or words. Undoubtedly, such methodological advances as time-interval measurement will refine both our description as well as measurement of those behaviors perceived as "stuttered."

The Role of Listener Judgments

We have seen that certain types of speech disfluency and behavior are more likely than others to be associated with listener perceptions of stuttering (see Young, 1984, for further review of this area), even though significant exceptions to this rule can and do occur. Most importantly, however, the reader will note the phrase "listener perceptions of stuttering." We should be clear that perceptions of stuttering involve listener evaluations. Some very interesting, important strides in the direction of computer- or machine-assisted recognition of stuttering have recently been made (Howell, Sackin, & Glenn, 1997a, 1997b). Despite such advances, we still lack, and will for some time, widely available, clinically usable "machines," whether analog or digital, that can analyze audio- or video-tapes of speech and related behaviors of suspected people who stutter and indicate (1) which sounds, syllables, words, phrases, or sentences are *stuttered* or contain instances of *stuttering*, and (2) whether the speaker who produces these speech events is a *person who stutters*. In the final analysis, we, the trained listener, still must decide, after careful and (hopefully) objective assessment, whether we judge a particular speech behavior as stuttering and whether the person who produced that behavior is or is not an individual who stutters.

Speakers Differ; So Do Listeners

Listeners, while central to the process of judging stuttering, are also part of the problem. Just like when two or more people observe and report an event such as an auto crash, such observations, evaluations, and reports are subjective, variable, and difficult to make. These differences in listener judgments, if we think about it for a moment, should not surprise us. Just as speakers differ in their speaking abilities, so too do listeners differ in their listening abilities. Recognizing the variability and difficulty of making such perceptual judgments should not discourage us from developing a reasonably complete listing of events that are *most apt* to be perceived as stuttered. Errors in judgment between as well as within listeners are to be expected. Indeed, such expectation should alert us to the fact that these judgments are not a simple undertaking and that definitive statements about presence, frequency, and location of stuttering should be accepted with due caution.

As the above suggests, any rules we make about what is and is not stuttering will be broken. Exceptions will always be found that do not fit the rule, no matter how cleverly we devise our rules. However, given our reasonable need to cautiously generalize, we can safely say that stuttering or stuttered speech usually involves *within-word* disfluencies (e.g., Boehmler, 1958; Schiavetti, 1975; Williams & Kent, 1958; Zebrowski & Conture, 1989), but sometimes can also involve effortful-sound disfluency perceived *between* words, such as hesitations between words (e.g., Curlee, 1981). Our notions of what is and is not stuttering will undoubtedly be refined by advances in measurement technology—for example, the development and refinement of time-interval measurements (e.g., Cordes et al., 1992), whereby stuttering is identified within specified time windows or epochs rather than associated with specific syllables or words, as well as the possibilities of machine- or auto-mated-recognition of stuttering (e.g., Howell et al., 1997a; 1997b). For the purposes of this text, however, the above, perceptually based descriptions and/or definitions of stuttering would seem to be quite adequate.

How Do We Measure Stuttering?

The measurement of stuttering, at this point in time, essentially involves listener judgment. Simply put, listeners must make a number of decisions, oftentimes very rapidly, to arrive at such judgments. In essence, the listener must make decisions about disfluency: (1) type; (2) duration (whether prolonged or reiterative); and (3) associated audible manifestations of physical tension, escape, and avoidance. If the disfluent event is of a type, duration, and tension the listener judges to be "stuttered," the listener may label the event as such. After that, the listener may, either in his or her head, on paper, or on computer, count the number of these judgments in a given sample and determine whether their frequency is sufficient to warrant labeling the individual as someone who stutters or someone at risk for continuing to stutter. In this section, we will explore how disfluency type, duration, frequency, and associated physical tension influence our measurement of stuttering.

For both clinical as well as research purposes, we often must make categorical judgments to distinguish stuttered from fluent speech (e.g., like separating football players into halfbacks, fullbacks, and quarterbacks). Despite the discrete nature of these judgments (e.g., this word is stuttered and that word is not), we are judging an event—(dis)fluent speech—that occurs along a continuum (e.g., like a thermometer). For example, on one occasion, listeners might judge the /p/ in the word "popcorn" to be "marginally fluent" if it contained a slightly longer than normal stop phase, for example, 100 milliseconds (ms; 1000 ms = 1 second). However, on another occasion, if the same speaker maintains the stop phase for a bit longer, for example, extending it to 200–250 ms, listeners might now judge the /p/ as a short sound prolongation, block, hesitation, or stuttering. We might analogize this to room temperature (as measured on a thermometer) that we initially judge to be "just right," but as the thermostat is turned up slightly, we judge the room to be "too warm." In other words, subtle changes along an objectively measured continuum of temporal aspects of speech (or room temperature!) might lead to fairly nonsubtle, categorical, or discrete differences in judgment. It is a bit curious to this author why more studies like Zebrowski and Conture (1989) haven't been reported whereby listeners judge the presence/absence of stuttering of sounds, syllables, or words that have been systematically altered acoustically, for example, the stop phase of sounds being lengthened along a continuum from typical to 1000 milliseconds (1 sec). Such research would help indicate where along the continuously varying continuum of acoustic events—for example, one, two, or three iterations of a sound—we are most likely to categorically judge sounds, syllables, or words as stuttering. Let us look at a few ways we can describe speech as stuttered versus nonstuttered.

Frequency of Disfluency as a Means of Differentiating

We might differentiate stuttered from nonstuttered speech on the basis of frequency of disfluency. Table 1.2 squares with our clinical experience and is based on data reported by Johnson and others (1959). This figure shows that very few, if any, of the children who produce, on the average, 3 or more *within-word* disfluencies per 100 words are *apt* to be called or judged to be a person who is normally fluent or a non-stutterer. However, as Table 1.2 also shows, the populations overlap—people who do and do not stutter—in terms of the number of their exhibited within-word speech disfluencies. Thus, there will always be some children described as "people who stutter" who produce 1 or 2 within-word disfluencies per 100 words as well as some children described as "normally fluent" who produce 1 or 2 within-word disfluencies per 100 words.

Yairi (1997a) recalculated only what he termed the "stuttered-like disfluencies" (SLDs) from Johnson and others (1959) data and reported that SLDs were (on average) 11.51 per 100 words for children who stutter but only 1.88 for children who did not stutter. Similarly, Yaruss, LaSalle, and Conture (1998) report, on the basis of a clinical sample of 100 2- to 6-year-old children, that the mean frequency of total speech disfluencies was 11.42 disfluencies per 100 words, a figure very similar to the 11.51 reported by Yairi in his recalculation of Johnson's earlier data. However, it should be pointed out, that the Yaruss and

TABLE 1.2　Decile Distribution of Frequency of Within-Word Disfluency for Children Who Stutter (CWS) and Children Who Do Not Stutter (CWNS)

Decile Distribution of Frequency of Within-Word Disfluency	Young Male CWS (N = 68)	Young Male CWNS (N = 68)	Young Female CWS (N = 21)	Young Female CWNS (N = 21)
1	0.43	0.00	0.50	0.00
2	0.93	0.00	0.64	0.25
3	1.68	0.22	1.53	0.26
4	2.84	0.40	2.38	0.29
5	3.77	0.55	2.80	0.53
6	5.04	0.60	4.47	0.55
7	7.06	0.95	6.01	0.95
8	10.07	1.22	7.29	1.60
9	17.47	2.16	11.95	2.37

(After Johnson et al. [1959], Tables 69 and 70).

colleagues' data are based on total not a subset of (i.e., "stuttered-like) disfluencies. Thus, their *clinical* sample may underestimate, to a degree, the total amount of stuttering that one might observe in a random or *experimental* sample of children known or suspected to be stuttering (i.e., a sample based on children brought to a research setting by a caregiver with no implied or expressed purpose of receiving clinical diagnosis or treatment). It is perhaps safest to assume that the Yaruss and colleagues' data are reflective of a representative clinical sample of 100 children observed at the time of initial clinical evaluation (i.e., a sample of children brought to a clinical setting by a caregiver with the express purpose of receiving a diagnostic and possible treatment). Of course, it could be argued the other way—that an experimental sample may overestimate the number and nature of stuttering typically observed in a clinical setting! Whatever the case, Yairi's observation is quite consistent with two of the Yaruss and colleagues' observations: (1) the mean number of total disfluencies or SLDs are appreciably greater for children who do than for children who do not stutter, and, probably more importantly; (2) children who produce two or fewer SLDs or within-word speech disfluencies per 100 words are generally not labeled as people who stutter.

Therefore, try as we might, it is quite difficult to differentiate between people who do and do not stutter *solely* on the basis of frequency of stuttering, within-word disfluencies, or total disfluencies. This is similar to the remark of Johnson and colleagues (1959) that "there are no 'natural' lines of demarcation between 'normal' and 'abnormal' degrees of nonfluency" (p. 205) Why? Well, a small percentage of normally fluent speakers will always be observed who produce a frequency of within-word disfluencies similar to that of people who stutter and vice versa. In essence, our decision rules for placing categorical boundaries at "fixed" points along a continuum of fluent/disfluent speech behavior will always cause us to make some errors in judgment. Thus, zero-tolerance for judgment error is an error in and of itself! The only debate we can have, in this writer's opinion, is the size and nature of the *error* (either false positive or *false negative*). Indeed, in the clinic, in the research lab, the presence of error is a certainty (see Thorner & Remein, 1982, for an excellent discussion of false positive, false negatives, and related issues). Figure 1.1 shows the various types of diagnostic decisions and errors that can be made when attempting to decide who is and who is not stuttering. However, there are no published data, to this writer's knowledge, specifying the number and percentage of times the average SLP makes each of these decisions or errors when deciding who is and who is not a person who stutters. We can say, however, based on the Yaruss and colleagues' clinical data, that clinicians who observe a child produce 10 or more total disfluencies per 100 words should, at least, look very carefully at the rest of the child's speech fluency and related speech and language behaviors (see Adams, 1980, for simular criteria). There is a fair chance that the child will require treatment, or at least a reevaluation.

Type of Speech Disfluency as a Means of Differentiating

We might also try to differentiate stuttered from nonstuttered speech by measuring within- versus between-word disfluencies. In other words, we might try to dichotomize stuttering and fluency into two separate camps or categories by assessing differences in the *type* of speech disfluencies. One typical way of doing this is to consider within-word disfluencies as stuttered and between-word disfluencies as normal disfluencies (see Conture 1982,

Diagnosis		
"Reality"	Positive (Child Who Stutters: CWS)	Negative (Child Who Does Not Stutter: CWNS)
Ture	(Hit) Categorized as CWS and actually is	(Correct Rejection) Catorized as CWNS and actually is
False	(False Positive) Categorized as CWS but actually is CWNS	(Miss) Categorized as CWNS but actually is CWS

FIGURE 1.1. Four possible relations between the diagnostic decision that (a) an individual is or is not a stutterer and (b) the "reality" of whether the person actually is or is not a stutterer. While many clinicians seem concerned about committing false positives relative to stuttering, it is the writer's experience that a "miss" or false negative is just as likely if not more likely to occur (adapted from Thorner & Remein, 1982).

1990b) (not at all dissimilar from Yairi's SLD categorization schema). However, as we mentioned earlier, some within-word disfluencies will be judged as "normal" or fluent; conversely, some between-word disfluencies will be judged as "stuttered." In attempts to clarify these issues, let us return to our previous example describing a person holding or prolonging the stop phase of /p/ in the word "popcorn."

As we previously described, a person might hold the stop phase of /p/ in the word "popcorn" (by pressing his or her lips together) a bit longer than typical (i.e., say 200 ms rather than the typical 60 ms). Some might judge this longer /p/ as prolonged, blocked, or stuttered; however, if the same speaker holds the stop phrase for only 100 ms, which is still longer than usual, some might judge this as fluent (if only marginally so). Thus, these two judgments—stuttered versus fluent—are related to differences in duration of the stop phase of /p/ rather than the fact that the two speech events represent two categorically or absolutely different kinds or types of speech events. Indeed, quantitative differences in speech behavior (e.g., changes in length, duration, or physical tension of articulatory contact) are just as likely to influence perceptual judgment as qualitative differences in speech behavior (e.g., sound/syllable repetition versus revisions). In some cases, the "quality" or "type" of disfluency may not change. Instead, the "quantity" of the disfluency may change—for example, the duration of the disfluency lengthens, beyond some as yet unknown *threshold of acceptability*; once having heard this, the listener judges the speech event as "stuttered."

Where does this all leave us? Well, even those speech disfluencies—for example, sound or syllable repetitions and sound prolongations—most apt to be considered stuttered (e.g., Boehmler, 1958; Schiavetti, 1975; Williams & Kent, 1958), or described as SLD

(Yairi, 1997a), will sometimes be judged to be fluent. Again, as hard as we may try, our definition of what is and what is not stuttered will have to remain relative, not absolute. We can create reasonably reliable (but not absolutely error-free) guidelines for judging what type and frequency of disfluency is most apt to be considered stuttered or might warrant us considering an individual speaker as a stutterer. These guidelines, however, are just that: guidelines. Exceptions to the rule, as in all areas of human behavior, can, will, and should be expected.

In reality, the wise researcher or clinician will consider the entirety of a person's speech fluency, for example, the frequency of total, within-, and between-word disfluencies, the duration of a representative sample of these disfluencies, the overall severity, and so forth. While one can capture much of what is important by looking at total frequency of disfluency together with frequency and type of SLD, one should always keep an eye open for the client or subject who doesn't fit the mold. Conversely, it is not wise to throw out useful rules merely because exceptions can be noted or found. Would we argue that the reported average height of 5′9″ for U.S.A. men is "bogus" merely because we observe a U.S.A. man who is 6′3″? Conversely, would we say that the 6′3″ male is not from the United States merely because his height doesn't agree with the U.S.A. average? To have an average or mean we *must* have a range of behavior around that mean. And, as researchers and clinicians, we *must* be prepared to deal not only with the average but the normal dispersion of behavior that ranges around that average.

Physical Effort, Tension, and Avoidance Associated with Stuttering: The "Effortless-Avoidance" Continuum

One part of the stuttering whole—associated physical effort, tension, and avoidance—is thought by some to significantly differentiate between stuttered and nonstuttered disfluencies. Undoubtedly, in this writer's opinion, some differences in our judgments of stuttering relate to the degree of physical effort, tension, and avoidance associated with stuttering AND the examiner's ability to quickly and accurately perceive the same. Indeed, if defining stuttering is problematic, defining the amount and nature of "effort," "tension," and "avoidance" associated with stuttering may be even more so. When discussing this topic, I am reminded of the person who supposedly said, when asked to define pornography, "I can't define it, but I certainly know it when I see it!" That is, observers have difficulties defining/describing the nature of physical tension and avoidant behavior associated with stuttering, although they frequently remark and/or react to tension and avoidance in association with stuttering when they observe it.

This "effortless-avoidance" continuum is, in this writer's opinion, a large part of the "it-is–it-is-not-a-stuttering" debate (for the time being, we will ignore the feelings of "unawareness," "frustration," and "fear" that probably underlie these observable behaviors). Judging this "effortless-avoidance" continuum is separate from identifying total as well as different disfluency types. Further, this judgment will not necessarily be made any easier by the use of different means for measuring stuttering (e.g., online versus manuscript-based assessments, see Yaruss, Max, Newman, & Campbell, 1998). While exceptions can and do occur, many children begin their instances of stuttering with little or no apparent physical effort or tension (i.e., effortless disfluencies). As the problem continues, and the child becomes increasingly frustrated trying to talk and tries to help him- or herself "get unstuck," more physical tension is typically employed, tension that may or may not be audible (i.e., effortful or tense disfluencies). Pitch rises, for example, may denote such increases in physical effort or tension. Finally, more and more physical tension, rather than helping, actually can hinder the forward flow of the child's speech; the child's frustration becomes increasingly mixed with, or shading into, actual concern, worry, or fear. The child may either abandon communication already started (i.e., escape) or change what and how he or she is going to talk (i.e., avoid).

The development of this sequence of events—effortless, effortful, avoidance—associated with stutterings may progress rather gradually in some children and in others progress quite rapidly within days, if not hours. However, in terms of our present discussion, rapidity of development is not an issue. Rather, it is the presence of visual and/or auditory indices of effort, tension, and avoidance AND our ability to recognize same that may influence our judgments of stuttering, regardless of our definitions of what disfluencies are stuttered and/or manner of assessing. While scales that attempt to judge naturalness (e.g., Martin, Haroldson, & Triden, 1984) and suitability (e.g., Franken, van Bezooijen, & Boves, 1997) may indirectly get at such events as tension and avoidance, clearly this is an area that needs further study.

It would seem that our ability to measure stuttering will probably be significantly improved, in terms of reliability and validity, if we can develop: (1) a clinically viable procedure, whether based on units of time (e.g., number of 1-second epochs containing a perceived instance of stuttering) or speech (e.g., % stuttered syllables) that reliably identifies instances of stuttering between and within listeners; (2) a data-based description of the types of speech disfluency that are relatively highly (not absolutely) associated with those judgments; and (3) a perceptually based scale of the degree of tension and/or effort associated with those judgments. The first (1) would have both clinical as well as research utility while the others (2 & 3) would have primarily research utility—for example, studying physiological differences among the parts (e.g., sound prolongations versus sound/syllable repetitions) of the stuttering whole (i.e., reliably judged instances of stuttering). While we have made excellent progress toward reaching these goals, more work continues to be needed. In particular, clinicians, as well as researchers, need to focus on the perceptually apparent tension-avoidance associates of stuttering. These associates, in this writer's opinion, are one of the stumbling blocks on the road to a universally accepted and usable means of assessing stuttering and people known or suspected of stuttering.

Norms to Establish Whether a Person Stutters

Although we might like to use group norms (for example, more than 10 speech disfluencies per 100 words = stuttering) to assist us in establishing who is and who is not a stutterer, existing data still do not appear sufficient to provide us with effective group norms. Recent studies, however, like that of Ambrose and Yairi (1999) move us in that direction, through the use of their "weighted stuttered-like disfluency" measure. Tests like the *Stuttering Severity Instrument-3* (Riley, 1994a) and the *Stuttering Prediction Instrument* (Riley, 1981) are also excellent beginning points. However, what is needed is more information, on a year-by-year or month-by-month basis, regarding the mean (plus range) number and type of speech disfluencies produced by children from say two to six years of age. Previous research in this area (for example, Davis, 1939, 1940; Johnson & et al., 1959; Williams, Silverman, & Kools 1969; Winitz 1961; Yairi 1981, 1982; Yairi & Clifton, 1972; Yairi & Jennings, 1974; Yairi & Lewis, 1984) has advanced our knowledge considerably.

In recent years in particular, longitudinal studies of early childhood speech (dis)fluency development reported by Yairi and colleagues (e.g., Yairi, 1997a; Yairi & Ambrose, 1992; Yairi et al., 1993) have significantly helped us understand the development of speech (dis)fluency in children. In this author's opinion, we cannot collect enough data in this area, for only by amassing more and more information about typical speech (dis)fluency in early childhood are we going to make more informed clinical decisions as well as refine our ability to appropriately select children who do and do not stutter for the purposes of research. Indeed, (1) continued massive exposure to and influence of television, computers, and other media on our children's language and cognitive development, as well as (2) changes in the traditional family structure, where both father and mother now work outside the home, strongly suggest that such research needs continual updating and expanding. Furthermore, if at all possible, such information should be based on *longitudinal* (several samples sequentially spaced out over time) versus cross-sectional (a sample taken at only one point in time; for further general discussion of longitudinal/cross-sectional studies see Schiavetti & Metz, 1997, pp. 55–58).

The One Constant About Stuttering Is Change

Clinicians, like researchers, must understand that people who stutter, just like people who do not stutter, *vary* in their behavior (this discussion relates, of course, to our earlier discussion about central tendencies or averages in behavior and ranges of behavior around the average). Clinicians, in their sampling of their clients' behavior, must try the best they can to capture quantitative and qualitative variations in stuttering. This decreases the chances that the clinician will be fooled into thinking that the client's change during therapy is due to therapy when it may be nothing more than "natural" variations in behavior. It is nice to know about the central tendency (average, median, or mode) of a person's stuttering. However, without knowing something about the dispersion of values around that central tendency (e.g., high and low values or the range, variance, standard deviation, or semi-interquartile range [i.e., 25th to 75th percentile]), the clinician will find it *very* difficult to interpret how representative the central tendency is of the person's behavior. Stuttering is a fluctuating, dynamically varying behavior, and no matter how static or fixed the terms we use to describe it, we cannot change the fact that it is highly variable, particularly in children.

To expect that a stutterer's average stuttering frequency reflects what would be observed from minute to minute or day to day would be like expecting to find the next ten people you meet to have an IQ of 100 because 100 is the mean for the population! To work with stuttering is to work with a variable commodity, a behavior whose frequency of occurrence is ever changing. All too often both clinicians and researchers alike ignore such change and thus overlook the fact that variability is a fundamental aspect of stuttering. Understanding the variable nature of stuttering is so important, so central to effective treatment and study of the problem, that it is fair to say that those who do not have such understanding do not understand stuttering!

What Nonspeech Behaviors Are Associated with Stuttering?

When observers see and hear speech events typically perceived as stuttering, these same observers may also see and hear at least two other events: (1) (non)speech movement and physical tension and (2) (non)verbal reports of psychosocial discomfort and concern (Bloodstein, 1995). During instances of stuttering, events (1) and (2), plus the speech behavior itself, make up a behavioral complex consisting of speech + nonspeech + psychosocial behaviors (the latter most likely, although not exclusively, observed when stuttering has become more habituated and/or existed for some time).

Indeed, many times beginning SLPs or student SLPs, when observing stuttering, may disregard the speech behavior associated with stuttering. Instead, they may focus on observing the more noticeable, relatively long duration (non)speech behaviors and reports of bodily movement, physical tension, and psychosocial discomfort and/or concern associated with instances of stuttering. In our opinion, SLPs who remediate stuttering should be able to do what I term *parallel process* (with all due apologies to my colleagues in speech science): simultaneously process or handle different types of information coming from different sources or modalities. In our opinion, the treatment of stuttering should not be undertaken by an SLP who cannot or will not simultaneously process different events, events that are perhaps related to each other but with each having its own seriated time course and meaning to the person's overall communication problem.

As early as 1940, Barr suggested that nonspeech behavior should be considered when evaluating the speech of people who stutter. While many clinicians, we think, would agree with Barr, it is interesting to note that there have been relatively few empirical studies of nonspeech behavior associated with stuttering (Conture & Kelly, 1991a; Krause, 1982; LaSalle & Conture, 1991; Prins & Lohr, 1972; Schwartz & Conture, 1988; Schwartz, Zebrowski, & Conture, 1990; Yairi et al., 1993). Thus, even though tests like the *Iowa Scale of Stuttering Severity* (Johnson, Darley, & Spriestersbach, 1963) or the *Stuttering Severity Instrument-3* (Riley, 1994b) attempt to assess the (non)speech behaviors, movements, and tension commonly observed in association with stuttering (e.g., Brutten & Shoemaker, 1967), the fact remains that we still do not fully understand the amount and nature of nonspeech behavior associated with instances of stuttering, particularly during typical parent–child communicative interaction.

In a detailed investigation of these associated nonspeech behaviors, we (Conture & Kelly, 1991a) studied the nonspeech behavior of 30 young (3- to 7-year-old) children who stutter (*prior* to any prescribed therapy) during stuttering and compared those of 30 age and sex-matched normally fluent peers during comparable fluent utterances. We reasoned that if nonspeech behavior associated with stuttering was appreciably different than the norm, such differences would be most apparent when compared to the fluent productions of people who do not stutter. As part of this study, we assessed over sixty different nonspeech "behaviors" and found that: (1) Young people who stutter produced more nonspeech behavior during their stutterings than their normally fluent peers did during comparable fluent productions; and (2) only three nonspeech behaviors significantly differentiated the two groups of children, that is, the young people who stutter were much more likely to: (a) move their eyeballs to the side (b) blink their eyelids and (c) raise their upper lip (the latter gesture sometimes seen as part of a sneer or disgust facial gesture). It was our impression that of these three behaviors, the movement of the eyeballs to the side and blinking was most apt to be associated with instances of stuttering. While it is not appropriate in this space to extensively theorize about these findings (for such a discussion see Conture & Kelly, 1991a, pp. 1051–1053), the following conclusions would seem reasonable: (1) Children who stutter, at or near the onset of their problem, are exhibiting a relatively large amount and variety of nonspeech behavior in association with their stutterings (i.e., these nonspeech behaviors do not necessarily develop only after the child has been stuttering for a while); and (2) many of these nonspeech behaviors would seem to briefly minimize or block the young stutterer's visual information about his or her listening partners' reactions to the speech behavior and/or the stutterers (an example of disruption in "oculesics," see Egolf & Chester, 1973).

Perhaps, the facial gestures and bodily movements and tensing associated with stuttering may suggest that the stutterer is trying to cope with the stuttering itself. (In a slightly different vein, Sheehan [1958] speculated that the nature of these associated behaviors is projective of the individual "behind" the stuttering; for example, "active" or "aggressive" individuals who stutter might produce a greater number and variety of associated behaviors than say a more "passive" individual who stutters.) It is also possible that, for example, a head turn to the right, neatly time-locked with the initiation of the articulatory contact of a feared sound or syllable, indicates the stutterer's belief that head turning may help "get the sound out." Maybe a person who stutters comes to feel that if a little bit of head movement and physical tensing of neck and shoulder muscles helps, then a great deal more should really help!

Indeed, we could say that these associated nonspeech behaviors actually do on occasion "work"! That is, by seemingly chance association with successful forward movement through a sound, syllable or word, these associated behaviors appear to become reinforced in much the same way that the green shirt the pitcher wore on the day he pitched a no-hitter takes on special properties (see Skinner, 1953; LeFrancois, 1972; Hill, 1997 for discussion of superstitious behavior). Both the green shirt and the head turning may be viewed by the pitcher and the person who stutters, respectively, as being something that helps or as something essential to successful completion of the task at hand. Unfortunately, for the person who stutters, this "superstitious" behavior cannot be discarded as easily as a shirt! In fact, all too often the associated nonspeech behaviors of people who stutter become just another part of rather than solution for their speaking problem.

What Are Some Basic Generalizations About Stuttering?

It is a strange twist of fate, but nonetheless true that speech-language clinicians are far more likely than theoreticians to be asked a highly theoretical question: What causes stuttering? This question is typically asked by: the parents of children known or suspected to be stuttering, people who stutter, the press, the lay public at cocktail parties, and so forth. And, often times, an SLP's ability to clearly, quickly, and persuasively articulate an answer to this question determines his or her *ethos* (believability) and clinical acumen in the eyes of the layperson asking the question. Think about it: If you asked a physician if he or she knew what caused middle ear infections and he or she hemmed, hawed, and was vague, what would be your assessment of their medical knowledge and/or ability to appropriately treat patients? Thus, both students and clinicians alike have a vested interest in knowing something about current information and speculation regarding the cause of stuttering. Simply put, clients' beliefs and opinions about an SLP may, from the very beginning, be significantly influenced by the SLP's ability to respond to the simple to ask but difficult to answer question: "What causes stuttering?" To provide both clinicians and students alike with more facility in responding to this question, as well as a better understanding of stuttering, in this section we will describe some basic facts about stuttering and in a later section describe some basic theories about stuttering.

Typically, when speech-language pathologists are often asked about the cause of stuttering, the question relates to the questioner's "favorite organ." For example, it's not uncommon to be asked: "Is the brain involved with stuttering?" Well, of course. The brain is always involved when we talk fluently, so why not when we talk disfluently? Or, "Is the larynx involved in stuttering"? Again, of course it is. When we talk fluently, the larynx is involved, so why not when we talk disfluently? It is not the mere involvement of the brain, larynx, tongue, and so forth in stuttering, but the *nature* of that involvement we are unclear about.

Again, this writer finds it very ironic that people charged with the applied or clinical assessment and treatment of stuttering (i.e., speech-language pathologists) are routinely confronted with a highly theoretical question: "What causes stuttering?" Indeed, to clearly and meaningfully answer such a question one needs to have a reasonable grasp of theoretical knowledge about stuttering as well as the ability to articulate it. Before exploring some theorizations, we will describe some facts and generalizations about stuttering as well as how it behaves. This description should help us better understand some of the more current theories used to explain the cause of stuttering. This, in turn, should assist us to answer the often asked question, "What causes stuttering?"

To begin, Table 1.3 lists some general facts about stuttering. These facts are self-explanatory and need little amplification in this space. However, as additional research becomes available, the number and nature of these facts may change. For example, the percentage of people who stutter who recover has been variously estimated to be as low as 50 percent to as high as 80 percent. Only further clinical observation and research can help clarify this matter.

Some Relatively Safe Generalizations About Stuttering

1. *Stuttering is most likely to occur during bidirectional communication.* We can safely say that stuttering is most likely to be observed when people are talking to someone else. As simple-minded as this may sound, it is not possible, with any degree of reliability, to observe a person who stutters, when he or she is not talking, and determine whether that

TABLE 1.3   Some Basic Facts About Stuttering

Prevalence:	About 1% of school-age population (lifetime incidence reported around 5%)
Sex Ratio:	3 boys for 1 girl, on average
Familial Incidence:	For 50% or more of people who stutter, some other family members also stutters.
Onset: Median	Typical range = 2-4 years, with most beginning by 7 years of age (a disorder of childhood)
Nature of Onset:	For about 70%, onset is gradual
Speech at Onset:	Typically, relatively physically non-tense repetitions of sounds and syllables, but can be physically tense sound prolongations and/or blocks
Spontaneous Recovery:	At least (some report as high as 85%) 50% exhibit improvement without formal treatment
An Instance of Stuttering Is Most Apt to Occur on:	Word-initial sounds; longer words; nouns, verbs, adjectives, and adverbs; longer, more grammatical complex utterances
Concomitant Speech and Language Problems:	In children, phonological concerns, in particular, commonly associated with stuttering

Note: While other "facts" exist—for example, children who stutter are more apt than their normally fluent peers to exhibit difficulties with speech sound articulation/disordered phonology—facts listed in this table are among those, that over time, appear to be the most well established. Also note that recent research (e.g., Howell, Au-Yeung, & Sackin, 1999) indicates that the type of word stuttered on changes as a function of age.

person may stutter. For stuttering to occur, the person who stutters is usually engaged in spoken communication that is *bidirectional* in nature. By "bidirectional" we mean spoken communication that goes back and forth between a speaker and listener. This explains, at least in part, why people who stutter exhibit very little stuttering when "talking" to an infant because the communication is unidirectional. That is, communication with an infant involves a minimal degree of bidirectional spoken interaction even though one might assume that certain psychosocial and other "messages" may be passed back and forth between baby and his or her admirer. Au-Yeung and Howell (1998) present a very interesting discussion about how conversational context may influence whether speech is produced more or less fluently. With children, for example, they speculate that the nature of the parents' utterances can make it more or less easy for the child to subsequently formulate responses to questions asked by parents. Au-Yeung and Howell suggest that a child might use less effort and exhibit more fluency when saying "It is red" in response to the question "Is the pencil red or blue?" but use more effort and exhibit less fluency when responding "It is red" to the question "What is the color of the pencil?" While stuttering can and does occur, on occasion, when the person who stutters talks to him- or herself, dogs, babies, and so forth; but the main "venue" for stuttering is bidirectional communication between a speaker and listener.

2.   *Stuttering generally begins and develops in childhood.* We can safely say that stuttering is a problem of childhood. Stuttering, which begins in childhood, is called *developmental* stuttering. That is, for the vast majority of people who stutter, they begin to do so by 7 years of age, with a few beginning in the years after that to about 12. Another far rarer form of stuttering, *acquired* stuttering, typically begins in adults, has a sudden onset and usually follows physical trauma (e.g., Ackermann, Hertrich, Ziegler, Bitzer, & Bien, 1996; Van Borsel, Van Lierde, Van Cauwenberge, Guldemont, & Van Orshoven, 1998). Acquired stuttering usually begins after a stroke or a cardiovascular accident (CVA) or a blow to the head during a car crash. However, acquired, sometimes called "neurogenic," stuttering (i.e., stuttering that typically begins in adulthood and secondary to damage to the nervous system) is the exception rather than the rule. (For completion's sake, we should also note that there are reports of stuttering beginning in adulthood for seemingly psychogenic purposes [Mahr & Leith, 1992]). Despite such a dramatic onset in a previously typically fluent adult, we want to stress that the number of individuals exhibiting acquired stuttering is significantly less than the number of individuals exhibiting developmental stuttering. In essence, for the vast majority of people who stutter, the origins of the problem are in childhood.

It seems safe to assume, however, that the quality and quantity of stuttering changes as the child grows older, becomes a teenager, and the teenager becomes an adult. For example, the rather long duration sound prolongations of an adult with a severe stuttering problem probably did not develop overnight (yes, a percentage of children may begin with such disfluencies, but these children are not among the majority of children who begin to stutter in childhood). Most likely, when this adult was a child, his or her instances of stuttering were somewhat shorter in duration, probably less frequently exhibited, and possessed less audible manifestations of physiological tension than the adult form of the problem. So although the problem begins in childhood, it can and often does change in form and frequency over time.

3.   *The relatively rapid coming and going of stuttering, the BEHAVIOR, during spoken utterance suggests that relatively fast changes in the state of communicative processes PRECIPITATE OR CAUSE stuttering.* Stuttering is more ephermal than evermore. The fact that stuttering *behavior* results from an online disruption in the state of fluency rather than an ongoing, pervasive *trait* is best exemplified by comparing stuttering to other speech and language disorders, for example, a phonological disorder. With a phonological disorder, the trait or number and type of phonological processes or speech sound errors can be reliably observed in the morning, noon, and night, and then similarly the next day (of course, some variation or inconsistency in phonological processes is apparent, but relative to stuttering, a phonological disorder is a constant characteristic of the child's speech at a particular period during the child's development). With stuttering, however, there are moment-to-moment changes in the state of the person's fluency. Thus, what is observed in the morning may have little relationship to what is observed in the afternoon. Thus, it seems safe to consider stuttering as an online change in the *state* of the person's fluent speech. Stuttering is not a trait that the person always possesses, but a state that the person sometimes exhibits. Indeed, this writer believes that somewhere within the rapidly changing, transient nature of stuttering lies the key to its cause and eventual solution.

4. *The relatively slow coming and going of stuttering, the PROBLEM, across days, weeks, and months suggests that relatively slowly changes in the state of extracommunicative processes (e.g., psychological excitement, temperament) AGGRAVATE, EXACERBATE, OR MAINTAIN stuttering.* It is a fact that the *problem* of stuttering varies, it waxes and wanes, cycling up and down, over hours, days and weeks. These rather slow changes in the person's fluency, this author speculates, are related to development (e.g., gradually improving abilities to rapidly, sequentially, and accurate move speech mechanism), temperamental reactions to environmental change, pervasive excitement in the person's environment, and so forth. These relatively slow changes in the *problem* of stuttering, although appreciable, are viewed by this author as exacerbating the more fundamental, rapid changes in state that he believes actually precipitate or causes instances of stuttering. In essence, and as previously mentioned, stuttering, the behavior, characteristically *varies* with time and place of communication. It is not static; it is ever changing, particularly in the speech of young children.

5. *Stuttering is more apparent within certain places within the utterance and on certain utterances (i.e., rapid changes in state).* Stuttering is most apt to occur on word-initial sounds or syllables, within low-frequency or low-usage words within longer, more grammatically complex utterances. In other words, stuttering appears most likely at certain places (e.g., on word-initial sounds) within an utterance and more often on some utterances (e.g., longer utterances) than others. Even though the frequency of stuttering changes considerably, stuttering IS NOT a random event any more than continual changes in verb inflection (e.g., from regular to irregular verbs, from past to present tense, etc.) reflect a random event. As mentioned above, normal, rapid changes in the state of the person's communicative processes are, in this writer's opinion, one of the keys to understanding the cause of stuttering. For example, unlike the aforementioned "slow" changes in state of fluency due to, for example, a developmental change in a child's speech motor control or a long-term raising of a child's excitement level (e.g., the child told about a trip to Disneyland three months before he or she will go!), these "rapid" changes in state of fluency are sound, syllable, word, phrase, or utterance-based. That is, these rather rapid changes in the state of fluency are believed by this author to be somehow associated with the complex processes that take place between our initiating thoughts and the resulting program that drives motor execution for speech. These changes are too rapid, too often occurring at certain places within the word (e.g., word-initial sounds), too highly correlated with certain (longer, more complex) utterances to be involved with anything other than formulative disruptions above the level of the motor system. In essence, we believe that these rapid changes in fluency must involve aspects above the level of the motor system (even if the motor system contributes) because the place within the utterance where stuttering occurs is not random; it is highly associated with certain syntactic, semantic, and/or phonologic variables. For example, the length (e.g., Bernstein Ratner & Sih, 1987; Logan & Conture, 1995) and grammatical complexity (e.g., Logan & Conture, 1997; Yaruss, 1999b) of the utterance are known to be associated with the frequency of stuttering. However, while Silverman and Bernstein Ratner (1997) found, for both adolescents who do and do not stutter, that normal disfluencies increase with increases in syntactic complexity, they did not find that stuttering frequency was influenced by increased syntactic complexity. Hence, as Silverman and Bernstein Ratner suggest, there may be a diminution in the influence of syntactic complexity on stuttering over the course of language acquisitions.

Indeed, one might make a reasonable case for the idea that much of the rapid variations in childhood stuttering, from utterance to utterance, relate to natural variations in length and complexity of utterances, variations that some children who stutter may find difficult to negotiate through in a smooth, error-free fashion, especially when they use faster than normal speaking rates. It is this writer's considered opinion that uncovering the mechanism that precipitates or causes stuttering will require an intense examination of the processes (i.e., syntactic, semantic, and phonological encoding) that rapidly transforms our concepts to a "program" that instructs the speech production mechanism. When instances of stuttering have such a rapid onset and offset within an utterance, it seems reasonable to assume that factors that precipitate stuttering must also involve rapidly change processes, for example, those processes involved with grammatical encoding.

6. *Stuttering is more common among males and in certain families.* Stuttering tends to be more prominent in males than females and "runs in families," although the exact percentage with which stuttering occurs in families is still less than clear. The gender issue, of course, should not surprise given the fact that boys exhibit more of almost all developmental problems than girls and the fact that boys tend to move through various speech and language developmental a bit less rapid and smoothly. Whatever, the fact that stuttering is more apt to occur in males and run in families suggests biological, inherited aspects, or at least an inherited predisposition toward exhibiting overly disfluent speech sometime during speech and language development. Recent years have witnessed a variety of attempts to describe the genetic components of stuttering (e.g., Ambrose, Yairi, & Cox, 1997; Cox, 1988; Felsenfeld, 1997; Kidd, 1983; Yairi, Ambrose, & Cox, 1996), work that will undoubtedly continue into the future. Among the many challenges in this area, is the fact that stuttering may not result from a single factor but several factors that interact in highly complex ways. Perhaps, we may find that some "causes" are more likely to be inherited while others less so. Further, once a plausible model of the genetics of stuttering is established, our biggest challenge will be to determine "what" is inherited, for example, a slow-to-develop Broca's area (i.e., the brain region situated within the third frontal convolution). Above all, it will be a challenge to figure out how the inheritance of a "fixed" deficit can create a "variable" behavioral problem like stuttering, where variation is not merely present but nearly the *sine qua non* of the problem.

7. *More children "outgrow" than continue to stutter.* About one or more of every five children who begins to stutter will probably continue on into later childhood and beyond. This indicates that as many as four out of every five children who being to stutter recover, with or without therapy. The trick, of course, and it's a big one (which we'll discuss extensively in the next chapter on assessment), is figuring out, at the time of initial evaluation, which of the children we are testing will and will not require treatment to improve. It is all well and good to say nearly four out of every five children recover without services. However, and this is most important, this statement still will not make apparent, at the time of initial evaluation, whether the child being assessed will be the one who continues to stutter or among the other four who will "outgrow stuttering."

8. *Certain conditions will make stuttering decrease, at least temporarily.* One of the more baffling observations, and one that SLPs are often asked about, is the fact that certain conditions, like singing, giving a memorized speech, or acting in a play, will help the person who stutters speak more fluently, at least temporarily. While the exact mechanism behind these temporary changes are not precisely known, the fact that stuttering can temporarily decrease (or increase), sometimes dramatically, remains a fundamental fact about this problem. Indeed, it is these sudden improvements in stuttering that some individuals have used to dupe the public into believing "the cure" was on hand. For example, some of these "procedures" require people who stutter to speak in time to rhythmic swinging of arms, speak while staring at lit candles, wear various devices that make the person concentrate more on the device than trying not to stuttering, and so forth. Ultimately, of course, these temporary "improvements" in stuttering are related, in some as yet unknown fashion, to the rapid changes in state of fluency previously noted. The hallmark of these changes in the state of fluency of the person who stutters is the relative (1) *speed* with which they can bring about change in the speech fluency of people who stutter, (2) *predictability* with which they change speech fluency across most people who stutter, and (3) *consistency* with which they change speech fluency within a person who stutters.

9. *The power of suggestion, as with the treatment of most human problems, is very much involved with the treatment of stuttering.* This topic was beautifully and fully explored by Van Riper (1973). As Van Riper accurately noted, the power of suggestion and/or placebo effect is just as influential when treating stuttering as it is when treating a wide variety of human conditions, for example, physical ailments, pain, psychological conditions, and so forth. Whether we like it or not, the power of suggestion and/or placebo effect is part of any treatment regimen. Too often, in fact, suggestion and placebo are the main ingredient in the cures and treatments sold by quacks. Furthermore, all too often, such treatments are purchased by an unsuspecting public quite ready to believe in the quick fix, the silver or magic bullet, the passive cure, the remedy requiring no pain or strain on their part. Generally speaking, a person's participation in speech-language therapy is not like putting on a pair of glasses or taking an aspirin for a headache. Instead, the client must DO something to receive maximal benefit from speech-language therapy. Stuttering does not result, as far as we know, from a virus or bacteria that can be defeated merely by swallowing a pill. The client must *actively* make changes in speech and speech-related behavior (not passively hope for the best) to receive benefit from speech-language therapy.

Cures Are for Hams and Other Edibles

Now is a good time, while we are discussing the power of suggestion, to mention "cures" for stuttering. Anyone who has treated the common cold or the problem of stuttering recognizes one reality: We are not yet at the point where we can meaningfully discuss *curing* most common colds or stuttering. Cures, outside those applied to hams and other edibles, suggest total, complete, and for all time recovery—something a bit short of miraculous, but nevertheless a remarkable event. While we cannot categorically deny the present existence of a cure for stuttering, it seems far more appropriate at this point in time to discuss our abilities, as speech-language pathologists, to facilitate positive change in the speech and related aspects of individuals who stutter. No, it is not my purpose in writing this book to discuss or tout a cure for stuttering. Instead, I'd like to keep as close as I can, both theoretically as well as therapeutically, to the facts of the matter, to ground my approach in the agony as well as the ecstasy of reality.

Certainly, therapeutic success of a particular method is important; however, success, because of its highly elusive nature, is extremely difficult to ascertain. For example, what is meant by and how does one define *success*? How long and how many times *after* formal therapy ended was stuttering behavior sampled and under what conditions? What was the nature of the problems exhibited by the clients who received the method? What was their behavior like *before* therapy began? These and similar questions quickly put into perspective, we think, the many claims that this or that therapy procedure with people who stutter typically results in 90 percent or greater success (see Bloodstein, 1995; Conture, 1996 for a more detailed overview of therapeutic success with people who stutter).

As we have seen, the problem of stuttering is most apt to be observed in males, especially in early childhood and while the person who stutters is communicating with other people. Most people who stutter begins to do so in childhood, before 7 years of age; however, a few adult individuals may suddenly begin to stutter, usually after some physical trauma. While the frequency of stuttering is continually changing, stuttering is not a random event. That is, it can be predicted that stuttering will occur on word-initial sounds or syllables, less frequently occurring words, and on longer, more grammatically complex utterances. The rapid changes in the state of fluency that constitute instances of stuttering may be associated with equally rapid changes in grammatical, semantic, and phonological processes that underlie speech and language production. For the approximately one out of five children who continue stuttering into later childhood and beyond, treatment can and is often recommended, as we'll discuss in Chapters 3 through 6. Most important, however, at present we still are a long way from determining, at the time of initial diagnostic, whether the child we are evaluating is among the four who will recover without therapy or is the one who needs therapy to recover. And, as with all human problems, the power of suggestion can have an appreciable effect over and beyond the fact that a particular treatment is effective.

What Are the Characteristics of People Who Stutter?

As clinicians, we must continually strive to recognize the central tendency or *average* among our clients who stutter as well as those behaviors of our clients that disperse or *range* above and below the central tendency. Just as the fact that the average IQ is 100 does not mean that the "average" individual has an IQ equal to 100, so we find that all people who stutter are not identical in terms of their problem and related concerns. Once again, stuttering is a behavior, a behavior that varies around some central tendency. To overgeneralize and expect all individuals who stutter to be the same, just because they stutter, is to oversimplify. Remember, people who stutter don't enter the doors of your clinical domain in a group, they walk in, one at a time, as individuals. Given these cautionary words, in general, what might we expect of people who stutter? The following is not an exhaustive review of this area—for a more detailed description of these characteristics see Bloodstein, 1995; Silverman, 1996—rather it is general overview to give the reader some appreciation for our current understanding of the characteristics of people who stutter.

First, let's consider the *psychosocial* adjustment of people who stutter. Perhaps Bloodstein (1995, p. 236) summarized it best, ". . . the weight of accumulated evidence does not appear to indicate that the average person who stutters is a distinctly neurotic or severely maladjusted individual in the usual meanings of these terms." He also suggests that "... people who stutter *on the average* are not quite as well adjusted as are typical normal speakers" (p. 236–237) but notes that such lack of "social adjustment" is probably a normal reaction to an abnormal situation (my phrase, not Bloodstein's!). That is, people who stutter, according to Bloodstein, may be "... socially maladjusted to the extent that they avoid contacts with others requiring speech." We will, in the next chapter, visit the area of *temperament* (e.g., Guitar, 1998; Oyler, 1996a, 1996b; Oyler & Ramig, 1995), a variable that would seem to influence psychosocial adjustment and/or reaction to stuttering. One area related to personality, temperament (e.g., Oyler, 1996a), which we now know is something we begin to exhibit right from birth, appears to be particularly germane. At present, we are just beginning to understand how a person's stuttering might relate to the fact that they are "behaviorally inhibited," for example, strong reactivity to novelty, change, objectively non-threatening events like the dark, or "slow to warm up," for example, stopping one's interactions when people unfamiliar approach, reluctance to answer the door, or separate from parents. For the present, therefore, we believe it safe to say that the average person who stutters is within normal limits in terms of psychosocial adjustment. However, these people may show a degree of social maladjustment relative to situations where they must talk—a logical reaction, we would suggest, and one more indicative of the fact that the psychological integrity of people who stutter is intact than it is awry.

Second, what of the *intelligence* of people who stutter? Silverman (1996, pp. 64–66) does a nice job of summarizing past and present research regarding the average IQ of people who stutter and suggests that people who stutter fall within the area of 100 (the average for the population as a whole). However, in studies that have directly compared people who do to those who do not stutter, the IQs of people who stutter is slightly lower, approximately half a standard deviation, a fact that may explain why they also lag about six months behind their peers educationally (e.g., Andrews, Craig, Feyer, Hoddinott, Howie, & Neilson, 1983). In this writer's experience, the intellectual abilities of people who stutter range across the spectrum similar to people who do not stutter, even though people who are mentally challenged can and do exhibit stuttering. Again, this author would caution against using central tendencies for the group of people who stutter to predict how any one individual who stutters might perform; at the risk of redundancy, clients come to a clinic one at a time, not as a group, and the wise clinician must remain ever open to the real possibility for individual differences. Obviously, if a person who was mentally challenged also stuttered, we would have to evaluate and treat the stuttering in the context of diminished intellectual abilities; but by and large, the average person who stutters who receives speech and language treatment in clinical settings other than those that serve the mentally challenged (e.g., the public schools) is roughly within normal limits intellectually.

Third, what about the *personality* of people who stutter? This has been extensively studied and suffice it to say that there is no personality trait common to all people who stutter. Naturally, of course, as suggested above, people who stutter will be more or less likely to enter and avoid any social situation that requires them to speak. Again, Silverman (1996, pp. 68–76) does a nice job of covering the various aspects of personality that at least some people who stutter seem to exhibit—for example, depression regarding their coping with stuttering, guilt about stuttering, and so forth. Again, as with intelligence, one can certainly find people who are, for example, very non-outgoing, and the stuttering of such people needs to be evaluated and treated within the context of this extreme reluctance to socially interact. However, to expect all people who stutter to exhibit such traits because some do is to operate on the basis of stereotypes rather than on the basis of the personal reality of each individual person who stutter.

Fourth, what would we expect to observe regarding the *speech* disfluencies of people who stutter? To a degree we have already covered this. In essence, the data shown in Table 1.1 provides a reasonable overview of the nature and frequency of the types of speech disfluencies one would expect to observe in children who do and do not stutter (Yairi, 1997a, updates this information, for example, see Yairi's Table 3.3). However, as we tried to make clear in preceding sections, we would not automatically label an individual as a person who stutters if they produce one or two stutterings, stuttered-like, or within-word disfluencies. Someone who has just experienced one bout of alcoholic intoxication does not immediately seek out the local AA chapter, neither should a temporary period of stuttering or within-word disfluencies mean that a person would or should immediately seek out therapy for stuttering. Just as the *frequency* and *predictability* of alcoholic consummation and intoxication, not just drinking itself, give cause for concern, we only start to become real concerned about a person's speech when the exhibited stutterings become *persistent*, *predictable*, and *consistent*, and not just merely occur on occasion when they speak.

Fifth, and finally, what about the *speech and language abilities* of people who stutter? In recent years, this area has received extensive review (e.g., Bernstein Ratner, 1997a; Louko, Conture & Edwards, 1999; Nippold, 1990; Tetnowski, 1998) as well as empirical study (e.g., Bernstein Ratner, 1997b; Logan & Conture, 1997; Louko, Edwards & Conture, 1990; Paden & Yairi, 1996; Paden, Yairi, & Ambrose, 1999; Throneburg, Yairi, & Paden, 1994; Yaruss & Conture, 1996). In general, as Bloodstein (1995, p. 250) notes, children who stutter appear to exhibit more articulation errors or phonological processes than do their normally fluent peers. With regard to the language abilities of people who stutter, Andrews and colleagues (1983) suggested that people who stutter perform poorly on some tests of language abilities. (While findings in this area are less than consistent, data supportive of Andrews and colleagues' suggestion have been reported by several researchers, e.g., Anderson & Conture, 2000; Murray & Reed, 1977; Williams, Melrose, & Woods, 1969.) However, Bernstein Ratner (1997b) suggests that the ". . . results of many recent studies have, for the most part, suggested that the language capabilities of individuals who stutter do not differ appreciably from those of nonstutterers" (p.103). Bernstein Ratner further suggests, however, that subtle, *subclinical* concerns with language abilities (i.e., less than clinically significant deficits in language knowledge or performance, deficits that neither warrant the label of language delay or disorder or warrant treatment to resolve) may be exhibited by adults who stutter (e.g., Bosshardt, 1993). Perhaps, these adults represent a subgroup within the population, that is, by definition, because they still stutter, they are the *persistent* not *recovered* people who stutter. Whatever the case, we have minimal understanding of whether these subtle differences are exhibited by children who stutter or whether those children who exhibit these subtle differences are more likely to persist. In the chapters that follow, we will discuss how knowing something about the language knowledge and performance of a person who stutters may help us more thoroughly and beneficially evaluate and treat that person. In the meantime, the jury is still out, way out, regarding the role that phonological, semantic, and syntactic knowledge and performance play in the onset, development, and maintenance of stuttering in children, teenagers, and adults.

Why Do People Stutter (Subtitled, What Causes Stuttering)?

To begin, let me say right up front: I simply do not know, in any precise way, what causes stuttering! Furthermore, all my professional and personal experience suggests that no one else does either. Likewise, I also don't know the best way to treat stuttering. And I really don't know if there is only *one* way. Again, I'm not sure if anyone else does either. Of one thing I am sure, however: The history of stuttering, both theory and therapy, reflects a multidimensional problem that has repeatedly and successfully defied unidimensional solutions. So, if readers of this book hope that I am going to reveal *the* cause of stuttering or the silver bullet for "curing" it, they are probably going to be disappointed.

The above said, I believe I know some of the things that probably don't typically cause *developmental* stuttering for *most* people—for example, physical and/or psychological trauma (yes, there are definitely cases where developmental stuttering seems to begin after some form of psychological or physical trauma, but these are more exceptions than the rule). Indeed, the case histories of most people who stutter look very similar to those of people who don't stutter (e.g., Adams, 1993; Yairi, 1997b, pp. 24–28, provides a nice review of the role of parents and home environment on childhood stuttering). However, there would appear to be some things that we might reasonably conclude about the causes of stuttering, given the large amount of research that has been conducted on this topic (e.g., Bloodstein, 1995).

Lay Opinion About Cause

Of course, besides the diversity of professional opinion on the matter, we must deal with a diversity of lay person thought on the matter. For example, I have had grandparents and friends tell the parents of young children that tickling a child will cause stuttering. We smile at such advice, but to the young parent, especially if the child subsequently begins to stutter, such advice may seem sage and/or to actually explain the child's behavior. Of course, if tickling caused stuttering, most of us would be stuttering, wouldn't we? No, the simple act of occasional tickling of a child will not cause that child to stutter; however, some people, whether they be professional or lay public, do not want information to cloud their judgment! The half-life of a theory, no matter how bad, is far greater than the most blatant fact. And while lay public mis- or disinformation may trouble us, we should not try to get the theoretical house of the lay public in order while the theoretical domain of our profession is still in a less than trivial state of disarray!

Professional Opinions About Cause

To begin, I believe it important that we, as students, clinicians, and researchers, be as tolerant as possible regarding the evolving nature of stuttering theory. In essence, the marketplace of ideas regarding theory development is mainly a seller's market. A theoretician puts his or her wares out on the market and waits to see how many will buy them. And, like any commodity, a fool and his or her money are soon parted! Truly, with regard to theories of stuttering, *caveat emptor* (let the buyer beware) is the best policy.

Be that as it may, at this point, we should be, in my opinion, willing to entertain *likely* rather than *certain* explanations for why people stutter. Furthermore, the more sources of theoretical input we receive, from as many different perspectives as possible, the greater the possibility that no relevant issue will be overlooked, although we can readily appreciate the sentiments of some (Smith & Webber, 1988) that we may be suffering from a surfeit of perspectives relative to stuttering.

Certainly the too-many-cooks-spoil-the-broth status of stuttering theory and therapy makes for confusion for students in training, workers in the field, as well as the lay public. Disagreements for disagreement's sake are, to put it mildly, ludicrous. However, it is only by offering different theories and therapies in the marketplace of ideas that the truth will emerge. Eventually. Disagreements, not agreements, typically foster and encourage new insights into old problems and are part of the stuff from which progress is made. However, while we may agree to disagree, we should be able to do so without becoming disagreeable.

Theories of Stuttering

Theories of stuttering can be traced back to antiquity (e.g., Rieber & Wollock, 1977). And while we can learn a good deal from the study of most theories about stuttering, some theoretical explanations have become part of rather than the solution for the problem. Indeed, some theoretical explanations adequately deal with one facet of stuttering while seemingly overlooking many others. Facts, it has been said, are pesky things; they seldom go away no matter how strong our theoretical cleanser. In this regard, I like to paraphrase Sinclair Lewis (1920) and suggest that the reality of our clinical days has all too often failed to live up to the dreams of our theoretical nights.

More recently, Bloodstein (1995, pp. 59–103), for example, has done an excellent job of sorting these theories into three interrelated groupings: (1) those that attempt to explain the discrete stuttering response itself; (2) those that attempt to explain the etiology of stuttering; and (3) those that attempt to explain stuttering by "shifting the frame of reference," that is, try to explain stuttering within some relatively new or different theoretical framework (e.g., stuttering as a learned behavior). We won't recapitulate (even if we could) Bloodstein's thorough overview of theories of stuttering (past and present). Rather, we will focus on a handful of relatively current theories that seem to be driving most recent research and therapy in the area of stuttering.

Nature, Nurture, or Interaction. The theoretical pendulum of stuttering never really stops in the middle. Instead, throughout the history of the study of stuttering, this theoretical pendulum has often careened in the direction of one of two extremes. One extreme can be characterized by theories heavily if not exclusively dependent upon "*nurture*" or environmental factors (e.g., stuttering as a learned behavior). The other extreme can be characterized by theories heavily if not exclusively dependent upon "*nature*" or organic factors (e.g., stuttering resulting from lack of cerebral dominance for control of activity of the speech mechanism). Unfortunately, in this writer's opinion, these theoretical extremes (i.e., pure nature vs. pure nurture), have often lead to 'tis-'taint dueling between extremists. For example, one group of "enthusiasts" who put all their eggs in the "nature" basket may duel with those who put all theirs in the "nurture" basket (and there are those who take a third extreme, that is, an atheoretical extreme or "who cares what causes stuttering as long as my treatment works"). And while dialogue between followers of these two considerably different points of view have helped highlight those issues most important to consider, it also sometimes generates more heat than it sheds light. Therefore, the present writer has taken what he believes to be a bit more tenable, middle-of-the-road approach. This approach considers *both* nature and nurture and, most importantly, we believe, their *interaction*. This type of approach has been described as an *interactionist* approach (see Purser, 1987, pp. 258–259). In its most general form, an interactionist point of view suggests that our external behavior influences our internal thinking and our internal thinking influences our external behavior; however, this perspective is a bit too general regarding interaction for our current purposes.

My Basic Assumption About the Cause of Stuttering.   Again, rather than taking a position supporting either nature or nurture, it is this writer's basic assumption that stuttering is caused by a complex mixing, meshing or interaction between nature and nurture. Put in other words, this writer believes that stuttering results from a complex interaction between the *environment* of a person who stutters and the *inherited* skills and abilities that the person who stutters brings to his or her environment. It is this writer's basic belief in interaction between environment and innate or inherent abilities that leads him to describe himself as an interactionist.

In an ideal world, things would be clean, simple, and straightforward; unfortunately, this is an imperfect world where things are often dirty, complex, and intertwined with one another. It might be nice, in some ways, if stuttering had a straightforward genetic (e.g., see Kidd, 1983, 1984) or environmental (e.g., see Johnson & Associates, 1959) origin. However, neither "pure" nature nor nurture models have been able to adequately explain stuttering (see Ambrose, et al., 1997; Cox, 1988; Felsenfeld, 1997 for more recent descriptions of genetic aspects of stuttering and how environmental variables may interact with these aspects). While these two polar opposite models—nature versus nurture—nicely describe selective acts, neither completely circumscribes the entire play.

In the Milieu or in the Mouth.   This writer, based on his experience, has difficulty putting the onus on one, supposedly defective, organ. Likewise, it is difficult for him to assign the blame solely to parental practices and rearing. Indeed, he feels strongly that a combination of ingredients must be included in the recipe that causes stuttering and exacerbates as well as maintains it. And, just like with a recipe, if each person who stutters has a little less of this but more of that, then the end product, while essentially similar to the original, may be different in subtle and not so subtle ways. For example, even though both Person X and Person Y are diagnosed as people who stutter, the proportion of Person X's environmental contributions to stuttering may be greater than for Person Y. Conversely, Person Y's speech-language production contribution to stuttering may be greater than for Person X. Indeed, we will assume that the proportion of these ingredients differs from one person who stutters to the next (for similar speculations, see Smith & Kelly, 1997, particularly Figure 10–2). Okay, we can accept, for argument's sake, that one person gets a pinch of ingredient X while another person gets one-fourth teaspoon, but what might be the specific ingredients to be included in the recipe?

Basic Ingredients of Most Modern-Day Theories. We will concentrate our discussion of ingredients on those most likely to be involved with the rapid changes in state of fluency previously described. Why? Because it is these changes, the rapid moment-to-moment changes in fluency, that we believe are at the heart of the riddle of stuttering. Granted, events that take longer to onset and offset, for example, a week of excitement prior to a big test may exacerbate the person's stuttering. However, we submit that such longer or relatively slow changes are *superimposed* or layered on the rapid changes in the state of fluency. The rapidity and variability of the onset and offset of instance of stuttering requires underlying, causal processes that are equally rapid, variable, and dynamically interactive. And while changing from a face-to-face conversation to talking to someone over the phone may exacerbate stuttering (e.g., make instances of stuttering longer or more physically tense), these factors are simply too slow to account for the rapid, moment-to-moment changes in the state of a person's speech fluency, particularly within a conversational situation that remains fairly constant. Neither can these relatively slow changes in tempermental reactions, emotional states, situations, and so forth easily explain why stuttering increases with increases in utterance length, tends to occur on nouns, verbs, adjectives, and adverbs with adults who stutter, and so forth. Thus, for the present discussion of ingredients, we will focus on variables seemingly capable of rapidly changing the state of a person's speech fluency.

Table 1.4 lists the basic ingredients that I believe are probably involved in the cause of instances of stuttering. First, I would expect that *syntactic encoding* (i.e., suffice it to say, the computational rules or calculations used by the speaker to generate sentence frames, for example, Noun Phrase [NP] + Verb Phrase [VP]) is involved with stuttering. Essentially, morphosyntactic construction, that is needed to produce a sentence frame, may be slow and/or inefficient for some people who stutter. Second, I would expect that semantic selection or lexical retrieval (i.e., suffice it to say, the selection of "fillers" [lexical items or words] from the lexicon or "catalogue" that need to be inserted into the "slots" within the syntactic "frame") is involved with stuttering. Essentially, retrieval of the so-called "lemma" or syntactic word (see Levelt, Roelofs, & Meyer, 1999, pp. 1-8, for further description of lemma and related concepts) may be slow and/or inefficient for some people who stutter. Third, I would expect that phonological encoding (i.e., suffice it to say, the ability to select phonemes and then insert them into a plan or program that would "drive" the speech mechanism) is involved with stuttering. Essentially, for more than a few people who stutter, there may be a slowness and/or inefficiency of "phonological spell-out" of the so-called "lexeme," or word form, once the lemma or syntactic word has been selected. Fourth, I would expect that motor execution (i.e., skilled, volitional movements, particularly of the oral/laryngeal area) is involved with stuttering at least for some people who stutter. While most of the above are *internal* (i.e., inherent to the person), I also assume that *external* (i.e., inherent to the person's surroundings) *environment* issues are involved with stuttering. However, these environmental events, in my opinion, have probably more

---

TABLE 1.4   Some Basic Ingredients Involved in Initiating and Exacerbating of Instances of Stuttering*

Initiating:
Syntactic encoding
Lexical, storage, and/or retrienal
Phonological encoding
Motor execution

Exacerbating/Perpetuating:
External environment
(e.g., inappropriate communication models, inappropriate communication interactions, etc.)

Internal environment
(e.g., temperamental reactions to mistakes, environmental change, differences, inappropriate communication "practices" [e.g., routinely using longer, more complex utterances])

*"Initiating" ingredients are those the author believes to have a high likelihood of initiating/causing instances of stuttering, and, hence, a stuttering problem. "Exacerbating" and "Perpetuating" ingredients are those the author believes to have a likelihood of aggravating or maintaining instances of stuttering, and, hence, a stuttering problem.

influence on the relatively slow (across days, weeks and months, rather than from one utterance to the next) changes in state of fluency and are, therefore, more involved with *exacerbating* than *precipitating* stuttering.

Finally, I would expect that the four variables noted above impact the person's speaking in a dynamic, online fashion that varies from speaking act to speaking act. In other words, these variables would produce an event, that is, stuttering, that is more reflective of a particular state of speaking than a trait of speaking. It would seem possible to combine these four variables—syntactic encoding, lexical retrieval, phonological encoding, and motor execution—in an infinite number and variety of ways (similar to the interactions depicted in Smith & Kelly's Figure 10.2). However, at this point for pedagogical reasons, I will restrict my discussion to a rather finite number of possible interactions, although I *definitely* assume that there are a variety of dynamic, nonlinear interactions among all of these ingredients. I also assume that these interactions differ among different individuals. To begin, however, are the "ingredients" that I've previously listed especially unique or new under the sun? Hardly, as we'll see immediately below.

Some Modern-Day Theories or Models of Stuttering That Seem Ingredient-Specific.
The beginning student of stuttering comes to quickly realize one thing: There is no dearth of models to explain stuttering! Certainly, in a book with an applied emphasis, it is neither appropriate nor possible to cover *all* such models (as we've said before, that is more appropriate for and done masterfully by Bloodstein [1995] in his classic textbook). However, it is quite possible to discuss some of the main, current theories and how they shape our theoretical as well as therapeutic thinking.

To do so, I have somewhat arbitrarily separated seven of the more current models (see Table 1.5) into two groupings: (1) those models that provide *ingredient-specificity* (I-S); and (2) those models that provide *mechanism-specificity* (M-S). The I-S models mainly

TABLE 1.5   Some Examples of Ingredient-Specific (IS) and Mechanism-Specific (M-S) Models of Stuttering*

I-S Models:
Wall & Meyers (1995)
  "three-factor" model
Adams (1990), Starkweather & Gottwald (1990)
  "demands and capacity" model
Smith & Kelly (1997)
  "dynamic, multifactorial" model

M-S Models:
MacKay & McDonald (1984)
  "slow to activate/deactivate nodes associated with speech muscle movement system" model
Wingate (1988)
  "fault line/dyssynchrony between utterance planning and assembly" model
Perkins, Kent, & Curlee (1991)
  "dyssynchronous syllable frames and segment content" model
Postma & Kolk (1993), Kolk & Postma (1997)
  "covert repair hypothesis/impairment in phonological encoding" model
Other example (not covered in detail in text)
  Karniol (1995), Howell, Au-Yeung, & Sackin (1999)

*"Ingredient-specific" models are those that, in the writer's opinion, appear to focus on the basic ingredients related to the initiating, exacerbation, and perpetuation of stuttering. "Mechanism-specific" models are those that, in the writer's opinion, appear to focus on the mechanism or means by which stuttering may be initiated, exacerbated, or perpetuated. Some models, for example, the Demands and Capacity Model, may fit both categorizations, but is listed in the category that it appears to most directly address. Note: Models are meant to be tested, and such testing may modify the model; therefore, if any of the models listed is empirically tested, the present version of the model may differ from its future version.

seem to provide insights into possible *ingredients* that may contribute to stuttering as well as how these ingredients interact among one another. The M–S models mainly seem to provide insights into the possible *mechanism(s)* that actually cause instances of stuttering. While no such dichotomy is totally satisfactory—for example, some I-S models do make some attempt to specify the mechanism—the I-S/M-S distinction provides us with one useful framework to examine the current state of the art relative to theories of stuttering.

Ingredient-Specific (I-S) Models. **1.** *Three-factor model.* Wall and Myers (1995), using what they call "a three-factor model," depict the interaction among three different, but interrelated "ingredients," that is, psycholinguistic, psychosocial, and physiological factors (p. 11) through appropriate use of three intersecting circles (i.e., a Venn diagram). Indeed, it would seem that some aspect of "language," "psychology," and "physiology" must be involved singularly or in combination with stuttering, especially if one takes, like this writer, an *interactionist* point of view.

As previously mentioned, this writer finds it difficult to contemplate *pure* (i.e., 100%) physiological or pure psychological explanations for the cause of stuttering; such explanations just don't square with the facts of stuttering as he knows them. For example, how could a *constant* motor difficulty mainly manifest itself on nouns and verbs or when speaking in the presence of the teacher but not a friend? Conversely, why would an individual with a *purely* psychological problem, for example, neurotic anxiety about communicating during stressful situations, exhibit significantly slower nonspeech movements of the tongue or lips? Again, as long as we view stutterings, the behavior, as a trait, as a constant, as something always there, ever present—a state of affairs (no pun intended) that clearly does not exist—we miss one fundamental aspect of stuttering, that is, instances of stuttering reflect rapid, moment-to-moment changes in the state of the person's fluency, changes that follow the continual fluctuations in the processes of speech and language production.

2. *Demands and capacity model.* Similar to Wall and Myers, another theory, the "demands and capacity" (D&C) model (e.g., Adams, 1990; Starkweather & Gottwald, 1990), suggests that stuttering relates to a variety of interactions between elements of nature as well as nurture. As this writer understands the situation, no one element(s) or interaction holds prominence in terms of cause, but some might seem more likely candidates than others (see Bernstein Ratner, 1997a, for critique of this model). This model appears to assume that, for example, *demands* within or between "domains" (e.g., language might be a domain, or speech motor control might be a domain), that exceed the *capacity* of another aspect of the same or different domain would lead to disruptions or disfluencies in speaking.

For example, let us assume that a child has an excellent capacity for generating long, complex utterances. This *capacity* may, however, place *demands* on the child for rapid, relatively complex articulatory adjustments (note: while there may be some *de facto* assumptions that demands are always external while capacities are always internal to the speaker, this is not necessarily the case, at least in theory). These demands for rapid, relatively complex articulatory adjustment could, in turn, exceed the child's inherent ability to quickly, precisely, and sequentially make needed adjustments in speech motor control. That is, the child would be at risk for stuttering, according to the D&C model, because the child's above-normal-limits language capacity placed demands on the child's speech motor control that far exceeded the child's capacity for quick, precise, and sequential control of speech production. Again, the possible D&C interactions are limitless, a fact that makes the model robust in terms of its ability to account for many different causal possibilities. Conversely, such seemingly endless ability to explain many possible causes of stuttering also spreads the model rather thin and difficult to test. For example, regarding stuttering, which D&C interactions does the D&C model suggest are the most fruitful for investigation, why, and under what circumstances?

3. *Multifactorial model.* Another fairly recent model, the dynamic, multifactorial model described by Smith and Kelly (1997), provides discussion of all the ingredients discussed by Wall and Myer. Furthermore, Smith and Kelly go one step further and describe the types of observations or level of analysis needed to assess these many ingredients or variables. What is particularly nice about Smith and Kelly's formulation, in this writer's opinion, is their Figure 10.2 that shows four different people. In this figure, a "stack" or collection of roughly circular areas represents each person, with each area relating to "factors" that contribute to stuttering. This figure helps us to see, I think, that different interactions among a collection of factors may contribute to stuttering in different ways for different people (something alluded to before by this writer). Such discussion is a bit reminiscent of Van Riper's (1971) widely cited four "tracks" of etiology and development, or as it has been said before "different paths to the same end." The Smith and Kelly model does a nice job of pointing out that individual variations among different variables may mean that we should be talking about causes rather than cause of stuttering. However, it leaves open whether the number of these "dynamic interactions" are infinite or finite and which of these interactions is of greatest import to the cause of stuttering.

Overview of I-S models. While difficult to empirically assess, it is interesting to consider Starkweather's notions about demands and capacities, Wall and Myers' idea about complex interactions among various factors, and Smith and Kelly's attempts to account for individual variations in number and nature of factors. These formulations seem to circumscribe almost all variables most likely to be involved with stuttering and present a variety of reasonable notions about how these variables might (in)appropriately interact. However, in my opinion, these models don't go quite far enough. They open the door, show us the many possible directions to consider, but don't quite suggest which route to take. Perhaps heavy on ingredients, they are light on mechanism. That is, I think they fall a bit short, and I assume purposively so, of providing enough specificity in terms of identifying what the precise mechanism that may cause stuttering. For example, how does a capacity that exceeds a demand actually result in an instance of stuttering? In other words, the I-S models provide less than full detail about the precise mechanism, within each model, that leads to sound prolongations, sound/syllable repetitions, monosyllabic whole-word repetitions, and so on (i.e., instances of stuttering). And, of course, as Smith and Kelly imply, with their individual variations shown in Figure 10.2 of their chapter, the precise mechanism that causes stuttering may differ among people who stutter. However, this may not be the most parsimonious way of thinking about the actual mechanism(s) that causes stuttering. Even though different ingredients in different amounts may contribute differently for different people, it would seem, in the end, that a finite number of mechanisms must be triggering the speech events we call stuttering. In subsequent paragraphs, we will examine just what those mechanisms might be.

Mechanism-Specific Models of Stuttering.   In contrast to the aforementioned I-S models, below are four fairly recent models (Kolk & Postma, 1997; MacKay & MacDonald, 1984; Perkins et al., 1991; Postma & Kolk, 1993; Wingate, 1988) that seem to be more specific about the possible mechanism that causes stuttering. Many of the "ingredients" discussed by these four M-S models are quite similar to those in the I-S models of Adams, Starkweather, and Gottwald, Wall and Myers, and Smith and Kelly. This writer neither endorses the following four theories nor refutes the preceding three previously discussed. All I am suggesting is that the following theories "go out on a limb" more in trying to specify the mechanism(s) that may cause stuttering (a limb that subsequent empirical evidence could easily saw off, but so be it, theory development and testing is not for the faint of heart!). And while the following brief review of modern-day theory greatly simplifies often elegant theorization, I hope my review will provide the reader with a skeleton or framework with which to begin to develop an understanding of some current theories of stuttering, the details of which will take further study than this clinically oriented text can provide.

1. *Slow-to-activate speech movement model.* MacKay and MacDonald (1984) seemingly concentrating on the *physiological* factor mentioned by the three I-S models, appear to suggest that stuttering results from difficulties at the motor or speech muscle movement level. In essence, MacKay and MacDonald assume that the "nodes" (i.e., theoretical constructs representing muscle-specific patterns of movement) of the speech muscle movement system are too slow to activate as well as too quick to recover after activation. Meaning: The muscle movement system of people who stutter, although slow to be activated, once activated for a particular sound or sound cluster, has a tendency to be quickly reactivated. This results in a repetition of the sound or sound clusters just "served" by that "node" controlling underlying muscle-specific patterns of movement. MacKay and MacDonald stay close to the basic observation that instances of stuttering typically consist of repetitions of sounds and syllables. Furthermore, they primarily focus on the muscle movement system, without a great deal of emphasis on processes above this level (e.g., syntactic or phonological encoding). In this writer's opinion, as a possible mechanism for explaining instances of stuttering, there is considerable merit to MacKay and MacDonald's notion of slowness of activation within the communication systems of people who stutter (indeed, we will see the notion of slowness of activation being central to another theory, that of Postma & Kolk). Where this writer has some difficulty is with the emphasis MacKay and MacDonald seem to place on the motor system, when considerable data and thought would suggest that the phonological, semantic, and syntactic processes above the motor system make important contributions to stuttering.

2. *Fault line hypothesis.* Wingate (1988), seemingly focusing on the *psycholinguistic* factor mentioned by Wall and Myers, albeit with more specificity, also attempted to specify the mechanism that causes instances of stuttering. However, Wingate appears to center or locate this mechanism "above" the level of the motor system. He suggests that stuttering relates to a dyssynchrony (a word we'll see again with the Perkins and colleagues' model to be discussed shortly) between utterance planning and assembly. Wingate seems to be assuming that stuttering relates to the ability of the person who stutters to quickly and fluently attach the nucleus of the syllable with the onset of the syllable. He describes a "fault line" between syllable onset (initial consonant cluster) and syllable nucleus (vowel). At this "fault," the "attachment" between syllable onset and nucleus does not take place. This is the reason we hear the person repeat or prolong the first syllable until the "attachment" occurs. Wingate puts forth a reasonable hypothesis about instances of stuttering occurring at the demarcation between syllable onset and nucleus. However, Postma (1991, pp. 18–19) justifiably questions whether the boundary between syllable onset and nucleus can account for the location of all or at least most instances of stutterings, for example, more than a few stutterings occur at the boundary between syllable nucleus and syllable coda (final consonant cluster).

3. *Dyssynchronous syllable frames and segment content model.* Perkins and colleagues (1991), employing all three factors (i.e., *psycholinguistic*, *psychosocial*, and *psychological*), mentioned by the previously discussed I-S models, suggest that stuttering occurs when integration of the syllable frame and segment content becomes dyssynchrous. Perkins and colleagues' speculation appears to relate, at least in part, to what are called frame-and-slot models of sentence production (e.g., Dell & Julliano, 1991). Perkins and colleagues appear to suggest that the syllable "slot" is improperly correlated in time with the segment (sound or sounds) "filler" that must go into the slot. When this dyssynchrony occurs, disruptions in speech, according to Perkins and colleagues, are likely to occur. They also mentions psychosocial contributors, something that few of the current M-S models discuss in any detail. In fact, Perkins and colleagues' model's main asset (i.e., few viable causation candidates are left out) is also its main liability (i.e., too many possible causation candidates are left in). That is, when a theory stands for everything, it may fall for anything. Thus, while there is much to applaud about Perkins and colleagues' model, particularly its notion of dyssynchrony between syllable slots and fillers, its obvious eclecticism makes it somewhat difficult to fully comprehend as well as empirically test salient aspects of the model.

4. *Covert repair hypothesis.* Most recently, Postma and Kolk (1993) and Kolk and Postma (1997), primarily concentrating on *psycholinguistic* variables describe what they term a "covert-repair hypothesis." With this hypothesis, Postma and Kolk suggest that people who stutter have an impairment in phonological encoding (i.e., the part of the speech production system that develops an articulatory plan or program for the speech motor system to carry out). (See Figure 1.2.)

Actually, Kolk and Postma (1997, Figures 9.4 & 9.5) appear to suggest at least two possible means by which speech errors might increase and, thus, lead to increased opportunities for self-repairs, speech disfluencies, and/or stuttering. First, *increased speaking rate, normal rate of activation*: Here the speaker's rate of activation of speech/target units is normal, but by increasing the rate of speaking, the speaker speeds up or moves the point of selection "forward" in time (from point S to S- in Figure 1.2a, after Kolk & Postma's, 1997, Figure 9.4); thus increasing the chances the speaker will make a misselection because both target and competing units have equal levels of activation at the point of selection. Second, *normal rate of speaking, lower/slower rate of activation*: Here the speaker uses a normal rate of speech, thus selecting at a normal point in time (S, in Figure 1.2b after Kolk & Postma, 1997, Figure 9.5); but because the speaker exhibits a slow or low rate activation of target and competing units, he or she is again likely to make a misselection because both target and competing speech units are equally activated at the point of selection. For people who stutter, however, we might ask: "Which is it, a faster rate of speaking or lower activation rate?" Well, Postma and Kolk seem to be suggesting that a combination of both factors—increased speaking rate and slower rate of activation—may contribute to instances of stuttering.

Thus, for people who stutter, according to Postma and Kolk, activation of intended sounds or "target (sound) units" are delayed or slow to activate for people who stutter. This is thought to result in a longer period of time during which their intended sounds are in competition with other sounds. That is, people who stutter experience a longer period of time during which the sound they intend to select is in competition for selection with other sounds. The problem arises for the person who stutters, according to Postma and Kolk, when the person initiates or maintains speech at a rate faster (i.e., tries to select sounds more rapidly) than the rate at which the slow-to-activate phonological encoding system makes

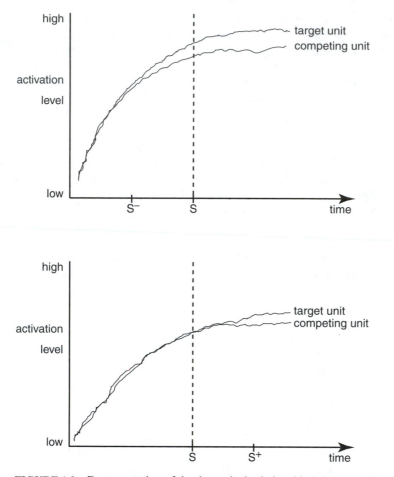

FIGURE 1.2 Demonstration of the theoretical relationship between activation of a "target" unit (e.g., "b" in the word "bean"), "competing" unit (e.g., "d" in word "dean"), and point of speaker selection of these units. (a) Normal rate of activation. Here, at the point the speaker selects (S) a sound to be inserted in his or her phonetic plan, the level of activation has risen higher than that for the competing unit, increasing chances of correct selection. (b) Low activation rate. Here, at the point in time when the speaker selects (S) a sound to be inserted into his or her phonetic plan, due to slow or impaired phonological encoding, both the target and competing units are at the same level of activation, increasing chances of errors in selection errors. Note: In (a), selecting at *earlier* points (S-), for example, by using faster speaking rate, would increase chances of errors, even though the individual's speech and language production system has, in general, normal rates of activation. In (b), selecting at a later (S+) point in time, for example, by using slower speaking rate, would decrease chances for errors, even though the individual's speech and language production system has, in general, slower rates of activation. (Adapted from Kolk & Postma, 1997, Figures 9.3 and 9.4, with permission)

available appropriate phonological targets. This "mismatch" increases the chances that speech sound selection errors will be made (i.e., sounds other than those intended will be selected). If these errors are detected by the person who stutters, according to this theory, such detection will result in a self-repair or correction, which, in turn, is perceived by the listener as stuttering.

This theory has much to recommend it. For example, the Postma and Kolk model makes a rigorous attempt to account for the stutterings that actually occur in conversation. Paraphrasing Bernstein Ratner (1997b, p. 101), the strength of a model can be assessed by how well it can predict or account for the type of errors that actually do as well as do not occur in spoken language. However, unless extended or modified, the current focus of the covert repair hypothesis on the phonological level, to the exclusion of syntactic and semantic variable as well as eschewing consideration of motor aspects of speech production, may limit its ultimate ability to account for stuttering in all situations. That is, it may have limited ability to handle the sort of individual variations that Smith and Kelly's multifactorial theory so aptly attempts to describe.

As the preceding discussion indicates, with the exception of MacKay and MacDonald, most mechanism-specific (M-S) theories of stuttering appear to focus on events *above* the level of motor speech production. Again, this does not imply that focus on "higher levels" is correct and consideration of "lower centers" incorrect (indeed, it is almost a certainty that some overarching theory that bridges between lower- and higher-center causes will be best able to account for a larger part of the whole of stuttering). It does suggest, however, that such focus on "higher centers—for example, phonological processing—makes sense to these workers and seemingly fits at least some existing objective information about stuttering. Many of these M-S (and some I-S) theories also seem to involve, in one way or another, *dyssynchronies*, *mismatches* or *temporal asynchronies* between processes that must be finely and exactly correlated in time and space to produce a fluent end product. However, while the D&C model of Adams and Starkweather focuses on a mismatch between demands and capacities, on a number of different levels, it does not focus on time. Time, however, is central to other models, for example, the dyssynchonous syllable frame/segment content model of Perkins and colleagues or covert-repair hypothesis of Postma and Kolk. Perhaps it is fair to say that mismatches among two or more variables appear to be *necessary* for modern M-S models, with temporal asynchronies or mismatches *sufficient* to disrupt processes known to require very rapid, exquisite coordination to achieve fluent speech.

Time is of the essence with most of these mechanism-specific models (i.e., increased speaking rate is assumed to exacerbate the mechanism hypothesized to cause stuttering). That is, many modern-day theories concerning the cause of stuttering implicate rate of initiation and/or production of speech as either an important originating or aggravating variable. It also seems fair to say, as Bernstein Ratner (1997b) suggests, that greater appreciation of linguistic and/or psycholinguistics is needed to fully grasp the implications of some of these models, for example, Wingate's (1988) "fault line" hypothesis or Postma and Kolk's (1993) covert repair hypothesis. While psychosocial factors play a role in one model (i.e., Perkins et al. model), most current M-S models do not place a great deal of emphasis on psychosocial variables (for a contrast, see Guitar's [1997] speculations about the importance of emotions in the treatment of at least some children who stutter). However, as we will try to make clear later on in this book, the person's temperament, in particular, would appear to be a variable that may exacerbate an already existing problem. And, perhaps it goes without saying, that all of these M-S, if not I-S, models await further testing with perhaps the Postma and Kolk model, at this point, receiving the most empirical testing (e.g., Postma, Kolk & Povel, 1990a; Yaruss & Conture, 1996).

Temporal Misalignment: One Essential Aspect of Many Modern-Day Theories of Stuttering

After reviewing the various modern-day theories of stuttering, the reader may be curious about my own theory of stuttering. To begin, as I've said before (Conture, 1990b), I believe that stuttering involves a complex interaction between the person's abilities and the person's environment. Likewise, Ambrose and colleagues (1997) provide intriguing statistical evidence that the "the skills and abilities" that underlie recovered as well as persistent stuttering have a genetic etiology but suggest that these factors more than likely interact with and are modified by environmental variables. However, as superficially attractive as a belief in interaction may be (at least to this writer), this notion also suffers from a vagueness or lack of specificity regarding the actual *mechanism* that may "cause" stuttering. For example, knowing what proportion of individual differences in the population of people who stutter (i.e., variance) can be accounted for by genetic factors, and that these genetic factors can *interact* with environment factors, does little to clarify what Au-Yeung and Howell (1998) call the "proximal" cause of stuttering (i.e., the actual factors that trigger instances of stuttering).

As mentioned above, one "key" aspect of most current theories of stuttering is a *mismatch* either: (1) *within* the person who stutters; and/or (2) *between* the person who stutters and his or her environment (e.g., listener). And, while some theories emphasize either (1) or (2), it is quite possible, within most modern-day theories, for people who stutter to experience both types of mismatches, although not necessarily to the same degree. To my way of thinking, however, the word *mismatch* is not quite specific enough. Instead, I would like to refine this word a bit and concentrate on what I believe precipitates instances of stuttering: *temporal misalignment*. A temporal misalignment or improper temporal alignment of one variable to another implies a mismatch (e.g., the train coming into the station before the passengers are there and ready to board). Figure 1.3, depicting three different scenarios of a car merging onto a busy highway between two cars, may help to give the reader some idea regarding temporal mismatches.

In Figure 1.3a, the car merges from the on-ramp onto the highway at 70 mph, 10 miles faster than the flow of traffic and hence hits the car in front. In Figure 1.3c, the car merges from the on-ramp onto the highway at 50 mph, 10 miles slower than the flow of traffic and gets hit by the car from the rear. In either case, by failing to match the speed of traffic, a disruption or accident occurs, as opposed to Figure 1.3b where the car merges from the on-ramp onto the highway at 60 mph, exactly the speed of the flow of traffic and slots itself neatly into the time window between the two cars.

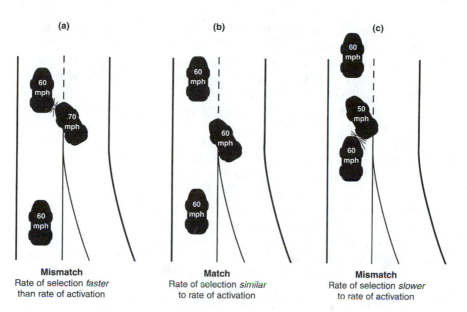

FIGURE 1.3   Merging cars analogy. This figure attempts to show, by analogy, how speed/timing (mis)matches between rate of selection (cars entering highway) and rate of internal activation (cars already traveling on highway) may result in accidents/errors. In "mismatch" (a), the car enters too fast relative to the flow of traffic, and an accident occurs (i.e., rate of selection is faster than rate of activation thus increasing likelihood of errors). In "match" (b), the car enters at a rate similar to the flow of traffic, the flow of traffic continues smoothly, no accidents occur at the point of entrance/selection (i.e., rate of selection is appropriate to the rate of activation thus minimizing errors). In "mismatch" (c), the car enters too slow relative to the flow of traffic, and an accident occurs (i.e., rate of selection is slower than rate of activation thus increasing the likelihood of errors).

Back to speech, however, the rapidity with which instances of stuttering come and go strongly suggests that whatever processes underlie instances of stuttering must also come and go rather rapidly. That is, sometimes the processes are temporally aligned and the resulting speech behavior is smooth and fluent. Other times, however, these processes are subtly to not-so-subtly misaligned and the resulting speech is hesitant, repetitious, or actually stopped until the underlying processes are temporally aligned. But I get ahead of myself.

First, I am inclined to believe that developmental stuttering, that is, stuttering that begins in childhood (generally before 7 years of age but clearly before 12) is related to one or more temporal misalignments in the processes that underlie speech and language production. One type of such temporal misalignment can be between *automatic* (i.e., an event that a person cannot directly regulate) and *controlled* (i.e., an event that a person can directly regulate) processes, for example, rate of activation of phonemes to be selected (i.e., automatic) versus rate of selection of phonemes to be inserted into a phonetic plan (i.e., controlled). For example, an "automatic" process, for the purposes of our present discussion, might consist of the rate at which words, syllables, or speech sounds become activated for selection (e.g., Kolk & Postma, 1997). Conversely, a "controlled" process might consist of the rate at which a person tries to initiate and/or produce speech. It may be also possible, theoretically, for two automatic processes to be temporally misaligned, for example, syntactic encoding and lexical retrieval.

These "internal" temporal misalignments may be exacerbated by external environmental factors, for example, a parent who continually talks over the end of the child's utterances forcing the child to rapidly plan for, initiate and produce spoken language. And while the following discussion is going to take a decided speech sound or phonological orientation, one could make similar arguments about other speech-language processes. For example, there may be temporal misalignments between lexical ("word") retrieval and morphosyntactical ("grammar") construction. Indeed, it may be possible—for example during early childhood development—that two automatic processes are more than occasionally temporally misaligned in such a way that sentence production is less than normally fluent. For instance, the child is able to more rapidly retrieve words from the mental lexicon or dictionary than these words are able to trigger appropriate syntactic or grammatical structures. This would lead to the prediction, for example, that a child who stutters can much more rapidly retrieve a verb than the child's grammatical encoder can construct an appropriate verb phrase.

The Assembly Line: An Analogy for Mismatches Within the Person Who Stutters

In essence, any time there is a temporal misalignment or temporal mismatch between processes involved with speech-language production, the speech and language production system of the person who stutters (or anyone, for that matter) may create an error. These errors, if detected by the person, may lead the person to repair them, which results in the person repeating, stalling, hesitating, or prolonging while making the repair. While the following is an admittedly less than ideal analogy, we present it in attempts to make our point a bit clearer. Here, we employ the classic comic routine in the old Charlie Chaplin movie or the "I Love Lucy" television series depicting a "temporal conflict" between assembly-line conveyor belt and assembly line worker.

Here, in Figure 1.4b, we see boxes moving along a conveyor belt, into which pies must be selected and then inserted by an assembly-line worker. Note that the rate the pies move along the conveyor belt (an "automatic" process) cannot be directly regulated by the assembly-line worker, but the assembly-line worker can try to match his or her rate of boxing each pie (a "controlled" process) to the rate of the conveyor belt. In this case, one pie is put into one box (e.g., phoneme slot in the phonetic plan that will "drive" the speech motor system) and the end product (e.g., the phonetic plan), a string of appropriately boxed pies, continues smoothly from left to right. That is, the factory worker tries to select an available or "activated" pie at the right rate to insert into the appropriate "box" of the phonetic plan. However, in Figure 1.4a, we see that if the assembly-line worker's own rate of boxing each pie is too fast relative to the pie-delivery rate of the conveyor belt (i.e., a temporal misalignment between automatic and controlled processes), the worker selects the wrong pie to insert into the box. And, finally, in Figure 1.4c, we see another form of tem-

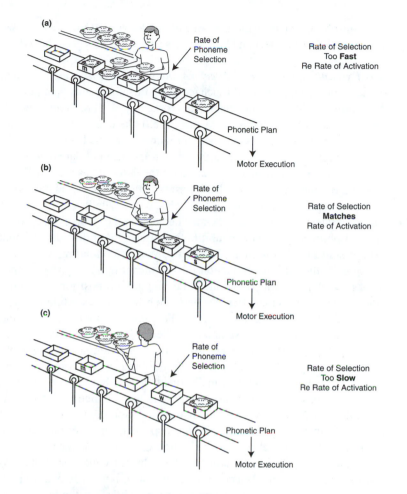

FIGURE 1.4 Assembly-line worker putting pies in box analogy for the word "swim." This figure attempts to show, by analogy, how speed/timing (mis)matches between rate of selection (man selecting and inserting pies in their respective boxes) and rate of activation (speed of conveyor belt containing pie boxes) may result in pie-box mismatches/errors. In "too fast" (a), the man selects and attempts to insert pies in box too fast relative to the rate of the conveyor belt, resulting in some pies not being boxed (i.e., the rate of selection is faster than the rate of activation, resulting in errors). In "match" (b), the man selects and inserts pies in boxes at a rate similar to that of the speed of the conveyor belt, resulting in all pies being correctly boxed (i.e., the rate of selection is similar to the rate of activation, minimizing errors). In "too slow" (c), the man selects and attempts to insert pies in boxes at a rate slower than speed of conveyor belt, resulting in some boxes not containing pies (i.e., the rate of selection is slower than the rate of activation, increasing likelihood of errors). In (a) and (c), the phonetic plan for the word "swim" will contain "errors," that is, too many or too few pies. The phonetic plans for (a) and (c), the supposed instructions to the motor system, may result in a speech error. The extent to which the speaker detects, stops the process of encoding (i.e., selecting, assembling, etc. the sound segments), and attempts to correct these errors before they are overt are thought by some (e.g., Postma & Kolk, 1993) to result in speech disfluency due to the speaker's attempts at correcting.

poral misalignment, only this time rate of pie delivery of the conveyor belt is faster than the worker's ability to select and box the pies and some pies go unboxed.

One Example of a Mismatch: Performance-Ability (P/A) Gap.   Moving out of the realm of pie manufacture, how could such temporal misalignments precipitate or cause stuttering? Also, how would environmental factors (or, using Wall & Myers' term, "psychosocial factors") interact with such misalignments? We'd like to discuss such possibilities through the means of the illustrations contained in Figures 1.5a and 1.5b.

In Figure 1.5, which represents an extrapolation of data reported by Wolk, Edwards, and Conture (1993), which were based on the essential aspects of Wolk's (1990) doctoral dissertation, the present writer has "normed" (using age-based norms) the diadochokinetic (i.e., how rapidly can one produce uni-, bi-, or tri-syllables in a given amount of time) and speaking rates of 21 age- and sex-matched children (7 who exhibit normal fluency but disordered phonology, 7 who exhibit both stuttering and disordered phonology, and 7 who exhibit stuttering but normal phonology). We are comparing here (i.e., looking for "mismatching") the rate of production during meaningful or propositional speech ("performance" or P) to the rate of production during nonpropositional speech ("ability" or A). In other words, what is the difference between how fast these children chose to speak (P) versus how fast they really can speak (A). These data are not presented as the definitive answer to these questions, but as exemplars of the types of comparisons that need to be made to uncover, if any exist, mismatches that may contribute to stuttering. Note that the so-called P/A "gap" is greatest for children who stutter but have no disordered phonology and smallest for children who exhibit normally fluent speech but disordered phonology.

We might take these data to suggest, at least in theory, that if we reduce the P/A gap for children who stuttered without disordered phonology, we might have a positive influence on their stuttering (again, this is just speculation, a notion that is in need of empirical verification). Conversely, and again in theory, we might make the children who exhibit disordered phonology with stuttering more disfluent by increasing their P/A gap! Does such speculation have merit? We don't honestly know, but we do believe that there is a need for more such research, carefully examining possible, no matter how subtle, mismatches between apparently related processes (either within the person who stutters or between the person who stutters and his or her environment). However, we believe that these temporal misalignments will *not* be a constant trait of the person's speech and language production but vary as the *state* of their speech and language production varies to meet the ever-changing needs of spoken communication. Most of us know and accept the fact that there are vast differences in how we communicate when we *write*: grocery lists, post-it notes, personal letters, business letters, letters of recommendation, term papers, journal articles, and textbooks. However, most of us give little thought to the fact that there are similar differences in how we communicate when we *talk* with: children, pets, babies, friends, at work, at school, at home, and at play!

Second Example of a Mismatch: Sound Activation Versus Sound Selection.   Borrowing from the theorization of Postma and Kolk (1993), as well as their graphic illustrations of same (seen in Figure 1.2), we would like to examine another possible temporal misalignment, this time a bit more theoretically. Figure 1.6 (after Yaruss & Conture, 1996) shows,

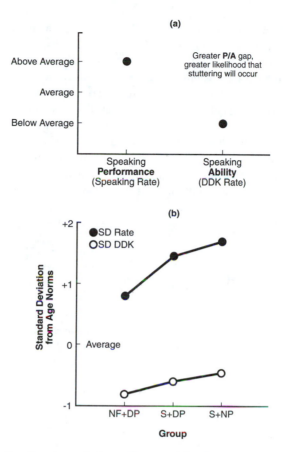

FIGURE 1.5 (a) Our first theoretical attempt to explain the S+DP Connection (with supporting data extrapolated from Wolk, 1990, with permission, shown in [b]). We conjectured (a) that when motor performance (P)—for example, rate of speaking during conversation—exceeded that of the person's motor ability, stuttering would be most likely and that this would be most apparent during the speech of children who stutter and exhibit disordered phonology. In a sense, this is a specific case of the Demands & Capacity Model. In (b) data are presented to support speculation represented in (a). Here, in (b) mean "normalized" speaking rate during conversation and diadochokinetic (alternating motion rates) rates are shown for children: with stuttering without disordered phonology (n = 7), stuttering with disordered phonology (n = 7), and normal fluency with disordered phonology (n = 7). Data was not collected for children with typical fluency and phonology. Articulatory speaking rate, in words per minute (WPM) based on a 300-word conversational sample, was converted to syllables per minute (SPM) by application of Ryan's (1974) formula (0.81*SPM = WPM), "normed" according to chronological age using Pindzola, Jenkins, and Lokken's (1989) data and converted into standard scores, that is, 05, 1.0, etc. standard deviations above or below the mean (0). Similarly, each child's average (averaged over 6 trials) diadokinetic (DDK) rate was "normed" according to age using data reported by Riley and Riley (1986) and converted into standardized scores similar to those used with articulation rate (adapted from Wolk, 1990). The "gap" between P (speaking rate) and A (diadokinetic rate), is greatest for children who stutter and exhibit disordered phonology and smallest for children who are normally fluent but exhibit disordered phonology.

in graphic form, how the rate of sound activation (an automatic process) could be in or out of synch with rates of sound selection (a controlled process). As Postma and Kolk suggest, stuttering may result, for example, with mismatches between a person's rate of *selecting* sounds and the person's ability to *activate* sounds for selecting. This would increase, in theory, the number of sounds in error in the speaker's phonetic plan (i.e., the plan or program that will drive the speaker's speech motor system). What does this all imply? Three things: First, in agreement with Postma and Kolk (1993), this writer believes that many people who stutter have either a developmental delay and/or an inherent impairment somewhere among the processes that ready or activate sounds, words, and so on for selection. Kolk and Postma (1997) make clear their speculation that this impairment resides at the level of phonological encoding. They base this speculation on the fact that stuttering is most typically exem-

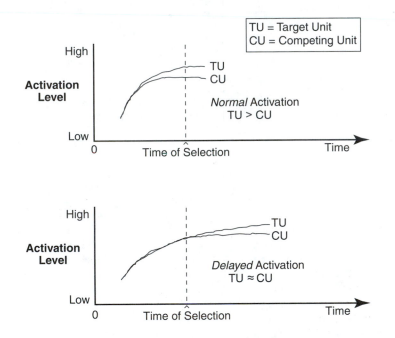

FIGURE 1.6   Normal versus delayed activation of phonological units (after Yaruss & Conture, 1996, with permission). With normal activation (top), the target unit (TU) achieves higher activation (expressed on the ordinate in arbitrary units of activation level) than the competing unit (CU) at the time of selection (TU > CU). With delayed activation (bottom), the target unit (TU) is in competition with competing units (CU) at the time of selection (TU = CU), increasing the likelihood that an inappropriate target will be selected. The rate of activation is considered an automatic process (i.e., an event that a person cannot regulate), whereas the time of selection is considered a controlled process (i.e., an event that a person can regulate). Adapted from Kolk, Conture, Postma, and Louko (1991). Note that this figure does not indicate decay of activation (the construct typically used in such models to account for the system's ability to keep from repeating the same act continuously).

plified by repetitions and prolongations at the sound or syllable level. However, this writer believes that impairments may also be possible at the levels of semantic and syntactic processing, given his observations that whole-word repetitions can be the most frequent type of disfluency in some children who stutter. Second, the person who stutters is selecting speech sounds (a "controlled" process) at a rate inappropriate for his or her system's ability to activate sounds for selection.

In this writer's opinion, it is the temporal misalignment between activation of sounds and the person's rate of selecting sounds that is one crucial variable, not the fact that the person who stutters speaks significantly faster than people who do not stutter. The important comparison, we are suggesting, is *within* the person who stutters not *between* people who do and do not stutter. To describe these issues, Kolk and Postma (1997) present figures similar to those of Yaruss and Conture (1996) with one important distinction: They also show (Kolk & Postma, 1997, Figure 9.4) what might happen if the rate of the speaker's selection remains the same or normal but the level of activation is low. Theoretically, the same concern as above would result, that is, the speaker or person who stutters should have an increased chance of misselection at a point where the target unit (e.g., "c" in the word "cat") and the competing unit (e.g., "b" in the word "bat") are about at the same level of activation.

Thus, whether people who stutter attempt an overly rapid rate of phoneme selection in relation to their rate of phoneme activation or a normally rapid rate of phoneme selection in relation to a low level of phoneme activation, the results in terms of their speech production should be the same: increased chances of sound misselections with increased chance of speech errors, resulting in increased chances of disfluency. Again, we are speculating that the most important mismatch to consider is *within* the person who stutters, even though the child's rate of sound selection could be influenced by external sources, for example, the perceived or real need to keep up with an excessively fast mother and/or father rate of conversation.

Mismatches Between People Who Stutter and Their Environments

Most of the above discussion, of course, focused on temporal misalignments within or internal to the person who stutters. However, it is also quite possible that mismatches occur between the person who stutters and his or her environment. What might such mismatches be? Well, the possibilities are seemingly limitless—for example, Yaruss and Conture (1995) reported a significant positive correlation between differences in speaking rate (in syllables) between mother and child who stutter and the child's stuttering severity. Perhaps, the greater the disparity or gap between mother and her child's speaking rate, the faster the child may need or feel he or she needs to select speech sounds. Here again, we are suggesting that the important comparison for our purposes here is *within* the mother-child dyad rather than the traditional comparison *between* groups of mothers—for example, comparing mothers of children who stutter to mothers of children who do not stutter.

To better understand the possible mismatches between parent and child, in terms of the onset and development of stuttering, we probably need to keep in mind three basic generalizations about developmental stuttering. First, stuttering typically occurs in *bidirectional conversational speech*, that is, situations where a speaker talks, a listener listens, then there is a shift in the speaking turn, the listener becomes the talker, the speaker becomes the listener, then the speaking turn shifts, and so forth. It is apparent that something about dialogic or bidirectional as opposed to monologic or unidirectional communication has a bearing on stuttering. Second, early childhood stuttering is *highly variable*, within and between speaking situations. Thus, some process or processes is rapidly varying within and between speaking situation. Finally, developmental stuttering begins in *childhood*. Thus, something about childhood, at least for some children, has a bearing on the onset and development of stuttering. Perhaps these three associates of developmental stuttering—dialogic communication, variation, and childhood—may give us insights into possible (mis)matches between parent and child behaviors in terms of the onset and development of stuttering. Why? Because common sense suggests that parents provide a large part of the communication sea the young children communicatively swim in. While it is essentially up to the child to learn and develop the ability to communicatively swim, the child's parents can create, no matter how unintentionally, a communicative ocean upon which the child flounders, speech- and language-wise, while trying to stay afloat talking.

But what of the other people—for example, older brothers and sisters, teachers—the child must deal with? While exceptions can and do occur, and individuals other than the parents can be influential, such individuals usually don't have the same relationship, socially, emotionally, communicatively, and so on, to the child who stutters that the child's mother or father might. Of course, with individuals besides the parents, the same principle of environmental exacerbation of inherent tendencies applies. For example, a teacher may continually talk over the end of the utterances produced by an 11-year-old child who stutters, the soccer coach may consistently expect quick, no-nonsense responses from an 8-year-old child who stutters, or a co-worker may rapidly speak in long, complex utterances, encouraging the 28-year-old colleague who stutters to do the same.

Nature Interacting with Nurture: One Source of Mismatches

In the second edition of this book (Conture, 1990b), we stated our belief that it takes a unique child being placed in an unique environment for the problem of stuttering to have its highest likelihood of occurring and continuing. Possibly a unique environment (e.g., one involving parents with an overly critical, perfectionistic attitude toward childhood speech and language development), all by itself, might be able to create such a mismatch between a child's attempts to live up to such external environmental standards versus the child's inherent abilities to do so. Figure 1.7 demonstrates several different ways a parent could be mismatched with his or her child—for example, speaking at a rate well beyond the child's ability to emulate, using utterances well beyond the child's ability to formulate, or responding to the child much faster than the child's system can readily tolerate (for further evidence of "mismatches" in parental behavior relative to child behavior, see Meyers & Freeman, 1985a, b, and c). A solely environmental cause for stuttering is possible, but not very probable. This is especially true if the child's inherent speech and language ability and devel-

Speaking Rate:

> Haveyoufinishedyourdinner?
> Have youfinishedyourdinner?
> Have you finishedyourdinner?
> Have   you finished yourdinner?
> Have   you   finished your dinner?

Utterance Length:

> When are you going to finish your dinner?
> Have you finished all your dinner?
> Have you finished your dinner?
> Have you finished dinner?
> All done?

Utterance Complexity:

> When I see that behavior, I wonder if you will finish your dinner?
> When do you think you will try to finish your dinner?
> When will you finish your dinner?
> Have you finished your dinner?
> Have you finished?
> All done?

Turn-Switching Pause (response time latency):

> Child → Can I go play?
>   Have you finished?←Mother
> Child → Can I go play?
>   Have you finished?←Mother
> Child → Can I go play?
>   Have you finished?←Mother
> Child → Can I go play?
>   ←1 sec →Have you finished? Mother

FIGURE 1.7   Changes in parents' speech (separately or together) that are NOT to be used *exclusively* when speaking with a child, but mainly when child appears to be exhibiting considerable speech disfluency. Rather, resisting a "one-size-fits-all" approach, parents are encouraged to maneuver according to the circumstances of their child's speech (dis)fluency. That is, the described changes in parental communicative behavior are to be used during a period when the child is exhibiting considerable speech disfluencies. During such a time period, some children may find it helpful, communicatively, to be exposed to an adult communicative model (not parental verbal instructions or teachings) that temporarily encourages the child to employ normally slower, shorter, and less complex communication, and minimizes parental talking for and/or interrupting the child.

opment are essentially typical. Likewise, it is possible that a unique child (e.g., a child with a delayed and/or deviantly developing neuromotor system), all by him- or herself, may develop stuttering in the presence of an otherwise typical environment. Again, possible, but not probable. If it was probable, the prevalence of stuttering among children with various delays and/or deviations of neuromotor control for speech would be considerably higher than it is.

Indeed, and as we will try to show in the assessment and treatment parts of this book, we believe that remediating stuttering, particularly in children, typically involves dealing with *interactions* between the child's unique abilities and the unique circumstances of the child's environment. (That such parent–child interactions, particularly communicative, may bear relationship to a child's stuttering severity can clearly be seen in Figure 1.8.) And such treatment, we believe, differs from treatment based on a conceptualization of a unique child speaking in a typical environment or a typical child speaking in an unique environment. Unfortunately, we are still not at a point where we can easily and readily discriminate among young people who stutter relative to their etiologies (e.g., discerning between those children whose home environments are and are not typical). However, we need to continually strive to develop such discriminatory abilities, in this writer's opinion, if we are ever to improve the long-term results of our therapy programs for people who stutter, to match our services with the actual needs of the people we serve.

The foregoing discussion attempted to provide some insights into essential aspects of stuttering: what it sounds and looks like, how it might be measured, what people who stutter are like, and what might cause and exacerbate the problem. I realize that this has been a lot of information for the reader to process, but this information is necessary for the speech-language pathologist, either pre-service student or in-service clinician, to understand as fully as possible. Why? In essence, speech-language pathology is a profession based on a body of knowledge that supposedly motivates and guides clinical assessment and treatment. Without that knowledge, the reasons for doing X, Y, and Z during assessment and treatment will be a mystery to the student or clinician, and, even more important, when a clinical procedure or approach does not work, or works poorly, neither student nor clinician will have the needed information to understand why and/or make necessary changes. As we have said before, one thing constant about stuttering is change. Thus, the successful clinician is someone who can: maneuver according to circumstances presented by real people who stutter, coping with variations in syntactic, semantic, phonological, and motoric processing created by variations in the real world of bidirectional communication. But before we begin in earnest to read how I might suggest assessing and treating such people, let's examine a little bit about my philosophy about people in general, and people who stutter and their behavior, specifically.

General Orientation Toward the Treatment of Stuttering and People Who Stutter

In the chapters that follow, I will discuss, in great detail, the assessment and treatment of stuttering in children, teenagers, and adults. And you are probably eager to get to those sections. However, to best understand my approach to assessment and treatment, it behooves

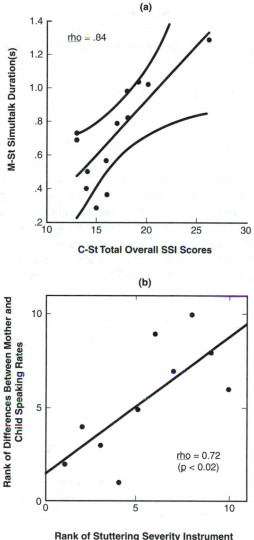

FIGURE 1.8. Data from two studies (Kelly & Conture, 1992; Yaruss & Conture, 1995, with permission) display some of the possible relationships between parent and child communication behavior. (a) Kelly and Conture (1992) reported a strong positive relationship between the total overall Stuttering Severity Instrument (SSI) scores of children who stutter (C-St) and their mothers' (M-St) simultalk (simultaneous, overlapping talking of speaker and listener) duration (in sec.); and (b) Yaruss and Conture (1995) show a strong positive relationship between the differences between child and mother speaking rate and the child's total overall SSI score. While more such work is needed, it is suggestive of one basic fact: that elements of parent-child communicative interactions are associated with the severity of the child's stuttering severity; certainly, there is no implication of causality here, but it would not be unreasonable to suggest that these interactions exacerbate and/or maintain the child's stuttering.

you to understand something about my general philosophy about stuttering, people who stutter, specifically, and people in general. In essence, just because people who stutter all share a common problem does not mean that they all share everything in common.

How to Talk About Stuttering When Speaking with Clients and/or Families

First, we need to talk about talking to our clients about talking. While the preceding parts of this chapter provide you a great deal of fundamental information about stuttering, it does little to help you figure out how to *talk about* or *verbally describe* those behaviors to your clients. Why? Well, remember that the individuals you will be assessing and treating will typically have no formal training in speech-language pathology. On the one hand, it is not really helpful for you to talk to yourself (and many times you have to do this!), fellow professionals, your clients, or their families employing the same terms your clients use. Rather, whether as practicing SLPs or student-clinician SLPs, we should make every attempt to insure that our description of our clients' concerns, problems, and so forth is as *descriptive*, *objective*, and *nonjudgmental* as possible. Yes, such terms as stuttering, stutterer, and blocks have their place in our oral and written discussions. But these terms should not be routinely substituted for terms that are more *behavioral*, *descriptive*, and *objective*. As much as possible, when talking with people who stutter and their families, we want to use terms that actually *describe* what they are *doing* rather than merely *label* their behavior in order to *categorize* it.

An Example Is in Order

Let us say you had a friend who had or who seems to have a significant weight problem, who had mentioned to you his or her concerns about the problem and had asked for your opinion. You might want to begin by talking with your friend about his or her weight problem and/or your observations. To do this, you might have to verbally describe your observation that you believe the person has inappropriate eating habits. You could do this in a variety of ways, but in terms of the types of words you use you would have two choices: (1) *Subjective labels* can be judgmental, can inappropriately stereotype, and many times can carry negative connotations versus (2) *objective behavioral descriptions* that describe what is being done or needs to be done—for example, frequently eating too much in too many situations increases the lower-fat and decreases the empty-calorie food you eat, and so forth.

Likewise, we can label someone as a stutterer or say that is an individual or person who stutters (see Conture, 1987c). Similarly, we can say that a person blocked, or we can say that the person pressed his lips together for too long and with too much physical tension. Granted, using subjective labels is a convenience and generally a shorter means of talking about people and their behavior; however, it is also a means of perpetuating negative stereotypes (see Woods & Williams, 1976, for discussion of traits typically assigned to people who stutter by SLPs). Most important, such labels do not clearly and directly describe what the person is *doing* or needs to *do*. In essence, many of the subjective terms commonly used by the lay public to describe stuttering actually don't! That is, these terms generally do not describe or tell the listener what the person who stutters is actually *doing*. Objective descriptions of the person who stutters and his or her behavior, on the other hand, while generally more verbose, are far less apt to carry negative connotations or be pejorative in nature. Most importantly, they are much more likely to clearly and explicitly tell the listener the nature of the behavior being discussed (i.e., what the behavior actually sounds, looks, and maybe even feels like).

All of the above, it may seem to the reader, sound like a semantic shell game, but a moment's reflection says otherwise. For example, would anyone of sensitivity and with an interest in really helping, when faced with a student doing "D" work in a course, tell the student he or she is "lazy"? Wouldn't it be more productive to ask the student to describe his or her in-class note taking, study habits, and what the student is studying? In other words, talk about what they are *doing* rather than who they *are*? While more verbose, is not the phrase "not working hard enough during the lectures trying to understand what is being said" a more effective way to communicate, to describe less pejoratively, than calling the person "lazy"? Such a listing can go on, and on but the point is that words do reflect the thoughts behind them. Unclear, subjective words can reflect unclear, subjective thoughts and understanding.

Words we use reflect the way we are thinking. Words can hurt the person discussing someone as well as the person being discussed. We would probably all profit by remembering the old saying that "our words should be soft because we never know when we'll have to eat them." Words can be used to communicate, describe, and provide insights or they can be used to inappropriately criticize, ostracize, or segregate. Words used by professionals in their professional practice should be, as much as possible: (1) *descriptive* in nature, (2) *objective* to the degree possible, and (3) carry *positive* or at least neutral *connotations*. Our words should be ones that contribute to a solution for the problem rather than become part of the problem itself.

Recognizing Differences in People and Behavior

As clinicians, we often forget to consider the person who stutters as a person first and a stutterer second. All too often in our sincere but sometimes overly eager rush to help, we tend to ignore the context of the person's life in our clinical dealings with that person. And, when we do so, we begin to attribute the person's problems and concerns to the fact that the person is stuttering. Would we, for example, think that all the problems a short person has are due to the fact that the person is shorter than the average? Instead, shouldn't we entertain the possible that these issues or concerns might just as well be related to other variables going on in the person's life?

People who stutter, just like people who do not stutter, have likes and dislikes, highs and lows, brothers and sisters, in-laws and bills to pay, dreams and schemes. They share in the same human condition that we all experience. To diagnose and remediate people who stutter as if they are isolates, living in a hermetically sealed environment free from concerns of family, society, and life is not only inappropriate, but just plain poor therapy. Speech-language pathologists need to consider the *context* of the life of the person who stutter's in order to see the individual as a person, as a functioning individual interacting on a number of levels with a number of people. The person who stutters is a person, like you and me, unique and without duplicate. These statements, we realize, border on platitudes, but they help us put into perspective the client's behavior as we go about evaluating and remediating that client.

Sometimes Cub Scouts Are More Important Than Speech-Language Therapy

When talking about the life that people who stutter lead outside the therapy setting, I like to use an example of one of my younger clients who exhibited a severe stuttering problem and who, without consulting us, opted to join Cub Scouts rather than continue to receive therapy from us. This young client was, right from the beginning, struggling for success in one of our weekly parent–child (P/C) fluency groups (Conture & Melnick, 1999; Kelly & Conture, 1991), groups that we'll discuss in detail in Chapter 3. He was developmentally behind his peers (communicatively and physically) and thus found it quite difficult to successfully participate in the P/C group containing children about his same age (chronologically similar but developmentally older). Conversely, when placed in another P/C group, with children a bit younger (chronologically younger but developmentally similar) than him, he reacted strongly that these younger children were "babies" and/or he didn't like the "baby games" used with this younger group of children (of course, he forgot the fact that he couldn't successfully handle the games of his chronological peers; whatever the case, his reaction is not all that uncommon in young children). A bit stymied, we shared the above information with his mother, who also had observed the same situation and seemed as perplexed as we in terms of how to proceed.

During our discussions with the mother, it became clear that this boy had really wanted to join a local Cub Scout troop ("all his classmates are"), but the weekly P/C group meeting was scheduled at the same time as the weekly Cub Scout meeting. A scheduled break from therapy ensued; when we next contacted the mother to resume therapy with her son, she informed us that she had enrolled her son in Cub Scouts rather than our P/C group. Our first, less than thoughtful reaction was "how could you" (or words to that effect); we explained the seriousness of her son's problem (it really was) and his need to continue therapy and the like. However, after calming down a bit and listening to the mother, it became clear that at this point in time Cub Scouts, its attendant socialization, and sense of being similar to one's peers was far more important for this child than our therapy. We supported the mother's continuing her son's participation with Cub Scouts and explained that sometime in the future he would need to resume speech-language therapy. We also suggested that once he got established with his Cub Scout troop that perhaps he could be late once in a while for the beginning of the meetings. After a four-month break from our P/C group, the boy resumed with our "younger" P/C group and continued attending his weekly Cub Scouts meetings. Over time he made excellent, if slow, progress. Whatever he received from joining and participating in Cub Scouts seemed to give him the security necessary to handle the approaches we use with the younger children and begin to receive much more benefit from the experience.

What is the Point?

Well, by assuming that the child's needs for our therapy outweighed his needs for the socialization associated with Cub Scouts, we would have been making a big mistake (and we've made more than our share of these!). As hard as it was at the time, luckily we were able to realize that there might be more to this client's life than just becoming more fluent (e.g., being liked and doing things with his peers) and we were able to resolve a clinical dilemma. We wish that all our clinical problems were so easily solved! All we are trying to say is that keeping the perspective that the person who stutters is a person first and a stutterer second helps us to understand, if not resolve, many such issues as they come up during assessment and treatment.

Tolerating Differences in People and Behavior

Intolerance for Individual Differences in the Ability to Communicate

It is my observation that speech fluency is one area of human behavior in which we have little tolerance for individual differences. We appear to accept the fact that some people can run, jump, climb, and calculate farther, faster, higher, and more accurately, and at earlier or later ages than other people. We are somewhat tolerant for differences in height and weight among people. We do not appear quite as tolerant, however, regarding differences among people in terms of speech fluency as well as speech and language behavior in general.

Many individuals implicitly or explicitly express their apparent unwillingness to accept the fact that some children go through periods of disfluency for longer durations than do other children, or that these periods of disfluency occur at later or earlier periods than exhibited by the child's peers. For example, my son, when nearing his ninth birthday, went through a period of about two weeks in which he produced a fair number of whole-word repetitions and more than his typical amount of part-word repetitions. Until that time, his speech (dis)fluency had never been something his mother, myself, or anyone else had ever thought particularly remarkable, especially different than other children his age. Other parents have reported to me similar increments in speech disfluency in the communication of their 8- to 10-year-old children.

Are these instances of disfluency peculiar to this age range of children? Are they indicative of particular pressures we parents or the schools or society place on this age child? Are these disfluencies related to sudden spurts in vocabulary growth or language or cognitive development? Do these disfluencies represent a discoordination in the timing and spatial movements of speech structures (e.g., Caruso, Abbs, & Gracco, 1988; Caruso, Conture, & Colton, 1988; Conture, Colton, & Gleason, 1988; Perkins, 1978; Perkins, Rudas, Johnson, & Bell, 1976) that may be related to some as yet unknown neuromotor or similar developmental change peculiar to this age child? Or, perhaps, to some complex, nonlinear interaction among many psychological, physiological, linguistic, and so on, factors (e.g., Smith & Kelly, 1997)? At present, based on our present level of understanding, we would be fairly vague if we tried to answer these questions. However, it is apparent that the speech fluency of *all* speakers, particularly children, is quite variable within as well as between speakers and speaking situations (e.g., Yaruss, LaSalle, & Conture, 1998). Undoubtedly, such differences among people are probably related, in a complex fashion, to a myriad of inherited as well as environmental factors.

Individuals Stutter but They Are Still Individuals

Similarly, when considering that people who stutter are people, we should also consider each such person's individuality (Van Riper, 1973). While there may be important commonalties among our clients, what may be appropriate in Sally's situation may not work with Marcus. Of course, it is not always easy, possible, or practical to gear therapy procedures to every individual need and ability of all of our clients. Nevertheless, we should at least recognize each client's individuality and not overly generalize.

Procedures that make good sense to Mr. and Mrs. Brown for their son Joey may totally baffle and confuse Mr. and Mrs. Garcia in their dealings with their daughter Consuela. Likewise, with some of our clients we will need to make explicit the rationale and reason for each and every step of our clinical attempts to change their stuttering (i.e., these are the relatively "active" clients). Conversely, others will simply want us to tell them what to do and when to do it, and we can skip most of the explanation (i.e., these are the relatively "passive" clients). (As an aside, we have relatively little information about which approach, an active vs. passive, is best for our clients' long term outcome; this author has seen both clients improve long-term). Reasons for these individual differences are not necessarily related to intelligence; such differences can also be related to the person who stutters or his or her family's (a) relative willingness to work at change, (b) different levels of motivation, (c) high degrees of emotionality surrounding the stuttering problem, making it difficult for the person to objectively deal with the problem, and so forth.

We Typically Don't See What We Typically See

Okay, you might ask, of what earthly good is it to make such an apparent, as-plain-as-the-nose-on-your-face observation about individual differences? We raise this issue because far too often, the apparent, the familiar, the everyday gets overlooked in our attempts to be creative and original. We need to continually revisit a basic fact: Not everyone is as fluent and articulate as Dan Rather, the television news announcer, at least most of the time. Recognizing this helps us appreciate that the individual we are evaluating may be developing, no matter how slowly or unevenly, in a "normal" fashion. Normal here means *variation* not *uniformity* in behavior. For example, Yairi and colleagues (1993), based on a *random* sample of children, report that recovery rates for children who stutter (who have received no indirect therapy), may range as high as 85 percent. Likewise, Yaruss, LaSalle, and Conture (1998), based on a *clinical* sample of children, report that as many as 40 to 50 percent of children who frequently exhibit instances of stuttering will probably eventually become fluent with or without therapeutic intervention. Thus, if we include on our clinical caseload (i.e., attempt to treat) *every* child who appears to be stuttering, how can we claim high degrees of success when at least 50 percent of our cases would probably have improved on their own? In essence, we must recognize one basic fact: Stuttering is, first and foremost, a behavior. And, as a behavior, stuttering varies within and between people and situations. Recognizing such variations, what we must strive for, it seems, is not merely determining the presence of stuttering in children, but the degree of risk that the child exhibits for *continuing* to stutter unless he or she receives treatment.

While a sizable proportion of the lay public may remain relatively intolerant of individual differences in fluent speech, we as speech-language pathologists must demonstrate our tolerance in word and deed for such differences in speech and language. Certainly, we want to recognize the importance of fluent, articulate, and coherent speech to a full and productive life, but we also need to stop trying to fix what may not be broken but merely different.

As Starkweather (1987) so aptly said, "The goal of therapy is not total fluency but normal disfluency." With this statement, Starkweather makes explicit the fact that people, no matter how apparently "normally fluent," are also sometimes disfluent, that their fluency varies across time and situations. Extending his comment a bit further, we might say that trying to make our clients who stutter *totally* fluent is about as realistic a goal as it is to make everyone *totally* perfect, happy, or contented. Individuals, particularly children who are still developing, have, are, and will continue to differ in terms of their speech fluency. Such differences do not mean that they are bad persons, just persons.

Enthusiasm for Changing People and Behavior

It is nice to be enthusiastic about helping people deal with and overcome their problems. It's great to feel great about helping someone help themselves become all he or she can be. It's wonderful to witness someone say or do something he or she has always wanted to do but was unable to do or thought he or she was unable to do. Enthusiasm, however, is not the same as realism.

Realism consists of understanding that changing human behavior, particularly in the long term, is a process fraught with ups and downs, setbacks and difficulties. What goes around comes around, and promising our clients simple solutions to complex problems eventually comes back to haunt us when the problems return, sometimes with a vengeance. We should be cautiously optimistic with our clients and ourselves while recognizing that there are many questions that still go unanswered. A recognition, we think, that should make even the most enthusiastic among us pause prior to promising an easy fix for a hard problem.

The Common Cold and Stuttering

Discussing the remediation of stuttering is a bit like discussing the remediation of the common cold. Many "remedies" exist for both stuttering and the common cold, with each remedy being backed by various forms of evidence. Some professionals enthusiastically advocate one form of remediation, while others support different forms with equal enthusiasm. Each approach has its enthusiasts *and* its skeptics. The enthusiasts claim tremendous success with their approach, while the skeptics continually jab away at the rationale and method of the enthusiasts, hoping to land a knockout punch. Oftentimes, unfortunately, the two groups fight on, oblivious to the fact that the rest of the field has moved to another arena and is now watching a different fight between the newly self-proclaimed champion and his or her contender for the title!

Whatever the case, one reason that so many different approaches work is that the terms like *common cold* and *stuttering* represent catchalls for a number of related but different problems with different causes. For example, symptoms of stuttering can "mingle" together with symptoms of a similar problem like "cluttering" (i.e., "a disorder of speech and language processing, resulting in rapid, dysrhythmic, sporadic, unorganized, and frequently unintelligible speech," Daly & Burnett, 1996, p. 238. For an excellent overview of the topic of cluttering, see St. Louis [1996], who edited an entire issue of *Journal of Fluency Disorders*, *21*, Numbers 3 & 4, devoted to this topic, and Daly & Burnett, 1999). Obviously, it would seem, treatment for clients whose fluency is influenced by both cluttering and stuttering should, in an ideal world, be different than for those clients who only exhibit stuttering. Conversely, others support the notion that common colds and stuttering have unitary symptoms and causes. Based on the work and speculation of ourselves and others (e.g., Daly, 1981; Preus, 1981; Prins & Lohr, 1972; Schwartz & Conture, 1988; Smith & Kelly, 1997), it seems quite possible that not only do the speech and related behaviors differ among people who stutter, but that the reasons for their problems may also differ.

Perhaps a poor analogy, but just like bananas, oranges, and apples are all called fruit, they nevertheless all come from different seeds and have somewhat different functions. Likewise, some of the things we label and react to as stuttering may have different etiologies and courses of development and may, in turn, be more or less responsive to different therapeutic approaches. While folk wisdom suggests that chicken soup helps people with colds, similar wisdom suggests that people who stutter may be helped by instructing them to "slow down, take a deep breath, and think about what you're saying." Of course, by chance alone, occasionally such unidimensional solutions get lucky and are actually associated with a "cure" for a multidimensional problem. Does this mean that chicken soup "cures" the common cold or that the aforementioned instructions "cure" stuttering? We think not.

Rationales Versus Recipes

We believe that clinicians should try to understand, as best they can, the reasons behind the method as well as the method itself. We, as clinicians, should try to understand why an advocated method is believed to work. This writer is not interested in simple recipes for clinical success that must be dutifully be followed step by step.

If a clinician does not know why a method is advocated (other than that it "cures stuttering"), why it is thought to work, and how it might be modified or adapted to suit the needs of each individual case, the clinician may blindly follow one set of instructions in all therapy situations. Granted, it is very important to know how to *efficiently*, *quickly*, and *cor-*

rectly follow the instructions in order to make the method work. However, if all we know is *the* method itself, then we become like poorly trained auto mechanics who wonder why their standard tools don't work with a car having metric fittings. In essence, the day usually dawns when the procedure does not work with this or that client. Without knowing *why* the procedure was supposed to work in the first place, what its basic rationale might be, the speech-language pathologist will find it difficult to adjust the procedure to meet the individual needs of the client.

Certainty in an Uncertain World

Tightly structured programs for the treatment of stuttering may give clinicians the impression that they know, or at least someone knows, what is going on, what needs to be done, and how to do it. Such programs can be, and many times are, suitable for certain people who stutter. However, difficulties arise when exceptions to the rule or new information occur that cast doubts on the prescribed program. One should not confuse the confident manner of the cookbook-oriented clinician who works with people who stutter with that clinician's expertise and ability to handle *all* clinical problems relative to stuttering. Clinicians who believe they have found *the* procedure or who uncritically follow one recipe for change with every client may, in my experience, quickly reject or vigorously disagree with information or approaches that fall outside the realm of their rigidly prescribed approach. Clinicians who seek and want to learn only *the program* seem to find it difficult to adjust to the clinical exception, to be flexible enough to deal with new information and changing approaches. The *recipe* or *cookbook* approach, particularly in view of the present state of the clinical art in stuttering, appears to hamper future growth in a clinician's ability to evaluate and remediate stuttering. As we've said before, with stuttering, as with life, change is apt to be constant.

Summary

Stuttering is a multidimensional problem that has and will continue to defy any unidimensional solution. And, in an ideal world, theories about, as well as therapies for, stuttering should contribute to a solution rather than become part of the problem. Recognizing that there is some behavioral overlap between the populations of people who do and do not stutter—in terms of the frequency and nature of exhibited disfluent behavior (e.g., Yairi, 1997a, Table 3.3)—our definitions of *stuttering* and who *stutters* must be *relative* rather than *absolute*. Otherwise, the use of absolute criteria will mean that some people who are and/or will become normally fluent speakers will be characterized as and considered to be a person who stutters and vice versa.

The better theoretical approaches, we believe, are those that recognize, at the outset, that: (1) No one currently knows what causes stuttering; (2) stuttering begins in childhood, is more apt to be exhibited by boys than girls, is highly variable, and occurs mainly in dialogic or bidirectional communication; and (3) stuttering behavior is more appropriately viewed as an online change in fluency, as a variable change in the state of fluent speech most likely related to the individual's inability to quickly and/or efficiently *plan for* as well as *execute* speech-language production—inabilities, we believe, that are most apt to disrupt speech fluency during the ever-changing, novel utterances that characterize unstructured, conversational, or propositional speech. Likewise, the better therapeutic approaches, we believe, are those that recognize, at the outset, that: (1) No one has developed a program that eradicates stuttering in all clients for all time despite all claims to the contrary; (2) there may not be a one-size-fits-all treatment approach that can effectively deal with the myriad of concerns one encounters with people who stutter; and (3) the goal of therapy, as Starkweather (1987) suggested ". . . is not total fluency but normal disfluency." And while we cannot, at present, resolve these nontrivial theoretical and therapeutic issues, if we can recognize their presence and importance, such recognition should eventually lead us to ask needed questions rather than be content with unsubstantiated answers.

Individuals who *persistently*, *predictably*, and *consistently* (PPC) produce instances of stuttering during bidirectional verbal communication are likely candidates for being characterized as people who stutter. Their candidacy becomes even more likely if we observe, associated with these speech disfluencies, speech and nonspeech indicators of bodily movement, physical tension, and psychosocial discomfort and concerns. Both students and clinicians should recognize that the previously mentioned PPC criteria are relative to both the observer and observed. The developmental and chronological age of the client, in particular, should be considered in making PPC judgments regarding the person's stuttering. Furthermore, particularly with older clients, an individual's opinion that he or she stutters and a clinician's opinion that he or she stutters may not always agree. Ascertaining who is and who is not a person who stutters is a complex decision based on many different considerations, a decision many times made relative to the particular person, his or her developmental and chronological age as well as their expressed and implied feelings, attitudes, and beliefs and those of their family.

In subsequent chapters, we will deal in more detail with the making of this clinical decision and the basis for making it. For now, we should recognize the challenge inherent in making such a decision while simultaneously understanding that such decisions can and, in many instances, must be made for the present and future benefit of the client and his or her family. We can clearly do harm by making rushes to judgment and conducting treatment in situations where, given enough time, and relatively simple changes in the person's environment, a problem might disappear. Conversely, we can do just as much harm by not wanting to hurt the client and inappropriately delay the delivery of needed clinical services.

What we must strive to develop, therefore, is the theoretical as well as informational base and clinical acumen/experience that will help us to discern the difference between (1) those individuals who truly stutter and/or will continue to stutter and who need our services and (2) those individuals who are truly not stuttering and/or will continue to improve in the future by themselves and are not in need of our services. Interwoven with these group differences are appreciable individual differences, the latter perhaps having significant impact on both our decision to recommend or not recommend treatment as well as the relative success of such treatment. Facts are bothersome things—they often resist theoretical cleansing. Lifting theoretical and therapeutic hammers to strike stuttering as if it was a nail, we may overlook the possibility that understanding and treating stuttering requires the use of several different theoretical and therapeutic tools, not merely those that can pound!

2

Assessment and Evaluation

"Ideas are not easily conquered by facts" (Kurlansky, 1998, p. 64). Indeed, many people seem to have the idea that diagnosing stuttering is simple—that is, the clinician merely listens and watches and, voila, it is crystal clear whether the person is someone who stutters. However, those of us who have embarked on the journey to better understand, assess, and treat stuttering recognize that if such diagnosis is "simple," we'd hate to see complex!

While much of our personal and professional lives are more about the journey than the destination, most of us forget or refuse to accept that fact. Instead, we often feel that the expert diagnostician or clinician has "arrived" at the clinical destination where he or she is all-knowing in terms of evaluation and treatment. The truth, however, is that even the expert is still embarking on the journey to ideal clinical practice. This journey started for the experienced clinician, just like it must for the less experienced clinician, with a single step. For the less clinically experienced reader of this book, perhaps reading and applying the contents of this chapter will constitute that first step, at least in terms of assessing stuttering.

Speech-language pathologists who remediate stuttering should have sufficient training and experience with the *assessment* and *evaluation* of stuttering in children and adults. While this training and experience is similar to that of other communicative problems—for example, phonological disorders, expressive language difficulties—it also has its unique aspects, aspects that are best learned and appreciated through experience. It is entirely appropriate that before considering the remediation of stuttering, we devote some time to considering its assessment and evaluation. Fortunately, there are several sources that interested readers can go to find out something about the assessment and evaluation of stuttering (Adams, 1977, 1980, 1991; Conture, 1997; Conture & Caruso, 1987; Conture & Yaruss, 1993; Costello & Ingham, 1984; Culatta & Goldberg, 1995; Curlee, 1980; Gordon & Luper, 1992a, 1992b; Guitar, 1998; Ham, 1986; Hayhow, 1983; Ingham, 1985; Johnson et al., 1963; Pindzola & White, 1986; Shapiro, 1999; Wall & Myers, 1995; Williams, 1978; Zebrowski, 1994). Thus, we will try not to unnecessarily duplicate previous efforts in this space. And, as we will try to point out, it is a false economy to short-change or skimp on assessment and evaluation. Oftentimes, what the clinician does not take the time to find out or uncover during the initial diagnostic, she will find herself using precious therapy time trying to assess, document, and understand.

Some Basic Beliefs That Guide Our Assessment Procedures

Instead, what we will try to do is to present assessment and evaluation procedures that we have found more or less useful. There are, however, three beliefs that we have about stuttering that heavily influence our assessment and evaluation procedures: (1) Stuttering relates to a complex interaction between the environment of the person who stutters and the skill and abilities the person who stutters brings to that environment; (2) stuttering rarely operates in an vacuum; it many times relates to subtle and not-so-subtle difficulties in other areas; and (3) individuals who stutter are individuals first and people who stutter second; there is more to their lives than stuttering (cf. Conture, 1987c).

With regard to the first belief—that stuttering relates to complex interaction between the person who stutters and his or her environment—we will not only discuss ways to assess the person who stutters but that person's environment as well. Regarding the second belief—that stuttering rarely operates in a vacuum—we will discuss assessment and evaluation of related behaviors such as speech articulation/phonology, expressive/receptive language and vocabulary, voice, neuromotor speech and nonspeech skills, nonverbal associates, reading and so forth. And in terms of the third belief—individuals who stutter are individuals first and people who stutter second—we will discuss ways and means by which we can gain perspective on the client's life by understanding the client's achievements and aspirations in school and work, parental standards for child raising and behavior, as well as many other aspects of his or her life.

Gaining Perspective on the Client's Unique Circumstances

Hopefully, all of the aforementioned considerations should help the SLP gain perspectives regarding the particular circumstances that surround each client's stuttering and related problems. For example, we gain this perspective when we consider that one person who stutters may have *limited* intellectual and employment capabilities while another may have *unlimited* intellectual and employment capabilities. As mentioned before, during assessment, as in remediation, the examiner should try to keep in mind that stuttering, in and of itself, does not encompass all of the client as a person nor the client's problems. Stuttering is but one of many components that make up an individual; some of these other components may play just as big a role as stuttering itself in terms of recovery from the problem.

Examining the Examiner

During the initial diagnostic, no matter how obvious it seems, it is nonetheless true that the client and associates will be evaluating the clinician! And, as the saying goes, first impressions are lasting (or, as an ad once stated, "one never gets a second chance to make a first impression"). It is therefore desirable that the clinician behave in such a way that the client regards him or her as: (1) a person concerned not only with the client's problems but also with the client as an individual; (2) a person who is nonjudgmental regarding both the client as a person and the client's problem; (3) a person who demonstrates a belief in the client's capacity for self-help; and (4) a person who demonstrates professional understanding and knowledge regarding the client's stuttering and related issues. Obviously, the SLP can't be all things to all people but, at the very least, the SLP should realize that his or her clients and their associates are also assessing the SLP! Many times what our clients perceive, be it right or wrong, has a powerful influence on whether they will listen to our advice and benefit from our therapy.

In general, the SLP's evaluation of people who stutter involves demonstrating to the client an understanding of stuttering while employing appropriate clinical affect and interpersonal skills. Haynes and Pindzola (1998, pp. 11–14) have discussed "the diagnostician as a factor," describing the general attributes needed to be an effective diagnostician. Shriberg and associates (1975) have detailed these professional, technical, and interpersonal skills, and Van Riper (1975) has discussed some clinician attributes thought to be of relevance to successful clinical intervention (see Schum, 1986, for further discussion of the client–clinician relationship). In our opinion, these professional and personal qualities of the clinician warrant consideration and study by any speech and language pathologist involved in the evaluation and remediation of stuttering and other communicative problems. (Beginning SLPs or student-clinicians at this point might want to read Appendix B which discusses some of the professional/personal qualities and concerns SLPs must consider in their daily work.)

Facilities

If first impressions are lasting, probably nothing is more influential, on the client and associates, as the setting for the diagnostic. While the busy SLP may see only the client and his or her needs, the client is generally scanning the total environment, trying to get a handle on who and what the SLP is all about. Some attention to detail on the part of the SLP is warranted and will help everybody focus on the client and his or her needs.

First, the ideal environment for evaluating stuttering (or any other communicative disorder, for that matter) should not possess auditory and visual stimuli that call *undue attention* to themselves. Distracting sights and sounds from outside as well as inside the evaluation room should be reasonably attenuated. A compromise is needed. While the evaluation room should not be overly cluttered, neither should it necessarily convey the sterility of a medical operating suite. Second, remember that for both you and your client the evaluation will take mental effort, concentration, and attention to detail, and the client, just like you and I, may find it difficult to recall some of this detail from the backroads of his or her mind. We can assist the client with this task and reduce, as much as possible, distractions in the environment so that both you and the client can concentrate on the business at hand. Third, as obvious as it might seem, try to insure that the chairs, tables, and nature of objects used in various tests are age-appropriate. The client doesn't know, in advance, the purpose of your procedures and can only assume on the basis of what is familiar to him or her (e.g., "play" versus "real" objects) what you might be thinking. Try to be as sensitive as you can to the older client's needs not to be patronized through the use of seemingly "juvenile" procedures, as well as the young client's feelings of intimidation when faced with seemingly "grown-up" chairs, tables, and objects.

Equipment

While obvious, it is this writer's clinical experience that SLPs need to be more aware of the single most important piece of equipment they use: the audio or video tape recorder and its associated microphones. Far too often, we observe professionals who seem insensitive to the fact that high-quality acoustic and/or videotape recordings are crucial in the establishment of adequate behavioral indexes (baseline, before treatment, or pretreatment measures) of stuttering and related behavior. The quality of these recordings will become even more important in years to come as computer-assisted acoustic analysis packages (e.g., see Read, Buder, & Kent's 1990, 1992 general survey and review of speech analysis systems) move from the research labs into the clinics.

Audio Recordings

Most poor quality audiotape recordings of stutterings (especially with children) result from one basic oversight: *inappropriate microphone placement*. To cut to the chase: *The microphone should be placed as close to the client's lips as possible*. This is especially true with children, who (1) inherently talk softer than adults and (2) often react to new settings, especially in the beginning, by producing less speech and/or minimally audible verbalizations. We can't emphasize the point strongly enough: Put the microphone as close as possible to the client's mouth!

Ideally, the recording surface of the microphone should be (1) placed perpendicular to the path or plane of the acoustic speech signal (for example, if the client is talking to a clinician across a table, the recording surface of the microphone should be pointed toward the ceiling or toward the wall to the client's immediate left or right); and (2) placed at a relatively constant distance from the client's lips and mouth. As mentioned above, with children, in particular, the *biggest* mistake most clinicians make is to place the microphone too far away from the child's mouth. In our experience, the microphone should be kept within inches of the child's mouth; a variety of small tie-tack, label, or lavalier microphones (e.g., Sony, Model ECM-50 or ECM-55) are available for this purpose and can be easily clipped on or fastened to the child's shirt or shirt collar (we've done this with hundreds of children). Again, no matter what brand of microphone is used, however, we have found that even the most expensive, sensitive microphone can't make up for one basic mistake: having too great a distance between the client's mouth and the microphone.

Put the microphone on the child's mother or father first. Using as matter-of-fact a tone of voice as possible, moving surely but slowly with our hands, as we clip the microphone on his or her shirt, collar, or sweater, we tell the child that he or she is going to wear a microphone just like an airplane pilot, an astronaut, and newscaster on TV. This gentle but sure approach with children helps most of them adjust and accept the wearing of a small clip-on or lapel microphone. However, no matter how we approach them, some young clients will resist the wearing of a tie tack or lapel microphone and/or seemingly be unable to forget about the microphone and continue to handle or touch it. One relatively easy way we've found to deal with this problem is for the clinician to fasten a similar microphone on the child's mother, father, or even on the clinician herself (this works, we suppose, on the premise that misery loves company). By clipping the microphone on the mother, father, or clinician first and having the child watch seems to help them adjust and accept the wearing of the microphone, particularly the slow-to-warm-up or behaviorally inhibited child. The microphone on the mother or clinician doesn't even have to be connected to a recorder, just as long as it is visible to the child on the parent or clinician. This procedure seems to help the child forget about the microphone and get on with the business at hand.

If both of the above requirements for microphone placement are met, the next thing the clinician should insure is that the record gain of the tape recorder be set or regulated so that the recorded level of the client's speech is neither too low (soft) nor high (loud). That is, the level of the VU meter is centered, during the recording, around the 0 mark. Not to put too fine a point on it, but if we seriously desire to achieve consistent, high-quality audio recordings of the speech behavior of people who stutter, then we should not employ tape recorders that have glow tubes for VU meters, that lack VU meters, or that have built-in (nondetectable) microphones. Speech-language pathologists who desire audio-tape recordings for the purposes of molecular and microscopic analysis of speech behavior (for example, narrow phonetic transcriptions, vocalized versus nonvocalized pauses, voice quality associated with stuttering, and so forth) are well advised to take the minimal time necessary to learn how to set up and implement proper audio recordings. It takes very little extra time and money to do it right, and with modest amounts of practice, these recording procedures become second nature; the resulting recordings are far and away superior (and are much easier for the clinician to listen to and analyze after the client leaves).

Video Recordings

Most poor-quality videotape recordings of people talking come from two sources: (1) low or inappropriate lighting of the subject and (2) relatively insensitive cameras or poor camera-to-subject position. Unfortunately, both issues—lighting and cameras—involve spending money, money that is frequently not part of clinicians' budgets. At the very least, however, the clinician can, without spending any extra money, do the following: (1) Insure that the room used for recording has reasonably decent overhead room lighting; and (2) insure that the area *behind* the client is neutral in color (e.g., beige, tan, etc.) and without a lot of distracting material, for example, toys, books, desks, and so forth. Spending a little money, the clinician can purchase a camera tripod (to maximize camera stability) with a smooth or fluid-filled pan tilt head (the head is the part, at the top of the tripod, that the camera rests on and permits side-to-side swiveling as well as up/down camera movement) so that the camera can be easily, smoothly and quickly adjusted to follow the ever-moving, ever-squirming child. Spending even more money, the clinician can purchase a low-priced light kit for illumination of the subject. (We have used such a lighting schema to videotape conversations of over 150 children between 2 and 7 years of age and their mothers. With very few exceptions, these lights were tolerated by these young children and their mothers.) Finally, if interest and budget permits, the clinician can purchase cameras that either operate in low-light situations (20 or less candlewatts of illumination) or have far greater sensitivity than the typical consumer-grade camera. Just as with audio recordings, a little attention to detail *prior* to video recording will make all the difference in terms of the brightness, contrast, and resolution of videotape recordings.

Informed Consent or the Client's Right-to-Know

A word or two is in order regarding clients' and their associates' right-to-know, or informed consent, regarding all of your clinical procedures and practice. In particular, if the client and associates are to be observed, taped (either audio or audiovideo), or otherwise scrutinized by yourself, your colleagues, or students-in-training, the client and associates should be so informed in as matter-of-fact a manner and tone as possible. Right from the beginning of the evaluation, providing the client an atmosphere of openness and honesty is important, in our opinion, because the atmosphere we send out to clients many times will be reflected in the atmosphere clients send back to us. Especially in a training situation, where supervisors and other student clinicians observe behind see-through mirrors, the client and family need to be told (1) that they are going to be observed and (2) who is doing the observing. Just recently, despite the present writer's over thirty years of working on both sides of the mirror, he forgot to mention to the families in one of his parent-child group that the groups would be observed by his doctoral assistant. One father, who finally couldn't contain himself, near the end of the group session blurted out, "I know someone has been observing us . . . I can see his outline through the mirror. . . . Who is watching us?" (apparently the door to the observation room had been left partially open, making the mirror more glass-like). The other parents quickly wanted to know as well. I quickly explained, with my point being that even though the see-through mirror is very familiar to me, it's not for the client and his or her relations, and we must constantly remember this.

Telling a client that such observational procedures are routine and essential to help you help him or her is not only an honest but a wise policy. Surely, such openness may make some clients more visibly concerned when they know they are being observed and taped (they may ask many lengthy questions about the observational procedure, the use to which the observed information will be put, and who is doing the observing), but it is clearly the right of the client to know such matters. Later, in this chapter, we will discuss our belief that clients and whoever they designate should get copies of our full-scale diagnostic reports. After all, it is more than likely that this is the way you would want to be dealt with if you were in your client's shoes.

Components of the Stuttering Evaluation

If we disregard, for the moment, the age of the client you will assess and evaluate, the *ideal* evaluation of stuttering should include the following components:

1. *An intake form*, filled out in advance of the evaluation by the client and/or parents, teacher, doctor, and so forth, providing identification plus basic information regarding history of the problem and related matters.

2. *An interview* with the client and, if available, associates, regarding history, current and possible future status of the problem plus motivation, need and desire for clinical services.

3. *Standardized and nonstandardized assessment* and evaluation of communicative and related skills.

4. Preparation and dissemination of a *written documentation* of findings and interpretations based on assessment.

While none of these four components is any more important than the other, it is my experience that those aspects of the evaluation that involve the clinician's interviewing and writing skills are those parts that seem the most difficult to master. Obviously, none of the skills needed to be a reasonably competent diagnostician develop overnight; beginning clinicians, in particular, should be cautioned not to expect to master interviewing and writing skills too quickly. With time, experience, and effort, however, beginning clinicians can learn to interview clients and their families in a productive manner and write about their observations and findings in a clear, succinct, and organized fashion.

The Intake Form

The first component, an *intake form*, should ideally have been completed *in advance* of the evaluation and should, at the very least, include information regarding identification of the client and associates, general information regarding history of problem and related matters, and *full* addresses of all parties to whom the client and associates want the written report sent. We hate to sound so picky, but it really is important to obtain complete and accurate identification information: addresses, zip codes, telephone numbers (home and office), complete birthdate and date of evaluation (day, month and year), present occupation, education, and so forth. It is our experience that this type of information is all too often neglected, missing or inaccurate; however, it often serves as the basis for the clinician's first remarks to the client. Besides, it is rather difficult to mail a client a copy of his or her diagnostic report if you have a partial or missing mailing address!

While perhaps obvious, the clinician should be encouraged to review the intake form *before* the client arrives, making note of any information that appears missing, unclear, or seemingly inaccurate. Thus, during the diagnostic itself, the clinician can ask the client to provide such missing, unclear, or inaccurate information. Even more important than the use of this information in the opening remarks to the client is its later use in the writing up of the diagnostic report, in making referrals, planning remediation, follow-up contacts, and the like. Furthermore, if the client or the client's parents, in the case of the child, take the time in advance to complete such forms, it suggests that the client or associates are at least willing to expend some effort in self-help. Conversely, when an evaluation begins *without* the client's having completed or only partially completing the form, we should ask ourselves the following question: "If this client is not willing and able to find the time and energy to fill out such forms, how willing and able will he or she be to put the necessary time and effort into speech therapy?" Of course, we might feel quite differently if the client has real difficulties reading/writing for reasons of illiteracy, speaking English as a second language, or other problems.

The Interview Procedure: Areas and Types of Inquiry

The second, and perhaps most important, component of the stuttering assessment is the *interview*. The interview involves a structured conversation between the clinician and client (and associates) whose purpose is to facilitate the clinician's ability to help the client. Generally, the interview consists of the clinician questioning the client and associates regarding past, present, and future events that directly or indirectly relate to the client's concerns. In this writer's opinion, no aspect of the evaluation requires more training, attention, listening, or observational skills than the interview. It is, therefore, very understandable that many beginning as well as experienced clinicians find this a challenging aspect of assessment and evaluation. Haynes and Pindzola (1998) do a nice job of overviewing the basic principles and procedures of diagnostic interviewing. Haynes and Pindzola suggest that the diagnostic has three interrelated goals: (1) to obtain information, (2) to give information, and (3) to provide release (for the frustrations and fears of the client) and support (for the client's strengths). These authors also describe and categorize both clinician and client questions and responses, and their discussion of clinical interviewing deserves study by serious students of assessment and evaluation. To begin, therefore, let us *generally* consider the number and variety of questions that Haynes and Pindzola, other authors, and the current writer typically use in a diagnostic interview.

Questions: Area and Style of Questions

Areas to Question.   The areas of inquiry and degree of specificity of questioning are probably the first consideration, especially for beginning clinicians. Haynes and Pindzola suggest that the clinician use an "interview guide" rather than a formal set of questions. For the more experienced clinician, we would agree that such a guide is sufficient and appropriate; however, for the beginning clinician, a bit more structure appears necessary. The general topics that Haynes and Pindzola suggest including in such a guide seem quite appropriate (e.g., "What is the respondent's perception of the problem?" "When and under what conditions did the communication disorder arise?" and so on). To address many of the topics Haynes and colleagues suggest assessing, we refer the reader to Appendix A, where they will find a listing of specific questions. Perhaps through a combination of general topics and specific questions addressing those topics, the beginning clinician can start his or her first several interviews with more comfort, direction, and support. Indeed, later on in this chapter, under "Questions: Some Specific Ones to Ask," we will provide our own "interview guide," which provides the frame that the clinician can fill with appropriate inquiry and questions.

Style of the Questioner.   Closely related to the areas of inquiry is the *style* of the interviewer. This can be as varied as there are clients; however, we agree that the "funneling" approach, as labeled by Haynes and Pindzola (1998, p. 39), is one excellent, useful style of interviewing during a variety of situations. Going from broad questions (e.g., "How does Mario do in school?") to more specific questions (e.g., "Does he speak well during oral reading?"), the interviewer gently and gradually helps the interviewee respond in a manner likely to provide useful, reliable information. Indeed, funneling is an interviewing skill very much worth developing, that is, knowing how to move from broad to specific questions within areas of important inquiry.

However, as I will say several places in these pages, it is an imperfect world. Knowing that we may question directly when indirectly is preferable or vice versa could lead us to experience paralysis through analysis. Taken to the extreme, this would be a situation whereby we cease helping people simply because we know that our help may be less than perfectly helpful! Instead, we must start somewhere, in some fashion, to help, even if our help is constantly evolving in terms of effectiveness. Suffice it to say, one very good, logical place to start is the interview, to inquire into the person's concerns, observations, perceptions, and understanding of his or her problem. And the vehicle for conducting this inquiry, after all is said and done, is the question. Of course, as we already know, not just any question will do. Indeed, different questions result in different answers; in the following section, we will examine some of those differences.

Questions: Specific Types. Flynn (1978, pp. 268–269) describes a number of specific questions or "elicitors" that may be used during the diagnostic (Flynn reportedly adapted these from Goyer, Reading, & Rickey, 1968. Flynn's questions used with permission.):

1. *Direct questions*—Ask for a reply on a specific topic
   Example: "What did you do last summer?"
   Closed questions—Direct but with greatly narrowed response field
   Example: "What did you do with Jim on the 4th of July?"
   Yes-No—The most restrictive direct questions
   Example: "Did you go to the parade?"
2. *Open-ended questions*—Specify only the topic and leave great latitude in replying
   Example: "Tell me about yourself."
   "Make up your own story about it."
3. *Leading questions*—Imply a specific kind of answer.
   Example: "You are a happy person, aren't you?"
   Loaded questions—Leading questions with emotional connotation.
   Example: To a loyal Republican: "Don't you agree that Ronald Reagan was a poor president?"
   Yes-response questions—Leading questions expressed in such a way as to encourage respondent to agree with statement.
   Example: "Of course you'll be the new group leader of the adult stuttering group, won't you?"
4. *Nondirective questions and statements*—Provide encouragement to the respondent to say more.
   Example: "I really like to watch hockey. You said you play hockey on the high school team?"
   Mirror question—Intended to get added comment on previous response.
   Example: "I feel real sad . . . You say that you are sad?"
   Verbal probes—"I see," "Tell me more," "Umhum," "Interesting," and "I'm not sure I understand." These "probes" generally get the client to talk more, but the content of the client's conversation can take a variety of directions, some more beneficial than others to the purposes of the diagnostic.

In our experience, the beginning clinician feels most comfortable with direct, closed, and yes-no questions, while the more experienced clinician more frequently employs nondirective questions. Ideally, the interview should be a constant blending and switching between these various types of questions: a direct question here, followed by an open-ended question, back to a yes-no question, then followed by a mirror question and a verbal probe or two. As mentioned above, the "funneling" or even "inverted funneling" (going from specific to general questions) described by Haynes and Pindzola are excellent ways to organize these disparate questions in a cohesive whole that leads to meaningful responses from the client and/or client's family. It is our experience that all of these types of questions have a place in the diagnostic and that the clinician should work on learning when each type of question is and is not appropriate to use. For example, when interviewing an older person who stutters who is, at the beginning of the diagnostic, having a great deal of trouble talking, you may find that a series of direct, closed, or yes-no questions, interspersed with a verbal probe or two, may be more preferable than asking a bunch of open-ended and/or loaded questions.

Questions: General Issues That Need to Be Addressed. The previously mentioned nine or ten specific questions can be related to three interdependent issues the examining clinician will want to consider:

1. *Questions leading to testing*: These are questions clinicians ask themselves about the client that lead them to test the client to find the answer(s), for example, "Is this client more or less fluent when he reads than when he speaks?"
2. *Questions directly asked of the client and associates*: These are questions clinicians directly ask the client, his or her parents, or associates—for example, "Why do you want to receive speech therapy at this time?"
3. *Questions answered by inference and guesstimation*: These are questions clinicians ask themselves about the client that require inferences in order to try to find the answer(s), for example, "What is the source of this person's desire to receive speech therapy (parental, peer, spouse, or employment pressure)?"

Questions that lead to testing are quite familiar to most clinicians: Is the client more fluent when reading than when speaking? On the average, how many of the client's words or syllables per 100 words or syllable spoken are stuttered? What is the client's most frequently produced disfluency type? Are the client's hearing, articulation, and language skills within normal limits? Can we get perceptual clues from client's voice quality during instances of stuttering that indicate how he or she is using the larynx during stuttering? Are the client's intellectual and reading skills of a nature to allow this person to derive sufficient benefit from remediation at this point in his or her life? These and other questions like them form the essence of what a speech-language pathologist will need and want to ask of the client who is suspected or known to stutter.

Questions directly asked of the client and associate are really most of what Flynn (1978), as previously described, was discussing. Such questions as the following are asked during the interview: How would you describe to me your or your child's stuttering speech behavior? Would you please show or demonstrate for me how you or your child stutter? What is your theory of why you or your child stutters? Did your stuttering (or your child's stuttering) begin with a sound prolongation or repeating of sounds and syllables? What types of therapy have you or your child previously received? Tell me more about why such therapies helped or did not help you or your child? What are your or your child's general strengths or weaknesses? Shortly, we will present a serial listing of questions that we use in the assessment and evaluation of stuttering that may serve as a guide to you in the development and implementation of your own interview procedure. By no means, however, should such a listing preclude or restrict you from developing different and additional questions to be used for your own interview procedure.

Questions that are answered by inference and guesstimation are also important to the diagnosis of stuttering. These types of questions require the SLP to develop the ability to judge but not be judgmental of people and their actions. Interestingly, clinicians frequently do not seem to even realize that they are asking or need to ask such questions. One important issue, relative to these types of questions, is the clinician's ability to judge whether the client has sufficient skills or potential for developing skills to make the necessary changes in speech and related behavior. To arrive at such judgments, clinicians will ask themselves the following types of questions: Is this person capable of expending the necessary mental and physical effort and time to change behavior? What seems to be the sources of motivation and desire for therapy (Prins, 1974; Starbuck, 1974)? Why is this person seeking services? How reliable, honest, and straightforward is this client in his or her responses to me? Does this person really appear to understand what I am saying and asking? Does this client appear to be assuming a *cure me* (passive consumer), or is he or she assuming a *self-effort with guidance* role (active producer)? Are these parents setting reasonable standards for child behavior and child raising?

Of course, all of the abovementioned questions are not asked independently of one another; they obviously dovetail and are at times redundant in terms of the information they provide. Redundancy, however, is not necessarily a vice—it may indeed be a virtue during the diagnostic because it provides a means for checking on the consistency and stability of the client's and associates' statements and behaviors. It should be clear, therefore, that the type of question the SLP asks is not restricted to this or that section of the evaluation. In fact, the answer to one type of question may partly or completely answer another type of question.

Questions: Some Specific Ones to Ask.   As mentioned above, Appendix A provides a series of questions that may be asked of the parents or associates of young children (they may be, as the wording in some of these questions suggests, adapted to use with older children, teenagers, and adults). As previously mentioned, these questions should be viewed as a *guide*, and in no way should they preclude or restrict the clinician from developing his or her own set of questions or variations of those currently presented. Tanner and Cannon (1978) developed a commercially available series of diagnostic questions that the clinician may ask the mother and/or father of a child who is (or who is suspected of being) a person who stutters. Likewise, Zwitman (1978) has presented a similar series of questions, and Thompson (1983) has developed similar questions that may be asked of a child's classroom teacher. Rather than go through each and every question, we will cover the groupings of questions and give an example of each and some rationale.

Introduction.   You've got to start somewhere and an open-ended question—for example, "What can we do to help you?"—helps clarify the purpose and set an appropriate "tone" to the interview. While some (Flynn, 1978) suggest avoiding the use of the word "problem" in the beginning of the interview, we have found that a few open-ended questions (like those given in Appendix A), stated in a matter-of-fact way, start the interview out in a positive direction and easily lead into subsequent questioning.

General Development.   After the beginning, we like to cover past history to the extent the person can and will remember such events and detail. Starting with the past does two things: (1) It provides you with perspective on the person, the person's associates, and/or the person's life; and (2) helps the person begin by thinking and talking about things that may not have the same degree of emotionality attached to them (i.e., time heals all wounds) that may be associated with present events. With parents, in particular, questions like "How does his general development from birth to present compare with his brother or sister or other children his age?" provides you perspective on their observational powers as well as understanding of general childhood development.

Family History.   Here are the first questions that directly deal with stuttering and/or speech-language-hearing problems. We have found that the general question "Are there any speech, hearing, or language problems in any other family members (living or deceased)?" is far more apt to uncover stuttering in the family than the simple question "Does anyone else (alive or deceased) stutter?" You can always follow up the general question with the stuttering question and sometimes, if you do, you'll be surprised at the responses you get (for example, a response of "No" to the general question but "Yes" to the question about stuttering and vice versa). Perhaps all this says is that the client wasn't listening, but we are inclined to think that it means that the client and associates attach different meaning to the words "speech problem" and "stuttering" and that some clients may even be trying *not* to reveal information about the past that they think may unduly influence your opinion about them or their child. Whatever the case, as we learn more about the genetics of stuttering (e.g., Ambrose et al., 1997; Howie, 1981), it may turn out to be very important diagnostically to know whether immediate family members or other relatives (alive or deceased) ever stuttered.

Speech/Language Development and History.   The rationale behind these types of questions, we believe, is fairly straightforward. However, responses to these types of questions are generally going to be more unclear when reported by teenagers and adults than when reported by, say, the parents of a 4-year-old (and for this reason the clinician might want to significantly truncate the number and variety of these questions when dealing with an older client). Like the other sections, this set of questions can be contracted or expanded according to the needs of the particular client and goals of the examining clinician. Of particular interest here are questions like "When did he or you begin to say his or your first words?" in relation to the question "When did he or you first begin to have difficulties speaking?" Many times, the parents, in particular, will report two or three years of remarkably fluent speech *prior* to the first observation of stuttering. This issue can be explored further in later sections.

Academic Information.   Obviously, parents of preschoolers are asked the most cursory question or two regarding schooling ("How does he seem to be doing in nursery school/the day-care center/prekindergarten program?"). For the school-age child through teenagers in high school, questions in this area can be very informative. Many times the problems you observe in the diagnostic—for example, difficulties with oral reading tasks, receptive and expressive language, attention span, and so forth—are also apparent in school. Sometimes it becomes apparent that stuttering is the least of the child's concerns and that therapy for same will have to be a lower priority to a number of issues that must be worked out through the school system—for example, hyperactivity in the classroom, chronically wandering attention and/or acting out against other children, social immaturity, autism, difficulties with reading and language to a point a where the child is required to repeat the grade, and so forth. The experienced clinician always wants to know something about the person's feelings toward and experiences with school, since these feelings/experiences may continue into the present and influence social, employment, and communication experiences.

History/Description of Problem (Past and Present).   By this point in the interview the rapport between client and clinician should be sufficient where the crux of the matter can be discussed: "Tell me about his or her speaking difficulties or problem." This question strikes at the core of the problem and the clinician shouldn't be surprised that like the center of the earth, this core, particularly for older clients, is going to be fairly hot. Questions here, although going back to the onset of the problem, deal with the here-and-now of the issue and are not things the client and associates particularly relish discussing. A delicate, supportive approach on the part of the clinician ("I know some of these questions are going to be tough, but just do the best job you can") will help.

There is a redundancy in the questioning here and it is for a purpose: to help the clinician get the clearest picture possible of the client's problem at present and from the beginning. Gathering this material is the SLP's job, this is what she or he is supposedly getting paid for. This is the type of material that will permit the SLP to say whether a problem exists and if so what course of action should be taken. Although previously discussed questions provide useful perspectives and supportive information, the SLP should try to keep in mind the purpose of the diagnostic and diagnostic interview: Does the person have a stuttering problem and if so what course of action should be taken?

Speech/Language Abilities.   Rationale for these questions would appear to be straightforward: Are there any other speech-hearing-language problems that contribute to or may need more immediate attention than stuttering? Although much is made of language development and difficulties with people who stutter, it is our experience that articulation/phonological problems occur in approximately one-third of all children who stutter. As the review by Louko and colleagues (1999) suggests, several studies (e.g., Louko et al., 1990; Riley & Riley, 1979; St. Louis & Hinzman, 1988; Thompson, 1983; Williams & Silverman, 1968), based on actual or direct examination of the speech behavior of young people who stutter, report that between 24 and 45 percent of young people who stutter exhibit some degree (e.g., mild, moderate, or severe) of articulation/phonology, which is a much higher percentage than typical for preschool children, of whom 2 to 6 percent reportedly exhibit mild to severe levels of articulation/phonological difficulties (Beitchman, Nair, Clegg, & Patel, 1986; Hull, Mielke, Timmons, & Willeford, 1971). At this point, the precise implications of the connection between speech articulation and speech fluency difficulties is unknown, but clinicians would be well advised to consider the implications of this connection on their diagnostic assessment and therapy plans when stuttering and articulation disorders are observed in the same child.

History/Description of Problem (Associated Behavior).   If a problem with fluency is apparent, this section permits the clinician to assess the degree to which the client is presenting overt reactions to the problem and, with children, the degree to which this is bothersome to the parent. Oftentimes, with children, it is their behavior—for example, head turning, eyes opening and closing, facial grimaces, and the like—*associated* with their stutterings, rather than their stutterings per se, that will convince the parents that the child needs help. As we have discussed elsewhere (Schwartz & Conture, 1988), while adults who stutter probably produce a larger number and greater variety of these associated behaviors than do children, young stutters definitively exhibit a number and variety of these associated behaviors (see Conture & Kelly, 1991a); it would seem that these differences are suggestive of different strategies for coping with stuttering.

Anxiety/Situational Hierarchy.   Brutten and Shoemaker (1967) were among the first to introduce the use of anxiety/situational hierarchies to stuttering theory and therapy. Erickson (1969) subsequently reported a scale for measuring the communication attitudes that distinguish people who stutter from people who do not stutter, and Andrews and Cutler (1974) revised this scale to measure change in these attitudes during the course of therapy. While the relation of the attitudes of people who stutter to changes in their speech as a result of therapy remains unclear (Ingham, 1984), Erickson's and Andrews' and Cutler's efforts in this area provide a solid beginning for the eventual development of an instrument for assessing these attitudes. More recently, Hanson, Gronhond, and Rice (1981) measured the speech-related attitudes of adult people who stutter with still another different but related form of a speech situation checklist; however, regarding children who stutter, only Guitar and Peters's (1980) experimental version of the Erickson scale and DeNil and Brutten's (1991) (see also Vanryckeghem & Brutten, 1997) *Speech Situation Checklist for Children* have seemingly been used to assess the self-reports of speech-related attitudes of school-age people who stutter. It is still unknown whether such a self-report questionnaire procedure could be readily and reliably administered to preschool/early elementary school-age children (between 2 and 7), the age period when most children actually begin to stutter.

While this writer's purpose for obtaining a "situational hierarchy" differs from those of individuals eventually interested in systematically desensitizing the client to various environmental stimuli, the procedure is roughly the same. At present, however, as mentioned above, this is most feasible to do with adults. When this is done with adults, an interesting observation may be made: Those adults who stutter who give the most detailed situational hierarchy—those who precisely describe and rank order in degree of strength of perceived emotionality a number of stimuli associated with stuttering—will often recover quicker from stuttering and results will be more lasting than those who provide a less detailed hierarchy. For most younger clients, though, some direct but simple questions like "When does he appear to stutter the most?" will elicit such parental responses as "When he is tired, excited, or in hurry and asking questions." Sometimes no such connection between environmental or child behavior and stuttering will be reported, and this observation is instructive, particularly if the clinician notices difference in the child's stuttering during different activities or when the child is feeling or behaving in certain ways. Also notice that this is the area where questions regarding avoidance of person, places, or things can be asked. Once again, avoidance is generally more pronounced or apparent in older people who stutter, but it is wise to get some idea if avoidance, in any form, is beginning to be part of the problem, even in children.

History/Description of Problem (or what people have been doing to "help").   There is a line on a Marlo Thomas' ("Free to Be You and Me") recording that goes "There is some kinda help which is the kinda help we can all do without." This is particularly true with people who stutter, and we, as clinicians, want to know as much about the past and present of these helping efforts as we can. In the main, suggestions to "Slow down and take a deep breath," "Speed it up, I don't have all day," or "Relax and think about what you are going to say" reflect expressions of sincere concern as well as frustration on the part of the listener.

Whatever the case, it helps to know what kind of reactions, suggestions, assistance, and so forth the people who stutter are routinely as well as occasionally exposed to. Having this sort of information is crucial in your attempts to help the client's associates adopt more facilatory reactions and minimize their apparently inhibitory reactions. It also gives you clues regarding what the client's associates as well as the client think cause as well as perpetuate the problem. This should be useful to you as you try to provide more objective, factual information about stuttering and what influences it.

Family Interaction.   While these types of questions are generally directed at the child or teenager living at home, they may also serve useful for the older client still living at home or one who is married. With the child, we want to know all we can about the role speech and language has in the home, that is, its relative importance, value, as well as the amount and kind routinely produced. It is not uncommon to find oral expression/speech highly prized in the home of people who stutter: The child may be encouraged to orally recite for family, friends, and neighbors saying such things as nursery rhymes, giving speeches, memorized stories, putting on little plays, or singing songs. We call this "performance" (as in command performance) speech. This is not unlike singing for one's supper or grandmother, as the case may be.

Routine "drill" with flash or cue cards where the child has to recite memorized numbers, objects, colors, sounds, words, or letters is also sometimes observed. These types of question on your part may also indicate that family dinners are spent with the television, radio, or stereo in the background in addition to mother, father, brother, sister and the young person who stutters talking. Once again, the client is a person, a person living in some environment, and it behooves the clinician to find out as much as possible about that environment in order to more clearly understand the person's stuttering and what may be done about it.

Social/Behavioral.   While tests like the *Vineland Test of Social Maturity* will help the clinician understand the child's social maturity, what we are after here is the client's ability to appropriately interact with individuals in and outside the home. Actually, this is very much related to questions regarding family interaction and academic experiences. Of particular note is the question "What does he/she do that particularly annoys you or anyone else?"

With an adult you might ask, "Do you know of anything that you do that might annoy your friends, relatives or fellow workers?" Usually, both parents and adults will respond,"You mean besides speech?" and we say "yes, besides speech." Oftentimes, particularly with parents, the thing or things that annoy them about the child's behavior, besides speech, are as much a reason to seek your advice as the speech itself! Further, with children, we are especially interested in knowing about the number and ages of friends they have in the neighborhood and, if they attend, in school.

Parental Fear of Childhood Independence.   It is not unusual for parents of children who stutter to say "We don't want her associating with this or that child," "We don't want him to get hurt, dirty, or in trouble playing outside," or words to the effect that they are having trouble letting the child have the normal amount of independence all children need in order to grow up and develop. Many of these parents will be particularly concerned about sending the child to nursery school, prekindergarten, day care, or even kindergarten or first grade ("people will pick on him . . . he is not ready . . . some of those children play real rough and Todd is so gentle"). One response I make to these parents, when it is apparent that their child has what it takes to absorb the slings and arrows of outrageous fortunes at the hands of peers, is something like "You want to know if it's all right if you keep her out of kindergarten and have her stay at home with you? Sure, as long as you plan on enrolling yourself in her school and sitting next to her in kindergarten, first grade, and beyond." This usually gets the point across: "Yes, I know its hard to let go, but let go you must, at least a little bit now, unless you plan on having your child lean on you for life."

Questions about the client's social life, maturity, and the like can provide the SLP with much-needed perspective. This is where the SLP will hear such things as the following: "frequently cries when he doesn't get his way," "is very much afraid of loud noise, fire, and the dark," "has no friends her own age," "seems to be much less mature than other children the same age," and "avoids conversations with people at all costs." While some of these observations can be attributed to a normal reaction to an abnormal situation, when a child *routinely* exhibits *strong* fears of the dark, loud noises, fire, or anything strange, the SLP may want to: (1) monitor the evolution of these fears and/or (2) make referral for psychosocial evaluation. A child who *routinely* exhibits *strong* fears of everyday events and objects may be a child whose sensitivities and emotional stability make it difficult for him or her to receive maximal benefit from speech therapy at least until such concerns are specifically addressed and mitigated.

The client's or associates' response to the question "Is there anything (other than speaking) that concerns you, in any way, about yourself or your child?" is particularly revealingly. Sometimes the answer to this question suggests one of the main reasons the client is seeking services: "I can't hold or find a job" or "Angie has no friends" or so forth. Any consistent and/or strong concerns expressed by the client or associates in this area bear further exploration, because they may be the "real" problem or at least significantly contribute to the person's inability to recovery from stuttering.

Wrap up.   As anyone knows who has attended a reception, leaving can almost be as awkward as arriving. The same is true of an interview. We have found that questions regarding things the client or client's associates think need to be or can be changed is a good way to end. Talking about past or present services for stuttering or other concerns the client has received gets people thinking about the role the present clinical services, if they are recommended, will play in their lives. Our last question is particularly instructive: "If you could wish for three things for yourself or your child (the sky is the limit), what would you wish for?" It is *not* unusual for speech language or any other aspect of communication to be excluded from this list. Such exclusion should tell the clinician something about priorities in the person's life. Although wishes do not necessarily reflect reality, wishes do tell us about a person's aspirations and desires and knowing something about these things is not to be lightly considered.

The Interview Procedure: General Issues and Concerns

Common Listening Problems.   In the beginning, clinicians often have trouble listening to their clients because they are too busy listening to themselves! That is, instead of listening to their client's responses they are too busy thinking of the next question they are going to ask (media interviewers are frequently guilty of this). As clinicians gain a bit more experience, they sometimes think they hear things or read things into their client's response that are probably best left unsaid. For example, a mother tells about her son's pet garter snake, to which the clinician responds by asking the mother, "Has Angus had any sexual adjustment problems that you know of?" Conversely, clinicians sometime hear the content of the question but not its attendant emotion (and vice versa). For example, a mother softly cries as she relates a story of a near drowning of one of her children that occurred shortly before her other child began to stutter, to which the clinician responds, "I bet you now know how to perform CPR, right?"

Sometimes, as mentioned above, the best response is no response, particularly if you start to feel that you are talking too much or asking too many questions. Silence is particularly golden when the client becomes upset, uncomfortable, or in other ways emotionally concerned. A simple gesture like handing the client a box of tissues makes it clear that you have nonjudgmentally recognized the person's feelings *and* that person's right to express him- or herself. On the other hand, as Flynn (1978) mentions, there is really no reason to remain silent when a client who has rambled on and on about interesting but ancillary issues finally decides to take a breath. In short, clinicians who interview must be as adept at listening to the client's answers to their questions as they are at asking the questions in the first place. The skill of knowing when and how to switch from speaker to listener and back to speaker during the diagnostic interview presents a challenging but most interesting part of the entire diagnostic. Haynes and Pindzola (1998) provide some excellent suggestions for how to improve interviewing skills, one of which is to "listen to all sorts of people." We couldn't agree more! The wider variety of people you listen to, the wider variety of ideas, emotions, thoughts, and adjustment/coping strategies you will be exposed to and the less likely you are going to miss or mishandle the incredible variety of clients you will need to interview during the course of your career.

Listening to and Following up on Answers.   Perhaps even more challenging than structuring the number and nature of your questions is knowing how to listen to and follow up on your clients' responses. Sometimes, as Flynn (1978) suggests, "an interested, attentive, relaxed silence" may be an appropriate way to respond to your client. We would agree with

Flynn, however, that frequent and prolonged use of such silence gives the client a less-than-positive image of you and/or may make the client somewhat uncomfortable. Most of the time, though, your followup to your client's responses will be verbal. Knowing when and how to follow up is a complex skill that needs to be mastered if one is to become a successful interviewer.

Following up on Questions.   A clinician's ability to follow up the client's responses to questions is based on his or her ability to listen and observe. Like a human form of an artificial intelligence program (an interesting metaphor if one stops to think about it), the clinician narrows down the possibilities with followup questions. For example, the clinician asks, "Did Damon start stuttering before or after the birth of your second child?" and the mother says "After." The clinician next asks, "Did you notice Damon stuttering before or after the second child began to speak?" and the mother says, "Shortly after the second child began to talk." The clinician next asks, "Was the second child talking more or less than Damon at that time?" and the mother says, "More. My second child has been a talkative motormouth right from the beginning." And so forth.

As we can see, the clinician rapidly—and hopefully fluidly—switches back and forth from listening to speaking: She listens to the client's responses to her questions and then asks a question or makes a comment based on that response. For an actual example of followup, consider the situation where we suspected a father of having unreasonably high standards for his daughter's verbal communication. The father said, in an extremely fluent, articulate fashion, that he had always had to sell himself through verbal communication. Following up on this comment, we asked the father about his boyhood and that of his relatives (an open-ended question), and he said that both he and his father had been champion debaters in school, having won many individual as well as team honors. We followed up on this by asking him to tell us more about his debating experience (a verbal probe), and the father stated that he had hoped the family tradition of debating would be carried on by his daughter and that he had been helping her learn to develop the necessary communication skills. Unfortunately, his daughter was only 8 years old, and it was our observation she was not exactly what we would consider an oral-laryngeal athlete. This information, developed from our followup, together with other observations, led us to strongly suspect that the father had somewhat unreasonable standards for his daughter's verbal communication.

It is not that the father was unwilling, unable, or reluctant to tell us about his debating days (although sometimes this is the case); it is just that he did not think it too relevant. And perhaps such information might not be too relevant for certain clients; however, we cannot consider the relevance of anything unless we have the thing to consider in the first place! Followup to client's responses, we have found, often provides this sort of information in the first place! We are not advocating, we hasten to add, that clinician use follow up as free license, carte blanche as it were, to snoop and poke through the stuttering client's and associates' dirty laundry. However, if the clinician believes the information is necessary to gain perspective on, derive better understanding of, and thus help the client, then the information is worthy of the clinician's attempts to retrieve it.

Deductive Reasoning During Clinical Interviewing.   The use of funneling should be distinguished from *deductive reasoning*, something that many interviewers often use and just as often misuse. We engage in deductive reasoning when we apply our basic *assumptions* to an individual behavior, person, or situation. When our assumptions are valid, our conclusions will be, too; however, all too often our basic assumptions are invalid or at least poorly validated. Typically, when an interviewer uses deductive reasoning in a clinical setting, he or she starts with some premises, ideas, or assumptions and draws conclusions about a specific individual or situation based on these premises. For example, say it is your general assumption, belief, or premise that rapid, long, and complex parental utterances exacerbate childhood stuttering as well as specific belief that the mother you are currently interviewing talks to her child using rapid, long, complex utterances. By putting these two believes or premises together, you conclude that the mother's communication exacerbates her child's stuttering. The mental process (i.e., reasoning) by which your conclusion was drawn from your assumptions is called an *inference*.

The weak link, however, was not your inference but your assumption. Indeed, if your assumptions are true, you *must* conclude that the mother's rate, length, and complexity of utterance exacerbates her child's stuttering. However, if your general as well as specific assumptions about the influence of parental utterance on childhood stuttering are untrue, your conclusion is also untrue, regardless of how logical your inference or reasoning. Thus, it's the validity of the basic assumptions, not the reasoning, that gets most interviewers in trouble. Indeed, many clinicians, beginning as well as advanced, worry more about the style of their interviewing technique than they do about the truthfulness of their basic assumptions.

Inductive Reasoning During Clinical Interviews.   We use *inductive* reasoning clinically when we try to derive general principles from individual facts. Again, like deductive reasoning, clinicians use as well as misuse inductive reasoning during clinical interviewing. For example, you observe that a child who stutters seems to be intolerant of all his mistakes (e.g., mistakes made while coloring, mistakes made while learning to throw a ball, mistakes made while playing a game, etc.). You then *infer* that all or most children who stutter are perfectionistic. From the behavior of an individual child, you derive a general principle about children who stutter as a whole. You have gone beyond the fact, however, because you have not observed enough children who stutter to know whether your general principle is correct.

In practice, deductive and inductive reasoning are inextricably related in a clinical interview. And, we hasten to point out, neither form of reasoning is superior to the other, nor should we avoid the use of such reasoning (we really couldn't, even if we wanted to, both are such engrained ways of thinking for most of us). Furthermore, in clinical and non-clinical settings, we move between these two forms of reasoning quickly and easily. And just as quickly and easily, we make mistakes in logic, mistakes that do not always help us help our clients. To deny, for even the most experienced clinician, the misuse of deductive and inductive reasoning is to join the flat earth society! Instead, all clinicians—both experienced and inexperienced—must carefully assess the role these forms of reasoning have on their clinical practice. In particular, clinicians need to make a conscious effort to minimize the misuse of either form of logical inference. In brief, the conclusions we draw from our basic assumptions or premises (deductive reasoning) and the generalizations we draw from facts (inductive reasoning) have as much if not more to do with the results of our evaluation than our particular style of questioning.

Assessing Communicative and Related Behaviors

With the intake form in hand and the results of the interview obtained, the speech-language pathologist may then turn to the third component of the evaluation: the actual assessment of communicative and related behavior. If the interview places a premium on appropriate questions and adequate followup, the actual assessment of communicative and related behavior places a premium on rapid but careful observations and clear, precise note taking. In the end, you will need and want to document all salient observations in written form (i.e., the diagnostic report), so when in doubt, write down your observations. After the client leaves, you will be glad you did.

Of particular importance to assessment and evaluation is the notion that behavior can be within normal limits but different from the mean. Again and again, the SLP will observe behavior that is different from the expected average or mean. The question, however, is whether this difference is appreciably or significantly different to warrant concern. Once again, I will call to the readers' attention that many of them will have an IQ that is different than 100, but is this cause for concern on their part? I think not. Most behavior seems to have a central tendency (mean, median, or mode) but "surrounding" that central tendency is a dispersion or spreading of values or scores (range, variance, standard deviation, etc.). Trying to understand and recognizing what would be a "normal" spread is a task that many clinicians will devote their lives to trying to understand, especially for behaviors that vary from one speaking situation to another, for example, stuttering.

Figure 2.1 shows a summary sheet listing results of all formal and informal tests that we routinely fill out during this portion of the diagnostic. Obviously, not every portion of this form will be filled out for every client, but we have found that having test results on *one* piece of paper makes the job of summarizing results much easier, quicker, and effective. Besides, when all information is gathered into one place, it significantly reduces the risk of losing information and better enables the clinician to relate findings from one area to those in another (for example, how does a child's expressive vocabulary relate to his or her expressive syntactic abilities?). Once again, the form presented in Figure 2.1 should in no way restrict or preclude the clinician from developing her own form; our form is presented as a guide rather than a prescription. However, whether clinicians use this or another form—we would encourage them to use such a form, it organizes, synthesizes, and rationalizes a lot of disparate, at times confusing, pieces of information.

Fluency

Assessing the fluency of speech requires that the clinician consider some or all of the following: (1) mean and range of frequency or number of *each* type of speech disfluency (for example, part-word repetition versus revisions) per 100 words or syllables spoken (more on the measurement of words versus syllables below); (2) mean and range of frequency of all or *total* speech disfluencies per 100 words or syllables spoken plus percentage of this total contributed by each disfluency type (for example, a client produces, on the average, a total of 10 disfluencies per 100 words and of these 10, on the average, 6 are sound prolongations, suggesting that 60% of all disfluencies are sound prolongations); (3) mean and range of *duration* of approximately 10 stuttered, stuttered-like within-word speech disfluencies (a digital stopwatch is most useful for recording this temporal measure), another related measure of duration is the average number of repetition per whole-word or sound/syllable repetition; (4) *consistency* of instances of stuttering (for example, on reading one the client stutters 10 times and on reading two, 6 times; how many stutterings on reading two were previously stuttered on reading one?); (5) average number and variety of *nonspeech* behaviors (for example, heading turning, eyeball turning, eyelid opening and closing, facial grimaces, and so forth) are associated with each stuttering; (6) results of such tests as the *Stocker Probe Technique* (Stocker, 1976), *Stuttering Severity Instrument-for Children and Adults–3* (SSI3) (Riley, 1994a), and *Stuttering Prediction Instrument* (Riley, 1981), as well as such severity rating procedures as *The Iowa Test for Stuttering Severity* (Johnson et al., 1963). While other behaviors such as attitudes of people who stutter (e.g., De Nil & Brutten, 1991), rates of utterance, turntaking skills, conversational overlaps between a person who stutters and listener (Kelly & Conture, 1992), differences in child–parent rates of utterance (e.g., Yaruss & Conture, 1995) are also important—and will subsequently be discussed—for now we will mainly concentrate on measuring speech fluency itself.

Frequency of Stuttering. While it is difficult to make hard and fast or absolute rules because we still lack adequate norms for speech fluency, our experience suggests that individuals who exhibit 3 or more stutterings or *within-word* disfluencies per 100 words spoken (averaged across various types and complexities of speaking situations) have some degree of fluency concern (however, this frequency of within-word disfluencies in and of itself does not mean that the person is an individual who stutters). The younger the client, of course, the less reliable any such absolute percentages become because of the still-developing nature of the young child's communicative skills. Readers should be aware that while other clinical guidelines exist with regard to frequency of stuttering, with one guideline suggesting 10 disfluencies (of all types) per 100 words (Adams, 1980), we are advocating the use of 3 *within-word disfluencies* per 100 words. These apparent differences are, we believe, fairly easily reconciled. In essence, individuals who produce 10 disfluencies, of all types, per 100 words of speech are more than likely producing 3 or more *within-word* disfluencies as part of that 10. We have chosen to mainly consider *within-word* disfluencies, since a great deal of research (e.g., Zebrowski & Conture, 1989) indicates that these are types of speech disfluencies that listeners are most apt to consider as stuttered and that people who stutter appear to produce much more often than normally fluent speakers (note exceptions mentioned on page 6). Therefore, we consider as stuttering any of the following behaviors: sound repetitions, syllable repetitions, whole-word repetitions (although not technically "within-word," research such as that of Yairi & Lewis, 1984, suggests that monosyllabic word repetitions are very much a part of childhood stuttering), audible and inaudible (so-called "blocks") sound prolongations (it is this writer's contention that what is being "prolonged" with a inaudible sound prolongation or block is the articulatory posture for the sound rather than the audible sound itself). A "count" rating sheet like that shown on Figure 2.2 is of value during on-line (while the client is speaking or reading) tabulation of number, type, and total of speech disfluency. Of course, the same rating sheet could be used with off-line or transcript-based measurement of speech disfluency (i.e., judging disfluencies from an audio or audio-videotape recording). A recent study (Yaruss,

Vanderbilt University -- Diagnostic Summary Sheet

Client's Name: _____

Client's Age: _____ DOB: _____

Clinician: _____ DOE: _____

Therapy: _____ Type: _____

Reevaluation Date: _____

STUTTERING:

Stuttering Frequency								
Judge	1	2	3	4	5	6	Mean	Range
Mean								
Range								

Rank order of Disfluency Types								
Type	1	2	3	4	5	6	Mean	Rank
SSR								
WWR								
A-SP								
I-SP								
PR								
INTJ								
REV								
Other								

Stuttering Duration								
Judge	1	2	3	4	5	6	Mean	Range
Mean								
Range								

Child's Articulatory Rate of Speech (without disfluencies, pauses, hesitations, etc.)								
Judge	1	2	3	4	5	6	Mean	Range
Mean								
Range								

Parents' Articulatory Rate of Speech (without disfluencies, pauses, hesitations, etc.)								
Judge	1	2	3	4	5	6	Mean	Range
Mother								
Father								

Stocker Probe
TOTAL Disfluencies:
Level   I   II   III   IV   V
#

Consistency/Adaptation
CI: Adapt:

Attitudes
Test: CAT-R
CAI
TCS
PPS
Score:

SSI
TOTAL:
Rating:
Frequency:
Duration:
Physical
Conc.:

SPI
TOTAL:
Rating:
Reactions:
Repetitions:
Prolongations:
Frequency:

SPEECH AND LANGUAGE:

Phonological Development
Word List: GFTA Weiss Hodson Other   Intell.: Excel. Good Fair Poor
Phonological Processes:
Percent of Consonants Correct (PCC):
1=typ; 2=del; 3=aty

DDK
Age Norms:

Grammatical Development
MLU/CU: TOLD:
Morphemes: TELD:
Syntax:

Receptive Vocabulary
Test: PPVT-III   Std. Score:
Age EQ: Percentile:
Notes:

Misc. Language

VOICE/ORAL PERIPHERAL/NEUROMOTOR:

Voice
Pitch:
Intensity:
Quality:

S/Z Ratio
Mean = 0.99; SD = 0.36

Oral Peripheral

SNTB

NOTES:

Max, Newman, & Campbell, 1998), assessing transcript-based versus real-time measurement of speech disfluency, showed that stuttering severity ratings were only substantially different (e.g., rated "mild" on basis of one measurement and "moderate" on basis of other) for 2 of 50 rated speech samples. Therefore, during-the-fact judgment of stuttering appears to be as reasonable a means for assessing stuttering as after-the-fact judgments, but there is no reason that both cannot be used, with the observer using either the average of the two forms of tabulating disfluencies, or assuming that after-the-fact judgments are the "gold standard," and filling in from during-the-fact judgments any speech disfluencies missed. To aid the observer in making on-line or during-the-fact judgments of stuttering, programs like Yaruss's (1999a) "counter" program may be of assistance. Freeing the observer from paper and pencil as well as tabulation of frequency, such programs will probably proliferate in the years to come. Figure 2.3 shows output of Yaruss's "counter" for two 4-year-old boys, one who does not stutter (CWNS) (see Bakker, 1999) and one who does stutter (CWS).

Recently, however, the usefulness of defining "stuttering" as *within-word* disfluencies has been questioned (e.g., Yairi, 1997a). Yairi points out that defining stutterings as within-word disfluencies excludes such between-word disfluency types as tense pause (i.e., barely audible manifestations of heavy breathing or muscular tightening between words, Williams, Silverman, & Kools, 1968), behaviors that, according to Yairi, are often produced by people who stutter. Yairi also believes that it is confusing if disfluency types considered as "stuttering" are also tabulated in the speech of people who do not stutter. In attempts to rectify this situation, Yairi and Ambrose (1992) introduced the *Stuttering-Like Disfluencies* (SLD) measure, which they believe has particular saliency for measuring childhood disfluency. The SLD measure includes sound/syllable repetitions, monosyllabic repetitions, tense pauses, and disrhythmic phonations (i.e., that kind of phonation that may or may not appear tense and disturbs or distorts the typical rhythm or flow of speech, Williams et al., 1968). Yairi's legitimate concerns aside, we still do not know whether the

FIGURE 2.1 Vanderbilt University Fluency Diagnostic Summary Sheet. This form is provided as an example or a model for clinicians interested in developing their own one-page diagnostic summary sheet. DOE=Date of Examination; DOB=Date of Birth; Re-eval=A re-evaluation assessment or diagnostic; SSR = Sound/syllable repetitions; Whole-Word Repetition = Whole-Word Repetitions; A-SP = Audible sound prolongations; I-SP = Inaudible sound prolongations (many times judged as "blocks"); PR = Phrase repetitions; INTJ = Interjections; REV = Revisions; and OTHER = "tense pauses," that is, audible instances of apparently physically tense articulatory contact, associated with a pause between words; Judges=Clinicians who are observing or assessing behavior; SSI=*Stuttering Severity Instrument*; SPI=*Stuttering Prediction Instrument*; CI = *Consistency Index*; CAT-R = *Communication Attitude Test—Revised* (for children; after DeNil & Brutten, 1991); CAI=*Communication Attitude Inventory* (for adults; after Andrews & Cutler, 1974); TCS = *Temperament Characteristics Scale* (for children; after Oyler, 1996); PPS = *Parents Perceptual Scale* (for children; after Oyler, 1996); MLU=Mean Length of Utterance; CU = Communication Units; TELD=*Test of Early Language Development*; TOLD=*Test of Language Development*; GFTA = *Goldman-Fristoe Test of Articulation*; PPVT=*Peabody Picture Vocabulary Test*; S/Z ratio=Length of sustained /s/ divided by length of sustained Z (after Eckel & Boone, 1981); DDK=Diadochokinetic or alternating motion rate assessment; SNTB = *Screening Neurological Test Battery* (after Wolk, 1990). Not listed in the QNST=*Quick Neurological Screening Test* (after Mutti, Sterling, & Spaulding, 1978), which is a reasonable means for screening the overall neuromotor development of children.

Vanderbilt University -- Disfluency Count Sheet

Client's Name: _____

Client's Age: _____   DOB: _____

Clinician: _____   DOE: _____

Overall	Mean	Range
Frequency		
Duration		
Client's Rate		

Sample #1 (100 words):

% of Total Disfluencies (%TD)		
Type	Freq	% TD
SSR		
WWR		
A-SP		
I-SP		
PR		
INTJ		
REV		
Other		
Total		

Sample #2 (100 words):

% of Total Disfluencies (%TD)		
Type	Freq	% TD
SSR		
WWR		
A-SP		
I-SP		
PR		
INTJ		
REV		
Other		
Total		

Sample #3 (100 words):

% of Total Disfluencies (%TD)		
Type	Freq	% TD
SSR		
WWR		
A-SP		
I-SP		
PR		
INTJ		
REV		
Other		
Total		

Speech Rat	Child	Mother	Father	Duration
Mean				
Range				

(do not count disfluencies, pauses, hesitations, etc.)

Notes:

Rank order of Disfluency Types						
Type	1	2	3	Mean	Range	Rank
SSR						
WWR						
A-SP						
I-SP						
PR						
INTJ						
REV						
Other						
Total						

SLD index is a (1) more reliable and/or (2) more valid means of documenting stuttering than within-word disfluencies. Likewise, we still do not know if using SLD rather than within-word disfluencies allows us to more accurately categorize someone as a person who stutters as well as document the severity and predict the chronicity of stuttering. Furthermore, and most important, we do not know whether the use of SLD versus within-word disfluencies would result in different clinical decisions—for example, SLD measurement suggesting treatment versus within-word disfluencies suggesting no treatment.

We do know, however, based on Yairi's (1997a) Table 3.3 comparison across eight different studies of childhood speech disfluencies, that the percent of total disfluencies that are SLD (%SLD) are considerably lower for children who do not stutter (Mean = 34%) than for children who do stutter (Mean = 72%). Thus, for the group, %SLD does seem to clearly discriminate between children who do versus do not stutter; however, the present author would caution that people who stutter do not come to the clinic in groups, they arrive individually. In fact, just a few days ago, this author evaluated a 4-year-6-month-old boy (who has been stuttering, according to his mother, for 17 months) that the author considered to be a severe person who stutters (e.g., scored a 31 on the Stuttering Prediction Instrument) whose %SLD = 34. This %SLD rating would put the child right on the mean for children who do not stutter and well out of the range for children who do stutter, according to Yairi's calculations! Thus, while such indexes as %SLD appear to offer promise for group assessment of stuttering, there will always be individual exceptions to the rule and clinicians must understand that and adjust their appraisal accordingly.

Sample Size. As Yairi (1997a) correctly pointed out, ". . . the size of a speech sample influences the representativeness of data describing subjects' disfluency" (p. 52). Unfortunately, clinicians, unlike researchers, do not always have adequate control over sample size. Be that as it may, the first issue that clinicians must consider with regard to the tabulation of stuttering frequency is *sample size* (i.e., number of spoken or read words). It is safe to say that the greater the size of the sample, the greater our confidence that we have adequately sampled the central tendency and variations in the person's behavior.

Practically, the sample size should be sufficient to permit averaging across several 100-word samples. We have found that a 300-word sample is sufficient for this purpose, but some might feel more comfortable obtaining 500 words. Indeed, in some clinical situations, for example, when assessing small groups of preschool children, getting 100 intelligible words per each child per session may be all that a clinician can legitimately hope to obtain in the usual 45–50-minute therapy session. Likewise, with a person who stutters very severely, the length of time he or she would take to produce 300 words is counterproductive to achieving the end-goals of the diagnostic ("Is there a problem or is there not a problem?") and a sample of 100 words might suffice (being supplemented, as soon as possible

FIGURE 2.2 Vanderbilt University Disfluency Frequency Count Sheet. This form is provided as an example or a model for clinicians interested in developing their own diagnostic disfluency frequency count sheet. SSR = Sound/syllable repetition; WWR = Whole-word repetition; PR=Phrase repetition; A-SP = Audible sound prolongation; I-SP = Inaudible prolongation; INTJ = Interjection; REV = Revision; and OTHER, for example, "tense pause"; Speech Rate = Syllables or words per minute, based on at least 10, preferably 30 utterances per speaker (mother, father, or person who stutters).

Disfluency Counter

(a)

Subject: CWNS - Age 4 - M   Situation: Clinic

WITHIN WORD		BETWEEN WORD		TOTALS	
SSR : 0	0%	PR : 1	50%	Words : 100	
WWR : 0	0%	INTJ : 1	50%	WW % :	0
A-SP : 0	0%	REV : 0	0%	BW % :	2
I-SP : 0	0%	Other : 0	0%	Total :	2

WITHIN WORD		BETWEEN WORD		TOTALS	
SSR : 0	0%	PR : 1	33%	Words : 100	
WWR : 1	33%	INTJ : 1	33%	WW % :	1
A-SP : 0	0%	REV : 0	0%	BW % :	2
I-SP : 0	0%	Other : 0	0%	Total :	3

WITHIN WORD		BETWEEN WORD		TOTALS	
SSR : 0	0%	PR : 1	50%	Words : 99	
WWR : 1	50%	INTJ : 0	0%	WW % :	1
A-SP : 0	0%	REV : 0	0%	BW % :	1
I-SP : 0	0%	Other : 0	0%	Total :	2

Disfluency Counter

(b)

Subject: CWS - Age 4 - M   Situation: Clinic

WITHIN WORD		BETWEEN WORD		TOTALS	
SSR : 3	38%	PR : 0	0%	Words : 100	
WWR : 1	13%	INTJ : 0	0%	WW % :	8
A-SP : 4	50%	REV : 0	0%	BW % :	0
I-SP : 0	0%	Other : 0	0%	Total :	8

WITHIN WORD		BETWEEN WORD		TOTALS	
SSR : 3	38%	PR : 2	25%	Words : 100	
WWR : 2	25%	INTJ : 0	0%	WW % :	6
A-SP : 1	13%	REV : 0	0%	BW % :	2
I-SP : 0	0%	Other : 0	0%	Total :	8

WITHIN WORD		BETWEEN WORD		TOTALS	
SSR : 1	10%	PR : 2	20%	Words : 100	
WWR : 4	40%	INTJ : 0	0%	WW % :	8
A-SP : 3	30%	REV : 0	0%	BW % :	2
I-SP : 0	0%	Other : 0	0%	Total :	10

FIGURE 2.3   Example of output of computer-assisted tabulation of speech disfluency (after Yaruss, 1999a, with permission) for (a) a child who does not stutter (CWNS) and (b) a child who does stutter (CWS) during 300 words of conversational speech in which the child is talking with his or her mother. R = Phrase repetition; W = Whole-word repetition; J = Interjection; A = Audible sound prolongations; I = Inaudible sound prolongations; S = Sound/syllable repetition.

after the beginning of therapy, with a sample based on a larger corpus of words). Once again, stuttering is a behavior, a behavior that varies. Indeed, the nature and extent of such variation can only be understood by the clinician if he or she collects a large enough sample to adequately assess variation. Granted, such a clinical sample is imperfect, but given the fact we live in an imperfect world, all we can do is strive to do our best within the confines of what we have and what we can possibly do.

Frequency Not the Only Measure.   The good news about stuttering frequency is that with a modicum of training, a clinician can learn to reliably count the number of times per conversation or reading passage a person will stutter. (It is, however, another matter how much agreement two different listeners will have on the *exact* sound, syllable, or word that was stuttered rather than the mere number of stutterings per conversation or reading [cf. Young, 1984 for review of this topic].) The bad news is that stuttering frequency, while certainly one of several factors used in judging stuttering severity, is less than perfectly correlated with other measures of speech fluency, for example, duration. Thus, to "capture" the totality of the speech disfluency problem of the person who stutters, several measures of disfluency, besides its mere frequency, must and should be simultaneously considered.

Stuttered Words Versus Syllables.   One other issue pertaining to the measurement of stuttering frequency is whether it should be computed in terms of percentage of stuttered *words* or *syllables*. At present, as far as we know, there is no conclusive evidence published in refereed journals that indicates that one procedure—words or syllables—surpasses the other in terms of accuracy or precision in estimating stuttering frequency. Yairi (1997a) suggests that ". . . a syllable-based metric more accurately reflects the amount of speech affected by disfluency" (p. 52), particularly when comparing the % of disfluencies per 100 words between, for example, 2- and 5-year-olds. As Yairi suggests, length of words most likely increases with age, as the child develops, and hence so do the number of syllables. Thus, basing our index of stuttering on words might be relatively reasonable in the 2- to 3-year-olds, where only 15 percent or so of their words are polysyllabic, it becomes somewhat problematic if basing our index of stuttering on words for 5- and 6-year-olds where 25 to 40 percent of their words are polysyllabic!

However, as the lady in the old hamburger commercial said, "Where's the beef?" It is incumbent on those who recommend the exclusive use of syllables and eschew the use of words, when counting stuttering, to demonstrate that theirs is the best or even a better system for distinguishing between those who do and do not stutter. At present, those who argue for a syllable metric have made reasoned appeals to our intuition—for example, there are more syllables than words, words get longer with age, and so on. But is there any proof that the decisions we make clinically (e.g., this child does and that child does not stutter) are significantly influenced by the use of syllables versus words? If there is, this writer has yet to hear about or see it. Indeed, Yaruss (in press), based on fifty 3- to 6-year-old children, found a ratio of 1.15 syllables per word for children between ages of 3 and 6; furthermore, this ratio wasn't significantly correlated with age, in other words, the 1.15 syllable per word ratio stayed relatively constant across age. Thus, while there is intuitive appeal to base fluency counts on a syllable versus word metric, available data do not suggest that there would be an appreciable difference in resulting classification and/or clinical decision. Furthermore, differences between stuttered syllables and words can be mathematically adjusted (e.g., if one counted the number of stutterings per word and wanted to know about stutterings per syllable, merely multiplying by 1.15 would produce a reasonable approximation). Likewise, Johnson and colleagues (1963) had suggested a 1.5 conversion ratio (words to syllables), but this appears to be based on adult speakers as does the 1.4 conversion ratio reported by Andrews and Ingham (1971). Clearly, there is a need for normative data here for children, in terms of the relationship of syllable per words across the life span. While the aforementioned conversion would only provide a rough approximation of stuttered syllables, given our current state of understanding in this area, it is probably sufficient for most clinical diagnostic assessment purposes. Ham (1986) provides an excellent discussion of this issue.

Disfluency Types.   Once the clinician knows something about the client's stuttering frequency, he or she should attempt to compute the relative proportion of total disfluencies contributed by each disfluency type. This, in our opinion, is a most important measure. For example, we have shown elsewhere (Schwartz & Conture, 1988) that the percentage of sound prolongations in a sample of stutterings is one important feature in distinguishing among youngsters who stutter. It will also be noted that the *Stuttering Prediction Instrument for Young Children-3* (Riley, 1994a) measures the presence of "blocks" (which are essentially audible or inaudible sound prolongations produced by stationary or fixed articulatory postures) to predict chronicity.

It is our belief that some stutterings, to paraphrase George Orwell, are more equal than others in terms of implications for severity and chronicity of stuttering. As more and more empirical investigations of the association between other behaviors and type of disfluency of people who stutter are undertaken, we expect to see *type* rather than *frequency* of disfluency become a very meaningful measure for both experimental and clinical purposes.

Typically, the client's disfluencies will consists of four to seven different types of disfluencies, with one or two of them accounting for most observed disfluencies. Computing and reporting the rank order, from most to least frequently occurring, of each observed disfluency type as well as its proportion (0 to 100%) of the total disfluencies is, we have found, quite an important measure. As we have shown (Yaruss, LaSalle, & Conture, 1998), based on a sample of 100 2- to 6-year-old children, the most frequently occurring type of speech disfluency is apt to be (a) sound syllable (47%) repetition, followed by (b) sound prolongation (26%), with (c) whole-word repetition (20%) coming in a close third. About 7 percent of children exhibited between-word disfluencies as their most common type of disfluency. As mentioned in Chapter 1, we believe that these differences in the type of speech disfluency that people who stutter most likely produce have implications for etiology and at the least for stages in development of the problem. We would really like to see basic and applied research address such possibilities.

In Chapter 3, which covers the remediation of stuttering in children, we will discuss how the most frequently occurring disfluency type is used as an index of where the child is in the development of the problem as well as what this means in terms of therapeutic approach. We typically consider a client who predominantly produces sound/syllable repetitions (i.e., the *Beta* phase of development, Conture, 1990b) to exhibit a less developed and established problem than a child who predominantly produces cessation or fixed articulatory type of disfluencies, for example, sound prolongations (i.e., the *Gamma* phase, Conture, 1990b). As our data shows (Yaruss, LaSalle, & Conture, 1998), there is yet another group of children who predominantly produce monosyllabic whole-word repetitions (we are uncertain, at this point, whether this finding can be extrapolated to teenagers and adults who stutter). Whether these differences in most commonly exhibited disfluency types suggest differences in the origin and course of development is an empirical question.

Our informal observations, at this point, after clinically evaluating and treating (as well descriptively and experimentally testing) hundreds of children, suggest the following:

1. If *all* we know about a child is that his or her most common disfluency is *sound-syllable repetition* and little or no sound prolongations, it is difficult to predict outcome. That is, seemingly equal percentages of these children recover with minimal therapeutic intervention while others require some period of indirect, direct, or combined treatment.

2. If *all* we know about a child is that his or her most common disfluency is *sound prolongations* and/or "*blocks*," such children generally require some period of therapy. Such children, in this author's experience, are generally more advanced in the problem of stuttering, regardless of their chronological age, and warrant, at the least, monitoring and reevaluation.

3. If *all* we know about a child is that his or her most common disfluency is monosyllabic *whole-word repetition*, we may observe that such children frequently also exhibit concerns with semantic or syntactic encoding or their interface. These children may require treatment, particularly if the child or child's family is strongly reacting to the disfluencies; however, as a general rule, treatment is successful with these children.

We hasten to add, however, that each additional piece of information we have about each of the three preceding groupings will influence our ability to predict as well as the client's prognosis. And more information does not necessarily mean that the resulting decision may be more favorable for the client; for example, a child with frequent monosyllabic whole-word repetitions and semantic abilities depressed relative to syntactic abilities may be extremely behaviorally inhibited, reacting to each mistake, error, or disfluency with tremendous anxiety, fear, and physical reactions that significantly exacerbate an underlying problem that is essentially benign.

Duration of Disfluency.   The "characteristics" of speech disfluencies of people who stutter have received considerable attention. One such characteristic, the extent—*duration* or length of stuttering—is often measured and thought to be one of several variables that contribute to perceived severity of stuttering (e.g., Ambrose & Yairi, 1999; Throneburg et al., 1994; Zebrowski, 1991). (For recent review of such literature, see Yairi, 1997a, pp. 66–68.) A related characteristic, the *number of units of repetition per sound/syllable repetition*, has also been studied (e.g., Ambrose & Yairi, 1995; Yairi & Lewis, 1985; Zebrowski, 1991). As Yairi (1997a) aptly points out, there is undoubtedly an interaction, or as he calls it "co-effect," between both of these measures and frequency of disfluency. For example, one child may typically repeat word-initial stops twice (e.g., "b-b-but") and do so 15 times per 100 words, whereas another child might repeat the same sounds once (e.g., "b-but") and do so 5 times per 100 words. Whereas the first child would exhibit 30 "extra" word-initial stops, the second child would only exhibit 5 "extra" word-initial stops, a difference that may, as Yairi suggests, significantly contribute to listeners' perceptions and judgment of normalcy for each of the two children.

It makes intuitive sense that the more units of repetition per sound/syllable repetition the longer the repetition, and Throneburg and colleagues (1994) provide data to support this intuitive notion. Throneburg and colleagues also provide some intriguing data to suggest that the duration of each element within the repetition may be diagnostic, a finding in need of replication by independent researchers (compare to findings of Yaruss & Conture, 1993 regarding Formant 2 (F2) transitions during sound/syllable repetitions).

Related to duration and number of iterations per repetition are the *rate* and *rhythmicity* of repetition. In theory, the *rate* of repetition could conceivable differ to the point where a three-unit repetition could take 1200 ms (400 ms per repetition) whereas another three-unit repetition could take only 600 ms (200 ms per repetition). Indeed, Yairi and Hall (1993) found that the silent interval between units of repetition was shorter in children who do than who don't stutter, suggesting that the rate of repetition for children who stutter is *faster* than for that of children who do not stutter. The *rhythmicity* (i.e., temporal regularity) of the units of repetition would seem to be a characteristic that listeners might react to, but to this author's knowledge, this variable has not been assessed. It is my conjecture that there would be greater variability in repetition (i.e., less rhythmicity) for children who are more severe and/or more likely to continue stuttering. Why? Because I assume that the more involved, severe, or persistent the stuttering, the more physical tension, physical reaction, and the like—behaviors that should make the person's speech all the less smooth, even-flowing, and rhythmic.

In terms of measuring duration, this author has typically measured the average (and range) of the child's stuttering duration across a randomly selected sample of 10 stutterings. The best way, in our experience, to become sensitive to differences in durations of various disfluency types is to measure them. This is best done using a digital stopwatch—they are a bit quieter (particularly those without an audible beep when the start/stop button is depressed) and easier to read than the "old-fashioned" analog stopwatch with its audible clicking and sweep second hand. If the clinician practices tabulating the duration of each client's stuttering (or at least a sub-sample of each), he or she will, after a while, be able to much better approximate, without the use of a stopwatch, the difference between a 250 and 750 ms instance of stuttering. Understanding such differences not only makes the clinician a better diagnostician, but also helps him or her assess behavioral changes in therapy because, in our experience, duration of stuttering is often one of the very first things to improve in therapy, even before frequency of stuttering and other such behavior. Becoming more sensitive to the temporal domain of each instance of stuttering also improves the clinician's ability to judge other aspects of timing relative to speech production—for example, number of syllables or words per minute and measures of alternating motion rate (diadochokinesis). As the clinician learns to appreciate the wide variety and number of fluent and disfluent events that occur under 1000 ms (1 second), he or she will be better able to quickly and precisely identify those behaviors of clients that need change in therapy. Assessment of stuttering requires more than merely counting instances of its occurrence—it also requires some ability to judge its type and duration as well.

Consistency of Disfluency.   Consistency of disfluency—the tendency for the loci of stuttering to be constant from reading to reading of the same material—can be judged on an informal as well as more formal basis described by Johnson and associates (1963, pp. 272–276, p. 292). Although we are still less than clear regarding the exact clinical significance of consistency of disfluency, we use this information as one more piece of data regarding the relative habituation and association of instances of stuttering with particular stimuli. Knowing something about the nature of the various types of stimuli that influence the consistency of stuttering, which has been thoroughly discussed elsewhere (Bloodstein, 1995, pp. 277–295), allows the clinician to show the client that stuttering has some degree of lawfulness—that it is not a random event behaving helter-skelter like so many kernels of corn popping in a popcorn popper (cf. Tate & Cullinan, 1962; Cullinan, 1988, for an excellent presentation of issues relating to the measurement of consistency).

Once again, however, we must caution: Be prepared for individual differences (Bloodstein, 1995, pp. 294–295 offered similar suggestions regarding individual differences in consistency). While this or that study may indicate that people who stutter, as a GROUP, are consistent in their stuttering, as we mentioned in Chapter 1, people who stutter don't enter your clinical doors in a group, they walk in as individuals. Individual behavior varies around the group's central tendency (e.g., mean), and it is not at all unlikely that one particular individual who stutters may show very little consistency (or minimal adaptation), but still be a person who stutters and needs your services. Another thing to consider is how to measure consistency in a nonreader, for example, a 4-year-old preschooler. Neelley and Timmons (1967) and Williams and colleagues (1969) utilized a procedure for collecting and measuring data on stuttering constancy in young children that we have used for years in our clinic. In essence, seven or so age-appropriate sentences (5 years and under = three- to five-word sentences; 5 years old and older = six- to eight-word sentences) containing age-appropriate vocabulary are read to the child, one at a time, and the child is instructed to immediately repeat back the sentence to the examining SLP. Most children can and will tolerate three readings/repetitions of these seven sentences; but, once again, individual differences in attention span, tendency to fatigue, memory for words, and the like may inhibit a child's ability to perform this task. Whatever the case, this procedure is easy to implement, takes very little time to complete, and may, for some younger clients, be the only time you get a reasonably adequate index of their fluency.

Number and Variety of Associated Nonspeech Behaviors.   Sometimes what is most apparent is what we know the least about. Although there is hardly a textbook on stuttering that doesn't mention *physical concomitants, secondary* or *associated* behaviors, there is actually very little objective information regarding these behaviors. While one can find no end to the number of clinical observations and anecdotes regarding these nonspeech, nonverbal behaviors, there are, to the best of our knowledge, only seven published, empirical studies of these behaviors (Conture & Kelly, 1991a; Krause, 1982; LaSalle & Conture, 1991; Prins & Lohr, 1972; Schwartz & Conture, 1988; Schwartz et al., 1990; Yairi et al.,

1993), with four of them being published in the last ten years. We suspect that the paucity of objective information regarding behavior associated with instances of stuttering relates to at least two factors: (1) Most such associated behavior is nonverbal, and it is far less than clear how such behavior can be systematically and objectively analyzed, particularly by speech-language clinicians whose interests and training lie in the realm of oral communication (see Ekman, 1982, for a discussion of such methodology); and (2) these associated behaviors are generally considered so idiosyncratic that little or no central tendency is assumed to exist.

While tests like the *Stuttering Severity Instrument* request, and rightfully so, the clinician to measure "physical concomitants," of each client's stuttering, it is far less than clear what numbers and varieties of these behaviors a clinician could expect to see across a number of people who stutter. It is entirely possible, as Schwartz and Conture's (1988) study of the associated behaviors of 43 young people who stutter indicate that there are commonalties in terms of the number and nature of these behaviors but only for "subtypes" or "subgroups" of people who stutter. That is, some people who stutter are very similar to one another but very different from all other people who stutter in terms of their associated behaviors. Thus, it is entirely possible that these similarities within a group and differences between groups, in terms of associated nonspeech behavior, have implications for (1) etiology of the problem and (2) remediation of the problem. It is also entirely possible that it is the number rather than the nature of associated behaviors of people who stutter that represents the main difference between them and the nonspeech behavior produced by their normally fluent peers during comparable fluent utterances. For example, a person who stutters may produce three nonspeech behaviors during a stuttering: a head turn, an eye blink, and raising of the upper lip, whereas a normally fluent speaker may only produce a head turn and an eye blink. Thus, much of what clinicians call "secondaries" may be nothing more frequent, exaggerated, or longer duration typical nonspeech behaviors rather than behaviors that are categorically different from typical nonspeech behaviors exhibited by people who do not stutter. Indeed, as the findings of Conture and Kelly (1991a) suggest, this seems to the case. That is, all but a handful of behaviors (i.e., eyeball movement to the side and eyelid blinking) significantly differentiate the stuttered speech of preschool children who stutter from fluent speech of their peers who do not stutter. In fact, in recent years, we and others (Conture & Kelly, 1991a; LaSalle & Conture, 1991; Schwartz et al., 1990; Yairi et al., 1993) have provided more documentation of these behaviors in young children than heretofore existed. However, at this point what is needed, in this author's opinion, is not more description of these behaviors. The number and nature, at least in preschool/early school-age children speech behavior, seems fairly apparent. Instead, we need more explanations for these behaviors that go beyond the mere anecdotal, emotional, psychological, and/or social without taking into consideration that the child is concomitantly thinking as well as receptively and expressively processing language. For example, it is quite possible that a child may look to the side during an instance of stuttering, not because he or she is avoiding eye contact or fearful, but because the child is thinking about what word to say or how to say it.

In essence, what makes these associated nonspeech behaviors all the more difficult to objectively assess is their interdependence with speech or verbal behavior (Beattie, 1983). While we might like to separate out, say, a speaker breaking eye contact with his or her listener from the speaker's words produced slightly before and during the break in eye contact, in reality these two events—verbal and nonverbal—are closely connected. Even if we greatly simplify the situation and assume that verbal behavior mainly conveys content while nonverbal behavior mainly conveys social/emotional message, we realize that the two messages—content and emotional—are inextricably related during most of our communications. For example, a father, with a steady gaze and lowered eyebrows, states "Helena, come in here, I want to talk to you about this stain on the coffee table." While the verbal message is relatively neutral, the speaker's associated nonverbal behavior gives Helena more than an adequate idea of how the father feels and what he might say. All of which leads me to my point: We are just beginning to understand the number and nature of nonverbal behavior associated with stuttering. What we are less certain about is the *reasons* for these behaviors, their significance for etiology and treatment and their relation to that produced during normally fluent speech. Further, we have very limited understanding of the role of a listener's nonverbal behavior in the problem of stuttering, particularly those of parents during the stutterings of their children. We don't know whether such behavior differs from that observed when listeners listen to fluent utterances and whether such behavior has potential for exacerbating or worsening the stuttering of the person who stutters. As I said at the beginning of this section, sometimes what is the most apparent is what is easiest to overlook.

Noticeable Nonspeech Behavior: The Straw That Breaks the Camel's Back. One of the more interesting phenomena with stuttering, in our experience, is parental reactions to their children's nonverbal behavior associated with stuttering. It is not unusual for parents to wait and only have their child evaluated *after* they notice that the child begins to produce nonspeech behavior during instances of stuttering. The child may have been "stuttering" for three to twelve months *before* the parent started to notice these associated nonspeech behaviors. It is our experience that parents react to these nonverbal behaviors for one or both of the following reasons: (1) The number and nature of the associated nonverbal behaviors appear, to the parent, to be different than that seen during fluency and thus "abnormal," unusual, and undesirable, something to be stopped, minimized, or eradicated; and (2) these associated nonverbal behaviors suggest to the parent that the child is "aware," "concerned," "bothered," or "frightened" by this problem and such a reaction on the part of the child concerns the parent. In the next section we will discuss how to deal (or should we say not to deal) with associated nonverbal behavior, but suffice it to say that it is a part of stuttering, a part that may provide us with a number of clues as to the severity, chronicity, and possible etiology of the problem.

(In)formal Tests of Stuttering

We have discussed elsewhere (e.g., Conture, 1997; Conture & Caruso, 1987) our diagnostic use of such tests as the *Iowa Scale for Rating the Severity of Stuttering* (Johnson et al., 1963), the *Stuttering Severity Instrument for Young Children-3* (Riley, 1994a), the *Stuttering Prediction Instrument* (Riley, 1981), the *Stocker Probe Instrument* (Stocker, 1976), and the *Children's Attitudes Towards Talking—Revised* (DeNil & Brutten, 1991). We typically use each of these instruments in our assessment of fluency but for very different purposes. For example, we (Conture & Caruso, 1987, p. 98 and Figure 1) showed how we use the *Iowa Scale* to provide loosely objective support for our "Tentative Diagnosis." In this case an individual described as a "moderate stutterer" would have an asterisk (*) after the word "stutterer" and at the bottom of the first page of the diagnostic report a footnote would say *Rating = 4 on the 0 (no stuttering) to 7 (very severe stuttering) *Iowa Scale for Rating the Severity of Stuttering* (Johnson et al., 1963). More recently (Yaruss, LaSalle, & Conture, 1998), we show how simultaneous consideration of the results of several of these tests are useful for differentiating among preschool children (1) who are most likely to require treatment, (2) who may require reevaluation, and (3) who are least likely to require treatment.

We are still a bit uncertain whether the aforementioned tests of stuttering severity are any more accurate than merely quantitatively as well as qualitatively assessing the client's frequency, duration, and type of disfluency. However, these tests are based on fairly representative samples of children known or suspected to be stuttering and thus provide the clinician with some sort of "norms" or values to which the clinician can compare the client under evaluation. Furthermore, the aforementioned tests are relatively easy and quick to use and appreciably help the clinician organize the salient measures of stuttering and related behaviors. One of these tests—the *Stuttering Prediction Instrument* (SPI)—is, in theory, an even more important test since it tries to predict the chronicity of the child's problem. That is, while a test of severity may tell us *today* about the severity of the client's stuttering problem, it really tells us very little with regard to *tomorrow*—that is, whether the client will continue to stutter into the future. For example, Yaruss and Conture (1993) used the SPI to help them determine whether children whose stuttering is more versus less chronic (i.e., high versus low SPI scores) differ in terms of speech production; however, without longitudinal data, it is really difficult to predict which children will become people who stutter chronically. For the present, however, the SPI and the other tests of stuttering severity provide us with the beginnings of an objective means for assessing the severity and chronicity of stuttering. All clinicians who manage people of any age who stutter should be familiar with the rationale behind administration, scoring, and interpretation of these tests. They are important adjuncts to the evaluation of stuttering in children, teenagers, and adults.

During the 1990s, the computer began to be employed to assist clinicians in the assessment and evaluation of childhood stuttering (Bahill & Curlee, 1993). This procedure—"a computer-based decision support system"—is based on the consensus assessment and evaluation judgments of five experienced clinicians and helps the clinician assess the probability the child needs treatment. These so-called "expert systems" are common in the field of medicine and, we believe, may become common in the field of audiology and speech-language pathology in the future. In essence, after (in)formal assessment of the child and the child's parents, the clinician answers a series of questions regarding parents' concerns and the child's behavior. The computer, by taking the answers to these questions and comparing them to criteria established by the five experienced clinicians, arrives at five different judgments from "no need for treatment" to "immediate need for treatment." Such computer-based testing systems will *augment*, not *replace* the judgment and decisions of the clinician.

Articulation / Phonological Behavior of Children Who Stutter

Thirteen studies that directly examined the articulation/phonologic disorders in children who do and do not stutter (see Table 7.1, Louko et al., 1999) strongly suggest that people who stutter exhibit more concerns with speech sound articulation or phonology than their peers who do not stutter. Examination of results from studies in this area (provided in both Louko et al. [1999], Table 1, and Bloodstein [1995], Table 18) show considerable range in the reported percentage of children who stutter and exhibit speech sound difficulties. (Conversely, but in a similar vein, Ragsdale & Sisterhen [1984] noted significantly more speech disfluencies in 20 children with mild to moderate articulation difficulties when compared to 20 age- and sex-matched children without articulation difficulties.) Indeed, Nippold (1990) has highlighted several methodological problems that undoubtedly contribute to this range in prevalence data; however, the overall tendency of evidence strongly supports Bloodstein's (1995) suggestion that, "There is hardly a finding more thoroughly confirmed in the whole range of comparative studies of people who stutter and people who do not stutter than the tendency of stutterers to have functional difficulties of articulation, 'immature' speech and the like" (p. 250). In fact, Paden and Yairi (1996) report significant differences on formal tests of phonology between children for whom stuttering is persistent and their peers who do not stutter, a finding confirming this author's observation that children who stutter and exhibit disordered phonology generally seem to take longer to recover from stuttering. Thus, phonological issues, both on theoretical as well as therapeutic grounds, need to be given more than a cursory consideration when assessing and evaluating stuttering in children. Again, we need to remind ourselves that children enter our clinic as individuals, not in groups. Our need to assess, evaluate, and treat their stuttering should not blur the clinician's view of the realities of the fact that children who stutter may have other speech and language problems, problems that may require treatment and/or influence our treatment of their stuttering. Suffice it to say that children who stutter have just as much right as children who do not stutter to have disordered phonology, disordered language, and the like!

While distinctions between *articulation disordered* and *phonologically disordered* are still less than clear, findings of the studies reviewed by Louko and colleagues (1999) indicate that between 7 percent to 45 percent of people who stutter also exhibit articulation difficulties. (We have removed from consideration two "outlier" studies that seem to appreciably under- as well as overestimate the prevalence of disordered phonology in children who stutter: Ryan [1992] reporting 0% at the time of testing but eventually 25% requiring "articulation therapy" and St. Louis & Hinzman [1988] reporting 67 to 96% of 48 children who stuttered also exhibited disordered phonology.) On average, therefore, approximately one-third of all people who stutter have some sort of difficulty—mild, moderate, or severe—with speech articulation. (While some of these people who stutter with articulation concerns certainly also exhibit difficulties with expressive/receptive language, we are unaware of any empirical findings that would suggest 24 to 45 percent of people who stutter also exhibit language problems.) Obviously, the nature and severity of these articulation concerns undoubtedly varies among people who stutter, just like it does in the normally fluent population. However, if we make the reasonable assumption that between 2 to 6 percent of the school-age population has some degree of a problem with speech articulation (Beitchman et al., 1986; Hull et al., 1971), then having approximately one-third of people who stutter also exhibiting articulation problems is several times higher than would be expected.

To provide the reader with some notion of what we are talking about, we present Table 2.1 (after Conture, Louko, & Edwards, 1993). Table 2.1 shows eight children who stutter, four with phonology within normal limits and four with clear phonological concerns. Study of the eight children depicted in this table points out the heterogeneity among children who stutter as well as the need to consider stuttering within the context of the entirety of the child's speech and language development. While it is clearly not necessary to exhibit a phonological disorder to stutter, neither does stuttering preclude an individual from also exhibiting a phonological disorder!

In essence, we would suggest to the clinician, particularly in the diagnosis of the school-age child suspected or known to be a person who stutters, to informally (or better yet formally) assess the child's speech sound productions. Typically, we use the "Sounds in Words" subtest of the *Goldman-Fristoe Test of Articulation* (Goldman & Fristoe, 1986) or the *Arizona Articulation Proficiency Scale* (Fudala, 1970) to assess the entirety of the child's phonology, not just the sounds we suspect are problematic. Besides noting the number and type of speech sounds in error, the clinician should also note the presence of any "unusual" phonological process, for example, glottal replacement (e.g., /bɛʔ/ for "bed"). Edwards and Shriberg (1983) have extensively discussed these and other phonological processes, and the clinician unfamiliar with phonological process analysis is well advised to read their discussion. In our experience, most (two out of three) school-age children who stutter will exhibit speech sound articulation and phonological processes *well within normal limits*. The remaining one child out of three will, however, exhibit *mild, moderate, or severe delays and/or deviancies in speech sound productions* that warrant further testing and documentation of the child's possible articulation or phonological difficulties.

As we will mention below with regard to expressive/receptive language concerns, it is not all unlikely to observe, as a young child who stutters becomes more fluent, for the child to exhibit concerns with articulation/phonology and vice versa. It is as if the child's previous stuttering problem obscured or made relatively unimportant the articulation concerns. A most important concern, in our opinion, is a child who begins to stutter after a period of time during which he or she exhibited articulation/phonological difficulties. In some cases, where the child was receiving treatment for the articulation problem, we have the growing suspicion that the therapy for correction or modification of the child's speech sound difficulties may have, in some as yet unknown way, contributed to the child's emerging speech disfluency problem. Given the possibility that some children seem to begin stuttering *after* therapeutic attention to their speech sound difficulties, we urge clinicians to use relatively low-key approaches to changing articulation (e.g., Conture, Louko, & Edwards, 1993; Louko et al., 1999). We also urge these clinicians to avoid employing therapies that emphasize a physically tense, posturally correct, and relatively rapid production of sounds in error. Indeed, at this point we are just beginning to understand the complex relation between speech sound articulation and speech fluency, and the clinician is best advised to proceed carefully, gently, and unhurriedly when correcting a child's speech sound problem, particularly when there are co-occurring speech disfluencies or the likelihood for such co-occurrence.

As mentioned above, we reported preliminary findings (Conture, Louko, & Edwards, 1993) from an experimental therapy program whereby we attempted to treat the two problems (i.e., stuttering and disordered phonology). What we were trying to do with this study was *not* to show that our program for stuttering was overly robust (indeed, it most likely can't be, given the difficulties of quickly remediating childhood stuttering when it is coupled with a clinically significant concomitant speech and language problem). Instead, we were trying to show that if treatment for a child's phonological difficulties is adjusted to

TABLE 2.1 Descriptive Examples of Children Who Stutter With (S+DP; $n = 4$) and Without (S+NP; $n = 4$) Disordered Phonology.

Subject & Group	Sex	Age (mos.)	Frequency of Stuttering per 100 words (range)	Duration of Stuttering (sec) (range)	S.S.I. (total overall score)	#PP	Specific PP
S+DP							
S1	M	56	13 (7–22)	.66 (.25–1.13)	Moderate (21)	14	INT, PV, ST, DEAF, FCD WSD, LAB, /s/CR, DEV, GL, LCR, AFF, VOC, EPEN
S2	M	60	10 (3–12)	.74 (.25–.87)	Moderate (17)	11	INT, VF, PAL, *LAT, ST ICD, DEP, PV, GL, AFF, VOC
S3	M	69	10 (6–15)	.60 (.25–1.3)	Moderate (17)	8	*LAT, GL, DEAF, VOC, LAB, VF, DEP, PV
S4	M	85	5 (2–9)	.30 (.20–.45)	Mild (9)	5	*LAT, VF, DEP, GL, VOC
S+NP							
S1	M	54	20 (11–28)	1.9 (.75–5.0)	Moderate (20)	1	GL
S2	M	75	23 (16–27)	1.2 (.25–2.6)	Moderate (22)	2	DP, *NEU
S3	F	78	17 (11–23)	1.2 (.32–3.0)	Severe (26)	2	GL, VOC
S4	M	79	12 (9–16)	.78 (.25–1.1)	Moderate (17)	1	INT

AFF	=	affrication		LAT	=	lateralization
DEAF	=	deaffrication		LCR	=	liquid cluster
DEP	=	depalatization		NEU	=	neutralization
DEV	=	devoicing		PV	=	prevocalic voicing
EPEN	=	epenthesis		/s/CR	=	cluster reduction
ICD	=	final consonant deletion		ST	=	stopping
GL	=	gliding of liquids		VF	=	velar fronting
ICD	=	initial consonant deletion		VOC	=	vocalization
INT	=	interdentalization		WSD	=	weak syllable deletion
LAB	=	labialization		*	=	processes are atypical

After Conture, Louko, & Edwards, 1993, with permission.

take into account and hopefully not exacerbate the child's stuttering, the treatment can be effective, and then over time both problems can be improved, albeit slower than either clinicians or parents might like.

Expressive/Receptive Language (Syntax)

Language difficulties can also accompany stuttering; however, as mentioned above, the frequency and nature of such language concerns with people who stutter is still unclear. Recently, Bernstein Ratner (1997b) provided an excellent review of findings and implications of studies of the content (semantics), form (syntax, morphology, and phonology), and use (pragmatics) of language relative to stuttering. Suffice it to say that people who stutter, as a group, do not grossly differ from their nonstuttering peers; indeed, as any clinician will tell you, there are more than a few children who stutter with very good to superior language abilities.

Anecdotally, from our clinical practice, we have occasionally observed people who stutter, particularly children, who exhibit a length and complexity of language structures that are *less than appropriate* for their age. Conversely, we have observed people who stutter, especially children, who exhibit a length and complexity of language structures that are *more*, far more, than necessary for them to communicate. Still other people who stutter seem less than adequate for their age in sequentially relating a story or event to a listener (this becomes, in our experience, more evident as the child grows older and telling such stories become commonplace as well as more complex). We have observed some other people who stutter, particularly those who seemingly have difficulties quickly and efficiently sequencing their communication, to persist in continuing to monologue ("to hog the floor") to the extreme frustration and boredom of their listeners. Some people who stutter, particularly preschool children, may also exhibit reductions in their expressive and/or receptive vocabulary—something we will discuss below—which, of course, places added strain on their ability to quickly and efficiently access or retrieve words during spontaneous conversation.

Even though the person or person's family is mainly concerned with stuttering, it is *very* important, in our experience, to thoroughly test as many facets of the person's speech and language system as possible. Why? It is not uncommon to find deficits and/or "mismatches" among aspects of language (e.g., very superior expressive language skills and very modest receptive vocabulary), difficulties that may need to be addressed simultaneously with the person's stuttering. Certainly, we would want to screen a child's expressive and receptive language abilities. Such screening could involve two observations: (1) assessment of our younger client's mean length of utterance (MLU) in morphemes and documenting the presence/absence of any and all grammatical morphemes, and (2) administration of the *Fluharty Preschool Speech and Language Screening Test* (Fluharty, 1974, 1978). (One might also use the *Clinical Evaluation of Language Fundamentals – 3, Screening Test* (Semel, Wiig, & Secord, 1996). If these relatively easy-to-obtain informal procedures suggest a problem, then we may also use formalized tests like the *Preschool Language Scale* (Zimmerman, Steiner, & Pond, 1979), *Test of Early Language Development-2* (Hresko, Reid, & Hammill, 1991), or *Test of Language Development: Primary 2* (Newcomer & Hammill, 1997). As we have mentioned elsewhere (Conture & Caruso, 1987), clinicians should try to distinguish between the receptive/expressive "language problems" that: (1) *perpetuate* (dis)fluency, for example, a client with a reduced MLU and a number of missing grammatical morphemes whose environment encourages inappropriately rapid production of long, complex utterances; and (2) *result from* or are *secondary to* a fluency problem—for example, a client who habitually uses subtly and some not so subtly incorrect vocabulary in attempts to avoid production of certain sounds, syllables, or words. As we continue to know more and more about the role language plays in stuttering (e.g., Bernstein Ratner, 1997b; Tetnowski, 1998; Wingate, 1988), we may come to see that all aspects of language influence speech fluency. For now, however, a thorough assessment of a client's language abilities, even though they are being assessed for known or suspected stuttering, is an appropriate, helpful, prudent, and wise procedure.

As we mentioned above with phonological concerns, sometimes, as a client who stutters becomes more fluent, a language concern appears (cf. Merits-Patterson & Reed, 1981). As with an "emerging" articulation problem, it would seem that the previously severe stuttering hid or drew attention away from an already apparent language difficulty. Therapeutically, this may mean a switch in emphasis from stuttering to language; however, a somewhat better approach, in our opinion, might be a blending, right from the beginning of therapy, of attention to fluency *and* attention to language issues. This is similar to what we have described and advocated (Conture et al., 1993; Louko et al., 1999) when stuttering and disordered phonology co-occur. More on this in the next chapter.

Expressive/Receptive Language (Vocabulary)

With regard to vocabulary, there are at least two tests that we routinely use that provide norm-referenced measures: the *Peabody Picture Vocabulary Test* (PPVT-III; Dunn & Dunn, 1997) and the *Expressive Vocabulary Test* (EVT; Williams, 1997). The PPVT-III (receptive vocabulary) and EVT (expressive vocabulary) can be appropriately used with children, teenagers, and adults. We have previously mentioned (Conture & Caruso, 1987) our use of the vocabulary tests as a rough index of a client's general intelligence. While we fully realize that informal/formal testing of intelligence is the province of the clinical psychologist, we need to know at the time of assessment whether the client's IQ is roughly within normal limits, hence, our use of the PPVT-III in this regard. We base our use of PPVT-III in this way on the fact that the PPVT-III as well as WISC vocabulary subtest are both highly correlated with the full-scale WISC IQ.

We have noticed three different "profiles" with regard to how preschool and early schoolage children who stutter score on vocabulary and syntactic tests:

- Both vocabulary and language scores are comparable—that is, they are both high, low, or mid-range (i.e., within 10 percentile points of one another).
- Vocabulary scores are lower than language scores—that is, they are 20 or more percentile points different).
- Vocabulary scores are higher than language scores—that is, they are 20 or more percentile points different).

To provide some support to the above, Table 2.2 shows the vocabulary and language test scores from ten preschool and early school-age children evaluated in our clinic during a twelve-month period. Of course, a larger sample is needed as well as a normally fluent comparison group (something we are developing, under more tightly controlled experimental conditions). However, there is nothing to suggest that these children are not representative of the children that we and others routinely evaluate. In this sample about eight of the ten children scored higher on the language than the vocabulary test, with two of the ten scoring comparably on the two tests.

Comparable Vocabulary and Language Scores.   In our experience, comparable vocabulary and language test scores are not as likely to be found with children who stutter as with their normally fluent peers. And when we do find such comparable scores, it has been our experience, therapy seems to proceed at a faster, more effective pace. This suggests, of course, that the child's speech and language production skills are all progressing simultaneously at about the same pace and that after a period of unsettled speech fluency, the child is going to develop into a reasonably fluent adult.

Vocabulary Lower Than Language Scores.   In our opinion, the second "profile" (low vocabulary, high language) is more apt to be seen in preschool children who stutter than their normally fluent peers (Anderson & Conture, 2000). Further, we believe that it precipitates, for some of these children, instances of stuttering. In essence, the language slots are ready before the vocabulary fillers. We also suspect, for many of these children, this vocabulary-syntactic disparity lessens with age and/or environment stimulation. These children, in our opinion, can be helped through a combination of treatment, parental counseling, and routine support for developmental processes, regardless of the slowness and/or unevenness of such processes.

Vocabulary Higher Than Language Scores.   The third profile, vocabulary higher than language, is a profile that we see with some of our clients who continue to stutter and/or require protracted treatment (although not apparent in the sample of children shown in Table 2.2). However, we do not know why this profile doesn't seem to change with development and generally requires, in our opinion, protracted forms of treatment that contain a strong component of language enrichment, stimulation, and treatment (see Hall, 1996; Hall, Yamashita, & Aram, 1993, for study of the relationship between better developed lexical than morphosyntactic skills in children with language disorders and increased disfluencies). At the end of the day, when we have a much better handle on the developmental cortical/subcortical processes of speech fluency, I believe we will find that these three "profiles" will be associated with different underlying developmental patterns in terms of the functioning of the brain and related structures.

Without getting into treatment at this point, suffice it to say, we want to help children who stutter retrieve and use words in as physically and mentally relaxed, unhurried, and gentle fashion as possible. Conversely, everything that the child, the child's environment, or the child's speech-language pathologist does to encourage the child to quickly retrieve words and to become frustrated, tense, fearful, and so on. when the word is not quickly retrieved or when the wrong word is retrieved, will be counterproductive to the child's development of reasonably fluent speech. We think it obvious that activities geared to enrich and stimulate vocabulary development should be helpful to all children, but particularly children exhibiting the second profile.

TABLE 2.2   Language, Vocabulary, and Disfluency Data Obtained for 10 Children (ages 40–63 months) Who Stutter Collected in a Clinical Setting. Percentile ranks and stanines (1 stanine—1/9 of total distributions) come from TELD & PPVT norms with deciles for total disfluency based on Yaruss, LaSalle, & Conture (1998) clinical sample of 100 children who stutter.

Children Who Stutter	Language (TELD)	Vocabulary (PPVT)	Total Disfluency
Male, 40 months	88th %, 7th Stanine	19th %, 3rd Stanine	Home: 18%, 9th Decile
Male, 40 months	92nd %, 8th Stanine	42nd %, 5th Stanine	Home: 13%, 6th Decile
Female, 42 months	99th %, 9th Stanine	87th %, 7th Stanine	Home: 10%, 5th Decile
Male, 44 months	99th %, 9th Stanine	66th %, 6th Stanine	Home: 20%, 9th Decile
Male, 45 months	58th %, 5th Stanine	32nd %, 4th Stanine	Home: 17%, 8th Decile
Female, 47 months	95th %, 8th Stanine	73rd %, 6th Stanine	Home: 16%, 7th Decile
Male, 47 months	92nd %, 8th Stanine	47th %, 5th Stanine	Home: 19%, 9th Decile
Male, 48 months	99th %, 9th Stanine	45th %, 5th Stanine	Home: 8%, 3rd Decile
Male, 51 months	99th %, 9th Stanine	90th %, 8th Stanine	Home: 9%, 4th Decile
Male, 63 months	99th %, 9th Stanine	77th %, 7th Stanine	Home: 14%, 7th Decile
	Mean = 92.0	Mean = 57.8	Mean = 14.4

Voice

In the 1970s and 1980s, perhaps no area in the field of stuttering received so much attention and stirred up so much controversy as speculation regarding how people who stutter use their larynx for speech production (e.g., Adams, Freeman, & Conture, 1984; Borden, Baer, & Kenney, 1995; Conture, McCall, & Brewer, 1977; Conture, Rothenberg, & Molitor, 1986; Conture, Schwartz, & Brewer, 1985). However, it must be noted that during speech, people who stutter and normally fluent speakers can use their larynx as either: (1) an *articulator*, for example, to adduct or abduct the vocal folds to or away from midline for the purposes of beginning or terminating voicing, respectively; or (2) a *phonatory vibrator*, for example, vibrating the approximated vocal folds for the purposes of voicing. While the articulatory and vibratory aspects of the larynx are interdependent, it is the latter, the larynx as a vibrator, that we are primarily concerned with when we discuss "voice" or "voice quality" and the former, the larynx as articulator, that we are mainly talking about when we mean "beginning with a hard attack" or "getting stuck on that sound."

With regard to voice quality, there is no published empirical research[1] that we are aware of that proves that the perceptually fluent speech of people who stutter, young or old,

---

[1]St. Louis and Hinzman (1988) report such differences; however, it is unclear from their published report whether the judgment of the voice quality of people who stutter was based on samples containing instances of stuttering. As will be mentioned below, the act of stuttering itself involves disruption in laryngeal behavior, which can, in turn, change perceived vocal quality. These changes during and surrounding instances of stuttering, however, should not be viewed like those of a voice problem that would be pervasive throughout most or all of the speech of people who stutter, the fluent as well as the stuttered aspects.

is more apt to be associated with a different sounding voice or voice quality than normally fluent speakers, or that people who stutter are more apt to have voice problems than normally fluent speakers—for example, hoarseness, harshness, breathiness, and so forth. This *does not* mean that vocal quality during instances of stuttering is similar to that observed during normally fluent speech. For example, it is not uncommon to observe sudden pitch rises during the stutterings of children whose problem is worsening. In fact, we believe that differences in vocal quality during stuttering are part or result of the act of stuttering, not something that precipitated the stuttering in the first place or an ongoing quality of voice throughout the entirety of the person's speech, the fluent as well as stuttered aspects. In essence, disruptions in voice quality *during* or *surrounding* an actual instance of stuttering should not be confused with disruptions in voice quality throughout all the speech of the person who stutters, the fluent parts as well as the disfluent. Oftentimes, the very act of stuttering involves laryngeal disturbances (cf. Conture, McCall, & Brewer, 1977; Conture, Schwartz, & Brewer, 1985), which result in changes in voice quality during the stuttering. These changes are not the same, however, as an ongoing problem of hoarseness, breathiness, diplophonia, inappropriately low pitch, monotonous voice, and the like. These vocal behaviors *must* be observed throughout the *entirety* of the client's utterances, the fluent and not just the stuttered parts, in order to diagnose the person as having a "voice disorder," in the traditional use of that diagnostic label.

Variations in Fundamental Frequency.   The first exception to the above rule involves several studies dating back to the 1930s whereby researchers assessed differences in variation of vocal fundamental frequency (pitch) between people who do and do not stutter. While Adams (1955) and Healey (1982) report the fundamental frequency of people who stutter is less variable than that of their normally fluent peers, these findings have not been subsequently replicated (see Bloodstein's [1995], p. 31). We must confess that these results of empirical studies are not consistent with our clinical experience that some people who stutter, young as well as older, seem to exhibit a rather monotonous, inappropriately low-pitched voice. Perhaps, in our clinical practice, we are listening to aspects of voice production other than fluctuations in pitch and, for some reason, we interpret this behavior as "monotone." Suffice it to say, that the low-pitched Johnny-one-note problem that we think we observe in children who stutter is not unique to people who stutter. Indeed, many people who do not stutter, for example, salespersons, teachers, business people, and so forth, also exhibit such voice use. Thus, it is probably safer to suggest that the presence of a low-pitched monotone voice is probably an individual rather than group phenomenon, perhaps resulting from rather than causing or even perpetuating stuttering.

Jitter, Shimmer, and Formant Frequency Fluctuations.   The second exception to the above rule appears to relate to a similar, but somewhat different line of research that has attempted to study "control of laryngeal-respiratory dynamics" (Newman, Harris, & Hilton, 1989) or "vocal tract stability" (Robb, Blomgren, & Chen, 1998). Newman and colleagues (1989) assessed pitch (jitter) and amplitude (shimmer) variations during the steady-state portion of sustained vowels, and Robb and colleagues (1998) assessed the steady-state portion of vowels in consonant–vowel-consonant (VC) words. Newman and colleagues found significantly more amplitude variations for people who stutter when compared to people who do not stutter, and Robb and colleagues found a significantly larger formant frequency fluctuation for untreated people who stutter when compared to controls. In essence, results from these two studies suggest that for older (subjects' mean age in the two studies ranged from 24 to 35 years with youngest subject being 12 and oldest 46 years of age) people who stutter, there may be some lack of laryngeal as well as supralaryngeal control during both sustained vowel and short CVC words. In terms of basic knowledge, finding "more" fluctuations in amplitude as well as formant frequency control seems to run contrary to earlier findings (e.g., Adams, 1955; Healey, 1982) that people who stutter exhibit less variation in fundamental frequency. Perhaps these contrary findings relate to differences in sample size and composition, but more than likely they are due to advancements and refinements in methodology in this area. Of course, replication, which generally takes years to complete, will help us understand the truth of the matter; however, the Newman and colleagues and Robb and colleagues findings suggest what most clinicians suspect: People who stutter have less than fully developed abilities to initiate and/or maintain laryngeal and supralaryngeal control during speech. In terms of diagnosis and treatment, the implications of these findings are unclear; however, at the least, it should lend support to those clinicians who assess the neuromotor control for speech of people who stutter.

Occasional Client with Hyperfunctional Voice Usage. The final exception to the rule that people who stutter do not have voice problems relates to the occasional observation that some people who stutter, typically a preschool or early school-age child, sometimes present a hoarse and/or breath vocal quality seemingly in relation to hyperfunctional voice usage. These are the clients who frequently "sing" with loud music or noise in the background, frequently imitate or use "monster," animal, car, truck, or machinery noises when playing; frequently and excessively yell inside and outside home; frequently engage in loud talking, and so forth. When such problems as inappropriately low-pitched, hoarse, or breathy voice do occur in a person who stutters, it usually justifies a referral to an ENT physician, particularly if the client or associates report that such voice quality is persistent.

Typically, we assess the voice of people who stutter through informal testing of their ability to change pitch from low to high (and vice versa) in both discrete and continuous steps. This may have to be modeled or demonstrated several times, since many naive speakers confuse changes in vocal level (loudness or volume) with changes in vocal fundamental frequency (pitch). Untrained speakers or singers may attempt to "go up and down the scale" by merely increasing or decreasing their vocal level (i.e., getting louder or softer). In our experience, the client's "flexibility" or variability of pitch is far more important than his or her modal or average value in terms of predicting whether the client will be able to, if required to do so, quickly and efficiently modify inappropriate aspects of laryngeal behavior. (Indeed, how often, during spontaneous speech, do we actually use "modal pitch"?) With younger clients, for whom low and high as well as pitch and loudness mean very little, we have found that using nonhuman or animal models (that they must imitate) works much better: "Make a sound like a like a baby kitty (or) Meow just like a baby kitty . . . Now just like the daddy kitty?" "Make a sound like a wolf howl. Like a siren." Having the client imitate these models permits the clinician to assess the client's ability to quickly, efficiently, and smoothly change from low to high pitch and back again, a crude but reasonable index of the client's ability to do this in running speech.

Another procedure we employ that we previously discussed (Conture & Caruso, 1987) is the s/z ratio (Eckel & Boone, 1981). Our experience indicates that youngsters below 7 to 8 years of age have difficulty understanding and/or cooperating with the task—they don't seem able to prolong the /s/ and /z/ for sufficient durations. However, even if these preschoolers shorten the duration of these prolonged fricatives to, say, 5 seconds in length, the clinician should be able to calculate the degree to which the client's s/z ratio approximates the norm: 1.00 (with approximately ± 1 $SD = 0.37$). The s/z ratio is computed by timing the duration (in seconds or milliseconds) that the client can sustain the /s/ on one exhalation and then dividing this duration by the duration /z/ was sustained on one exhalation. The client is given several chances to sustain the /s/ and the /z/ with the longest duration of each used to figure the duration and the resulting s/z ratio representing a "rough" means of determining the client's efficiency of vocal fold approximation or functioning during phonation.

Before leaving this area, we should add a word or two about technological approaches. With the increased use of computers and hardware/software specifically designed to analyze speech, there have been significantly more use of such devices as the electroglottograph or EGG (see Childers & Krishnamurthy, 1984; Childers, Naik, Larar, Krishnamurthy, & Moore, 1983; and Colton & Conture, 1990, for discussion of practical/theoretical aspects of EGG usage and interpretation), which may become increasingly useful for both diagnostic and therapeutic purposes. For example, one such early attempt was that of Conture, Rothenberg, and Molitor (1986), who reported that children who stutter are less apt (than their normally fluent peers) to use typical vocal fold adjustments during their transitions from consonants to vowel and vowel to consonant (it is quite unclear, at this point, whether these differences are perceptible to listeners but many, we suspect, aren't). At present, we interpret this to mean that children who stutter are using one of several different available means—albeit less efficient and perhaps more susceptible to disruption under stress—to make vocal fold adjustments for speech production. Again, our use of the EGG and other such devices (for example, the Visi-Pitch) for the assessment and remediation of laryngeal behavior in stuttering and other disordered populations will surely increase in the years to come, particular as researchers develop means to reliably digitize the EGG signal, thus making EGG information analyzable through convenient and reasonably priced desktop and laptop computers. One caution: SLPs should consider these devices as adjuncts or supplements to rather than replacements for their trained perceptual judgments. However, these same SLPs should try to keep abreast of these sort of technological developments, since they will have important implications for the types of diagnostic assessments and therapy programs some SLPs are already performing in cutting-edge clinical situations.

Hearing

While there is a great deal of empirical investigation as well as speculation regarding the role audition plays in stuttering (e.g., Conture, 1974; Neilson, 1980; Neilson & Neilson, 1987), most clinicians do not seem to place a great deal of emphasis on the assessment of audition with the stuttering population. This is unfortunate, because people who stutter have just as much right as people who do not stutter to have hearing difficulties! Ideally, a full-scale diagnostic for stuttering should include pure-tone screening (air and bone) as well as speech discrimination testing or at least obtain records of the most recent testing in this area.

For children in particular, middle-ear status should be, if at all possible, assessed by means of tympanometry—for example, static acoustic impedance measures (single peak tympanograms) reported in acoustic ohms. Of course, for some clients, it may not be possible to obtain "normal" tympanograms if the client appears to exhibit a cold, upper respiratory infection, or an allergy or if the client lacks sufficient cooperation to permit completion of testing. In those situations where further testing, at a later date, is not possible, the speech-language pathologist should at least try to record the presence or the history of any such middle-ear concerns as frequent earaches, eardrum rupture, persistent fluid in the ear, surgically inserted pressure-equalizing tubes, frequency and kinds of medications used to treat these concerns, and so forth.

The SLP should be aware of these concerns because they may mean that the client who stutters, who also has chronic middle-ear problems, will not always have the best auditory sensitivity discrimination. It may also mean that the child may be more tired and/or more prone to rapidly fatigue as a result of frequent middle-ear infections (and associated upper respiratory infections) in addition to the various medications used to remediate such infections or the excessive postnasal secretion brought about by a client's allergy.

A reasonable body of information is now available regarding: (1) the relationship between phonological difficulties and middle ear difficulties; (2) how we might best assess and treat these phonological difficulties; and (3) something about how parents perceive the impact of otitis media on their children's speech-language behavior (e.g., Paden, 1998; Paden, Matthies, & Novak, 1989; Paden, Novak, & Beiter, 1987; Shriberg & Kwiatkowski, 1982; Shriberg & Smith, 1983; Thielke & Shriberg, 1990; Thurnes & Caruso, 1994). Thus, when assessing a child whose phonological concerns appear intertwined with stuttering and who also exhibits persistent hearing and/or middle ear problems, we should be familiar with such information. It is entirely possible that for some of these children, persistent difficulties with hearing and/or otitis media may delay recovery and/or actually contribute to difficulties these children may be having with speech sound articulation and speech fluency.

Reading

It is interesting to note that while reading material is frequently used in the assessment and treatment of stuttering, speech-language pathologists often have little objective information about how, in general, a person's speaking behavior during conversational speech compares to oral reading. For example, how many clinicians realize that speaking rate is typically faster during oral reading than conversational speech? That is, Wingate's (1988, pp. 250–251) review of speaking rate during spontaneous speech versus oral reading suggests that speaking rate during spontaneous speaking is, in general, slower than during oral reading. Wingate goes on to suggest that this difference is due to the ". . . . demands that rise in the process of generating spontaneous speech" (p. 251). In essence, Wingate suggests that oral reading places fewer demands on our language system than the act of spontaneous speech, a suggestion clinicians may want to keep in mind both during assessment as well as treatment. In other words, the use of a book is not the only thing that differentiates oral reading from oral conversational speaking.

It is also interesting that reading material is frequently used in the assessment and treatment of stuttering even though the clinician may have little or no understanding of the reading abilities of the person who stutters. It seems obvious, however, if a person who stutters has oral reading difficulties, these difficulties may contribute to the person's stuttering during reading. While some of us (e.g., Conture & van Naerssen, 1977; Janssen, Kraaimaat, & van der Meulen, 1983), using standardized tests of reading abilities, reported no significant difference between the reading abilities of people who stutter and people who do not stutter, others have reported differences between people who do and do not stutter in terms of silent and oral reading (e.g., Bosshardt & Nandyal, 1988). Still others—for example, Brutten, Bakker, Janssen, and van der Meulen (1984), studying eyeball movement associated with silent reading—reported that people who stutter produced more eyeball "regressions" (eyeball moving back over previously read material) than normal speakers. Where do these apparent differences in empirical findings leave us clinically? Uncertain. That is, it is entirely possible during a diagnostic evaluation, although probably not the rule, that any one individual who stutters—particularly adults, based on Bosshardt and Nandyal's data—may also demonstrate reading concerns that warrant attention from a reading specialist before or at least during the time speech therapy is undertaken. As always, the SLP needs to coordinate speech-language services with the reading specialist so that the two services—remediation of reading and speech/language—*complement* rather than *compete* with one another. For example, any reading program that places emphasis on quick, precise, and physically tense articulation of reading material is not going to be in the best interests of a child who stutters. At the least, the SLP should understand that a child who stutters who also has a reading problem might find speech therapy difficult if reading material is used as a means of remediating speech behavior.

Academic Abilities and Status

Related to reading concerns are the school-age client's academic development and achievement. Academic concerns can be a problem in speech therapy with a child who stutters if the child is having so much trouble with school subjects that he or she feels discouraged or lacking in confidence and regards any new seemingly "academic-like" situation such as speech therapy sessions as a threat. Further, a child struggling with school work, particularly if that child is still doing poorly, is a child who may be tired at the end of the school day. Likewise, if the parents are struggling to assist the child and must frequently interact with the child's teachers over the phone or at school, they may have reduced levels of psychic energy to deal with the child's stuttering. Such fatigue needs to be taken into consideration by the SLP planning therapy for that child.

When the child's parents and/or the SLP's observations suggest that schoolwork and school progress are problematic, the SLP has several options. First, the SLP can assess whether the type and severity of academic difficulties impact the child's recovery. For example, difficulties in one subject, like math, while of concern to the child and the child's parents, are probably not overly relevant to the child's participation or progress in speech-language therapy. However, if the child has difficulties across a number of subjects, in particular in subjects directly relating to communication, like English and reading, the probability is much greater that the child's academic difficulties may interfere with the child's recovery from stuttering. Second, if the child's difficulties do seem to be interfering with his or her abilities to focus on speech therapy and/or diminish the child's energy for therapy, the SLP may want to obtain general as well as specific knowledge of academic performance to date through records and discussions with the client's teachers. Particularly with a school-age child, administering speech therapy without knowledge of the child's academic abilities, progress, and performance is like traveling through a strange land without a map. Third, if the child is really struggling with school, and that problem is utmost on his or her mind as well as on the parents' minds, it might be best to take a break from speech therapy, or at least reduce the number of sessions per week or month to allow the child to concentrate on the task he or she has selected as job one: schoolwork. The author has had children essentially ignore all therapy homework because of focusing on their schoolwork, schoolwork that was very difficult for them but mattered the most for them at that point in their lives.

Attention Deficit Hyperactivity Disorder (ADHD)

Interacting in a major way with academic performance as well as performance in speech therapy is attention deficit hyperactivity disorder (ADHD) (see Riley & Riley, 1988 for discussion of its possible relation to recovery from stuttering). Although there is still some level of unclarity and lack of agreement regarding the etiology, symptomatology, and management of ADHD (see Baumgaertel & Wolraich, 1998; Krupski, 1986; Shaywitz & Shaywitz, 1985, 1988, for excellent reviews of clinical and research findings relating to ADHD), the experienced SLP will recognize some of its more common symptoms: (1) failure to finish tasks once started; (2) inattention, easily distracted; (3) restless, overactive, and unpredictable behavior; and (4) disturbing other children (see Table 2.3, adapted from Baumgaertel & Wolraich, 1998, listing the basic or core behavioral symptoms associated with ADHD).

Shaywitz and Shaywitz (1985, p. 6) suggest the presence of ADHD if three to four interrelated symptoms occur for more than six months duration and have begun before the child is 7 years age: *inattention* (e.g., does not finish what is started), *impulsivity* (e.g., is extremely excitable), and *hyperactivity* (e.g., always on the go; would run rather than walk). According to Shaywitz and Shaywitz, there are three to four criteria for diagnosing each of these symptoms (inattention, impulsitivity, and hyperactivity). For example, impulsivity is diagnosed when at least three of the following are observed: (1) the child calls out in class, makes noises in class; (2) is extremely excitable; (3) has trouble waiting his or her turn; (4) talks excessively; and (5) disrupts other children. Evidence continues to mount that ADHD/learning disability (LD) probably has some form of neurological origin, with workers in this field attempting to resolve or treat the problem through educational and/or pharmacological means.

In this writer's clinical experience, it isn't that a child exhibiting ADHD doesn't observe what is going on around him or her as much as the fact that the child is observing everything around him or her, unfortunately, all at once! These children, in our experience,

---

TABLE 2.3   Core Symptoms of "Developmentally Discrepant Attention Control, Hyperactivity and Impulsivity" Behaviors Associated with Attention Deficit Hyperactivity Disorder (ADHD)

Inattention

- Careless mistakes
- Difficulty sustaining attention
- Seems not to listen
- Fails to finish tasks
- Difficulty organizing
- Avoids tasks requiring sustained attention
- Loses things
- Easily distracted
- Forgetful

Hyperactivity

- Fidgeting
- Unable to stay seated
- Moving excessively (restless)
- Difficulty engaging in leisure activities quietly
- "On the go"
- Talking excessively

Impulsivity

- Blurting answers before questions completed
- Difficulty awaiting turn
- Interrupting/intruding upon others

Adapted from Baumgaertel & Wolraich, 1998, with permission.

seem to lack the ability to selectively attend to the task at hand for a sufficient period of time before they are off onto a new and different task but for only a short while before they switch to yet another task. Obviously, if this sort of behavior persists in school and/or in therapy, the child is going to have trouble being successful. Wherever possible, referral to a clinical psychologist, child psychiatrist, or pediatrician *familiar* with this problem (and its behavioral, educational, and pharmaceutical management) is clearly in order if the SLP suspects ADHD. However, and this is very important, the SLP should realize that ALL children sometimes fidget, get distracted, become restless, disturb other children, and so forth.

Thus, it is not the mere presence of such ADHD-like behaviors that warrant referral but their chronicity and predictability—that is, their frequent and consistent occurrence across a wide variety of situations. Furthermore, the SLP should realize that there is no published, empirical evidence to suggest that children or adults who stutter are more apt to exhibit ADHD than their normally fluent peers; however, there is also no evidence to suggest that people who stutter *never* exhibit ADHD. It seems reasonable to suggest that a young person who stutters as well as chronically exhibits disruptions in attention regulation and activity modulation may, at the least, take a protracted period of time to recover from stuttering and, at the worst, unless ADHD is ameliorated, exhibit little or no improvement in stuttering. In closing this section, we hasten to point out: Most children who stutter do not seem to exhibit ADHD, but the SLP should try to recognize those who do and plan management strategies accordingly.

Tourette's Syndrome

Interestingly, Attention Deficit Disorder is a relatively common aspect of another disorder, Tourette's syndrome (TS), which shares common features with developmental stuttering. For example, TS onsets during childhood, typically more boys than girls exhibit TS, and TS tends to wax and wane over time. Tourette's syndrome is often thought to be associated with disturbances of the extrapyramidal motor system, in particular the basal ganglia (Abwender, Trinidad, Jones, Como, Hymes, & Kurlan, 1998). Indeed, Abwender and colleagues (1998) recently attempted to assess the relationship between TS and developmental stuttering by examining twenty-two people from ages 8 to 48 who stutter. They assessed these subjects by means of standardized clinical interviews as well as various psychometric instruments (e.g., *Leyton Obsessional Inventory—Child Version* [Berg, Rapoport, & Flament, 1986]). These researchers were reportedly interested in whether the group of people who stuttered exhibited neuropsychiatric features commonly seen in TS—for example, tics, attention deficit disorder, and obsessive-compulsive behaviors (OCB, e.g., persistent thoughts experienced, at least some time during the disturbance, as intrusive and inappropriate, causing marked anxiety or distress; for further description see Frances, First, & Pincus, 1995). While 40 percent (children) to 58 percent (adults) were observed exhibiting "definite or probable motor tics," the study did not explicate how "motor tics" were operationally disambiguated from the "associated nonspeech behavior" commonly occurring during stuttering. Perhaps more interesting, Abwender and colleagues reported, based on their clinical interviews and tests for OCB, that as many as 75 percent of the adults who reported/exhibited behavior consistent with OCB, with a lesser, but still clinically significant, percentage of children (50%) reporting OCB-like behavior.

Does this mean that TS causes stuttering or vice versa? Hardly. Indeed, a few words of caution are in order. First, such research, like any research, requires replication by independent investigators. Second, like so much of what we know about stuttering, even if many people who stutter exhibit a particular concomitant problem, there will be a significant number who will not exhibit the concomitant problem. Third, it is quite problematic to suggest that overlap, no matter how great, between a seemingly extrapyramidally driven problem like TS and developmental stuttering indicates that stuttering also results from an extrapyramidal problem. Such reasoning does little to explain the *sine qua non* of stuttering, that is, sound/syllable repetitions, sound prolongations, single-syllable word repetitions, and so on. These caveats aside, however, results of works like Abwender and colleagues are quite intriguing. At the least, such findings should be considered when initially evaluating people who stutter, for if ADHD, OCB, and the like, even in milder versions, are exhibited by some people who stutter, the presence of such concerns should be factored into any treatment plan purporting to consider the entirety of a person's abilities, behaviors, and needs into account when designing and conducting therapy.

To date, the writer has seen, in his clinical practice, at least three clients who stutter, each of whom had been clearly diagnosed by a clinical neurologist as exhibiting Tourette's syndrome. With each of these individuals, to greater or lesser degrees, the author noted facial tics seemingly having nothing to do with instances of stuttering—that is, "quick but brief contraction of one or more facial muscles during silence, and/or when the person was seemingly not planning for speech." Also apparent were subtle to not-so-subtle disruptions in pragmatic language skills—for example, seemingly ignoring the conversational topic under discussion, indulging in off-task behavior, playing apart/isolating from peers, and/or inappropriately changing the topic. While there are few guidelines here, the author received some success with these clients by referring to a SLP specializing in the assessment as well as treatment of pragmatic language concerns.

Neuromotor Speech and Nonspeech Behavior

Like some of the symptoms of ADHD, many children who do not stutter, on occasion, exhibit what some would call neuromaturational signs or "soft signs" of minimal brain dysfunction (MBD), for example, slow and/or asynchronous difficulties with some or many fine and gross motor tasks and so forth. All too often, in our experience, professionals, when observing these so-called "soft signs," are quick to apply the label of MBD, which implies structural central nervous system abnormality. And yet, even with a problem like ADHD, which would seem to clearly be related to MBD or structural CNS abnormality, computed tomography (CT scanning) studies of ADHD youngsters' cortical anatomy has proven normal (Shaywitz, Shaywitz, & Byrne, 1983). In other words, let us continue to assess the neuromotor abilities of people who stutter but at the same time be cautious when we interpret what "causes" the problems we observe in this area.

It is not uncommon for a child, teenager, or adult who stutters to demonstrate marginal skills in certain fine and/or gross motor tasks, particularly tasks that require rapid sequential and coordinated touching tip of thumb to each finger tip). Some clients who stutter will exhibit difficulty touching their tongue tip to either the middle of their upper lip or the middle of their chin, just below their lower lip. Some people who stutter may show slow and/or awkward movements when trying to rapidly move their tongue from side to side. They also may demonstrate "overflow" in that their mandible moves with their tongue instead remaining fixed or stationary, that is, they cannot maintain the necessary stabilizing "background" behavior, in this case a stationary mandible, to allow for the fastest and most precise "foreground" behavior, in this case, rapid side-to-side tongue movements. However, none of these skills, even for the normally fluent population, have been shown to relate to speech difficulties (see Hardy, 1970, 1978). Once again, we are not denying the existence of neuromotor difficulties in people who stutter, but we are urging caution in terms of how we interpret their etiology and relation to stuttering.

Diadochokinesis (Alternating Motion Rate).   Rates of alternating oral motor movements or diadochokinesis form one practical means for quantitatively and qualitatively assessing oral motor control. Diadochokinetic (DDK) movements can be assessed for uni-, bi-, and trisyllabic productions and then compared to published norms (e.g., Fletcher, 1972; Robbins & Klee, 1987). Indeed, DDK has been studied rather extensively in populations of children who do not stutter (e.g., Canning & Rose, 1974; Fletcher, 1972; Robbins & Klee, 1987). Interestingly, DDK studies of individuals with neuromotor difficulties like cerebral palsy (Hixon & Hardy, 1964) and Parkinson's disease (Canter, 1965) indicate that syllable repetition rates were more strongly related to the severity of speaking difficulties than rates of simple repetitive tongue, lip, or jaw movements.

In 1986, Riley and Riley introduced the *Oral Motor Assessment Scale* (OMAS), which provides some norms against which to compare the client as well as means to assess various aspects of oral motor coordination, that is, "accuracy" (precise and production, of target speech sounds), "smooth flow" (evenly spaced, correctly sequenced, coarticulated flow of syllable production) and "rate." At this point, it is still uncertain which of the three aspects—accuracy, smooth flow, or rate—of the OMAS are the most central to the diagnosis and management of youngsters' oral motor problems; but this test is a clear step in the direction of more quantitative, comprehensive testing of youngsters' speech motor abilities and development (see Peters, Romine, & Dykman, 1975, for examples of such clinical tests of youngsters' neuromotor development).

While the DDK abilities of people who stutter have long been studied (e.g., Rickenberg, 1956), more recently, Yaruss and colleagues (e.g., Yaruss, Logan, & Conture, 1995; Yaruss, LaSalle, & Conture, 1998) have explored the complex relationship between articulatory speaking rate in conversation, DDK rate for speech, and nonspeech movement of the oral structures in children who stutter. Results of these studies with children who stutter are far from complete, but the findings of Yaruss and colleagues suggest that as many as 40 percent of preschool children who stutter may exhibit DDK rates below normal limits for their chronological age (a finding consistent with Rickenberg [1956] who reported that DDK rate was significantly slower for adults who stutter than adults who do not stutter). So, clinicians should not be surprised to observe *some* children or adults who stutter exhibiting slow, inaccurate, and/or asynchronous DDK productions. Whether these problematic DDK performances suggest that the etiology, diagnosis, and treatment of stuttering has a neuromotor base is, of course, still an open question. In fact, the very means by which we measure DDK—that is, speech versus nonspeech stimuli—is also open to question. Yaruss (1998b) suggests, based on his preliminary analysis of DDK data derived from about 50 children who do not stutter, that DDK with speech ("puppy") is faster and more accurate that with nonspeech ("puh-puh") stimuli.

Thus, based on what we presently know, if we want to determine the rapidity and accuracy of a young child's speech production, it seems safe to suggest that we should use speech (e.g.,"daddy") rather than nonspeech (e.g., "duh-duh") stimuli during DDK testing. Obviously, we would want to factor out any units on a speech DDK trial that were stuttered, for example, a child who holds the "b" posture at the beginning of a DDK trial on "buttercup," like "bbbbbbuttercup-buttercup-buttercup . . . ." We would only calculate DDK rate for this child based on the fluent not stuttered or disfluent aspects of his or her DDK productions of "buttercup." In other words, the clinician excludes the time taken up by this initial stuttered syllable and computes the diadochokinetic rates based on the remaining fluent syllables.

Stuttering on DDK, Naming, or Single-Word Responses.   Clinicians will observe, with some people who stutter—particularly those who seem to have a more habituated, severe problem—some stuttering on the first mono-, bi-, or trisyllable produced in either an alternate or sequential diadochokinetic task. This stuttering usually takes the form of an audible or silent prolongation of the syllable-initial sound of the first syllable in the string, after which the client generally produces the remaining syllables in a fluent manner. Based on our experience, we believe that stuttering during the initial sound/syllable of these various diadochokinetic tasks suggests a very habituated problem as well as a less than positive prognosis (such stuttering may also occur on the *Goldman Fristoe Test of Articulation*, the Word Attack, as well as other subtests of the *Woodstock* reading test and can be similarly interpreted).

Screening Tests for Neuromotor Functioning.   Another, more general test of neurological functioning, is the *Quick Neurological Screening Test* (QNST; Mutti et al., 1978). The QNST assesses gross and fine motor movement, balance, coordination, and related abilities. QNST scores individuals as "normal" (0–24), "suspicious" (26–35), and "impaired" (35 and above); however, the QNST can be a difficult test to administer in whole or in part because the tasks it requires the client to perform require a good deal of cooperation, attention, and energy—variables that are often in short supply in children under 7 years of age, particularly at the end of a diagnostic.

A less formal neuromotor screening test was developed by Wolk and colleagues (1993) for the purposes of assessing the neuromotor function in pre-school children. This screening test, the *Selected Neuromotor Task Battery* (SNTB; for details, see Wolk, 1990, Appendix G), is a criterion-referenced test that requires the child to perform a series of simple motor acts, at the examiner's verbal request or in imitation of the examiner's model. The SNTB was a modified version of Peters and colleagues' (1975) "A Special Neurological Examination of Children with Learning Disabilities." The clinician merely checks off the child's performance on each of 8 items (0 = no difficulty/adequate performance and 1 = difficulty/poor quality of performance/nonperformance). The SNTB provides a gross overview of the child's neuromotor development and should be considered a screening rather than diagnostic test.

The OMAS, QNST, and SNTB should be viewed by the clinician as supplements to, rather than replacements for, the clinician's ability to judge oral motor proficiency. It should also be noted that the QNST's assessment of oral and/or speech motor movements is limited, although it provides a fairly extensive assessment of basic hand coordination and movement and the client's ability to "translate" auditory and visual information/instructions into hand movement. Of the three tests, perhaps the QNST provides the best "norms"; however, it is safe to say that most tests in this area are criterion- rather than norm-referenced.

Word Finding

Background.   The role of words—their storage, retrieval, and encoding—relative to stuttering is an area that has received, in the past ten-plus years, a considerable amount of attention. For example, Wingate (1988) reported that the scores on a test of "word fluency" (i.e., how many words an individual can write in a set period of time) were significantly less for adults who stutter than for adults who do not stutter, a finding taken by Wingate to suggest that stuttering relates to "more central functions" of the language production system. In a similar vein, Prins, Main, and Wampler (1997), in a study of lexicalization (i.e., the process by which speakers retrieve and encode words for expression), reported that adults who stutter exhibited significantly slower naming latencies than did adults who did not stutter. Prins and colleagues. interpreted these findings to suggest that slower processing of words could possibly disrupt speech fluency in some people who stutter. Most recently, Au-Yeung, Howell, and Pilgrim (1999) demonstrated that words, function words, have a far more significant role in stuttering, particularly in children below 9 years of age, than had been heretofore considered (for further studies of this interesting line of inquiry, see Howell, Au-Yeung, & Sackin, 1999; Howell, Au-Yeung, & Sackin, 2000). We firmly believe that of the various avenues of research currently being explored in the area of stuttering, studies of the word-finding, lexicalization, and expressive/receptive vocabulary of people who stutter will bear fruit of considerable theoretical as well as therapeutic import.

Testing. The general relation of word-finding to language abilities has been adequately explored elsewhere (Kail & Leonard, 1986) and we will not repeat this coverage here. It should be noted, however, that intervention studies of word-finding difficulties in children (e.g., McGregor & Leonard, 1989) suggest that word-storage encoding may be more central to word-finding difficulties than word-retrieval processes. Clinically, McGregor (1997) suggests that progress in word-finding difficulties (e.g., when measuring treatment outcome) may be indicated by reductions in single-word and discourse word-finding errors and an increase in semantically related errors (e.g., "lion" for "tiger"). In this writer's opinion, it behooves individuals interested in treating and researching stuttering to follow research in the area of word-finding, for many of the basic issues that need to be considered, assessed, and treated in terms of word-finding are being illuminated by such research.

We have discussed elsewhere (Conture & Caruso, 1987) the difficulties of separating out, in clients who stutter, those "latencies" of responding that are due to "word-finding" difficulties and those that are related to the act of stuttering itself. Indeed, in 1989, German introduced the *Test of Word Finding*, which is an objective means of assessing word finding and related abilities and, to date, this test appears to be the best way of assessing word-finding abilities in children that we have used (subsequently, German [1991] introduced the *Test of Word Finding in Discourse*). However, we are still not sure that any test can readily and reliably distinguish the response latencies of people who stutter due to difficulties with word finding from those due hesitating or pausing because of reluctance to say a particular sound, syllable, or word. What most of us collect, in our clinical assessment of people who stutter, are *treatment outcome measures* (e.g., % rankings on the PPVT) rather than *process measures* (e.g., response latencies when naming pictures) of lexicalization. While the former (outcome) is the direct or indirect result of the latter (process), a moment's consideration suggests that it is the process—for example, how fast a person can retrieve words—that might have its greatest influence on the person's speech fluency.

Psychosocial Adjustment

The overwhelming evidence suggests that the psychosocial adjustment of people who stutter is within normal limits (Sheehan, 1970a); however, this does not mean that any one individual who stutters might not have psychological concerns. In our experience, psychological factors that should be considered during the evaluation typically involve one or more of the following: (1) motivation for seeking services (a difficult but important variable to assess); (2) psychological aspects that may hinder or facilitate therapeutic progress; (3) psychological considerations that warrant referral to other professionals, for example, a clinical psychologist or a psychiatrist; and (4) temperamental characteristics of slow-to-warm-up and/or behavioral inhibition. (For useful overview of procedures to help parents deal with attitudinal and emotional factors in CWS, see Logan & Yaruss, 1999.)

Motivation.   It is not particularly easy to assess a client's motivation for seeking services. One essential aspect of motivation is this: Is the client seeking help for him- or herself (internal prodding) or because others have told the client to get help (external prodding)? External prodding, as from a parent or spouse, may get a person in the therapy door, but it will not provide the effort level, initiative, and insight necessary to successfully complete therapy. Internal-prodding motivation may result from a variety of factors, for example, lack of satisfaction with employment ("If I could only speak more fluently, then I could get a better job") or dissatisfaction with the social status quo ("If I could speak more fluently, I could meet more people, have more friends, do more things"). Occasionally, external prodding comes from an employer—for example, "Lois, if you want to become sales rep for the district, you've got to stop stuttering. We'll help you pay for the services, but you are not going to go any further in this company until you speak better." With parents, external-prodding motivation comes from their sincere concern for the child's future in school ("We want to get this cleared up before he begins school and it becomes a problem and gets in the way of his schoolwork.") and/or employability ("No one is going to hire him if he talks that way . . . he'll have real trouble finding a job."). In terms of parental motivation, as mentioned previously, parents seek help for their child when the child's problem continues for longer than they think it should, when the child starts to exhibit nonspeech behavior in association with his or her stuttering, and when the parent believes the child is starting to become "aware" of his or her speaking difficulties. In truth, the SLP can only guess at these various forms of motivation; however, the guess can be quite educated and should help in the planning of therapy and information sharing that must take place during the diagnostic and during therapy itself.

Psychosocial Concerns That May Hinder Speech Therapy.   Psychological concerns that hinder therapeutic progress can consist of such things as being overly subjective about the problem (or unable to be relatively objective about the problem even with the SLP's help); overly nonassertive, passive, and/or consumer-oriented (looking for the cure); overly argumentative-intellectual about the problem (deny emotions and explanations for behavior), projection ("Every time I open my mouth you think I'm stupid"), and so forth.

We become particularly concerned, during the diagnostic, if during some preliminary exploring with the client or his or her parents, we broach a seemingly reasonable explanation of a behavior or aspect of behavior that needs changing; and the client or parent does one or both of the following: (1) categorically or flatly denies that the reason or explanation has any validity or relation to their problem, or (2) provides a myriad of excuses for why the behavior occurred or is necessary or important. Our experience suggests to us that such strong denial and/or excuses represent a means for coping with problems that is a very counterproductive mechanism and is, in our opinion, an indicator of less-than-positive prognosis.

Healey, Grossman, and Ellis (1988) conducted an interesting study where they had a psychologist observe the psychological characteristics and associated behaviors of fifteen adult people who stutter who exhibited minimal improvement in speech fluency through a variety of therapies. Some of the common traits observed among these people who stutter were: (1) self-critical behavior, (2) perfectionistic attitudes toward performance, (3) extreme resistance to change, (4) low self-esteem and self-confidence, and (5) denial of increased fluency. While these observations are of interest, we still do not know whether these traits would also be exhibited in adult people who stutter who *did* increase their speech fluency as a result of therapy. Andrews and colleagues (Andrews & Craig, 1988; Craig & Andrews, 1985; Craig, Franklin, & Andrews, 1984) have tried to do just that: study differences in psychological and related characteristics between those adult people who stutter and who do and do not relapse after therapy. Among other variables, they assessed locus of control, that is, the extent to which a person perceives events as being a consequence of his or her own behavior (internal control) and, therefore, potentially under personal control versus the extent to which a person perceives events as resulting from luck or environmental influences outside his or her control (external control). Andrews and Craig's (1988) measures of locus of control, taken together with indexes of stuttering frequency and attitudes toward communication (Andrews & Cutler, 1974) indicated that 97 percent of those adult people who stutter and did not relapse (relapse = stuttering greater than 2% stuttered syllables at 10 months post-treatment) exhibited internal locus of control, "normal" communication attitudes, and no hint of stuttering on a telephone task at the end of therapy. Conversely, there were no adult people who stutter who were fluent 10 months post-treatment who obtained none of these goals—internal locus of control, "normal" communication attitudes, and no stuttering on telephone task—at the end of therapy. Hence, we have some evidence that certain psychological constructs, in this case locus of control, when taken together with other more typical measures of fluency and related attitudes, might help us predict long-term recovery from stuttering, an observation that bears continued investigation with people who stutter of other ages and in different therapy settings.

As Vaillant (1977) shows, *all* people have problems (see Schwartz's [1999, pp. 68-71] discussion of Vaillant's work relative to counseling people who stutter). What differs among people is the means—the psychological coping mechanisms—they use to deal with these problems. These differences in coping mechanisms make all the difference in the world in terms of people's satisfaction and success in dealing with personal as well as work-related issues. In later chapters we will discuss the relevance of these coping mechanisms to stuttering therapy, but for now suffice it to say that during the evaluation it is as important to understand the nature and number of psychological coping strategies as it is to understand the nature and number of problems the person who stutters and his or her associates are coping with.

Psychosocial Adjustment Issues That Warrant Concerns to Mental Health Professionals.
Some people who stutter (we estimate 5 to 10% of all people who stutter) exhibit psychological concerns of a kind and severity that may warrant professional evaluation and coun-

seling by trained psychiatrists or psychologists. Some of these clients, as Van Riper (1973) so aptly put it, seem to stutter ". . . with a gleam in their eye," with our only problem, as clinicians, being able to recognize that gleam. For these clients, who only seem to represent a very small percentage of all people who stutter, the stuttering problem and all its manifold aspects seem to fulfill unmet needs; and this group of clients would appear to need referral to a professional counselor.

With children, who cannot as easily articulate their psychosocial concerns, one may have to look for behavioral indexes. The following is a partial listing of some of these indexes: (1) a child who other children routinely shun or avoid; (2) a child who other adults report that they can't or won't manage or allow in their home; (3) a child who refuses to speak to the SLP, no matter what the topic or approach, after 30 to 90 minutes of trying but who readily talks to mother/father once SLP leaves the room; (4) a child who routinely acts out against other children; (5) a child whose strong fear of fire, loud noises, the dark, and anything strange is so routine and long-term as to be disruptive to home life; (6) a child who has been observed or known to hit, kick, or in other ways physically abuse animals such as cats or dogs; (7) a child who frequently, to the point of obsession, discusses guns, knives, or fire; (8) a child who routinely continues to wet the bed beyond 4 years of age, and (6) any combination of (1) through (8). Once again, it is the frequency and predictability of these behaviors, not their mere presence once in a while, that is of concern. And, while perhaps obvious, the more of these variables noted by a clinician, the more cause the clinician would have to make a referral to an appropriate mental health professional for at least a screening for psychosocial adjustment concerns.

It should also be recognized that it is not uncommon for a person who stutters, who is already receiving psychological counseling for other concerns such as depression or compulsive-obsessive behavior, to also seek out the services of a SLP; however, it is important to understand the reasons such a client might want the services of an SLP. Again, it is important to make sure that the two forms of therapy *complement* rather than *compete* with each other. While there is little objective evidence to suggest that psychosocial concerns (as a general rule) *cause* stuttering, it is quite possible that stuttering itself might lead to psychosocial adjustment problems, and psychosocial difficulties may exacerbate an already existing stuttering problem and/or make recovery from stuttering more difficult. As previously discussed, we feel it is unwise to view stuttering from either a nature *or* nurture perspective but rather one that views it as resulting from nature interacting with nurture.

Oppositional-Defiant Behavior.   While little is known about the frequency of oppositional disorder among people who stutter, the author believes that he has observed this problem, to greater or lesser degrees, in a few clients who stutter. When such behavior is present, this author believes it can significantly impede the progress of the client in treatment. Typically, what the author has observed, particularly when therapy has been less than successful or protracted, is that the child will frequently argue with adults, lose his or her temper, refuse to comply with adult requests, seem to deliberately annoy people, seemingly blame others for his or her mistakes, and become easily annoyed by others. Typically, parents will report frequent arguments with the client (see Frances et al., 1995, for further description). Again, little is known about the relationship between oppositional-defiant behavior and stuttering, and *certainly* it is not a frequent concomitant of stuttering. However, it does occur, this author believes, in some clients. When such behaviors as those listed above are *persistent* and *frequent*, it behooves the clinician, this author believes, to refer to appropriate mental health care professionals for assessment and/or possible treatment.

Again, as with ADHD, obsessive-compulsive disorders, and Tourette's syndrome, there is NO evidence that persistent and frequent oppositional defiant behavior CAUSES stuttering. However, its presence in a client will undoubtedly impede rapid, successful progress in speech-language therapy. With that in mind, the SLP is wise to cultivate relationships with clinical psychologists, especially those who specialize in treating children, for making necessary referrals for appropriate assessment and treatment.

Temperament

Temperament has been described as inherited personality traits that appear early in life (for excellent reviews see Goldsmith, Buss, Plomin, Rothbart, Thomas, Chess, Hinde, & McCall, 1987; Kagan & Snidman, 1991). More specifically, "temperament is an attribute of the child that mediates the influence of the environment" (Goldsmith et al., 1987, p. 509). Like many variables in the area of personality, temperament is a multifaceted construct used to describe a person's general disposition; it involves the range of moods that typifies the person's emotional life. Among some of the more important facets, workers in this field mention *reactivity* (e.g., the excitability or arousability of the autonomic nervous system, central nervous system, or behavioral responses to external stimuli), *activity* (i.e., lethargic to energetic levels of activity), *emotionality* (e.g., minimal to maximal response to novel stimuli), and *sociability* (e.g., preference for being alone versus being with others). When all these facets are considered as a whole, a person's temperament can be considered to be within normal limits, slow-to-warm-up, or behaviorally inhibited.

Testing. In recent years, the role temperament may play in the onset, development, and treatment of stuttering has received increased attention (e.g., Conture, 1991, pp. 380–381; Conture & Melnick, 1999; Guitar, 1997, 1998; Oyler, 1996a, 1996b; Oyler & Ramig, 1995; Rustin & Purser, 1991, pp. 13–24; Zebrowski & Conture, 1998). No one, to this author's knowledge, appears to be suggesting that temperamental variables *cause* stuttering; however, several, including this author, feel that temperamental characteristics may *maintain*, *perpetuate*, or even *exacerbate* stuttering. For example, Felsenfeld (1997) suggests that ". . . fast parental speech has deleterious consequences for fluency only for those children having a highly reactive temperament during a specific developmental period (e.g., 2 to 4 years)" (p. 18).

For the most part, at present, assessments of temperament are within the realm of clinical psychologists, however, we, as SLPs, need some sort of screening device to determine whether a child's temperament is significantly behaviorally inhibited and/or slow to warm up. In other words, if we are going to refer the child and family for assessment and possibly treatment of a child for temperamental variables that may get in the way of our speech-language therapy, we need more than just mere speculation and observations. Routinely, parents will tell the examining clinician that the child is "sensitive, has strong fears,

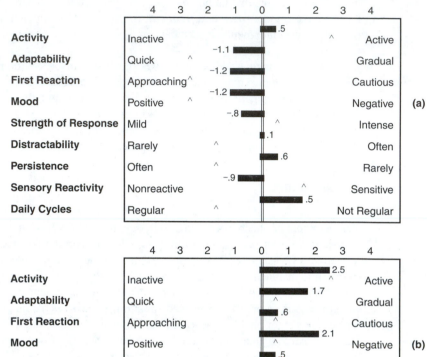

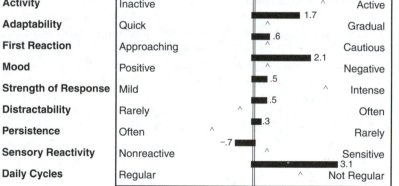

Bar shows questionnaire results. ^ shows rater's general impression on 9 facets of temperament for abbreviated version of the BSQ.

Scale: 0 = mean performance for 3- to 7-year-old child. 1 on this graph indicates 17 children in 100 have more extreme scores than this child. (2 = 3 in 100   3 = 1 in 100   4 = 1 in 1000).

Activity: The amount of physical motion during sleep, eating, play, dressing, bathing, etc.

Adaptability: The ease or difficulty with which reactions to stimuli can be modified in a desired way.

Approach/Withdrawal: The nature of initial responses to new stimuli – people, situations, places, foods, toys, procedures.

Mood: The amount of pleasant or unpleasant behavior in various situations.

Intensity: The energy level of responses regardless of quality or direction.

Distractibility: The effectiveness of extraneous environmental stimuli in interfering with ongoing behaviors.

Persistence/Attention Span: The length of time particular activities are pursued by the child with or without obstacles.

Sensory Threshold: The amount of stimulation, such as sounds, light, taste, smell or feel, necessary to evoke discernable responses in the child.

Rhythmicity: The regularity of physiological functions such as hunger, sleep, and elimination.

doesn't like changes in routine, is difficult to separate," and so forth. For example, this writer recently evaluated a 6-year-10-month-old boy who both stuttered and exhibited disordered phonology. When asked, the mother said that any correction, reprimand, punishment, or discipline of the child for any acts or behaviors was strongly reacted to by the child with apparent physical tension, pulling back bodily, and strong displeasure.

One test we have found useful to screen a child's temperament is Oyler's *Temperament Characteristics Scale* (TCS). When we administered the TCS, a test ranging from 7 (behaviorally inhibited) to 35 (behaviorally expressive), with the above child's mother and father jointly responding, the child received a score of 20 (similar to Oyler's reported mean score of 19 for children who stutter and appreciatively lower than the TCS score of 24 reported by Oyler). The parents referred to the child as "very sensitive" and quite "moral," wanting to be sure that everything and everybody was treated fairly, at all times. Such children, in our experience, react to any and all "attention" to their disfluencies in physically tense, worried, concerned, and even, in some cases, fearful ways. In our experience, children who score 15 to 20 on the TCS are at least slow to warm up, with children scoring 14 and below clearly exhibiting behaviors of the behaviorally inhibited (i.e., putting hands over ears when people in the room clap for joy, being extremely fearful of bugs, dark, strangers, baths, etc.)

Within the past two years, in attempts to further understand the role of temperament in stuttering, the writer has been using the *Behavioral Style Questionnaire* (BSQ; McDevitt & Carey, 1995), a paper-and-pencil test that parents respond to regarding their 3- to 7-year-old child. The BSQ, a norm-referenced test, provides insights into a variety of temperamental variables (e.g., activity level, ability to quickly versus gradually react/adjust to stimuli). Figure 2.4a shows a BSQ profile that reflects what this writer has found to be a reasonably typical profile for a behaviorally *expressive* child (in this case, a 3-year-old child who does not stutter). The BSQ profile in Figure 2.4b, in contrast, reflects what this writer has found to be a reasonably typical profile for a slow-to-warm-up, perhaps behaviorally *inhibited*, child (in this case, a 3-year-old child who stutters). A few cautions are in order here: (1) Some children who stutter can and do exhibit BSQ profiles that suggest they are behaviorally expressive; (2) some children who do not stutter can and do exhibit BSQ profiles that suggest they are behaviorally inhibited; and (3) more than the BSQ, although it is one helpful indicator, should be used, we believe, to determine the nature of a child's temperament.

FIGURE 2.4 Clinical assessment of temperament. Graphic display of results of the 100-question *Behavior Style Questionnaire* (BSQ) with two children: (a) 3-year-9-month-old child who does not stutter (CWNS), who appears to exhibit a *behaviorally expressive* temperament, and (b) 3-year-5-month-old child who does stutter (CWS), who appears to exhibit a slow-to-warm-up, possibly *behaviorally inhibited* temperament. Each child was rated by his mother. In general, lines or bars to the right indicate less positive temperamental characteristics (e.g., gradual or difficult adaptation to stimuli), whereas bars to the left indicate more positive temperamental characteristics (e.g., quick or easy adaption to stimuli).

At the least, we suggest, the clinician should strive to obtain results from such sources as the: TCS (previously mentioned) plus the BSQ plus informal, behavioral observations by the clinicians and/or parents, in order to determine if the child relatively routinely exhibits: (1) sensitivity to novelty; (2) continued reaction to novelty long after a typical child would have adjusted and/or "moved on"; (3) consistent, sometimes exaggerated, difficulties separating from parents; (4) lessened verbal output, particularly when confronted with change, novel or stress; (5) strong, pers°istent fears of the dark, loud noises, insects, nursery school, taking a bath, and so on. Given the above cautions, after using the BSQ on approximately 20 children and the TCS with approximately 50 children, we believe that childen who stutter (when compared to children who do not stutter): (1) score higher on activity level, (2) are more gradual in their adaptation, (3) are more cautious with their first reaction, (4) are more sensitive to external stimuli, (5) have more difficulties separating from their parents, and (6) exhibit strong fears of a variety of objectively nonfearful events, for example, the dark or taking a bath. Figure 2.4 shows typical BSQ profiles for CWNS(a) and CWS(b), based on the author's experience. Again, there are CWNS who are quite behaviorally inhibited and CWS who are quite behaviorally expressive. At present, Figure 2.4 should be judged as representing the author's preliminary notions of central *group* tendencies. Individual children, both CWNS and CWS, can and will differ from these central tendencies.

Whether systematic, controlled studies will support these preliminary, informal observations will hold up is an empirical question requiring further study by independent investigators. We do believe, however, that while the surface in this area is just beginning to be scratched, in the future, the temperamental characteristics of children who stutter will be more thoroughly and objectively assessed, providing rich insights into this important psychodynamic aspect seemingly involved with the onset and development of stuttering.

Bluntly stated, the time has come for SLPs to put their data where their mouth is. If temperament *is* an important variable, which I think it is, then SLPs should begin to document its nature and relationship to stuttering. In essence, clinicians and researchers alike should begin to collect data to support our notions about how temperament interacts with stuttering in children, teenagers, and adults. We must also be very, very clear that introversion, behavioral inhibition, and/or slow-to-warm-up temperaments are *not* the exclusive domain of people who stutter. Indeed, as part of this writer's research, he has been studying children who do not stutter and has found that some children who do not stutter score some of the lowest (i.e., behaviorally inhibited, introverted, shy/sensitive, and slow-to-warm-up temperaments) scores on Oyler's TCS that he has observed.

Who Is and Who Is Not Referred for Therapy

After collecting some or all of the above information, we come to the moment of truth: does the client have a problem and if so is therapy warranted and what should be its form. Figure 2.5 shows the three possible decisions and their resulting consequences: (1) Yes, the client has a problem (i.e., client most likely to require treatment); (2) uncertain, we are uncertain if the client has a problem (i.e., client may require reevaluation); and (3) no, the client does not have a problem (i.e., client least likely to require treatment). With category

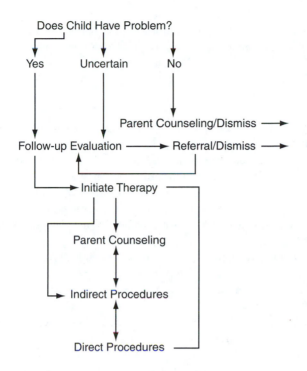

FIGURE 2.5   Diagnostic decision flowchart. A flowchart depicting the threefold diagnostic decisions—yes, no, or uncertain (an individual stutters—and the possible relation these have to management strategies. Note that therapy does not always follow a "yes" decision; a follow-up evaluation may occur first. There is nothing fixed about the number of these decisions—they could be expanded into five: yes, probably yes, uncertain, probably no, and no; or even seven: yes, probably yes, maybe yes, uncertain, maybe no, probably no, and no. Parent Counseling refers to counseling and/or information sharing about their child's problem and/or what they can do to help.

(2), in particular, we are suggesting, for many of these cases, a follow-up evaluation (we typically request such reevaluations within six months after initial assessment). This suggestion implies that some clients, particularly children, even those with obvious speech fluency concerns, may improve significantly enough within six months, simply as a result of developmental information sharing and counseling at the time of initial diagnostic, to preclude actual therapy. If, of course, the client still has a concern at the second diagnostic, then therapy is clearly recommended. However, fools can rush in where angels fear to tread! That is, the mere presence of stuttering, particularly in younger clients, is not, in and of itself, sufficient to warrant the time, energy, and expense of speech therapy until the clinician knows more about how long the person has been stuttering and the nature of the stuttering—in brief, much more about the entirety of the client's abilities and environmental interactions—and is able to observe these over a modest length of time (say three to six months). While we clearly do not want to deny services to anyone who needs them, we certainly don't want to make rushes to judgment and administer therapy to everybody who says or who others say needs help. We have an obligation to our clients to be as discriminating as possible in delivering our services, because if anyone can get them, no one really needs them.

General

We begin considering the possibility that an individual is at *high risk* for continuing to stutter when he or she exhibits stutterings, stuttered-like, or within-word disfluencies as relatively *predictable* parts of their speech; when these disfluencies *persist* over sufficiently long periods of time (no matter how cyclical their appearance may be); and when these disfluencies are *consistently* associated with certain sound-syllables, words, or speaking situations. A person may be safely considered to be a person who stutters or at high risk for becoming one when we know, with a relatively high degree of certainty, that a person will stutter when they talk (*prediction*), when they continue to do so for some time (*persistent*), and when their disfluencies regularly occur in association with observable events (*consistent*).

We must remember, however, that the terms *persistent*, *predictable*, and *consistent* (PPC), for all their soundings of definitiveness and absoluteness, are still terms whose meanings is relative to the person who has stated them. We know that we can go to extremes in stating that this or that is relative to its surrounds, that there appear to be very few or no absolutes regarding stuttering (mainly due to the rapid as well as slow changes in the state of fluency that underlie stuttering); however, we have had too many experiences with stuttering where one person's *persistent* behavior is another person's *occasional* behavior. Even in the presence of reports, particularly verbal ones based on second-hand information, that a particular person is consistently stuttering, we should proceed with caution and avoid making a rush to judgment. I am not going to advocate a see-no-evil-hear-no-evil stance, but blasting onto the scene with plans for remediating stuttering on the basis of one person's report of chronic or seemingly chronic stuttering is not particularly appropriate.

Those at Moderate Risk for Continuing Stuttering

Where the PPC criteria falls down, however, is with the person at less than "high risk" for continuing to stutter, a person who is usually, although not exclusively, a child under 10 years of age. With a child who may appear moderately "at risk" for continuing to stutter, we cannot nor should not wait until his or her stutterings become *consistently* associated with stimuli. Likewise, we may also want to begin therapeutic intervention before the child's stuttering becomes *predictable* every time the child speaks. Instead, with a person "at moderate risk" for stuttering, we must generally rely on the observation that the *frequency of stuttered disfluencies* has been *persistent* over a sufficiently long enough period of time to warrant our attention. For most children, this period of time will be between three and six months; however, for some, particularly those whose outset was associated with relatively long, fixed articulatory posturing (i.e., audible and inaudible sound prolongations of relatively long duration), this period of time may be days or weeks. Surely, as clinicians, we need and want to know, as soon as possible, whether an individual's problem is going to "fade into the sunset" with or without therapy. Such clinical knowledge, we might add, is something that all individuals who work in the field of stuttering would like to develop.

Those at Low to No Risk

A person is probably of little or no risk for continuing to stutter if his or her frequency and type of within-word disfluency has been highly variable over a three- to six-month period of time or longer, exhibits little predictability of speech fluency (may or not be disfluent when he or she talks), and appears unrelated to other events or stimuli. Of course, any person who, at one point, appears at no or low risk for stuttering can become at moderate to high risk for same, but the probability is generally low that such a change will take place. Other variables—for example, concomitant speech/language problems (e.g., Conture, Louko, & Edwards, 1993), attentional deficits (e.g., Riley & Riley, 1988), and temperamental variables (Guitar, 1997)—can also play a factor in determining whether a person is highly likely to continue stuttering. What we are trying to do here is make the point that it takes much, much more than the mere presence of stuttered-like or stuttered disfluencies in the speech of a person who stutters to determine that he or she has or will have a problem with stuttering. These decisions, while not easy, are nevertheless important if we are to improve our chances of delivering services to those people who would benefit the most from receiving them. Many times, judgments of persistency, predictability, and consistency of speech disfluency and related events involve a person-by-person decision.

TABLE 2.4   Suggested Guidelines for Diagnosing Preschool to Early Elementary School Children Most to Least Likely to Require Treatment

Presumed Likelihood that child Will Require Treatment	Total Frequency of Disfluencies	Sound Prolongation Index	Iowa Scale	Stuttering Severity Instrument	Stuttering Prediction Instrument
Most likely to require treatment	More than 10%	More than 30%	More than 3	More than 18	More than 16
May require reevaluation	6% to 10%	12% to 30%	2 to 3	12 to 18	10 to 16
Least likely to require treatment	Less than 6%	Less than 12%	Less than 2	Less than 12	Less than 10

Suggested guidelines for diagnosing preschool to early elementary school children most to least likely to require treatment, after Yaruss, LaSalle, and Conture (1998). It is very strongly suggested that several, rather than one, (in)formal test or measure be used to make such an assessment and arrive at such a diagnosis. It is further suggested that the clinician, after obtaining results from several means of observing/testing the child's speech fluency in attempts to determine whether a relatively high degree of "congruence" has been achieved among three or more observations/tests, relative to the ranges listed in this table, for each diagnostic category. If no such congruence is apparent, the clinician may want to consider: (1) other forms of testing, for example, in the home or school setting; (2) different guidelines; or (3) further evaluation, at a later date.

After Yaruss, LaSalle, & Conture, 1998, with permission.

Children

Recently, we (Yaruss, LaSalle, & Conture, 1998) provided some diagnostic data on 100 2- to 6-year-old children who are known or suspected to be at risk for stuttering. Our benchmarks for each of the above categories are given in Table 2.4. While not everyone necessarily agrees with our recommendations (see exchange between Cordes, 2000, and Yaruss, LaSalle, & Conture, 2000), we want to make clear that these benchmarks are suggestive not prescriptive. These treatment-recommendation benchmarks may be compared to the distribution of children's actual scores (Yaruss et al., Table 2) across a variety of commonly employed clinical procedures. In this way, you, the clinician, can better determine how our treatment recommendations co-concur with the type of data you and others typically collect during diagnostic assessments of preschool and early elementary school children suspected or known to be stuttering.

With children who stutter, as with adults who stutter, there seems to be no *one* behavior or test result that we use to decide on therapy or no therapy. Usually, arriving at a diagnosis as well as treatment recommendation is an additive process. That is, the more behaviors of concern we can stack up or add together, the higher the probability the child will require some form of treatment. Typically, we'll recommend therapy if we note two or more of the following: (1) the child's total frequency of disfluencies reach more than 10 percent; (2) the child exhibits sound prolongations (audible and/or inaudible) that constitute more than 30 percent of the total within-word disfluencies produced by the child; (3) the child scores 19 or higher on *Stuttering Severity Instrument*; (4) the child scores 17 or higher on *Stuttering Prediction Instrument*; (5) the child exhibits eyeball movements to the side and/or eyelid blinking during stuttering; (6) the child exhibits stuttering—stuttering clusters (e.g., "Mmmmmommy c-c-c-can I go out?") particularly if these clusters constitute 25 percent or more of the child's total disfluencies (LaSalle & Conture, 1995); and (7) the child's stuttering has been known to exist for 18 months or longer (Yairi, 1997a). Ancillary concerns that we would consider to increase the probability that treatment is warranted are: (1) frequent and/or unusual phonological processes; (2) instances of sound/syllable repetitions or sound prolongation (silent or audible) on the first mono-, bi-, or trisyllabic production of diadochokinesis tasks; (3) OMAS scores and/or QNST scores that indicate delays in speech and nonspeech neuromotor development; (4) parental speaking rates in excess of 235 words per minute; and (5) parents whose speech frequently overlaps (i.e., "simultalk") the speech of their child (see Figure 1.8a). We also note whether parents frequently use complex vocabulary/ linguistic structures that are too sophisticated for the child's level of development and frequently exhibit brief (0.5 s or 500 ms) "turn-switching" (Jaffe & Feldstein, 1970) or turn-taking pauses. Such parental behavior does (and did) not "cause" the child's stuttering; but it is quite likely that such parental communication behavior may exacerbate, aggravate, perpetuate, or worsen the child's speech disfluencies and/or make it difficult for the child to become more fluent.

Parents and Relatives of Children

Regardless of what we recommend—immediate therapy, reevaluation, or no therapy—we counsel or information-share with the parents. At the end of the diagnostic, we spend some time talking with the parents, even the parents of children who are doing nothing more than what is typical for their chronological and developmental level. We have found that with all parents, time spent at the time of the diagnostic, in counseling and information sharing regarding normal childhood development and behavior, is well spent. With some of the parents, particularly where no apparent stuttering problem exists, other concerns are the real concern, for example, inability to tell time and be punctual; inability to keep a tidy room; inability to read, write, and count; inability to be as athletic as Dad or an older brother or sister; the you-can't-sit-down syndrome, which may or may not indicate ADHD; and so forth.

Some of these parental concerns, we have observed, indicate that the parents are trying to speed of the pace of their child's developmental clock, as if they could bring about maturity and adult-like behavior in a 5-year-old! This parental concern is not helped as parents continue to "look laterally" at their relative's or neighbor's child, who is always going to do this or that earlier or better than their child. Sometimes, stuttering may be the name of what the parents say is their concern, but the real game is that they are worried that their child is "less than perfect." Le Shan (1963), in a marvelous book discussing such typical parental concerns, says much that is of assistance to clinicians and parents alike in understanding and dealing with these matters. It's not easy being a parent. There are the most minimal entrance requirements, and it is little wonder that parents become concerned. We want the parents of the child who stutters to become part of the solution rather than problem. To do that, we have to spend time information sharing and counseling parents on what stuttering is and is not, as well as those things that will facilitate change in their child's speech and related behavior.

Older Clients: Those Who Need Therapy

With older clients (say 16 years and older), the decision trilogy mentioned above—yes, uncertain, and no—becomes confounded with the notion of "benefit." Even with the older client who definitely appears to stutter, the SLP must consider whether the client can actually "benefit" from speech therapy. And if he or she can benefit, will that benefit last for more than a few weeks or months after the termination of therapy? While some might say it doesn't matter because therapy can't hurt, we would like to see more SLPs ask the question: "Can therapy, of any form, actually help?" There are no straightforward, simple answers to this question. It is a challenge to decide who might benefit from our services.

As in all matters, honesty is truly the best policy, but particularly with the older clients, who may have experienced several other forms of therapy before coming to you, it is important to lay all your cards out on the table:

> "Yes, you have a problem. And, yes, you are going to need help to change that problem. There are many things that can be done to help you become as fluent as it is possible for you to become. But let's be clear, you have been doing this for many years now. Some of these behaviors and attitudes are well-learned, well-ingrained, and established. Changing these behaviors and attitudes will neither be easy nor quick. We are happy to be your guide as you make these changes, but you'll be the one who has to do the changing. It can be done and we'll help and support you as much as we can, but you're the one who'll have to do the work . . . " And so forth.

Older Clients: Those for Whom Treatment Is Uncertain

With the uncertain category of older clients, those whose problem and need for therapy is uncertain, you'll find individuals who are fluent or relatively fluent. The presence of such individuals is an everyday reality in a college or hospital clinic. Although some of these clients appear essentially fluent, they are very concerned about their speech and their ability to interact with others, particularly through verbal communication. These individuals will frequently complain that speech is not automatic for them (like they feel it is for other people), that they have to think about speaking all the time, and that this lack of automaticity is one of the main reasons they want therapy. Sometimes, if the clinician makes careful, detailed visual and auditory observations of these individuals while they are talking, the clinician can spot or hear the brief, subtle things they seem to do to avoid, change, or stop saying particular sounds, syllables, or words—for example, the use of subtly inappropriate vocabulary. Some of these individuals have no apparent speech-language problem(s) but because they adamantly believe they have a problem, they have one! I have found that adult group therapy is beneficial for this type of client. It provides a forum to compare and contrast other problems as well as learn more about speaking and to gain more reasonable standards for fluent verbal communication. Some clients, with situation-specific fears and/or difficulties—for example, public speaking—may also benefit from groups like Toastmaster's International and, like many adult people who stutter, find the contact and colleaguality of self-help groups to be of benefit (more about self-help groups in the chapter on adults).

Those Who Appear to Stutter in Their Heads Not Their Mouths

Clinicians who have worked with children, teenagers, and adults who stutter will recognize that some individuals consider themselves to be people who stutter despite objective evidence to the contrary. These individuals are typically adults, and anyone who has clinically served these people knows the difficulties of dealing with people who are objectively fluent but who subjectively feel they stutter and that they should be considered as people who stutter (Douglas & Quarrington, 1952; Prins, 1974). These clients point out the fact that besides what we can hear and see (speech disfluencies, bodily movement, tension, and psychosocial discomfort and/or concerns), we must also consider aspects of the individual's self-concept (for lack of a better phrase) that are not as easily viewed and heard.

If an individual considers him- or herself to be a person who stutters, despite what the person sounds or looks like when they talk, this should not be ignored by the speech-language pathologist. In a way, these clients are like those clients Daly (1988) describes who, after a period of therapy, are " . . . fluent in the mouth but not the head." Many times, careful observation by the SLP of the so-called "fluent" person who stutters will reveal a wide variety of subtle behavior that the person is producing to get the sound or word out, to avoid saying the word, to get the listener to fill in or complete the utterance, or to circumlocute the situation, sound, or word. When asked, these people, like their more obviously disfluent peers, seem to universally complain that speech is a chore, that it is not automatic ("like everyone else"), and that they have to spend too much time thinking about *how* they are going to say something rather than *what* they are going to say (we will discuss these concerns in some detail in Chapter 5). Sometimes, if brought into a group of other people who stutter, they will express feelings of uneasiness or guilt that they "don't stutter as much as the rest of group" and that they are wasting or taking up the group's time with their problem, which is real to them while nearly invisible to external observers. Although some of these people also have other concerns, suffice it to say at this point that the SLP should be able to assess the nonobservable as well as the observable (particularly the *subtly* observable) in order to determine who is and who is not a person who stutters.

Older Clients: Those Who Have Problems Other Than Stuttering

A third category of older clients (and this also applies to younger clients as well) may have a problem, but it is neither stuttering nor other speech-language production concerns. Their problem may be speech apraxia, dialectical speech and language usage, psychoneurotic concerns, employment concerns, and so forth. We should not dismiss these other concerns out of hand but instead make the proper referrals to agencies and professionals more equipped and trained to deal with them. Obviously, building up a pool of agencies and professionals to whom you can make such referrals takes time, effort, and experimentation, but there is no way we can overestimate the importance of making appropriate referrals to agencies that can help your client with problems that are outside your professional purview and expertise.

Some Parting Thoughts

Thus, we can see that for both the child and the adult who stutter, deciding who is a person who stutters, whether the person, once labeled a stutterer, needs therapy, and what form the therapy should take is not a black-and-white decision. There appear to be three points on the diagnostic continuum for dealing with this challenge: (1) few clients receive therapy: recommending therapy for very few clients, instead concentrating on thorough information sharing at the time of evaluation where the client and associates are essentially told not to be concerned, that many "normally fluent" people do the same thing, and so on; (2) some clients receive therapy: recommending therapy on the basis of a differential diagnosis whereby a certain percent receive therapy immediately, another percent is reevaluated until it becomes clear whether therapy is appropriate, and another percent receives no therapy; and (3) all clients receive therapy: recommending therapy on the basis that it is good, can do little harm, and for some clients acts as a preventive measure. We are advocating the middle position—(2) some clients receive therapy—since it is our experience that not infrequently there is the marginal situation where therapy may or may not be of assistance. Furthermore, we believe that if anyone and everyone can get our services, then no one actually needs them, a situation that is clearly not the case.

We would like to see, particularly for the marginal client, more recommendations for "trial therapy" of three to six weeks in duration to see if remediation has a chance of being beneficial. Particularly with children, who are constantly changing along so many different dimensions, therapy immediately after the diagnostic may have little chance of being successful, but perhaps in three to six months it might be more effective. However, to make these sorts of decisions the SLP must have conducted a thorough evaluation. Indeed, remediation presupposes a thorough evaluation, and only by so doing can the SLP understand and weigh all factors in coming to an informed decision for or against therapy.

In this chapter we have tried to explore and share with you some of these factors, their relative importance to the evaluation of stuttering, and how they may influence our decision about whether therapy is needed and if so what kind. In subsequent chapters we'll discuss the remediation of stuttering. We hope that the reader will come to better appreciate how our regimens for remediation flow or follow from our approaches to evaluation. We take the first step down the road to remediating stuttering when at the beginning of the diagnostic we ask our client or his or her associates "What can we do to help you?"

We should not view evaluation as a messy detail that must be gotten through prior to the good stuff called therapy. Rather, the diagnostic is part of therapy, the investigatory part, but a part nonetheless. To begin therapy with little or no attempt to evaluate is like setting out to sea without knowing a great deal about the waters upon which you are going to be sailing, perhaps like the captain of the Titanic. Better, as the Boy Scouts would say, to "Be prepared." In particular, letting information cloud our judgment, letting facts challenge our ideas, is the sum and substance of the diagnostician who maneuvers according to the circumstances of the individual in front of them rather than follow the sweet refrain of ideas played by a Pied Piper ideologue.

Summary

If we assume that stuttering is a multidimensional problem, then we can also reasonably assume, in an ideal world, that the assessment and evaluation of stuttering is multidimensional. Unfortunately, however, our assessments of stuttering are more often unidimensional than they are multidimensional. In essence, in focusing on the client's frequency, duration, type, severity, and so on of speech (dis)fluency, we sometimes lose sight of the fact that concomitant issues—for example, disruptions of syntactic, semantic, phonologic, and motoric processes—significantly contribute to the person's problem. Indeed, too often we are lured away from such consideration by a tunnel-vision view of stuttering, turning what should be multidimensional considerations into a unidimensional focusing on speech disfluency, and only speech disfluency! As we have said before in this space, the fact that an individual is or is *suspected* of being a person who stutters should *not* distract the clinician from considering other speech, behavior, psychological, developmental, and so on behaviors and their possible contributing role to stuttering and/or successful recovery from stuttering. For example, even the most appropriate, correctly and carefully applied treatment procedures will not "make" someone more normally disfluent if during the application of such treatment, the person is inattentive 50 to 75 percent of the time!

Starting from the premise that the nature of the client's problem oftentimes dictates the nature of procedures used to remediate the problem, it is trite, but nonetheless true, to say that evaluation is the first stage of treatment and should be neither casually nor quickly undertaken. Such assessment and evaluation of stuttering typically involves two general procedures: (1) interview of client and associates regarding attitudes, feelings, beliefs, and history concerning the problem and related matters—for example, familial history of stuttering; time since onset of stuttering; nature of professional and/or parental "assistance" the client may have already received; academic development, progress, and status; and so forth—and (2) objective and subjective assessment of speech fluency and related behavior—for example, frequency, type, duration, severity of stuttering (if at all possible, assessed in several speaking situations); speaking rate as well as audiometric issues such as middle ear problems; articulation/phonological development; pragmatic use of language; expressive and receptive syntactic and semantic abilities; gross and fine motor skills for speech and nonspeech behaviors; voice quality; and so forth. Important ancillary issues should also be assessed (according to the dictates of each individual case)—for example, persistent and frequent inattention, impulsivity or hyperactivity (suggesting attention deficit disorder and a possible referral to a clinical psychologist), slow-to-warm-up and/or behaviorally inhibited temperamental characteristics, difficulties with academic achievement and progress, especially reading (if reading materials are to be used during treatment), cognitive abilities, psychosocial adjustment, and so forth.

While most clinicians realize and attempt to carefully interview parents, far less often do we find clinicians observing the speech and language behavior of parents. As we have shown (Figure 1.8), certain parental behaviors are associated with the stuttering severity of children's stuttering. Again, such association does not imply causation, but it may suggest that some parental communicative behaviors may exacerbate and/or maintain a child's already existing stuttering problem. At the least, therefore, clinicians should try to assess the parents' speaking rate (particularly in relationship to that of their child's), their tendency to talk for or over the child, the routine length and complexity of the parents' utterances when conversing with their children, the length of time between the end of a child's utterance and the beginning of the parent's, the parents' tendency to mono- rather than dialogue, and the like. If the SLP is attempting to help a child be more patient and wait when he or she has forgotten a particular word or how to say same, it will not help if that child routinely re-enters a home environment where parents rush the child to talk, interrupt the child during his or her utterance, are explicitly or implicitly impatient and corrective of any pauses or speaking errors made by the child during communication, and so forth. The only way to assess such parental behaviors, in this writer's opinion and experience, is to assess them! This can be accomplished by the clinician observing 300 to 500 words spoken by the child during a 15 to 30 minute parent–child conversation. Obviously, of course, the more such samples of parent–child conversations, obtained across as many different situations as possible, the more stable, at least in theory, the SLP's estimate of the child's central tendency of speech (dis)fluency during conversational speech.

Although during assessment, we want to keep in mind what stuttering is and/or what may be importantly related to it, we also want to keep in mind what stuttering is not. Stuttering is *typically* not a problem of speech intelligibility, cognitive problems, marked psychological disturbance or voice quality. Further, despite parental feelings to contrary, we have little or no evidence that parents *cause* stuttering. This is not to suggest that parents, or any other adult or even child listener, do not do things to *exacerbate* or maintain a child's speech disfluencies—for example, parents who persistently and frequently interrupt the child as he or she begins to speak. While the jury is still out whether the *planning for* versus *execution of* speech-language production is more important to the onset and development of stuttering, it is highly likely that one or both somehow contribute to instances of stuttering. Therefore, during the diagnostic for stuttering, the clinician should be able to assess and evaluate, as best possible, the client's abilities that seem to be related to the planning and execution of speech–language production. For example, when assessing a client's abilities that relate to the *planning* of speech–language production, the clinician might employ the *Patterned Elicitation Syntax Test* (PEST; Young & Perachio, 1993) or the *Expressive Vocabulary Test* (EVT; Williams, 1997) to assess syntactic and semantic abilities, respectively. Likewise, when trying to assess abilities that may relate to rapid and/or correct *execution* of speech production, the clinician might assess oral and/or speech diadochokinesis as well as compare the child's rate of repetitive nonsense syllables to that of the child's syllable rate during conversational speech (see Figure 1.5b, this text). And it should not be assumed that just because the client is an adult who stutters that these concerns with planning and execution of speech–language production are of no concern. For example, of two adults who stutter whom this author recently assessed (both college-educated and gainfully employed), one had a clinically significant reduction in receptive and expressive vocabulary while the other scored only at the 30th to 40th percentile rank on these tests, even though both adults' phonology as well as syntactic abilities were in upper ends of normal limits for their ages!

In brief, assessment and evaluation of stuttering often requires the clinician to examine other problems—for example, delayed phonological development—that may co-occur with stuttering and require significant adjustment to therapy. This means, therefore, that the clinician must simultaneously take several different perspectives on stuttering to ensure the most complete understanding and hence develop the most appropriate treatment. Such multifaceted observations should, in turn, be developed into a written document (e.g., Appendix C provides an example of such documentation) that provides the foundation upon which any treatment plan is erected. From initial greeting of the client to final signature on the written diagnostic report, assessment and evaluation should be viewed by the clinician as not only a vehicle to gather and disseminate knowledge, but as a means to *orient* and *educate* the client and the client's family about the clinician's philosophy of approach to treatment.

CHAPTER

3

Remediation: Children Who Stutter

Stuttering Is a Disorder of Childhood

Between the sometimes dark of adolescence and the relative light of infancy lies childhood. During this period of dependence, day-care centers, and dolls, the roots of stuttering grow and, for some, take a firm hold. In fact, the onset of stuttering is often reported at about the time of one classic childhood milestone: switching from a single-word vocabulary to noun + verb construction. Perhaps, for these reasons and more, stuttering is appropriately considered a disorder of childhood (Bloodstein, 1995).

In fact, stuttering not only begins, for most individuals, during the early years of childhood development, but the number of individuals who continue to stutter into their teenage years and beyond drops off by 50 percent or more (Ingham, 1985; Sheehan & Martyn, 1970). Indeed, recent research (Yairi & Ambrose, 1992; Yairi et al., 1993) shows that within the first two years of the onset of stuttering, recovery rates for children range between 65 percent and 75 percent, within as many as 85 percent of children recovering within the next several years. This suggests that about four out of five (about 85%) of those children who begin to stutter recover sometime in childhood. Why some children recover from stuttering and some do not goes well beyond the scope of the present chapter, but the possibility for recovery must always be considered when we first diagnose and then agree to treat a child for stuttering. At the least, it would seem, our treatment should facilitate, speed up, and support recovery from stuttering.

These facts, as well as common sense, would seem to suggest that much of our research and remedial efforts with stuttering should be directed toward children who stutter; however, common sense is not all that common both among clients and clinicians.

The Clinician

In our zeal to learn the technical-professional and interpersonal skills of a speech–language pathologist, we often fail to examine who we are and what we need to be in order to assess and treat people with communication disorders. Such factors as intelligence, maturity, and stability are all germane, but by themselves they do not automatically translate into making someone a skilled SLP. I mean, we can hope that the pilot of the next plane we fly is intelligent, mature, and stable. But do we want him or her to assess and treat people who stutter? Do we want you to fly the airplane? No, there is obviously more, much more, to being a successful clinician. It behooves us, therefore, before we get into the nitty gritty of treatment, to examine some of the characteristics of effective clinicians.

Six Characteristics of Successful Clinicians

In essence, besides our specific approach to the evaluation and remediation of stuttering, we need to understand something about the SLP's knowledge, motivation, and personal characteristics as they pertain to clinical involvement with people who stutter and their associates. Van Riper (1975) described three personal characteristics that successful clinicians appear to possess: accurate empathy, nonpossessive warmth, and genuineness (see Appendix B for more general discussion of clinician concerns and characteristics). We would like to add three of our own: the ability to listen, the ability to adjust to changing circumstances ("maneuver according to circumstances"), and the ability to make quick, accurate behavioral observations.

Briefly, *empathy* relates to our ability to understand or imagine how other individuals feel about themselves and events that surround them. It is the ability to "walk a mile in my shoes," to view events as others do, that successful clinicians make so apparent. Being able to take the perspective of the other person is key to understanding how he or she is reacting and coping with his or her circumstances. The second characteristic, *warmth*, is something we all feel, to greater or lesser degrees, in our daily interactions with people; it is another feature that successful clinicians seem to exude and establish in their clinical relations. Warmth relates to our ability to imply or make explicit our desire to help our clients, to make them know we care and that we think they are O.K. (perhaps, best done when we ourselves can say, "I'm O.K.—You're O.K." [Harris, 1967]). The third characteristic, *genuineness*, relates to the clinicians' openness, the ability to expose their unique human traits, and be, in essence, themselves. It is difficult to like your clients when you demonstrate in one way or another that you do not like yourself (before you love others, first you have to love yourself). Clients don't expect a superhero for a clinician, but they do expect clinicians to be honest and straightforward with them regarding their assets and liabilities.

The fourth characteristic, *listening*, is very much related to the first (empathy). Listening involves attending and responding to the denotative aspects of communication but even more, the connotative as well—the message behind the message, the message that is written between as well as on the lines. Clients want a clinician who can listen to them, a clinician who can attend and respond to the subtleties of their verbal and nonverbal communication. If a client feels that there is "no use talking when nobody is listening," there is little chance that therapy will be successful. The fifth characteristic, the ability to *adjust* or be *flexible* ("maneuver according to circumstances"), is required in order to deal with the dynamics of the constantly changing circumstances of therapy. A clinician can be well prepared, like a coach with a game plan; but within minutes after therapy begins (or shortly after the game begins), circumstances change and the clinician must adjust (the coach must scrap the game plan). For example, the clinician must adjust and be flexible when the client is not feeling well, the client has regressed, the client hasn't done his or her homework, the client doesn't understand or can't seem to deal with today's lesson plan, the therapy plan is obviously inappropriate, and so forth. These are situations requiring a clinician to work smarter not harder. Successful clinicians roll with the punches and go where the client takes them. Unsuccessful clinicians, to paraphrase an old proverb, are a bit like swimmers who continue to fight their way upstream, seemingly expecting that at any moment the river will change direction for them. In short, in my opinion, the inflexible clinician is the unsuccessful clinician. The sixth characteristic, *quick, accurate behavioral observations*, is a attribute/skill that definitely improves with age but only if, as the person ages, he or she tries to improve the skill (and, going along with these observational skills is the need to collect and document our observations; see Olswang & Bain, 1994, for a good overview of data collection for purposes of monitoring the client's behavior)! The clinician who is a keen observer of behavior is able to readily "ballpark" the client's stuttering frequency, duration, most common disfluency type, and severity. This skill comes from recognizing the need to be accurate but quick in observing and assessing the client and the client's behavior. While few clinicians can be like the observant Sherlock Holmes or Columbo (the latter, of course, of TV and the former of novel fame), many more could be far better at observing what is in front of them if they would apply themselves more and concentrate their efforts on learning how to recognize behavior. All too often, clinicians, particularly beginning clinicians, focus on "what to do" rather than on "what to see." The successful clinician recognizes that the slowing down, getting prepared "silences" before speech initiation are part of the stutterings of the person who stutters; the unsuccessful clinician only understands that the client appears "nervous."

Certainly, other attributes exist that are correlated with successful clinical practice. For example, clear and consistent charting of observations, for example, through the use of such devices as the so-called SOAP notes, where the clinician daily/weekly charts his or her subjective (S), objective (O), assessment (A), and plan (P) impressions, observations, and goals. The above six attributes seem to among the most common we've observed exhibited by those clinicians we think are successful. While it is not the purpose of this book to help clinicians develop the above six attributes and skills, it does seem appropriate to spend some time discussing how some of these clinician skills interact with the clinical process.

Problem-Specific Empathy

Of the three personal characteristics of a successful therapist who treats stuttering, the one that seems the biggest challenge for normally fluent SLPs to obtain is that of empathy. Here I refer to problem-specific empathy: what it physically feels like to actually stutter and to be a person who stutters (on that note, Jezer's, 1997 book is a wonderful introduction for anyone with interest in knowing what it is like to stutter and be a person who stutters). This is a particularly challenging attribute for the normally fluent SLP to develop, but if the SLP has decent general empathetic listening skills and is a keen behavioral observer, problem-specific empathy can be readily developed.

The old classroom practice of having undergraduates go out and stutter openly for a day or two in front of ten different strangers was a small step in the direction of developing this problem-specific empathy. We can, to greater or lesser degrees, empathize with people who have various problems that we do not have ourselves. However, as SLPs, we are not called upon to professionally help these various people; instead, it is our responsibility to assist people (people who stutter, in this case) who feel that they are unable to move forward when speaking. How do you, as a normally fluent speaker, get the feeling of what it is like to be "stuck" when you talk? Clearly, the ideal way to appreciate this feeling is by doing it yourself; however, this is not to suggest that people who stutter are the only ones who can do stuttering therapy (any more than it says that heart attack victims make the best cardiovascular surgeons or bank robbers the best criminal lawyers). What we are saying, though, is that normally fluent speakers must realize that problem-specific empathy is not going to "happen" to them (normally fluent speakers with problem-specific empathy for stuttering are made not born). They will have to work diligently to grasp some of the behaviors, feelings, and thoughts that people who stutter experience when they stutter.

I, therefore, in attempt to develop and refine my problem-specific empathy, frequently ask the client who stutters (in as kind, gentle, and supportive fashion as possible): "Tell me what it feels like to you—in your own words—to stutter. Do you feel terror? embarrassment? anger? fear? pain? fright? hurt? frustration? a numb sensation? Do you feel a tightness in your chest? your throat? your mouth? Is there anything else you do, for example, lift weights, hold your breath, try to open a hard-to-open jar top, that makes you feel the same sort of tightness or constriction in your upper torso and neck? Is it anything like having a close accident in your car? Is it anything like suddenly touching a hot stove burner you thought was off (demonstrating the quick pulling back of the hand/arm and the quick, forced inspiration of breath)? Do you ever want to run out of the room and hide? Do you wish that speech was more 'automatic,' like it seems to be with your friends?" and so forth.

In this way, over the years, asking these questions of a number of people who stutter, I have gained a measure of appreciation for the feelings of individuals when they stutter. I say *measure* because truly no one can totally understand what it feels like to be someone else. We can come close to such understanding, we can get a pretty decent idea, but we never fully know, and we should know when we don't know. Indeed, one of the hallmarks of clinicians who fail is that they don't know that they don't know. They simply don't comprehend that their listening skills are less than they should be, that their general as well as problem-specific empathy is less than ideal. Far better that they can't do these things but at least know that they can't do these things! The latter individual will at least attempt to make some effort to learn what they don't know.

An Analogy to Help with Empathy.   One way we have found that seems to closely describe the feelings that people who stutter experience when they stutter is to analogize it to the momentary panic, terror, and fear people encounter when they pull back from a ledge or high place from which they almost fell. During the physical maneuver back from the ledge, people attend to emotional elements and have little awareness of what they did that got them safely back from the edge. We've discussed this before and described it as a *mental whiteout*. Ironically, this whiteout is the worst time for people who stutter to objectively concentrate on what they are doing that interferes with their speech production. Rather, they are trying to "blast through" the sound, syllable, or word, full speed ahead and damn the torpedoes! Like verbal dynamite, they try to blast through the feeling of being stuck. At this point in time, they aren't analytical or objective, they are subjective, they want out of the instant of stuttering, by whatever means possible! However, it is precisely at this very point in time—that is, during the whiteout—that we need to help them more objectively concentrate on their behavior. We try such analogies out on our clients—and invite them to develop their own—and listen to what they say. We are using these analogies in attempts, albeit a bit artificial, to "walk a mile in their shoes."

Clinical Art Interacts with Clinical Science.   On our better days, when we are hitting on all eight cylinders, we try to be as honest with our clients as possible when they ask us questions about stuttering. We try to make it clear that we don't totally understand everything about stuttering (an example of genuineness) but also try to make clear that we really want to know about the clients' feelings so we can understand their problem and help clients help themselves (an example of warmth). We hear the client out when discussing a routine problem he has with ordering coffee at a diner (an example of listening) and essentially scrap large parts of our lesson plan, trying to help the client problem solve a situation—ordering a cup of coffee—that, although it seems relatively trivial, is of major daily consequence for the client (an example of flexibility).

It should be clear, however, that the aforementioned personal characteristics and skills are necessary but not sufficient for successful therapy. As Van Riper (1975) mentioned in some detail, the personal characteristics of the SLPs who work with people who stutter must be built upon a solid foundation of knowledge about stuttering and then refined through a series of experiences with people who stutter. What good, for example, is it to be the most genuine, warm and empathetic SLP alive and then turn around and teach the person who stutters to take a deep breath and hold it for two seconds each and every time he talks? Our technical-professional and interpersonal skills are like yin and yang, interweaving together in the whole we refer to as our "clinical abilities."

Perhaps, describing the clinician's personal characteristics and skills is just another way of talking about the *art* of stuttering therapy. Likewise, describing the clinician's knowledge of and experience with stuttering is simply another means of discussing the *science* of stuttering therapy. When the art and science of stuttering therapy are viewed from this perspective, it is a bit easier to see that each is necessary, but only taken together are they sufficient for successful remediation of stuttering. All the warmth, empathy, and listening skills in the world won't help the clinician who doesn't understand what stuttering is about; conversely, all the knowledge in the world about stuttering won't help the clinician remediating stuttering who doesn't understand that he or she is dealing with humans not automatons.

Clinician/Client Reluctance to Deal with Childhood Stuttering

First, speech-language pathologists, until the past ten years or so, have directed much of their research attention to adults (cf. Conture 1987b for further discussion of this topic). While there are numerous reasons for this, one major reason is that adults who stutter are simply more cooperative and can participate in more complicated studies than young children. A second reason is that one can be fairly certain that a 20-year-old with a history of ten to fifteen years of stuttering *is* a person who stutters. However, it is far less clear that a 4-year-old with a six-month history is or will become a person who stutters. And finally, the caution that parents shouldn't openly discuss or call undue attention to the child's disfluent speech left many SLPs very hesitant to rush in where angels apparently were afraid of treading.

Second, the clients themselves may certainly be reluctant as well. We daresay that when the reader was 3, 4, or 5 years old, the last place on earth he or she wanted to spend a sunny afternoon was in a clinician's office! Playing was next to godliness for all of us as children, and "working on our speech" was not particularly high on our priority list. Further, while adults who stutter generally seek out our services on their own, children are typically brought by their parents. Indeed, the problem is generally a problem for the parents long before it is a concern for the child. So, it is not surprising that some young children who stutter are eager and ready for speech therapy, while others hang back and appear to resist the SLP's every effort. Some of these youngsters appear receptive to our therapeutic efforts and readily make and implement necessary change, while others appear uncertain and confused about almost everything that goes on in therapy. Likewise, some children who stutter easily leave mom and dad and proceed into the therapy room, while others kick and scream as if being led to the gallows! It is no small wonder, therefore, that beginning clinicians encountering such experiences with children who stutter are less than eager to repeat the experience and may be more comfortable with the relative cooperation of older clients, who at least seem more motivated than the average 4-year-old to sit down and work. However, children who stutter and their families can and should be helped, even though understanding the dynamics of which children who stutter are helpable, motivated, and able to benefit from speech and language remediation is as complicated as it is with older individuals who stutter.

Knowing Literature Pertinent to Children Who Stutter

SLPs who manage young children should be aware of literature specifically addressed to remediation of young children who stutter (e.g., Ainsworth & Fraser, 1988; Conture, 1982; Conture & Caruso, 1987; Conture & Melnick, 1999; Cooper, 1978, 1979; Guitar, 1984, 1997, 1998; Kelly & Conture, 1991; Luper, 1982; Luper & Mulder, 1964; Onslow & Packman, 1999; Rustin, 1987; Rustin, Botterill & Kelman, 1996; Van Riper, 1973; Wall & Myers, 1995; Williams, 1971; Zwitman, 1978). Likewise, the SLP should be aware of and be prepared to share with parents the publications and videos that explain stuttering and what can be done about it that are specifically addressed to parents (Ainsworth & Fraser, 1988; Conture, 1994; Conture & Fraser, 1989; Conture, Guitar, & Fraser, 1997; Cooper, 1979; Guitar & Conture, 1988; Johnson, 1946). These latter publications and videos can be given to parents to elaborate upon, reinforce, and clarify points made by the speech-language pathologist in counseling sessions. Of course, such publications and videos are not always completely read, viewed, or understood by the parents, but with the SLP's encouragement and guidance, as well as further or repeated explanation and answering of questions, parents can be helped to gain valuable insights from reading this material. Whatever the case, we have found that the SLP should be thoroughly familiar with the contents of these self-help publications—these publications should *never* be handed out until read by the SLP—and the SLP should be ready and willing to help parents grasp, critique, as well as implement their contents.

Similarly, since many children who stutter will be initially assessed and/or referred by the family doctor or pediatrician (see Yairi & Carrico, 1992 for survey of pediatricians' attitudes/practices regarding childhood stuttering). Thus, the SLP should be aware of articles on stuttering published in medical journals (Conture, 1982; Cooper, 1980; Guitar, 1988) as well as literature regarding stuttering specifically addressed to physicians (Guitar & Conture, 1991). The SLP can cite these medical journal publications when interacting with pediatricians or family practitioners, and the contents of these publications can provide a basis for informed discussion between the SLP and the physician.

Remediating Children May Mean Involvement with Their Parents

Over forty years ago, Johnson and associates (1959) made the well-known statement that ". . . the problem [i.e., stuttering] involves an interaction of at least two persons, a speaker and listener. At the moment of onset of the problem the speaker is typically a child . . . and the listener is nearly always one of the child's parents, usually the mother" (p. 236). Thus, while perhaps obvious, another reason that remediating stuttering in children differs from remediating stuttering in adults is that the SLP will many times have or want to deal with the child's parents (see Conture, Louko, & Edwards, 1993; Conture & Melnick, 1999; Kelly & Conture, 1991; Louko et al., 1999). And parents, like their children, come in a variety of sizes and shapes, and their personal idiosyncrasies will influence therapeutic success. To make the situation even more challenging, parents are often unclear regarding their role in remediating young people who stutter; some parents see little if any purpose being served by their involvement (for example, a mother might say "Bobby is the one with the problem not me"). Parents themselves, of course, are *not* the only problem; sometimes the SLP is responsible for unduly engendering guilt, concern, or confusion in parents regarding their contributions to their child's speech and language problems. Parents of children who stutter need support, encouragement, and advice on ways to explore and make changes that will facilitate their child's speech fluency. What they don't need are additional lectures, sermons, reprimands, and chastisements for past and present, real and imagined transgressions against their children—many of them already feel bad enough—they don't need our help to feel any worse (see Gregory & Gregory, 1999 for a good overview of basic issues to consider when counseling children who stutter and their parents).

Le Shan (1963) discusses the role of parental guilt in the upbringing of children, and Le Shan's thoughts are well worth reading by SLPs who may need to consider parental guilt and what should and should not be done about it. While the SLP will strive to do nothing to increase and everything to decrease parental guilt regarding their child's stuttering, the SLP will need to recognize that in many cases all the good that is done in therapy can be offset, in a relatively short time, by parents who cannot or will not understand their role in their child's speech and language development. This does not imply that the child's parents *cause* stuttering but that some of the things they do may be *maintaining*, *perpetuating*, *aggravating*, or *exacerbating* the child's problem.

Variables That Initiate Versus Exacerbate Stuttering. In this writer's opinion, no distinction could be more important, in terms of theory and treatment, than that between variables that *initiate* versus *exacerbate* stuttering. For example, evidence mounts that perfectionistic, highly reactive, behaviorally inhibited, and the like temperamental characteristics are often observed in children who stutter (Oyler, 1996a, 1996b; Oyler & Ramig, 1995); however, it is just as clear that such characteristics also occur in normally fluent children (e.g., Kagan, 1994). Therefore, if such temperamental variables do play a role in stuttering, they must exacerbate or maintain the duration and nature of as well as associated reactions to instances of stuttering rather than initiate stuttering. Why? Well, these behaviorally inhibited temperamental characteristics are thought to occur in 15 to 20 percent of children; therefore, if these characteristics initiated or caused stuttering, the prevalence of stuttering would be far greater than the approximately 1 percent typically reported in the population (see Bloodstein, 1995, Tables 3 and 4).

Talking to Parents About the Cause of Stuttering

Their Own Behavior as Causal Versus Maintaining Agent   The SLP wants the parent as an ally not a foe in the fight to improve the child's fluency. As the above discussion suggests, one of the better ways to make an enemy out of the parent is to explicitly or implicitly indicate that the parents *cause* their child's stuttering. Once this is done, the war is generally lost before the first battle has even begun.

Again, the SLP should help the parents understand the difference between agents (behaviors, factors, or variables) that may *cause* versus *maintain* stuttering. This is no intellectual shell game—there is a difference. To begin, we tell the parents, no one knows what *causes* stuttering. We may discuss some of the possible causes but repeatedly explain that no one can be sure, with their child, which one, if any, of these possibilities applies. However, we go on to explain that there appear to be a variety of things that parents do that may contribute to a child's speaking difficulties once they begin and that these *maintaining* (or aggravating, contributing, or perpetuating) factors may need to be explored and possibly changed. One means we use to explain these concepts to parents is something we call the *knife and salt analogy* (Figure 3.1). The knife blade is the *cause* of wound, while the salt rubbed in the wound *aggravates* or *contributes* to the discomfort. The salt may hurt, but it didn't cause the wound. The knife is the reason for the wound and, as we say to parents, we are not sure what knife caused their child to stutter, but we do have some information about the types of salt that may be perpetuating the problem. Likewise, if the child falls out of the tree and breaks his or her leg, it's the fall that broke the leg. However, if the child comes to the parent, noticeably limping and complaining of severe pain in the leg and the parent encourages the child to "run it off" in a quick game of touch football rather than drive the child to the nearest emergency room for physician consultation, the parent has exacerbated the child's problem, perhaps even worsening the initial break in the leg bone.

Nature Versus Nurture.   Very much related to parents' concern that they, by something they did, "caused" their child to stutter is the issue of inheritance. It has become increasingly clear (e.g., Ambrose et al., 1997; Cox, 1988; Felsenfeld, 1997; Kidd, 1983) that genetics plays some sort of as yet imprecisely defined role in stuttering. However, if, for some people who stutter, stuttering is "inherited," it does not happen in a straightforward Mendelian genetic way as with eye or hair color or height. Furthermore, if 50 percent of the

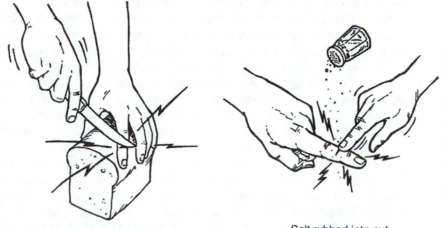

Knife **causes** cut and pain

Salt rubbed into cut
maintains the pain

FIGURE 3.1. Knife and salt analogy. Here the knife originally caused the cut and pain while salt rubbed into the cut maintains the pain. Just as the child's abilities may originally cause too frequent production of within-word disfluencies, environmental issues (for example, parents who expect and demand quick, precise and mature speech from a 4-year-old) may maintain or aggravate the child's speech disfluencies.

relatives of people who stutter also stutter, this means that 50 percent of the relatives don't! Perhaps, what is inherited is not only or even necessarily an "anomalous speech and language system" (e.g., Guitar, 1998) but temperament. That is, temperament is often described as *inherited* personality traits that appear early in life (e.g., Goldsmith et al., 1987). Whether partially or completely inherited, temperament is clearly influenced by, and malleable to, environmental variables. And if the environment influences a supposedly inherited variable like temperament, why couldn't the environment influence stuttering, whether it is partially or completely inherited? Indeed, as we have said elsewhere (Conture & Zebrowski, 1992): "[I]f children and their behavior are *immutable* to the influences and behaviors of their parents, why should we, as SLPs, believe that these same children and their behavior are *mutable* to our therapeutic administrations?" (p. 127). Clearly, therefore, environmental or nongenetic factors must play a role (Cox, 1988), if only a partial one, and it will be some time before we know the relative contributions nature and nurture make to the onset, development, and perpetuation of stuttering for people who stutter as a group as well as for any one individual person who stutters.

Indeed, knowing that their child may be predisposed to react to psychosocial or communicative stress by ceasing or reiterating speech sound production (that is, stuttering) should make the parents work all the harder to minimize those elements in their interactions with the child that may be contributing to their child's tendency to stutter. The possibility that a child is predisposed to stutter should not mean that the parents and SLP must throw up their hands, give in and "let nature take its course"! For example, let's assume that what is inherited is a generally slow-to-develop system for fluent speech production. Knowing this, the parents can be more supportive of and tolerant for the longer-than-normal time it will take their child to reach fully mature speech production. Whatever the case, the SLP should be prepared to discuss with the parents the possibility that genetics plays a role in stuttering (and at this point in our knowledge this is mainly a strong possibility, not an absolute certainty) and present evidence that would support and refute such a possibility. The outcome of such a discussion should neither panic the parents into having tubular ligations or vasectomies, nor should it absolve them from their responsibilities to change behaviors of their own that may be exacerbating their child's problem.

While lay people may believe that stuttering has either a nature *or* nurture cause, the SLP should realize that the probability is much greater that nature *interacts* with nurture to cause and perpetuate the problem. The SLP should also realize that predispositions to behave in a certain way do not mean that such behavior *cannot* be mitigated or modified or that the child is preordained to behave that way for life. Furthermore, many times, by the time the SLP meets the child who stutters, the causal agents have long since disappeared— instead, what probably remains are a host of perpetuating events that are now much more salient to the child's remediation. It is the SLP's job to help the parent focus on the present and future while understanding, but not unduly dwelling on, the past.

Parents Generally Want to Do the Right Thing

Shortly, we are going to discuss our approach to remediating stuttering in young children. Some of this approach, as will be seen, involves talking and working with parents. Because of this, some preliminary words are in order. Previously, we have discussed the issue of parental attitudes and behavior as *causal* versus *exacerbating* factors, and we won't reiterate that discussion in this space. However, we do want to stress that it is our experience, despite the impression one gets from reading the daily newspaper, that the vast majority of parents love their children. Most parents care about and want to do the right thing by their child, but sometimes they just don't know how to go about doing it. For the most part, parents' *intentions* are excellent—it is just their *methods* that need modification.

Parents, like all of us, want to do the right thing; and with our expressed respect, support, and a little guidance, they can be helped to do more and more of the right things for their child and themselves. Parents need respect and support for their attempts to understand and deal with their children, not reprimands, lectures, and threats. Some parents will take longer than others to see the error of their ways, but few will cooperate if they feel they aren't being treated with respect or are being told that their intentions are all wrong. Just like their children, parents respond best when it is their *behavior* rather than *themselves* that is being critiqued.

Therapy

When to Start, How Long, and How Often

Once the clinician decides that the child has a stuttering problem or a high probability for developing one *and* that the child needs therapy, the clinician must decide about the nature of the therapeutic intervention. Bound up in this latter decision are three nitty-gritty questions: (1) When should therapy start? (2) How long will it take? and (3) How often per week? Unfortunately, there are, at least to this writer's knowledge, no fixed guidelines to help the clinician decide.

Starting therapy with preschool and school-age children generally involves some compromise between the parents' urgency to begin therapy yesterday and the clinician's ability and/or willingness to begin immediately. It must be remembered that many times the parents have, for one reason or another, waited six, twelve, twenty-four months and (many times) even longer to bring the child in for services. Thus, in many of these cases an additional wait of one to six months is probably going to be of little consequence. Reevaluating *prior* to the start of therapy is many times a viable alternative. And, we hasten to point out, reevaluation does not preclude the clinician from talking with the parents in some detail (at the time of initial evaluation or during subsequent phone calls) about the child's problem, things parents can do at home to help, things they might change that would help their child, providing the parents with appropriate literature, and so forth.

Suggested Guidelines

Beginning Therapy with Young Children. In Yaruss, LaSalle, and Conture (1998) we provided a number of guidelines for deciding whether treatment is warranted. Table 2.6 described these guidelines. As mentioned above, we would suggest that if the child meets three or more of the criteria we describe in the "most likely to require treatment" category, he or she would seem to be a likely candidate for treatment (e.g., the child exhibits at least 12% total disfluencies, at least 40% of stutterings are sound prolongations [sound prolongation index], and their SSI score is at least 22). To these suggestions we would add the following as indicators that the child should receive treatment as soon as possible: (1) The child has been stuttering for eighteen months or longer (Yairi, 1997a); (2) more than 33 percent of the child's disfluency clusters are of the stuttering–stuttering variety (LaSalle & Conture, 1995); (3) the child exhibits eyeball movements to the side and/or eyelid blinking during stuttering (Conture & Kelly, 1991a). If the child also exhibits concomitant speech sound articulation problems (particularly if exhibited phonological processes are indicative of delays or deviations in phonological development), the therapy plot may thicken, something we will discuss later in this chapter. The above variables, as far as we can tell, are additive, with the more of these exhibited by the child, the greater the chances that treatment is warranted. Children who appear to stutter but who exhibit none or only one of the above probably can be more appropriately put on a waiting list and/or diagnostically reevaluated, but this period of time should probably not exceed six months.

Suggested Guidelines for Length of Treatment. While it would be nice to have a one-size-fits-all length of treatment (certainly, funding agencies would appreciate this), the reality of humans and their behavior suggests otherwise. Indeed, the length of time therapy takes depends as much on the child and his or her parents as it does on the therapy he or she receives. Our experience indicates that most children take approximately 24 weeks of once-a-week therapy before they are ready to be dismissed. Some children are quite successful after only 12 weeks, and some still require therapy for 36 or more weeks. It has been our experience that parents need to be told—right in the beginning—of the average length of time therapy may take, the low end (e.g., 12 weeks) as well as the high end (e.g., 36 or more weeks) possibilities. For a variety of reasons, most parents think there is a one-size-fits-all length of treatment and they must learn, right from the beginning, that that is not the case (indeed, with a moment's reflection they would realize that this is not realistic—e.g., the length of time it takes children to learn their ABCs, numbers, how to print, etc. varies widely). While some youngsters who stutter will improve simply with parent counseling (either in person or over the phone), many will require visits to a SLP for some period of time. The length of therapy will also be influenced by the inclusion of maintenance or follow-up sessions; once again, the parents should be informed, right from the beginning, of the approximate number and nature of these maintenance or transfer sessions.

How Often per Week the Child Should Receive Treatment.   How often therapy occurs (on a weekly basis) is a question open to debate. There are pros and cons, in our opinion, to both intensive (e.g., everyday, all day, for three weeks) and extensive (e.g., once a week for a six-month period) approaches to therapy. There can be little doubt that intensive therapy brings about relatively quick behavioral change, but we question whether there is enough time for parents and children to make the type of attitude, feeling, and lifestyle changes that are sometimes necessary to support long-term behavioral change. Conversely, extensive therapy provides the time necessary to make needed attitudinal, feeling, and lifestyle changes; but behavioral change is relatively slow, occurring over a matter of weeks and months rather than days. At present, we have little empirical data that would allow us to answer one of the most important questions regarding this topic: Are there significant differences between intensive and extensive therapy with regard to *long-term* improvement or transfer? Until we know that children who stutter are more likely to *remain* fluent not just *become* fluent as a result of intensive versus extensive therapy, clinicians will select one or the other approach based on their experience, philosophy, and clinical schedules.

Know When to Let Go and Change Therapy Tactics.   One important caution: Let the child and the child's data talk to you! That is, if, after four to six treatment sessions, the child makes little or no change in the target behaviors, for example, using shorter, simpler sentences or using less physical tension during stutterings, the clinician *must* reassess his or her approach with the child. Don't persist with the unsuccessful. Get a second opinion. Call someone with expertise in the area. Reassess the child. Whatever, don't merely try to help by continually treating the child. Rather, actively search for the treatment that actually helps the child! In this writer's opinion, one of the more common errors of clinicians is continuing with the same treatment when it is apparent the treatment is having little or no benefit for the client. Often this occurs when the clinician has not done a sufficiently thorough diagnostic and doesn't have a real clear idea about the child's fundamental problems and needs. And like parents, the clinicians' *intentions* are the best—it's just the *method* that is less than ideal and/or appropriate.

Three Issues All Clinicians Encounter

No matter what the approach, the SLP who services youngsters who stutter will, sooner or later, have to deal with three issues in the earlier stages of therapeutic intervention: (1) mentioning the label *stuttering* in the presence of the child and/or the parents of the child; (2) talking to the young child, in clear, nonpejorative, but nevertheless direct terms, about talking in general and his or her talking in specific (e.g., Williams, 1971, 1985); and (3) the age of the child. The first two issues, we are cautioned by some, are better not broached since they are counterproductive to successful remediation. Conversely, some appear to feel that little or no harm will be done by calling the child a stutterer and directly talking and dealing with the child about talking. Once again, there is little empirical evidence to support either approach, and the clinician must sort out for him- or herself which of the two competing theories makes most sense.

Saying the "S" Word

Our experience suggests the following: When trying to *describe* the child's speech, we want to do just that! And the only effective means to describe something is to use the most descriptive terms you know that you think the client and associates will understand and relate to, for example, descriptive terms like "hard," "easy," "smooth," "gentle," "bumpy," "skidding," "repeating," or "stopping." A term like stuttering, for all its common use by the lay public, is simply not as descriptive—it tells neither the child nor parents what the child is *doing* and thus doesn't tell them what must be *done* to change. However, putting a bell and cowl on the word "stuttering" and treating it like a leperous entity is patently silly. It makes little sense to go out of your way not to say the "s" words if the parents and/or child have already being using "stuttering" or "stutterer" to talk about the child or his or her speech. Instead, recognize reality, and try to help the parents understand the difference between descriptive and nondescriptive terms and how their usage can help or hinder therapeutic progress. When the nondescriptive "s" words come up, deal with them as matter-of-factly as possible but resume usage of their more descriptive counterparts as soon as possible.

Talking to the Child About Talking in General and the Child's Talking in Specific

This is a variation on the concerns about saying the "s" words. Here, however, we are not only concerned about making the child's problem worse but whether the young child can understand what we are saying. At the least, we would hope that our words are (1) as descriptive as possible and (2) of a level that the child can understand and relate to. While it may be most parsimonious and correct to describe the things the child does as "cessation" and "reiteration" of speech production, it is probably better to use terms like "stuck" and "bouncing."

We'll come back to this issue later when we discuss the specifics of indirect and direct therapy. However, for the present, let us briefly examine the essence of Williams' (1985) "talking about talking" procedure that he used to change the child's beliefs about speech and related behavior. Let me say at the outset that this procedure would *not* be used with a child receiving indirect treatment, for example, in the context of a parent–child treatment group. Rather, this would more likely be employed with a child for whom indirect treatment has been minimally successful and/or who needs direct treatment.

Williams (1985) stated that this approach was *not* designed to "work on speech" or to show the child that he or she should talk in a certain way. Instead, Williams conceptualized this approach as a "set of structured experiences" thought to guide the child's observations, to help the child confront and eventually change beliefs. Williams suggested that the child's *external* behavior was motivated by what the child *internally* believed. Or, as Williams put it, ". . . the child's beliefs create strong motivations for (the) ways they [sic] behave." To change the external, Williams (1985) appeared to believe, one must change the internal. And his *talking-about-talking* procedure was Williams' attempt to bring about such change. Below is this writer's distillation of Williams' (1985) classic approach to the changing of children's beliefs about speech and related behaviors (listed in the rough order in which Williams employed them):

- *What's Wrong?* The clinician would begin by exploring what the child thinks "is wrong." Some children have (a) fragmented/vague notions (b) no idea or (c) imaginative and specific ideas about what is wrong.
- *What Are You Doing to Help?* The clinician then helps the child explore what the child is doing to help him- or herself. Again, what the child is doing to help is based on what he or she thinks is wrong, Typically, the child will describe, with the clinician's help at articulating the situation, that he is trying to "blast out" the sound, syllable, or word that he feels is "stuck." When what the child does to help doesn't work, the child may feel, in whole or in part, one or more of the following emotions: (1) frustration, (2) embarrassment, and (3) helplessness.
- *What's Going On?* The clinician then helps the child understand what is going on when she begins to talk and what she can do about it. In particular, the clinician tries to help the child recognize the difference between what the child is trying to accomplish and the actual result of his or her efforts.
- *When We Learn, We Make Mistakes.* Basically, the clinician is helping the child realize that making mistakes is a natural part of learning, that it is okay to make mistakes and that by decreasing attempts to avoid or stop making mistakes, stuttering can actually become better. Perhaps paraphrasing Williams' words is best: "When we learn to talk, we all make mistakes . . . maybe you made more mistakes then some others . . . you didn't want to make so many so you began to fight them. The harder you fought, the more mistakes you made . . ."
- *Changing Behavior Depends on What the Child DOES.* The clinician helps the child realize that he or she must change DOING not FEELING. In other words, the child is helped to learn to change the way he or she does things in the presence of emotions—for example, feeling pressured to respond to questions. The child is helped to learn that stuttering consists of things he or she *does* to interfere with talking. Stuttering does not erupt, stuttering is something the child does.

In essence, Williams' (1985) *talking about talking* helps the child bridge the gap between what the child *intends* to do and the *actual* way he or she *behaves*. This is directed at giving the child internal resources to change, not external recipes to "suppress" stuttering. The clinician is trying to help the child understand that he or she has a choice in terms of the way he or she behaves and the time needed to change in desired ways. Again, Williams' *talking-about-talking* is probably best employed within the context of direct treatment.

The Child's Age in Relation to the Type of Therapy Prescribed

It is our experience that the longer the time since onset, the greater the chance the child and/or his or her family will need some form of treatment. Likewise, it is our experience that the child's chronological age is an important consideration when planning the length and type of therapy. However, it is *not* our experience that chronological age is significantly related to the frequency, duration, or severity of stuttering in preschool/early school-age stuttering (see Yaruss, LaSalle, & Conture, 1998, Table 3). That is, it is our experience that a 4-year-old has just as much right as a 6-year-old to exhibit a severe stuttering problem.

While stuttering seems to follow an as yet poorly understood developmental sequence, the *rate* and *nature* of progress of this development vary widely from one young stutterer to another. Further, the child's chronological age at the time of onset—for example, an onset at 4 years versus 6 years of age—interacts in a complex way with the speed and type of development of stuttering. Some children rapidly move from producing mainly sound/syllable repetitions to sound prolongations while others take several months, if not years, to do the same thing. Indeed, some begin almost immediately with sound prolongations and/or blocks (Yairi, 1997a). Still other children steadily increase the frequency and duration of their instances of stuttering while others exhibit a herky-jerky progression, now more and longer stutterings, now fewer and shorter stutterings. Age, therefore, is a variable in planning therapy. For example, with very few exceptions, we have found it unwise to group 7-year-olds with 4-year-olds; however, chronological age *per se* has a far less than perfect relation to the quantity and quality of the child's stuttering problem.

Direct Versus Indirect Approaches

One general consideration is whether speech therapy with the child who stutters should be *direct* or *indirect*. Van Riper (1973), Ramig and Bennett (1997), and others have already covered this topic; but it is a topic that continually seems to concern and confuse SLPs who treat preschool and school-age children who stutter. At the outset, let us point out one truth: There is considerable variation within *both* indirect and direct therapies. As we have said elsewhere (Conture & Melnick, 1999, p. 17), ". . . there is as much variety among different 'indirect' methods as there is among different 'direct' approaches."

By *indirect* we mean any approach that does not explicitly, overtly, or directly try to manipulate, modify, or change the child's speech fluency in specific, and oral communication skills in general. With *indirect* therapy, the clinician tries to push both ends towards the middle! That is, the clinician simultaneously focuses on the child and the child's environment, particularly parents. In essence, with the child the clinician *models* desired behaviors and with the child's parents *encourages* (through modeling, instruction, and counseling) desired behaviors. Thus, indirect therapy many times also involves information sharing and/or counseling of the parents in addition to remediating the child's behavior through a variety of relatively low-key, play-oriented activities where desired speech and speech-related activities are clearly modeled but not the obvious focus. With an *indirect* approach, explicitly talking about the child's actual talking behavior is kept to a minimum, and the focus is more on relatively relaxed, enjoyable communication between clinician and child.

Ideally, a portion of each session of indirect therapy involves the parents interacting with the child, using a similar communicative model demonstrated by the clinician, for example, normally slow speaking rate and minimizing interrupting the child.

Conversely, a *direct* approach involves explicit, overt, and direct attempts to modify the child's speech and related behavior. While direct therapy can involve the child's parents, it usually does not involve to the same degree as with the indirect approach. More explicit, direct talking to the child about his or her talking (e.g., "Billy, you tensed up when you said that sound, let's see if we can try to change that . . ."), the "bad" as well as "good" parts, can and often is part of a direct approach.

Now that we are now a bit clearer on the distinctions between *direct* and *indirect* therapy approaches to childhood stuttering, which approach do we take? Once again, we find there is no easy or simple answer to what seems to be a rather straightforward question, no one-size-fits-all solution to a world whose problems come in many different sizes and shapes! While the indirect approach may be quite feasible for some, the direct procedure makes more sense for others. It is not too hard to decide about children at the extremes: indirect approaches for a child who is just beginning to stutter versus probably a more direct approach for a child who has been stuttering for three or four years. But how to decide about the many, many children in between these two extremes? Clearly, an indirect approach will have minimal impact on a 4-year-old's stuttering if that child is producing 30 percent disfluent speech with 90 percent or more of those disfluencies being sound prolongations. However, even with this child, direct therapy may not necessarily be the best approach if the child's parents are *consistently* and *continually* correcting the child's stuttering (e.g., "No, say it this way, Billy, without all that stuttering . . . stop, slow down, take a deep breath"); interrupting the child; speaking over the child's utterances; using long, complex utterances at extremely rapid rates of speech; and routinely making a series of verbal demands or requests of the child, especially when he or she is tired, without really waiting for the child's response before asking the next request.

One of the things we are trying to say here is that the child's chronological age is not as significant a factor in making the indirect/direct decision as the nature of the child's problem and both his and his environment's awareness/reaction to it. This does not mean chronological age is of no consequence in the planning of our therapy. Indeed, we would not want to use the *exact* direct procedures for a 4-year-old that we would employ with an 18-year-old; we would want to temper, modify, or drastically change certain of these procedures to make them more suitable for the younger client.

Age Grouping for Therapy

After many years experience evaluating (e.g., Yaruss, LaSalle, & Conture, 1998) and treating (e.g., Conture & Melnick, 1999) children known or suspected to be stuttering, we have come to the conclusion that the nature of therapy—that is, *indirect* versus *direct*,—is more related to the nature of the child's problem than to the child's chronological age. (As I write this, we have just evaluated a 5.5-year-old girl whose problem is easily as severe as that of the typical 10-year-old!) Certainly, experience has shown us, we don't want to group 7-year-olds with 4-year-olds, but we also don't want to assume that the 4-year-old's problem is less than that of the 7-year-old. There is a fine balancing act the clinician must perform here: gearing the approach so that the older child isn't underwhelmed or put off by the seemingly "juvenile" nature of the therapy versus overwhelming the younger child with tasks that he or she perceives to be or actually are beyond his or her level of development. Again, for the children at the chronological extremes, for example, a 3-year-old, it is easy to group the child in with social and intellectual peers; however, figuring out the best grouping for a child who is about 5 might be more problematic, especially if he or she is relatively socially mature. With all children, but especially with "gray zone" children—children on the cusps between a younger versus older group of children—adequate placement is empirical, trial and error. And if the parents are involved, as they should be with many of these children, the clinician is wise, right from the beginning, to explicitly express her uncertainty about which group will work best with the child, that some experience with both groups may be necessary before final placement in the group that works best for the particular child.

Four Categories of Children Who Receive Services

In our first version of this book (Conture, 1982, pp. 42–44) we discussed three groupings of children whom we typically remediate. We have expanded this trilogy somewhat to include the following four groupings: (1) children having no objective-subjective-communication whose parents are reasonably to quite concerned; (2) children who exhibit stuttering but whose parents are minimally or completely unconcerned; (3) children with some stuttering whose parents are also concerned; and (4) children having some to a great deal objective-subjective-communication problem whose parents are reasonably to quite concerned. In reality, we know that more than these four child-parent combinations are possible, but for the present, they seem to cover the bulk of the children we assess and treat and provide one reasonable means of organizing and overviewing this area.

Young Children with No Communicative Problems Whose Parents Are Reasonably to Quite Concerned

When a child is essentially fluent, that is, when the child's type and frequency of speech disfluency is within normal limits for the child's chronological and developmental age level, remediation of the child's speech fluency is contraindicated. Figure 3.2 typifies the frequency of total, between-word, and stuttered disfluencies exhibited by such a child (i.e., "minimal risk"; for sake of comparison, Figure 3.2 also provides similar data for a child at high as well as low risk for continuing to stutter). While this may seem like a reasonable decision based on the facts of the matter, sometimes the child's parents see things otherwise (especially, in our opinion, if one or both of the parents stuttered or had a close relative who stuttered and are, therefore, overly sensitized to stuttering and its implications). With these children, the child's parents or other important adult listeners explicitly, insistently, and/or strongly state their belief that the child has a stuttering problem, that the child is a stutterer. In many (but not all) of these cases, the parents are raising their first child; they are generally, but not exclusively, younger parents (30 years old and younger). Parents who deny the "normalcy" of their child's fluency are the exact opposite of a different group of parents

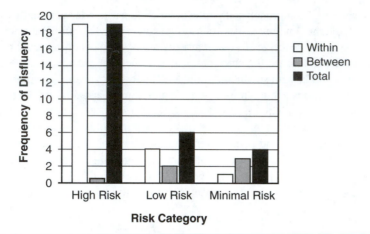

FIGURE 3.2.   Examples of total, between- and within-word disfluencies exhibited by three different children. Each of these three 4-year-old children was judged by the author, after extensive behavioral observations (in the home and in the clinic) as well as parental interviewing, as (1) being a high risk for *continuing* to stutter, (2) being at low risk for *continuing* to stutter, and (3) being a normally fluent speaker, with little or no risk for *developing* a stuttering problem. NONE of these children had been, at the time of the author's assessment/ evaluation, previously evaluated or treated for stuttering or any other speech, hearing, language, or voice problem.

(who we will discuss later on in this chapter) who deny the "abnormalcy" of their child's fluency. Both parent groups provide the clinician with a challenge.

Before going any further, one caution is in order: It is quite possible that the parents are seeing and hearing aspects of the child's behavior that you, the SLP, have not or cannot observe during the diagnostic. For example, Yaruss (1997a) has provided ample evidence about how childhood stuttering differs according to speaking task and/or communicative context. Indeed, we recently began treating for stuttering a 3;6-year-old-girl whose identical twin apparently did not stutter. The child's stuttering was apparent, but barely so, during therapy, although the parents still expressed concern. In a fairly brief time the child's fluency got to and stayed well within normal limits (1 to 2% stutterings per 100 words) and we began to question: (1) our original assessment, and (2) the feasibility of continuing the child and her parents in our weekly parent-child stuttering group. So, as part of a ongoing research project, we went to the child's home and there, when talking to the child, noticed about the same level of fluency, that is, 2 percent stuttering per 100 words (this is quite fluent speech and only the highly vigilant and observant will notice such disfluency). However, the mother reported, quite clearly and with detail, how the preceding night, when she and the twins were trying to make a pie together that the little girl was quite disfluent! Was the mother overly critical or did the little girl actually have an afternoon where she was highly disfluent? We, of course, will never know for sure but, given my experience with parents, I am more than inclined to believe the mother.

The above example with the 3;6-year-old girl points out at least three important things: (1) Parents can and do have opportunities to observe their child in speaking situations where the child's fluency differs from that of the speech-language pathology clinic; (2) SLPs need to sample the child's fluency in as many different situations as possible (e.g., Ingham & Riley, 1998); and (3) SLPs need to conduct their own independent assessments of the child but also take into careful consideration the parents' or other lay persons' diagnosis and observation. It is important for the SLP to realize that she doesn't have to observe the child at his or her worst (this needs to be said clearly and explicitly to the parents); she only has to observe the child speaking in enough different situations during the diagnostic to answer the question: "Would the observed speech disfluencies increase in frequency and duration (and perhaps change in type) given different and/or more environmental stressors?" If the answer is yes, then the child needs some form of intervention; however, if the answer is no, then intervention may not required. Whichever evaluation applies, before disregarding a parent's claim that his or her child stutters, the SLP should be as sure as possible that his or her sampling procedure was as varied and thorough as possible. If there are doubts (e.g., the child's fatigue at the time of assessment limited the breadth and depth of sampling), it is very reasonable and prudent to reevaluate the child in three to six months and see if the child's behavior has changed and/or whether the parents are still concerned.

Parents who seemingly insist, despite evidence to the contrary, that their child stutters generally appear to want the best for their child. They also seem to expect, in a number of areas, that the child will achieve at high levels of performance, regardless of the child's present abilities. As we've said before, we believe that the intentions and motivations of many of these parents are fine; it is just their methods of interacting or dealing with their child that may need some modification. Or as Johnson, Brown, Curtis, Edney, and Keaster (1967) suggested, "Parents are usually well-intentioned persons who have a great deal of love and affection for their children. The difficulty is that sometimes they do not understand the problems their children face. Their well-intentioned efforts to help are sometimes misdirected" (p. 144). Such parents seem to fall into three different, but not necessarily mutually exclusive, camps:

1. Why can't my child be perfect (like I was)?
2. My husband (wife) is wrong and he (she) thinks I'm wrong about how we raise our child.
3. These problems run in the family.

Parents' Concerns

Why Can't My Child Be Perfect (Like I Was)? The first camp, why can't my child be perfect, involves the situation where the parent(s) seem to want their child to be perfect and they are frustrated because the child, like most humans, cannot achieve such perfection. These parents may tell you that they want their 5-year-old son to be a doctor, a rocket scientist, or some other professional. These parents often see the world in black and white terms: either all good or all bad. And because of this, they may consider their child and his or her behavior to be either all right or all wrong. That is, they appear to believe that either their child's behavior is all right or their child and their child's development are all wrong. These parents seem to have trouble believing that their standards for their child may need modification; rather, they tend to see the problem as being produced or caused by the child.

Such parents have never heard or, if they did, believed the phrase: If you can't change the facts, change your attitude!

Many times these children are heavily monitored by the parents in terms of communication and social and academic development, and these parents may be less than flexible in their standards for child behavior (see Amster's 1995 discussion of relation of perfectionism between parents and child). First and foremost, these parents must be provided with clear, succinct, and nontechnically expressed information about what to typically expect from children of the same chronological and developmental age as their child. Second, these parents need to objectively assess their own standards for their child's development and performance in light of what is typically expected for children the same chronological and developmental age as their child. Third, these parents must be patiently and, in some cases, repeatedly and firmly instructed to evaluate and adjust their expectations for their child's behavior in general and speech and language development in specific. Many of these parents are also apt to do a lot of telling rather than showing the child what they want. Or, as Bettleheim (1985) states, many parents are "... ready to teach their child (but) ... are less ready to accept the idea that they can teach only by example" (p. 57) and that children "... are influenced less by what (parents) tell them than they are by what (parents) do" (p. 57). Getting across to the parent that it's the model not the lecture that instructs is one of the greatest challenges SLPs will have with such parents.

These parents, like many others, can be helped by discussing with them booklets and videos like those developed by Cooper (1979), Conture and Fraser (1989), Conture, Fraser, Guitar, and Williams (1995), and Conture, Guitar, and Fraser (1997) so that they will have a better understanding of typical speech and language development as well as stuttering. We have found that these parents can be helped if they will listen to reason: If they will entertain the notion that their standards for their child are less (or more) than desirable and, most importantly, that these standards need reevaluation and change. Sometimes, referrals to psychologists and psychiatrists who specialize in child–family counseling may be the only way such change can be made. We have more often observed, however, that the child's "problem" is generally resolved when the parents' concerns and standards for the child's behavior are modified and brought into line with what is considered reasonable for a child of the chronological and developmental age of theirs.

My Husband (Wife) Is Wrong and He (She) Thinks I'm Wrong. Related to the why-can't-my-child-be-perfect situation is the situation where one or both parents thinks the other is wrong. This is most commonly manifested where the mother *frequently* and *consistently* states that the father is "too strict" with the child and/or the father just as *frequently* and *consistently* states that the mother is "too lenient" with the child or "lets the kid get away with murder." Neither parent seems to agree with the other in terms of the way in which the child should be raised (such disagreements are generally noticed when discipline is an issue) or how a child the age of their son or daughter should speak, think, read, write, behave, play, and so forth. In its worse case, the parents are so polarized that nothing short of psychological/marital counseling will suffice. However, most parents are not so polarized but they do disagree, not only in private but openly and frequently, about the raising of the child in front of the child. This particular parental situation, like most other parental concerns, is only a *dilemma* if it occurs frequently and consistently.

Again, if arguments between parents are the rule, rather than the exception, then the parents may need more than simple information sharing and informal counseling by the SLP. Perhaps the child is the focal point for difficulties the mother and father have between themselves. They may be taking out their frustrations and anger with each other on the child. As mentioned above, in some of these cases referral to appropriate psychological services may be appropriate (interestingly, we think, that mothers seem to be somewhat more receptive to such referrals than fathers). Remember though that reasonable people, even parents (!), can disagree with one another, such disagreement is not cause for signing up teams of opposing divorce lawyers, but merely an indication that the two "combatants" need to explore the dreaded "c" word—compromise—for the good of the child that they both clearly love.

In most cases, however, we have found that parents *will* listen to reason and seriously try to minimize their differences when they are helped to realize that their difficulties may be adversely influencing the child. As we said above, the vast majority of parents love their children, have excellent intentions, but just need to reconsider and modify their actual approaches to the raising of their children. In such cases, where one of the parents is quite convinced that the child has a communicative problem, whereas the other is just as firmly convinced that no problem exists, the clinician should avoid giving the appearance of choosing sides. Persistence on the part of the clinician in helping the parents to see their child as he or she really is, not as they idealize him or her to be, is important. Helping parents more closely *match* their perceptions of their child to the *realities* of their child will go a long way to helping the parents become part of the solution rather than part of the problem! Continued reiteration of basic child development information is important: Just becoming a parent does not mean that someone is automatically bestowed with deep, rich clinical insights as well as full understanding of the complexities and long-term process of child behavior and development. The SLP must persevere in these matters if he or she expects to move these parents in the right direction.

The plain truth of the matter, as we will discuss throughout this and subsequent chapters on remediation, is that *real* changes in such parental attitudes and behavior may take more time than any of us would like. The clinician should try to: (1) be as persistent as possible without being obnoxiously repetitive; (2) convey respect for and listen to the opinions and ideas of parents—they have perspectives that any clinician, no matter how wise or experienced, can learn a great deal from; and (3) explicitly express to the parents the fact that the clinician knows that the parents love their child, that they have the best of intentions for the raising of their child. If the SLP can do all three of these things, at least some of the time, it is amazing the change parents can and do make and the degree to which the parents can come to see the realities of their child's behavior.

Stuttering Runs in the Family.   Once you've experienced a car accident, you realize they can happen to even you. You become a bit more cautious, a bit more wary when you drive, a bit more likely to quickly and routinely buckle up your seatbelt. The old saying of once bitten, twice shy applies here. Likewise, in a family where the parents of the child stuttered themselves or knew an Uncle Fred who stuttered, is it not hard to see why parents would be on the lookout for their offspring to begin doing the same thing. In essence, the parents, through exposure and experience with stuttering exhibited by relatives and/or themselves, have become sensitized to the problem. There is nothing particularly new about this observation/interpretation—it was made previously by Gray (1940) and Johnson (1961). Bloodstein (1995), summarizing these observations, said that Johnson and his students believed that in situations where stuttering "runs in the family," what occurs is a ". . . handing down of a 'climate of anxiety' about the hesitant speech of children" (p. 124), that these families were "stuttering conscious" and seemed to ". . . watch their children anxiously for signs of it" (p. 125). We are not suggesting here that inheritance of a predisposition for stuttering does occur, merely that the possibility definitely exists for individuals with experience with and exposure to stuttering to be sensitized to, aware of, and concerned about the problem. In essence, the influence of inheritance *does not* preclude the influence of environment.

The SLP must walk a thin line with these cases and their families. While the SLP doesn't want to deny the real possibility that stuttering tends to "run in families" (for example, at least 50% of the relatives of people who stutter also stutter, Johnson & Associates, 1959), the SLP must realize that this tendency doesn't absolutely dictate the fact that the child will also stutter. Yes, there may be an increased probability that the child may be and will continue to stutter but not an absolute certainty that this will be the case. The sun coming up tomorrow is a *certainty*, picking the winner of the Kentucky Derby based on bloodlines, trial runs, and the like involves *probability*.

Look and They Shall Find.   Many times these parents give the appearance of waiting for the other shoe to drop; they sometimes seem to have been looking since the child began to speak for signs of stuttering and, to paraphrase an old saying, "look and they shall find." Many times one or both parents will mention the horrible stuttering problem of themselves, Uncle Ralph, or Sister Daphne and how they hope that their child does not end up the same way they or their poor relative did. Some of these parents also seem to have high, relatively unreasonable expectations for their child's speech, language, fluency, and behavioral development, even when confronted with the fact that their child is developing at his or her own normal, albeit slow, pace. Like many parents, these parents will have numerous old persons' tales about what causes stuttering and/or what makes it better or worse. They are likely to bring up the issue and want to know your opinion of whether stuttering results from (1) a physical flaw *or* (2) a psychological problem ("Is this something he was born with or did we cause the problem?"). Some of these parents may begin to shop around from one SLP to another until they find one who will agree that their child has a stuttering problem. It is important, particularly with this type of parent, to quickly establish your credibility and concern for their child while at the same time conveying your respect for and willingness to listen to their opinions. You may find your patience being tested since you will have to continually reiterate what you believe the facts of the matter are and what you think the parents need to consider to make appropriate change.

Counseling the Parents and Keeping in Touch

When all is said and done, counseling parents about their child's apparently nonexistent, subclinical, or very mild stuttering problem is both remedial as well as preventive. You try, through information sharing, discussion, and counseling, to help the parents provide for their child a home environment conducive to optimal development of speech fluency and related behavior. For example, parents may need to assess and change their own speech behaviors (e.g., routinely using long complex sentences while rapid-fire questioning him or her about the child's school day), communicative interactional styles, emotions, feelings, attitudes, and so forth. During this time, the parents may want you to "therapize" the child and the degree to which they insist on this therapy may be an indirect measure of the degree to which they are abdicating their responsibilities for helping their child. Perhaps, if you bring the child in for informal play therapy (for example, Axline, 1947; Murphy & FitzSimons, 1960; Van Riper, 1973) or for general speech and language "enrichment" or "stimulation," you may assuage the parents while you continue to discuss with them what they may do to change their interactions with and expectations of their child.

Many times, immediately after the initial evaluation, when the parents have just been interviewed and the problem is fresh in their minds, is a good time for a thirty- to sixty-minute information sharing session. Sometimes, as we and others (for example, Johnson & Associates, 1959) have found, this initial post- evaluation findings and recommendations session is all these parents need to significantly diminish their concerns. At the risk of being overly detail conscious, it really helps to make sure, before these parents leave the first time, that they have written down somewhere your office phone number and address and that they truly feel that that they can call you (we specifically tell them, "Feel free to write or call me") if they have further questions or concerns. It is very important to give these parents the impression that the door to your clinic, office, or school is always open, wide open, to them. Do whatever you can to minimize any parental feelings that they are "locked" out from further contact. Instead, let them know that you want to and expect to maintain contact with them and will welcome their calls. (Since some parents are not aware of how busy the average SLP's schedule may be, I tell them that sometimes, when they call, they won't be able to get me immediately and will have to leave a message on my voicemail. However, I tell them, at the time of the evaluation, that if they do leave the message on my voicemail that I'll get back in touch with them, as soon as possible, if they leave their name, number and a time when it is best for me to get back in touch with them. If you have email, are comfortable with clients contacting you through this mode, give them your email address as well.) Whatever we do, we try to provide these parents with a sense that someone is available to help and that the parents themselves have the ability to positively change.

Parental Guilt. As mentioned above, when counseling parents, one point that most authorities seem to agree on is the need NOT to make parents feel guilty (or at least any more guilty than they already feel) about their child's behavior or problem(s). No issue, in this writer's opinion, is more salient to effective remediation of the child as well as counseling of the parents. A guilty parent, particularly an uninformed one, is going to be an uncooperative, even resistant, and overly concerned parent. In essence, increase parental guilt if you are interested in lowering your effectiveness in helping them and their child!

Le Shan (1963) writes about this point (i.e., parental guilt) in length, and we believe it is important to remember and consider in parent counseling. Instead of engendering feelings of parental guilt, we, as SLPs, should try to provide parents with objective information about speech and language behavior in general and stuttering in specific. Of course, this requires you to listen and thoughtfully respond to their questions about same. We should try to support parents in their attempts to understand and explore their feelings, concerns, and thinking about their child and their role in their child's general and communicative development. Such exploration may take many meetings with you, depending on the nature and type of parent feelings and concerns.

Parents Are Individuals Just Like Their Children.   While much is written about the individual nature of the child, we often forget that parents are also individuals. Too often, because of the frantic nature and relative brevity of the clinical day and our many clients, we tend to deal with each parent in fairly similar ways. That is, we tend to gloss over individual differences and try to talk to and handle each parent as though the parent was the "typical" parent of a "typical" child who stutters. This is not an inherently evil practice; indeed, some degree of commonality must exist among these parents for us to develop an effective remediation regimen. However, when we routinely and consistently counsel each and every parent in the same manner, we run the risk of overlooking some individual parent differences that may make a significant difference in terms of the particular child's progress. Behaviorally, this may be seen on when SLPs, with all good intentions, have a signal or knee-jerk reaction to the denotation of particular words without considering variations in the word's connotations and/or underlying feelings of the speaker.

For example, we, as SLPs, may become concerned if the parent routinely uses the "s" word (see p. 141, this chapter) when talking to his or her child about talking but become more relaxed when another parent talks about talking to the child using such terms as "hard" and "easy" speech. And yet, the specific words used may not be as important as the manner in which the parent uses them. As Neill (1960) suggests, ". . . it doesn't matter what a parent says to a child as long as the parent's feelings towards the child are correct," and, we might add, the child recognizes the appropriateness of such feelings. The point here is that we (and this writer is including himself) sometimes give patented or standard responses and recommendations to parents without carefully considering the individual nature, needs, and concerns of parents and their child. It is the wise clinician who can detect and differentially respond to those aspects of the parents of young people who stutter that are typical as well as those that are unique. Suffice it to say that if children are individuals, then logically so are their parents.

Recognizing the uniqueness of each parent and attempting to avoid increasing parental guilt must be done within the broader construct that these parents are raising children in a highly technical, competitive, information-driven economy and society (and becoming more so with each passing year). Too often, clinicians, particularly clinicians without sufficient experience interacting with a variety of parents, misinterpret a parent's remarks that "Buddy can do better in school" or "Maria isn't very careful in her work" as meaning the parent is too demanding, perfectionistic, rigid, insensitive, or sets too high standards. While recognizing that some parents of people who stutter do seem, as Neill (1960) puts it, to ". . . want to speed up the pace," this does not mean that *all* such parents are overly demanding or time urgent or that even those parents who are somewhat demanding are necessarily demanding regarding every aspect of their child's behavior every hour of the day. Clinicians should work to understand the difference between normal parental concern and those concerns that frequently and consistently occur and seem to be less than desirable in terms of fostering the type of environment where a child's speech fluency can positively develop.

Finally, and at the risk of stating the obvious, parents are people, and as the song goes, "people with children" (Thomas et al., 1972). Many of us will eventually become or already are parents, and we should recognized that parents encounter many of the same problems that SLPs, as people, encounter in daily living. When we clinically interact with the parents of people who stutter, we try to do so within the perspective that we are dealing with people who happen to be parents. We try not to be too willing to cast the first stone at parents who, after all, are people like the rest of us, with all our human foibles and fortes.

Reevaluation of the Child and Keeping in Touch with the Parents

With the child with no apparent problem but whose parents are quite concerned, we generally set up, at the end of the initial evaluation, a diagnostic reevaluation. Indeed, reevaluation is one of the clear suggestions that can result from application of *Second Opinion* (Bahill & Curlee, 1993), a computer-based decision support system for evaluating incipient stuttering in children. Such reevaluations permit us to maintain contact with the parent, monitor the parents' actual ability to positively change, and assess changes in the child's speech and related behaviors over time. Try to maintain contact with these parents, not as a means of extending your professional control, but as a way for these parents to contact you at times when *they* are concerned. If parents have a scheduled reevaluation that they are told they can cancel any time, this seems to give them the security that something is being done, while at the same time, it makes it easier for them to call in with "interim" reports. Keeping in touch with these parents reduces their feeling of helplessness, frustration, and "being alone in the boat"; your suggestions and insights may well be the only voice of reason the parents hear, and, as this writer can attest, these parents need that, especially if they are routinely receiving old wives' tales and other forms of misinformation from well-intended but misinformed relatives and friends. Besides, the parents know, at some level, that you are not emotionally involved with their child and that you can be as objective in your suggestions.

Know Something About Parenting Books. When helping these parents we also may feel it important for the SLP to know and understand what parenting books the parents have and/or are reading. The young parent raising a first child usually reads such books as those by Spock and Rothenberg (1985), Brazelton (1974, 1983), those published by Gesell and associates (for example, Ilg & Ames, 1960), or one of the many "how to" parenting books like that of Dodson (1970). The SLP should read and be familiar with these books and develop an understanding of the types of written inputs many parents routinely turn to when they have questions and concerns about the general well being of their child.

Children with Some Stuttering Whose Parents Are Unconcerned

If you establish that the child is producing a frequency, duration, and type of speech disfluency that puts the child at risk for becoming a stutterer, then you have to tell this to the child's parents, guardians, or adult associates. However, no matter how patiently, clearly, and sensitively you express your belief, some parents are simply not going to accept, believe, or understand your findings. While some of these parents may appear as if they don't respect your opinion, clinical acumen, and experience, most of them are actually are hoping against hope that (1) the child's problem will go away with time and/or (2) denying the reality of the situation. And for some of them, to be frank about it, the decision to deal with their child's problem comes down to finances in that the parent may justify, in whole or in part, their apparent lack of concern or action on the basis that the treatment is simply too expensive. We should not quickly judge or react to these parents, especially those where finances play a role. Why? Well, if we examine our own lives we can see how, for merely monetary reasons, we frequently delay, postpone, or simply avoid a brake job that would make our car safer, dental work that would make our teeth less apt to further decay, or home repairs that would make our home less hazardous.

Some of these parents may shop around until they find some professional who agrees with their feeling that the problem will resolve with time and/or that there is no problem. Others will simply wait several years and eventually come back to you with the simple statement, "I guess he didn't outgrow it." The most difficult of this group of parents are those who intellectually know that there is a problem but emotionally seem to deny its existence. These latter parents find a variety of reasons why they can't meet scheduled appointments, why scheduled appointments conflict with the all-important tuba lessons, and why therapy, although necessary, may actually be "harming" the child. And, this writer hastens to add, the reader is cautioned not to think that these are the concerns of the uneducated parents. No, some of the worse offenders are highly educated parents whose own personal and professional agendas are so full, demanding, and stressful that they exhibit little interest in, willingness, or time to get involved with treatment of their child. Such parents need time to think the situation through, and most of them, with sufficient support and the right kind of gentle but firm advice that the child's problem is not getting any better, can come to see the reality of the situation. Remember: *Most parents want to do the right thing, it is generally only their approach or methods that need change.*

Who Knows Who Will Become Fluent and Who Will Continue to Stutter?

To make this situation even more of a challenge, the child's actual speech behavior appears, to the parents, to support their belief that the child will get better by him- or herself or that there is no problem. It is not hard to see why parents think this way when we consider the following types of behaviors exhibited by many of these youngsters. First, these children generally, but not always, exhibit no apparent awareness of a speech disfluency problem. Second, the child's disfluencies are marked by fairly unpredictable cyclical changes of indeterminate length; one day (or week or month) the child is "good" (that is, the child does not stutter) and the next, "bad" (that, the child stutters quite frequently). Third, most of these youngsters' speech disfluencies are relatively relaxed or "easy" in that they are associated with little sign of physical tension and are generally only 250 to 1000 milliseconds in duration. Fourth, the child is still relatively willing to talk in a variety of situations about a variety of topics. And, of course, it has been shown (Yairi & Ambrose, 1992; Yairi, Ambrose, & Niermann, 1993) that within the first two years from the onset of stuttering, recovery rates (i.e., rates of improvement without treatment) for children range between 65 percent and 75 percent, with as many as 85 percent of children recovering within the next several years; that is, more than four of five (85%) children who begin to stutter eventually recover. In essence, the child is just as often fluent as disfluent, seems to have little awareness of a problem or concern about talking, exhibits disfluencies that are generally short in duration and associated with minimal physical tension, and many times improves without treatment. Given this sort of picture, it is small wonder that some parents believe that there is no problem and/or that the problem will resolve itself. And, of course, a percentage of these children do become better with time, with or without therapy.

The Problem May Improve, but Who Knows for Whom?   The only problem with all this is that no one, to this writer's knowledge, can accurately and reliably determine which children, initially diagnosed as stuttering, will and will not resolve with time. Remember, clinically this is an individual, not a group, decision. In this writer's opinion, the two, extreme ways of dealing with this uncertainty are: (1) telling *all* such parents that their child will "outgrow" the problem; and (2) telling *all* such parents that their child has a problem and needs remediation as soon as possible. Both approaches would appear to be playing the odds. With option (1), the he'll-outgrow-it approach, a percentage of the children will improve; but for another percentage, therapy will eventually be necessary. With option (2), the everybody-gets-therapy approach, treatment will certainly be provided for those who need it, but probably needlessly remediate a percentage who don't. Instead of these two one-size-fits-all approaches, what is needed, in this writer's opinion, is more clinical investigations that try to uncover reliable indicators, no matter how subtle, that a child: (1) has a stuttering problem, and (2) that the problem will probably not resolve with time. At present, no such indicators exist; however, many are working in this direction (e.g., Ambrose & Yairi, 1999; Yaruss, LaSalle, & Conture, 1998), and someday this area will be far clearer than it is at present. Above ("suggested guidelines for beginning therapy . . ."), we provided some data-based suggestions for behaviors to watch for when trying to decide whether treatment is necessary. However, much, much more needs to be known about these behaviors in relationship to long-term improvement or lack thereof in stuttering.

We explain these findings to the parents in as clear terms as we can, but some of these parents still disregard these observations. Sad to say, but you are going to lose a percentage of these "discussions" with parents. That is, some of these parents will keep their child out of therapy until such a time that the child's stuttering has become so habituated, obvious, and pervasive as to make its remediation very problematic. Likewise, some of these parents, for a variety of reasons, will not follow up on your suggestion that the child needs help from other professionals—for example, a psychologist—and wait until related problems become far more pronounced or pervasive. Fortunately, in our experience, the percentage of parents who continually deny or disregard our assessment or referral is relatively small, while most of the rest of these parents, after some degree of discussion with us, begin to see that their child indeed needs some form of professional intervention.

Concomitant Speech and/or Language Problems Exhibited by Children Who Stutter Somewhat

Since the preceding edition of this book, much has been researched and written about the concomitant problems of children who stutter (e.g., Conture, Louko & Edwards, 1993;

Louko et al., 1999; Louko, 1990; Nippold, 1990; Paden & Yairi, 1996; Ryan, 1992; Throneburg et al., 1994; Wolk et al., 1993; Yaruss & Conture, 1996). What have we learned from this research? Several things. First, without a doubt, even given differences in methodology, subject selection criteria, and the like across many different studies (see Nippold, 1990 for excellent critical appraisal of this area of study), the prevalence of phonological concerns in the population of children who stutter is greater than that in the population of children who don't stutter. Second, that there may be some differences in the nature and persistence of stuttering among children who both stutter and exhibit disordered phonology when compared to those who only stutter. Third, while phonological processes and/or speech-sound misarticulations may be more prevalent in the speech of children who stutter, these same children are more apt to stutter on slips of the tongue than the systematic speech-sound errors we call phonological processes. Fourth, it is possible to simultaneously remediate phonological processes and stuttering, given due consideration to both problems and how one might influence the other, without increasing stuttering—in fact, in some children, actually improving it considerably. Where does this leave us? Uncertain about the exact nature of the relationship between stuttering and concomitant problems, but quite certain that one exists (at least for a sizable portion of children who stutter) and that our diagnosis and treatment of stuttering in young children must take this into consideration.

Quite obviously, therefore, it is not uncommon that a child with an incipient stuttering problem, whose parents believe has "no problem," may also exhibit other concerns (e.g., language delays, phonological difficulties). Such co-occurrence obviously confounds the situation, but, with some consideration, patience, and thought on the part of the SLP, can be dealt with quite constructively (see Conture, Louko, & Edwards, 1993, for an example of one such treatment approach). Patience, however, is the watchword here, and it is particularly unwise to rush in and remediate one part *without* considering its influence on the whole of the child's speech and language abilities and development. It must be emphasized: Development of speech fluency is not an isolated phenomenon but is intricately interconnected, if in poorly understood ways, to the child's overall development of morphosyntactic construction, phonology, semantics, pragmatics, as well as related processes. If, for example, one were to remediate phonological difficulties of a young person who stutters by employing repetitive drill and flash cards, which emphasize overly correct, precise, rapid, and physically tense articulatory postures and gestures, the child's speech "sounds" may indeed improve, but this procedure would have a less than desirable, long-term influence on the child's fluency problem. Similarly, it does not help a child become more fluent, as Van Riper (1963, p. 319) observed, if parents try to "speed up" the pace of normal speech and language development by overtly correcting and attempting to modify and change the child's speech and language that are well within normal limits. This is especially true, in our experience and opinion, if the child's temperament is on the slow-to-warm-up, behaviorally inhibited, overly worried about mistakes end of the spectrum. In our opinion, such temperamental characteristics, on the child's part, make changes in environmental input or interaction with the child all the more important, if not complex.

Using a Concomitant Problem to Get Therapy Going

Sometimes the concomitant problems of a young child with incipient stuttering can be used to advantage, particularly if the parent believes there is no concern. It is not uncommon that these parents may be more receptive to therapy focused on language or articulation concerns. We would still tell the parents that the child is or has potential for developing a stuttering problem but that other problems co-occur and probably need more attention at this point. If the parents agree to such a strategy, then we proceed to "work" on the child's language and/or articulation problem while at the same time discussing with the parents their behaviors (and changes in same) just like we would if the child was being remediated for stuttering! If asked by the parents why they have to, for example, decrease the amount they interrupt their child, decrease their rate to normal/slow normal when talking to or in the presence of the child, we explain that this sort of change makes it easy for the child to verbally interact with the parent and puts less time pressure on the child to communicate—changes that should help every aspect of the child's verbal communication, not just fluency.

Dealing with Delays in Language in a Child Who Stutters

Delays and/or deviance in language development (e.g., Bernstein Ratner, 1993) do occur with some children who stutter (e.g., Murray & Reed, 1977; Ryan, 1992)—whether or not their parents think they stutter—and when present, these concerns with language need to be assessed and possibly remediated (Watson, Freeman, Chapman, Miller, Finitzo, Pool, & Devous, 1991, have also reported "linguistic impairment" in 11 of 19 adults who stutter). Sometimes a child's speech disfluency problem seems secondary to delays and deviance in expressive as well as receptive language development. When this is the case, the child's language skills need attention prior to remediation of fluency. I would say this is particularly true when the speech disfluency is of the physically easy (i.e., physically nontense), relatively brief duration part- and whole-word repetition, as well as phrase repetition, variety. However, we have noticed that some children whose language seems delayed and/or deviant in development may actually become *more* disfluent when their language actually improves. This observation supported by an empirical study of the impact of language therapy on a child's speech disfluencies (Merits-Patterson & Reed 1981). We have noticed this association between positive change in language and increases in speech disfluency to be particularly apparent in children around 5 to 6 years of age. We are not sure what this means or its long-term implications for recovery from disfluency, but we are inclined to speculate that increases in the length and complexity of verbally expressed languages increase the opportunities for instances of disfluency to emerge. Thus, this is probably a natural by-product of improved but still unstable expressive language skills. While there are some mixed findings in this area (in part due to differing methodologies), the bulk of the research suggests that stuttering is more apt to occur on utterances that are longer (e.g., Gaines, Runyan, & Meyers, 1991; Logan & Conture, 1997; Melnick & Conture, 2000; Weiss & Zebrowski, 1992) and more complex (e.g., Bernstein Ratner & Sih, 1987; Gaines et al., 1991; Kadi-Hanifi & Howell, 1992; Weiss & Zebrowski, 1992). Again, speech (dis)fluency cannot be disentangled from the syntactic, semantic, and phonologic web within which it is woven.

Some children who stutter may have a mean length of utterance (MLU) (Brown, 1973) roughly appropriate for their chronological age, but exhibit mastery of particular grammatical morphemes (i.e., morphemes whose main purpose is to modify the meaning of content words or to more specifically indicate relation of content words) that is less than appropriate for this stage of language development. For example, the use of *be* as a copula verb (the *is* of "She is tired" and the *are* of "You are captain") may be omitted by some children who stutter who are at Brown's stage IV of language development. It should be clear, however, that we are not saying that *all* of these children who stutter have language problems, or that they all exhibit the same type and severity of language difficulties, or that language problems cause stuttering. It is a challenge to decide which problem—a language delay or stuttering—needs most immediate attention; however, therapy oriented to modification of language seems most appropriate if the child's speech disfluencies are of a physically easy, relatively short duration and consist mainly of part- and whole-word repetitions. Conversely, therapy should probably be more oriented to modification of stuttering if the speech disfluencies are associated with visible and audible signs of physical and psychological tension, are relatively longer in duration, and mainly of a blocking or sound prolongation (audible and inaudible) type. Of course, there is nothing that says that both problems—language difficulties and stuttering—can't be simultaneously dealt with in the same session. However, it is probably the case that the clinician will focus at least 60 percent of his or her attention on one problem and 40 percent on the other but can also change these proportions when improvement in one area or changes in the overall problem dictate.

Dealing with Articulation/Phonological Concerns in a Child Who Stutters Somewhat

A recent review of this area (Louko et al., 1999), particularly as it relates to the diagnosis and treatment of stuttering, makes it quite clear, on the basis of thirteen studies that directly examined the articulation/phonological disorders of children who stutter (see Table 3.1), that prevalence of these disorders in these children far exceeds that of the normally fluent population (with the recent findings of Paden, Yairi, & Ambrose, 1999, being consistent with studies shown in Table 3.1). For example, Williams and Silverman (1968) reported that 24 percent of 115 elementary school-aged people who stutter had associated articulation defects compared to 9 percent of their normally fluent peers. Riley and Riley (1979) reported that 33 percent of 100 young people who stutter also exhibited articulation difficulties. Daly (1981) reported that 58 percent of a subgroup ($n = 25$) of young people who stutter—taken from a larger sample ($n = 138$)—evidenced articulation disorders. Thompson (1983) observed a 35 to 45 percent incidence of "suspected (articulation) deficits" in two samples ($n = 31$ and ($n = 17$) of young people who stutter. Cantwell and Baker (1985), in a large clinical investigation of the psychiatric and learning disabilities in 600 children with speech and/or language disorders, reported that 30 percent of the 40 people who stutter in their sample also exhibited an articulation disorder. Thus, from a low of 19 percent to a high of 96 percent (Mean = 41%), thirteen studies, of relatively large sample sizes, indicate that stuttering and "articulation" difficulties co-occur for a sizable proportion of children who stutter (quite obviously, 41% is far greater than the approximately 2 percent to 6 percent of the school-age population who have articulation concerns [Beitchman et al., 1986; Hull et al., 1971]). These findings do not mean that one problem causes the other but that the two problems frequently—we guess that about one-third of the children we assess and/or treat for stuttering exhibit some form of articulation concern—co-occur and that the SLP should be prepared to handle such co-occurrence.

TABLE 3.1. Fourteen Studies that *Directly* Examine Articulation/Phonological Disorders Exhibited by Children Who Do/Do Not Stutter. (The number of children in each of two groups is provided: Children who stutter and who do not stutter.) Paden, Yairi, and Ambrose (1999) added to original table by author (Conture).

Author	Number of Stutterers	Number of Nonstutterers	% of Stutterers with Articulation Disorders	% of Nonstutterers with Articulation Disorders	Summary
McDowell (1928)	33	33	19	16	Articulation difficulties; significant differences between groups
Schindler (1955)	126	252	49	15	"Other speech disorders"
Morley (1957)	37	113	50	31	"Other speech disorders"
Williams & Silverman (1968)	115	115	24	9	Associated articulation difficulties
Riley & Riley (1979)	100	—	33	—	Associated articulation difficulties
Daly (1981)	138	—	58	—	Articulation disorders
Thompson (1983)	48	—	35–45	—	"Suspected articulation difficulties"
Cantwell & Baker (1985)	40	—	30	—	—
St. Louis & Hinzman (1988)	48	24	67–96	—	—
Louko, Edwards, & Conture (1990)	30	30	40	7	Greater number and variety of phonological processes, more /s/-- cluster reduction for children who stutter
Ryan (1992)	20	20	0	0	No significant difference on formal articulation test; but 5/20 (25%) of stutterers eventually required articulation therapy
Throneburg, Yairi, & Paden (1994)	75	—	7	—	Reported "severe phonological deficits," no report of mild/moderate phonologic deficits
Paden & Yairi (1996)	36	36	22/36 (61%) (moderate severe-phonological deficits)	14/36 (39%) (moderate severe-phonological deficits)	Significant differences on formal test of phonology between persistent stutterers and their controls
Paden, Yairi & Ambrose (1999)	22 persistent 62 recovered		Persistent stutterers scored lower on measures of phonological development than recovered stutterers		Recovered most apt to be mild; persistent more apt to be moderate or severe in terms of mean error score

Source: After Louko, Conture, & Edwards; Paden, Yairi, & Ambrose (1999)

One Guideline for Establishing the Presence of an Articulation/Phonology Problem.
Of course, there are articulatory problems, and then there are articulatory problems. A slight distortion of an /s/, or perhaps an /l/, is probably no real problem and can generally be ignored as the SLP proceeds to help the child modify his or her disfluencies. However, reduced intelligibility in association with multiple articulation errors with omissions and substitutions, as well as distortions, are problematic, particularly if the child also exhibits any "unusual" phonological processes (for example, glottal replacement: /be?/ for "bed") (Louko et al., 1990). One clinical guideline SLPs might consider is whether the child scored below the 30th percentile on the sounds-in-words subtest of the *Goldman-Fristoe Test of Articulation* (GFTA; Goldman & Fristoe, 1986). If the child scored below the 30th percentile on the GFTA, and certainly if below the 20th percentile, this child's speech sound development is, at the minimum, at the low end of normal limits (which is roughly one standard deviation below the mean), and further clinical consideration of this fact is probably warranted. And while evidence of frequent, multiple articulation errors, with or without unusual phonological processes, in a child who is also stuttering is not cause to panic, it is cause for caution, to adjust therapy to the needs and abilities of the particular child.

The Child Who Begins to Stutter AFTER Therapy for Articulation Problems

SLPs who work with children have, sooner or later, heard about or actually observed a child who began to stutter AFTER therapy for remediation of a speech misarticulation problem (such situations have been previously noted by Hall, 1977; Van Riper, 1963, p. 318). While no one, at this point, knows what the precise relation between articulation/phonology and stuttering is and whether therapy for one helps or hinders the other, it is apparent that some, albeit unclear, relation exists between speech fluency and speech sound production. What often seems to happen with these children, in this writer's experience, is that the child begins therapy too early for his or her "articulation problem." This seemingly leads the child, even though the articulation concerns improved, to learn what sounds are his or her *problem sounds* and that the child has to "work" or be careful or cautious to correctly, precisely, and quickly produce these sounds. This sort of approach is, in our opinion, counterproductive to long-term facilitation of the child's speech fluency and, in some cases, may actually exacerbate the child's stuttering problem.

As one apparent antidote, these children need experience with speaking in a physically relaxed, relatively slow-paced atmosphere where communication is made an enjoyable, interesting, and shared activity. Phonetic placement drills or direct remediation of these youngsters' speech fluency and articulation is secondary; first, the SLP must help the child come to realize that speech isn't such a chore, that it can be fun and done in a relatively physically easy, unhurried manner. In essence, the child needs to be encouraged to learn that the reason for speaking is *communication*! No child—indeed none of us—speaks to be fluent or flawlessly correct in pronunciation. We speak to communicate, first and foremost! Or as Johnson (in Johnson, Brown, Curtis, Edney & Keaster, 1967) nicely put it, "Assume he's (the speaker) is doing the best he can and that it is more important for him to want to talk to you than to sound correct" (p. v).

The Young Child Who Stutters and Exhibits
Speech Sound Problems

A child, who hasn't had any form of therapy, exhibiting both stuttering and articulation concerns presents a slightly different problem. First, the SLP should carefully think thorough the *relative* importance of modifying the child's articulation problem versus his or her stuttering problem. While the child may indeed be misarticulating some sounds, is it not possible that, although delayed, these problems will gradually resolve by themselves? If this doesn't seem to be the case, than remediation of these sounds-in-error may be necessary. Second, realize that these children do not need further instruction in which sounds are problems or difficult for them to produce. That is, no matter what the approach to their articulation concerns, children who both stutter and exhibit clinically significant speech sound errors *do not* need further instruction in how to work at, force out, or be careful, cautious, hesitant, or uncertain about the production of their "problem" sounds. They *do not* need to learn or be encouraged to learn concern, fear, fright, avoidance, and struggle when confronted with the production of certain sounds. Indeed, some of these children already seem to have these ideas or are at least on the road to developing such notions! Third, it is better that these children receive no speech therapy rather than one that exaggerates, emphasizes, or stresses "overarticulation" of speech sounds and/or physically tense speech articulatory musculature and posturing. Too many of these children, without our help, are unfortunately developing (at a greater or lesser rate), what Bloodstein (1975, p. 29) referred to as "certain convictions, preconceptions or expectations" that people who stutter may have or develop regarding speech and language production. Bloodstein (1975, p. 29) further suggested that, over time, the "tension and fragmentation" in speech, which Bloodstein appeared to regard as the essence of stuttering, are based ". . . on beliefs the speaker holds about the difficulty of speech." If, therefore, the child is directly or indirectly encouraged, by adults in his or her environment, to view certain of his or her "mispronounced" sounds as "difficult," such "encouragement" may lead to further "tension and fragmentation" rather than improved communication.

It seems that sometimes our good intentions to assist some of these children with their articulation/phonological difficulties backfire on us when the youngsters just learn more sounds to fear and more and better ways to physically tense up and push out speech segments (see Dell, 1980 for further discussion of ways to deal with these issues with the school-age people who stutter). In essence, what appears to be needed for these children is assistance in helping them develop more physically easy, less hurried, less hesitant or rushed means of initiating and maintaining speech rather than overly careful, cautious, physically precise, and overarticulated productions of sounds.

Young People Who Stutter Who Are Almost or
Completely Unintelligible

Assuming that about three young people who stutter out of ten have some level of articulation concerns, we speculate, based on our clinical experience, that about one of these three children will be quite unintelligible. Here, of course, "working on articulation" is not a question—something needs to be done to help these youngsters become better understood by their listeners. However, all the cautions raised above—when remediating the articulation concerns of children who stutter—still need to be considered. These children also need experience with physically easy, unhurried, and enjoyable forms of communications. Of course, it is difficult for these children to experience "enjoyable" communication when their listener is continually asking them, "Say that again" or "What did you say?" or "Huh?" We have also found that some of these children may begin to stutter for a while as their articulation improves. We are not sure why but suspect with these cases that the entirety of their speech sound production development is delayed and that the "normal" period of disfluency that many children experience is also delayed in terms of its onset. Thus, the period of disfluency typically observed around 3 or 4 is now being produced by these children when they are about 5 or 6 years of age. Much more needs to be explored in this area, but for the present, the SLPs should approach these children somewhat differently than the typical child who stutters.

Dealing with Voice Problems in Children Who Stutter

As mentioned in the previous chapter, as a rule, children who stutter exhibit voice usage roughly or grossly within normal limits. When concerns with voice usage are present, however, the two most common, based on our experience, are (1) inappropriate low-pitched, monotonous, or restricted pitch range (see Adams, 1955; Healey, 1982 for support of this clinical observation, but, for example, Ramig, Krieger, & Adams, 1982; Healey, 1984; Sacco & Metz, 1989 for contrary evidence) and/or (2) hoarseness related to hyperfunctional voice use. The former—low-pitched, sometimes referred to as Johnny-one-note behavior—seems to be far more common than the latter—hoarseness. While this is an area in need of a great deal of empirical study, we can share some of our clinical observations regarding how to best handle these problems.

As mentioned in the previous chapter, it should be noted that the very act of stuttering, for example, tensely posturing the vocal folds in either an adducted or overly abducted position, influences the vocal quality associated with the instance of stuttering. We are not here discussing changes in vocal quality associated with the actual instance of stuttering; rather we are discussing differences or changes in vocal quality throughout the entirety of the child's speech, the fluent as well as disfluent aspects.

Low-Pitched, Monotone (Johnny-One-Note) Children Who Stutter.   We have no empirical evidence to support us, but we speculate that the low-pitched, monotonous voice of some children (and teenagers and adults as well) is somehow related to the child's stuttering problem. That is, the child may be lowering his or her pitch and restricting pitch variations in an attempt, albeit seemingly maladaptive, to avoid, minimize, or reduce the duration and frequency of stuttering. This would suggest that the stuttering precedes the low-pitched, monotone; however, as we said, we have no evidence that this is the case, but we think it is highly likely. It is also possible that the low-pitched monotone reflects overall delays and/or difficulties the child is having with speech motor control (see Conture, Rothenberg, & Molitor, 1986), which is also reflected in the child's stuttering. Whatever the cause, we have found that the stutterings of a child who also exhibits a low-pitched, monotonous voice can be readily remediated—providing there are no other concerns—with the "voice problem" being essentially ignored. We don't know what influence increased fluency would have on the child's voice usage, but we think that we have observed children begin to use a wider range of pitch as they become more fluent. Once again, however, this is an empirical issue in need of investigation.

Hoarseness in Children Who Stutter.   The other kind of voice problem—hoarseness—presents us with a slightly different challenge. Frequently, upon questioning, the parents will tell you that the child who is hoarse does one or more of the following: (1) excessive yelling inside and outside of the home; (2) habitual loud talking inside and outside the home; (3) frequently imitating animal, machine (e.g., trucks, cars, planes, and so forth), or "monster" noises; (4) frequent singing in accompaniment to loud background music or noise; and/or (5) incessant talking, even under conditions where talking can be appropriately minimized, for example, while riding a bike. Of course, one might naturally expect and not be overly concerned if one noticed some hoarseness or change in vocal quality associated with a child's cold, laryngitis, flu, or upper respiratory infection; such changes are usually temporary and resolve with the illness and should not generally be of much concern, at least long term. However, in the absence of such illnesses and/or where the hoarseness becomes or seems to be more persistent and chronic in nature, a referral to an ENT specialist would appear justified. Asking the parents to have the ENT send you, the SLP, a copy of his or her findings and recommendations would be very helpful in planning speech-language therapy. Sometimes these children will be asked to (1) minimize the kinds of vocal abuse mentioned above and/or (2) give their voice some degree of vocal rest. However, it is our experience that both the parents and child will need more, much more, than a one-time lecture in this regard and will need the help and support of the SLP in making such changes and making these changes consistently. Therapy for stuttering can be conducted concomitantly with therapy for voice problems as long as the cautions described above (e.g., emphasizing physically relaxed, relatively unhurried, and enjoyable forms of verbal communication) are heeded.

Dealing with Other Problems in Children Who Stutter

Some Children with Special Needs May Become Overly Dependent.   While an occasional child with cerebral palsy or cleft palate will also stutter, this writer has not had enough repeated experience with these types of children to warrant any meaningful generalizations. What appears to be the case is that each of these children presents a relatively unique situation that must be dealt with accordingly. Furthermore, the relation between the other problem and stuttering is not particularly clear; what is needed, it seems, are published reports of detailed case studies of these children to increase our understanding of the nature and means of remediating the special problems and needs these youngsters appear to have.

What I will say, however, is that with some of the children, especially those with more involved problems like cerebral palsy, this writer has observed some children that were seemingly overprotected by the adults in their environment. This is a natural consequence, I believe, when parents deal with a child who in many cases does seem frailer than the norm, does need more custodial care, and does need special services and attention. The parents, consciously or unconsciously, through their care and concern for the child with special need, foster a greater level of dependence of the child on the parents than is probably good for the child's development. In essence, because the child is actually more *dependent* on the parents than typical, some parents inadvertently and inappropriately increase the child's dependence by reducing the quantity and/or quality of what opportunities are available to the child for developing more independence. As a result of increased dependence on the parents, the child does not seem to develop the internal resources to handle situations that require self-initiative and independence, such as speech-language therapy on his or her own. The child may appear immature, with a low tolerance for frustration and an inability to work reasonably independently, without a lot of input from the clinician. In severe cases, referral to a child psychologist may be necessary before the SLP can effectively treat the child and the child's family.

Psychosocial Adjustment: Normal Reaction to Abnormal Situation. A seemingly more common "other" problem is psychosocial adjustment. However, in our experience, there are very few children who stutter who also exhibit clinically significant and apparent psychosocial adjustment concerns. This does not mean that youngsters who stutter and their families don't have psychosocial concerns, but the *origin* or *cause* of such concerns for different people who stutter may be quite different. Clinicians must try to distinguish between young children who stutter whose emotional concerns are seemingly normal reactions to abnormal situations (i.e., being unable to produce speech fluently) from those children whose stuttering appears related to a more basic psychosocial adjustment problem. We believe that it is a sign of psychological intactness for a child to become concerned about and hesitant to do what he or she cannot do very well. Of course, such concerns, on the part of the child, increase the complexity of the child's stuttering problem, but these concerns relate directly to the child's speaking difficulties and are not caused by other, more deep-seated psychological issues. Generally, many of these concerns will disappear or at least significantly diminish as these children become more fluent. These children need support and understanding for their concerns, but basically they need assistance in becoming more fluent.

Psychosocial Adjustment: Basic Disturbances. As mentioned in Chapter 2, another group of children, whose numbers, we estimate, only involve 5 to 10 percent of the stuttering population, have *real* psychosocial adjustment problems. Some of the behaviors we believe suggest at least a referral for a psychological evaluation are the following (it is possible that a child can exhibit one or more of these behaviors in a variety of permutations):

1. *Children who routinely demonstrate strong and persistent fears of fires, loud noises, the dark, and anything strange.* Many children do this on occasion or for brief periods of time during their development, but when the fears are chronic, strong, and predictable, when the child spends parts of every day or week openly discussing, worrying, and asking parental reassurance that, for example, his bedroom won't catch on fire, a psychological evaluation is not inappropriate (i.e., when the child is obsessed with these concerns and compulsively repeats activities in relation to them,

a referral for psychosocial evaluation would appear appropriate). While this can be an issue related to the child's temperament, if such worry unduly intrudes in the child's daily life activities, then referral to a mental health professional may be warranted. Again, these concerns may reflect behavioral inhibition or temperamental issues, but whatever they reflect, these children probably need to be evaluated by a child psychologist knowledgeable about such concerns and what can be done about them.

2. *Children who are acting out physically against other children either at home, at play, or at school.* Once again it is the frequency and persistence of these physical acts that are important. An occasional slap or punch is one thing—*daily* punching, kicking, pushing/pulling, slapping, or pinching small animals and/or other children, particularly for no apparent reason, is something that should not be overlooked. This problem is particularly noticeable in the child who is not getting any positive attention for school achievement, i.e., he is failing or not mastering his or her school assignments (and attempts to "master" others by physically acting out). These children seem to opt for the idea that attention, of any type, is better than no attention at all.

3. *Children who other parents routinely refuse to let their children play with, or other adults or school personnel report they are having trouble controlling or dealing with.* Some of these children are also acting out physically against other children.

4. *Children who appear to have large amounts of anger and hostility stored within them that they cannot appropriately channel or express.* These children may be quite tenacious in their refusal to discuss themselves or their feelings, even when such discussion would appear to be an appropriate part of therapy.

5. *Children who refuse to talk to the examining clinician (after 30 plus minutes of trying) but readily talk to parents once the clinician is outside of the room.* Here we are *not* talking about 5 to 15 minutes reticence to communicate with the clinician because of shyness, separation anxiety, or the like. We are also *not* talking about a child who stops talking because of momentary embarrassment or fatigue or temperamental reactivity. What we are referring to here is the child who will not talk to us *after* 45 to 90 minutes of our trying, the child who seems to be purposely refusing to talk to us but will readily talk to mother and father when we are not in the room. While the examining psychologist may have little better luck than us at getting such a child to talk, it is our experience that the reasons these children refuse to talk are not solely related to stuttering and that family counseling may be a better place to begin than therapy for stuttering.

Which Comes First: Stuttering or Disturbance in Psychosocial Adjustment? Many times, with a child who stutters and who exhibits real or apparent psychosocial adjustment problems, the question comes up: Which came first, the stuttering or the psychological problem? In reality, this is often difficult to tell; but most of the time, even as the child becomes more psychologically intact, the child's stuttering remains. Both the parents and psychological professional should be made aware of such a possibility at the beginning of psychotherapy, so that their efforts can be focused on helping the child to develop in a more appropriate fashion psychologically and not be overly concerned that the child's fluency is not also improving.

Down Syndrome.   There is considerable evidence (see Bloodstein, 1995, pp. 260–261) to suggest that the prevalence of stuttering is uncommonly high in individuals with Down syndrome (a type of developmental or cognitive disorder). Thus, it is not surprising that clinicians who treat people who stutter may encounter people with Down syndrome who stutter (indeed, one such individual was recently added to the caseload in the clinic where this author works). No one, as far as this author knows, has been able to explain the connection between Down syndrome and stuttering. In the largest study (Preus, 1981) to date (n = 47) of the connection between Down's syndrome and stuttering, approximately 34 percent were found to be stuttering, but also 31 percent of the sample were exhibiting cluttering or cluttering-like behavior. Farmer and Brayton (1979) subsequently made the observation that the disfluency of people with Down syndrome was more of a cluttering than stuttering variety. Clearly, more, much more is needed to be known about this population in terms of the onset, nature, and causes of disfluency. It is this writer's opinion that the clinician should first try to discern if the disfluency tends to be more cluttering in nature (little apparent awareness of the problem, minimal apparent reaction to the disfluency, marginal intelligibility, a rapid rate of speech that often gets faster, and the speech less intelligible as the utterance progresses). If cluttering, obviously, the clinician will want to direct his or her attentions more in that area than for stuttering. Second, the therapy is probably going to have to be direct, with a lot of "doing it to" the client, rather than the client readily engaging with the clinician, due to their often limited level of cognitive development. This would involve clear, unambiguous reinforcement for changes in disfluency that are repeatedly and clearly modeled for the child. If the child is young, the parents can learn many of the skills we teach the parents of typical children to do (e.g., minimize interrupting, talking for the child, telling the child to slow down and take a deep breath). Clearly, more needs to be known about the best way to assess and subsequently treat individuals with Down syndrome who also exhibit stuttering. What treatment we have done with these children suggests that indirect approaches with them are not very powerful, although parental counseling can help; instead, the approach should be more direct albeit patient, gentle, and supportive because children with Down syndrome have the potential for learning to inappropriately physically react to and avoid disfluency, just like their typically developing peers.

Modifying the Stuttering of Children Who Exhibit Some Stuttering but Whose Parents Are Minimally or Completely Unconcerned

When confronted with these children and their parents, the writer has found that he has three choices: (1) observe the child through periodic reevaluations until such time as the child has no problem and/or the parents change their minds; (2) bring the child in for individual speech therapy; and (3) bring the child in for parent/child fluency group. Initially, we have found for most of these children that neither options (1) nor (2) are completely satisfactory. Thus, at present we tend towards option (3), the parent/child fluency group, an option we have detailed elsewhere (e.g., Conture & Melnick, 1999; Kelly & Conture, 1991) and will discuss, to some degree, in the next section.

With the first approach—periodic reevaluation—the SLP runs the risk of having the child's fluency problem and/or environment deteriorate; however, with the second approach—individual speech therapy—the SLP runs the risk of boring the child and the parents with therapy, since improvement may not come fast enough or be of sufficient quality and quantity to maintain motivation and satisfaction with therapy. If a parent/child fluency group is not a realistic or desired approach, one compromise between options (1) and (2) is to bring the child and/or his or her parents in for a period of trial speech therapy of, say, three to six weeks.

It must be stressed, however, that BEFORE this trial period begins, the parents must be clearly and explicitly told that this will be "trial" therapy that may only last for, say, three to six weeks. Thus, if the child and parents seem to benefit from this trial therapy, fine, the length of treatment can be further extended and/or modified as need be; if not, we cancel the trial therapy and put the client and family into a hold pattern during which time we observe through periodic reevaluations, phone calls to parents and school, or school and home visits (if possible). Even when parents are relatively unconcerned about the child's problem, it is all too easy to make a rush to judgment and initiate therapy with the child. Before we begin therapy with *any* child (or teenager or adult, too, for that matter), in addition to assessing whether the person will benefit from therapy, we must also try to make professional decisions whether the child is emotionally, socially, physically, communicatively, and otherwise ready for therapy. Therapy begun *before* the client is ready to benefit from same is not only counter-productive in the short run but in the long run has the real potential for turning the client off from therapy at a point when he or she is ready to benefit ("I already had speech therapy, and it didn't help").

The Parent/Child Fluency Group

We and others (e.g., Bailey & Bailey, 1982; Botterill, Kelman, & Rustin, 1991; Conture & Melnick, 1999; Kelly & Conture, 1991; Rustin, 1987) believe that involving parents in the therapy process, while adding to the complexities of the process, also increases our effectiveness and the child's chances for long-term recovery. There is, of course, nothing new about parental involvement in speech-language therapy. Again, Johnson and colleagues' (1967) remarks, made over thirty years ago, regarding parental involvement in speech-language therapy, were as true then as they are now:

> Parents are usually well-intentioned persons who have a great deal of love and affection for their children. The difficulty is that sometimes they do not understand the problems their children face. Their well-intentioned efforts to help are sometimes misdirected. . . . Absorbed in their own interests, they are sometimes neglectful or impatient of their children without the slightest intention of being so—indeed without knowing that they are. The conscientious speech clinician will, therefore, make a point of seeing the parents of the children with whom she works. . . . Both clinical experience and research studies have demonstrated the importance of enlisting the active cooperation of parents. (p. 144)

Not only has it been the long-standing clinical opinion of some (e.g., Rustin, 1987) the parental involvement in speech-language treatment is very important to long-term improvement, but over forty years ago researchers like Sommers et al. (1959) reported more rapid improvement in articulation abilities of children when parents were active members to treatment (e.g., attending lectures, observing treatment) than when they were not.

Do we know, in any definitive way, whether such parental involvement will have similar benefit when trying to remediate stuttering? No, we certainly do not. However, it seems reasonable to suggest that if a child's articulation/phonological behavior benefited from parental involvement, similar benefits might occur if parents were involved with therapy for stuttering. This is, of course, an empirical question, the answers to which, we suggest, will eventually provide support for the role of parents in treatment and long-term recovery in childhood stuttering.

Of course, if parents are unconcerned and/or resistant to therapy in any form, then they will not be actively involved with a parent/child (P/C) fluency group or any other form of treatment. While we are presently talking about parents who are unconcerned, the P/C group, we have found, is equally effective for children whose parents DO express concerns about their child's speech and related issues (these children and their parents will be extensively discussed in the next section).

The rationale, logistics, and difficulties of conducting such groups have been discussed elsewhere (e.g., Conture & Melnick, 1999; Kelly & Conture, 1991); however, we will, in this space, cover the essential aspects of these groups. In our opinion, the logic behind as well as the conducting of these groups is relatively straightforward and it can be modified, simplified, or made more complex as the need arises! Typically, the parent/child group meets once a week for approximately 45 to 60 minutes with the parents meeting in one room and the children in another. Groups generally meet in the late afternoon (3:00 to 6:00 PM), near the end of or after school is over, and weekly sessions are arranged in ten- to twelve-week blocks with about three blocks arranged per calendar year. The typical child is involved with the P/C group for two ten- to twelve-week blocks with some children only requiring one block and some four or more blocks. We are beginning to find that ten-week blocks are maybe a bit better for the child and parent: Twelve weeks seems to be two weeks too many, and both parents and child seem to get stale and/or bored with the process. In a university setting, there are typically breaks between blocks of treatment. While some might be concerned that are approximately four- to eight-week breaks between each ten-week block, a strong case can be made that these breaks are an excellent "living laboratory" for assessing the child's ability to transfer change during a period of nontreatment. If a child cannot maintain his or her improved fluency during scheduled breaks from active therapy, it is our experience that there is little chance that the child will maintain improvement once therapy is discontinued.

Arranging Groups by Age.   Before proceeding with details of the P/C group, the ages of the clients within each group should be discussed. While this topic was mentioned above, it is quite crucial when bringing children together as a group. Children, if at all possible, should be grouped together with other children of a comparable chronological and developmental age. In this way, the clinician maximizes the chances that the children will neither feel patronized nor overwhelmed by the level of activities. Once again, with children, the *form* of the activity is many times more important than its *content*. While the content, rationale, and purpose of activities may be the same for a group of 5-year-olds versus a group of 7-year-olds, the form should be adapted to the two groups' levels of development.

Logistics.   A typical group session begins with the parents and children being separated into two rooms. While we try to arrange some time each session for the parents to watch and participate with their children, sometimes the best laid plans of mice and SLPs go awry! Sometimes the parents and a clinician spend the entire session discussing parental questions and concerns and the parents minimally observe their children. Conversely, other times, the parents observe the entirety of their children's group, only entering the children's' group in the last 10 minutes of its functioning. Again, we have found it beneficial to try to include the parents in each and every group during the last 10 minutes of its functioning; however, if parents are really involved in their parent group discussion, it is difficult to get parents to terminate their own group discussions in time to participate in their child's group!

The Child's Group. After separating the children from their parents, the children, two to six age-comparable youngsters, are paired with one or two clinicians. In the two settings where I have conducted these groups (Syracuse and Vanderbilt Universities), one clinician acts as group facilitator while a second clinician (if available) can assist with the demonstration of group activities, helps the facilitator with "crowd control," and collects pertinent data (e.g., frequency of stuttering per 100 words of conversation speech). However, we believe that one *experienced* clinician should be able to run such a group just as effectively, although such groups should probably not exceed four or perhaps five children.

Each child sits on his or her own small rug; these are arranged in a semicircle around the clinician. In some situations, particularly during the first few therapy sessions, the clinician may want to label each rug with the child's name to avoid bickering over whose rug is whose and wasting precious therapy time. If chairs are used, each chair would likewise be labeled with each child's name. While we don't want the children to feel that they are in church, neither do we want them to develop the relatively laissez-faire attitude typically exhibited on the school playground. They are in the group to have a good time and to enjoy themselves, but they must be reasonably behaved and attentive during the activities. Indeed, some children have such poor pragmatic, attention, or social skills that, after this trial period, they have to be switched to individual therapy whereby hopefully these skills can be improved so that group treatment is eventually possible. Two types of children are not appropriate for group treatment: (1) children who interfere with the interactions of other children and who require so much of the clinician's time that she cannot deal with the other children; and (2) children who do not interfere with the interactions of other children but who "drift," lose focus, and attention in a group setting when they are the listeners and not the speakers, requiring one-on-one attention, in an individual setting, to achieve maximum benefit.

In essence, the child's group has two goals: (1) help the children change speech production behaviors that inhibit fluency and increase those behaviors that facilitate fluency, and (2) help the children change those communicative interactive behaviors that inhibit fluency and increase those communicative interactive behaviors that facilitate fluency. Each group session, therefore, combines therapy approaches that try to help the child speak more fluently as well as to develop communicative interaction behaviors that will facilitate this fluency. As mentioned in Chapter 1, we believe that stuttering relates to a complex interaction between the child's abilities and the child's environment. Some of that environment is "created" by things the child does during speaking that are not directly related to speech production, for example, interrupting people when they talk. Again, this is an indirect method. Changes are repeatedly modeled by the clinician in the presence of the child; rules for talking (e.g., "don't talk for others") are repeatedly explained; and the child's changes or approximations to change are gently but clearly rewarded verbally by the clinician. *No* attempts are made to directly change, modify, or manipulate the child's speech (dis)fluency. Why? Well, perhaps I can best shed some light on this rationale by citing a recent case that I have begun to evaluate.

Juan, a 4.5-year-old-child, was brought to our clinic by his mother and father. Suffice it to say, Juan is a severe stutterer (e.g., his total overall score on the *Stuttering Severity Instrument-3* [SSI-3] was 34, in the very severe range). In the course of the evaluation, the examiner was told that Juan strongly dislikes having his mistakes brought to his attention. Subsequently, the mother explained that she "has worked with" Juan (I've seen fathers as well as mothers and fathers together do this) to "get him to talk faster" and "help him finish his sentences." Juan also said during the evaluation that "mommy helps me talk fast to make my stuttering go away." The mother asked me if she should continue, to which I responded as nicely as but as firmly as I could: If what you did helped, you and your child wouldn't be in our clinic! Clearly, in Juan's case, some kind of help is the kind of help he could do without! My point: Juan, and more than a few children we see, are somewhat sensitive, reactive, and easily frustrated and fearful about their mistakes and/or environmental changes/differences (which include differences in their own as well as others' spoken communication). Thus, why would one want to point out, highlight, or focus on these children's "mistakes," when the child is already overly sensitized and/or reactive to them? My answer: We don't want to, to put it simply! Of course, the *fact* of "pointing out" may not the problem as much as the *manner* of the pointing out, the tone, the inflections and attitudes of the parent or clinician while mentioning or pointing out the mistake. In our opinion and experience, however, modeling rather than telling, instructing, or lecturing is the preferred way to go with these children, at least until the parent understands how to deliver neutral-affect comments and corrections of the child, a feat few if any parents, because of their emotional involvement with the child, can achieve, at least to begin.

Changing Speech Production Behavior.   As pointed out above, on the whole our approach to changing stuttering with our child's group approach is indirect—the clinician is not directly, by word or by deed, trying to modify the way the child talks. Instead, the clinician is trying, through play- or game-oriented activities, and frequent and repetitive modeling, to get the child to employ more pragmatically appropriate communication (e.g., not speaking for others, interrupting others, etc.) and speak with more appropriate levels of physical tension and at rates of production that are reasonable given the child's level of development. We do this through demonstrating, identifying, modeling, and trying, for example, to produce the temporal difference between "turtle" (slow) versus "rabbit" (fast) speech and the physical tension difference between "scarecrow" (relaxed) and "tinwoodsman" (tense) speech. However, one caution: Some of these children, regardless of apparent intellectual and social readiness, may not understand the concept of same/different (especially the 3- to 5-year-old children). Thus, it is not a bad idea to include examples of same/different (e.g., various colors, textures, and lengths of cloth) throughout the first two to five group sessions, so that children get a more concrete example of this concept. Another caution: The clinician should be ready and willing to demonstrate and use rabbit, turtle, scarecrow (Raggedy Ann), or tinwoodsman speech (see Figure 4.3). The clinician should be adept at *showing* and should minimize *telling* the children what she wants them to do. This is also true with the parents. And while the following will suggest that we try to change X (speech production) or Y (associated pragmatic, social, or communicative skills such as turntaking), nothing could be further from the truth. Both X and Y can be and are routinely, in our child groups, simultaneously addressed. We have to, in this space, deal with one and then the other to most clearly explain the relevant issues and the means for addressing each.

Reason for Changing Communicative Interaction (Pragmatic) Behaviors. Although becoming more fluent is the ultimate goal of any therapy with people who stutter, there are a number of related behaviors that, in our opinion, if left unchanged have the real potential for making it difficult for the child to maintain his or her fluency. Once again, speech fluency is not isolated, standing alone by itself, with no connection to other facets of the child's communication—for example, syntax, semantics, phonology and pragmatics. Especially with children, where their communicative abilities are evolving—often at different rates across the spectrum of skills they need to speak—we need, for optimal long-term improvement, to consider a variety of other behaviors besides fluency to help the child become fluent and maintain his or her fluency.

Typical Pragmatic Difficulties. It is not at all unusual to observe children who stutter to frequently interrupt people while they are talking, talk for others, talk out of turn or exhibit difficulty waiting their turn to talk, begin their speaking turn with little clear idea how to say what they want or even to have anything to say, and in general be less-than-attentive listeners. Likewise, some of these children will be unable to clearly, sequentially, and succinctly relay a story to listeners, especially if the topic of conversation is outside the room where the child and the child's listener are situated. In essence, they will monologue with the clinician or their parents, rambling from disjointed point of discussion to another, with no apparent beginning, middle, or end of their thoughts or communication. Such monologues, the parents will tell you, are often annoying to the other family members and the source of frustration on the part of the listeners, who, try as they might, are not able to understand the purpose and thrust of the child's monologue. To allow children to continually or frequently monopolize family or clinical sessions, with long-winded, disjointed, and off-task monologues is simply not appropriately socializing the child. No one, perhaps other than some of our politicians, is afforded the luxury of being allowed to ramble on and on with no apparent beginning, middle, or end, while listeners patiently sit and wait. It is not reality to allow children to frequently indulge in such practices and, if allowed to continue, these practices make children people who are less than desirable as conversational partners.

Means of Changing Pragmatic Skills. Accordingly, we use a number of play-oriented activities, games, and models to show the children how to: (1) LISTEN (when someone else is talking); (2) WAIT (your turn); and (3) DON'T TALK (when someone else is talking). Sometimes, getting children who stutter to obey or at least more frequently observe these rules is all that is necessary for them to become more fluent.

It would seem that it is difficult for anyone to speak with optimal amounts of fluency if they are always trying to "get a word in edgewise" and reluctant to wait to talk until it is their turn. Our clinical experience suggests to us that speaking rapidly, using long, complex sentences, exhibiting minimal or very short turn-switching pauses, interrupting and/or not listening to speakers when they talk are behaviors that stress the abilities of people who stutter to achieve and/or maintain fluent speech.

The Parents' Group.   The parents of the children are seen separately but simultaneously with group therapy for their children. While the group has a variety of functions, each group is a mix of (1) discussing concerns general to all parents and their children and (2) discussing concerns specific to one or two parents and their children. As in all groups, some parents are better than others at understanding how general concerns relate to their own situation or how someone else's problem, seemingly different on the surface, may actually be similar to theirs. For the SLP, the hardest skill to learn is the ability to walk the fine line between closing one's mouth and listening versus opening one's mouth and conversing. Neither too much listening nor talking will be effective, but there is a need for some mix of both.

When One Lives in the Past, It Is Hard to Exist in the Present and Prepare for the Future. Parents have a natural curiosity regarding the past, what may have caused their child to stutter, and their role in same. Indeed, it is a rare parent who doesn't start treatment with the classic question: "What causes stuttering?" We have, at the beginning of this chapter, already discussed this issue and won't repeat ourselves in this space. All we will say is to politely and respectfully answer their questions in this regard but to steer them, as best you can, away from a relatively fruitless dwelling on the *past* and concentrate on how things can be or can change in the *present* and *future*. While we can understand their curiosity and desire to make sense of the past, once it has been made clear to them that the past is over and done, that we have told them our best guess about what may have happened, and that we can only change the present, it is time to move on. Unfortunately, some parents remain *fixated* on the past and their possible role in their child's stuttering, failing to come to grips with what they may be able to do to change the present. For these parents, group therapy, while not a waste, probably will take longer and have less than optimal influence.

Peer Advisement.   Parents learn many things in a group setting, and not just from the SLP. From the other parents they learn that they are "not alone in the boat," that other parents share some but not all of their same concerns, that other parents can and do change, and that such changes do help their children. Indeed, the not-alone-in-the-boat feelings that many of these parents share lead some of these parents into making friendships with the other parents, friendships that involve socializing together outside the confines of the clinic.

From the SLP, the parents are provided with objective information about children in general and stuttering in specific. The SLP attempts to provide the parents with up-to-date and hopefully more accurate, rational perspectives with which to view themselves and their children regarding stuttering and related concerns. And, especially for the "hands-on" or "I-want-to-do-something" parents, the SLP tries to provide a variety of simple, effective means by which they can change their own speech behavior as well as related behaviors in order to facilitate their child's speech fluency. Each parent group session involves a lot of talking, either by the parents or the SLP or both. While these discussions can and do take the form of information sharing and counseling, they can take the form of parental venting and even one parent instructing or challenging another parent. That is, one or two parents will raise a concern or problem that is particularly vexing or frustrating to them, and other parents will identify with the problem and add their own feelings. In these situations, it is best for the SLP to listen and try not to get overly directive nor defensive, particularly when parents are being critical over apparent slowness or lack of progress in their child's fluency. Sometimes these parental venting sessions are based on misinformation on the parents' part about what should be taking place at a particular point in therapy. However, other times a parent's concerns are based on accurate perceptions that things are not going as well nor as quickly as they should for their child. If the clinician believes that a particular parent is getting out of hand with his or her critique, then that parent should be gently but firmly told so but, and this is extremely important, out of earshot of the other parents. One of our *cardinal rules* for conducting this or any group is as follows: *Praise in public and criticize in private*. A group leader violates this rule at his or her own peril. Throughout each parent group session, the SLP will find him- or herself rapidly shifting roles, first listener, then instructor, now supporter of what parents said, then challenger of what they say, and so forth. A healthy mix of listening, talking, supporting, challenging, guiding, and instruction is necessary for the SLP who conducts parent groups.

Maintenance Therapy.   In our earlier days, once a child had successfully maintained normal or near-normal fluency for the last half (4 to 6 weeks in length) of a block of the P/C group, we would dismiss (i.e., no therapy at all) and have the child and parents return in about six months for a reevaluation. While a number of these children maintained or transferred their fluency, a disturbing number of them didn't. For the past ten to fifteen years, to alleviate that problem, once a child achieves normal or near-normal fluency during the P/C group, we set up a "maintenance program." No single procedure, in our opinion, is more important to the *long-term* success of the child and family than a well-conducted, well-thought-through maintenance program. And the emphasis is on *gradual* rather than *abrupt* termination of treatment, to intentionally blur the edges between being in and out of treatment, for both child and parents.

Naturally, the specifics of this maintenance program vary somewhat from child to child, but, in general, from the time of initial treatment, the parent and child come to the P/C therapy group for approximately one calendar year. A typical sequence might look like this: first, once a week, for ten to twenty weeks, then twice a month for the first ten-week block, once a month for the second ten-week block, and one or two times for the last block. Using this *gradual* means of fading treatment out, we have found, we can better monitor the child's ability to transfer and at the same time get the child and particularly the parents gradually used to doing things on their own. Again, at the risk of putting too fine a point on the situation: we have found our gradual means of terminating, of providing maintenance treatment, to be a very important facet of our overall P/C group approach.

Parent/Child Therapy Group: Preliminary Treatment Outcome Data   There is considerable information about treatment outcome for more direct approaches to changing stuttering in children (e.g., Bloodstein, 1995, Appendix, pp. 453–472); however, there is far less treatment outcome data pertaining to parent/child stuttering groups, like ours. In attempts to rectify this situation, over about two and a half years, we have begun and recently completed a preliminary treatment outcome study with our various parent–child groups (Pellowski, Conture, Roos, Adkins, & Ask, 2000). This pilot study is, this writer hopes, the first in a series of studies we will conduct regarding treatment outcome for our parent/child stuttering groups.

In essence, Pellowski and colleagues (2000) studied 26 3- to 8-year-old children who, along with their parents, were participating in our weekly parent/child fluency groups. While we plan, with subsequent studies, to report on changes in pragmatic skills (e.g., percent of conversational turns that were interrupted by child and/or parent) as well as "customer satisfaction" (e.g., parental responses to standardized questionnaires) associated with these parent/child groups, the Pellowski and colleagues study concentrated on changes in stuttering frequency, one crucial element, we believe, in documenting change in stuttering related treatment. Again, these are *preliminary* data, but we believe that they provide insights into this approach to therapy with young children and an impetus for further, more refined intervention as well as analysis methodology (see Conture, 1999a, for further discussion of this issue).

To be a subject in this study, each child had to have participated in therapy for at least twelve sessions, but some had participated longer (range = 12 to 36 sessions). We began with 32 possible subjects, but for various reasons, data from 6 children was not available (e.g., a child who did not attend sufficient sessions), leaving us with 26 children (21 boys and 5 girls), ranging in age from 33 to 99 months. The average time between onset (TSO) of stuttering and beginning of treatment was 23 months (range = 3 to 63 months). The stuttering frequency data we report were collected across a variety of speaking situations in the clinical setting (e.g., clinician to child, child to child, parent to child), but were only collected within the clinical setting (see Ingham & Riley, 1998 for discussion of the desirability to base treatment outcome data on more than one speaking situation or setting). Below, we will return to the implications of "brief TSO" on treatment outcome data for young children.

Figure 3.3 shows that there was a significant group mean difference (related samples $t(25) = 3.33$, $p<0.01$) between the first four sessions and the last four sessions. In other words, for the group of 26 children who stutter, there was a significant decrease in stuttering frequency from the beginning to end of a reasonable period of evaluation (approximately three months of intervention). However, when we look below the surface of the group central tendency, we find that while approximately 65 percent of the subjects followed the tendency of the group to significantly decrease, approximately 35 percent did not, either exhibiting no appreciable change or even slight increases in stuttering frequency. Obviously, this one-size-fits-all approach needs adjustment, adjustment that must begin with the diagnostic, we believe, to match child with the treatment that seems best suited. This requires, with this project, retrospective review of initial diagnostic information to see how specific diagnostic data match with treatment outcome. Furthermore, the Pellowski and colleagues' data does not talk to maintenance/transfer, of which we are quite aware, but it is a beginning of that process that will take many years of effort to complete.

In the meantime, it is instructive, we believe, to look at results from some of the individual subjects to better understand the challenges that lie in front of us when assessing treatment outcome with young children. Figure 3.4 shows stuttering frequency data for four children, two of which we believe would be considered reasonably successful by most rea-

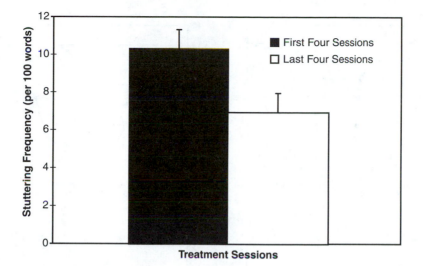

FIGURE 3.3   Treatment outcome for parent-child stuttering group. Average stuttering frequency of first four versus last four treatment sessions [related-samples t(25)=3.33, p<.01]. N=26 three- to eight-year-old children who stutter.
After Pellowski et al. (2000)

sonable individuals and two who showed little or no change, even a slight increase in stuttering frequency (on each graph is listed "% change," which is calculated by taking an average of the first four sessions [T1] then subtracting it from the average of the last four sessions [T2] and then dividing by T2 + T1, or expressed as a formula, % change = T2 − T1/T2 + T1). Child A, upper left graph, shows an appreciable decrease in treatment, a decrease we believe is "real" and related to intervention, particularly given that he had been stuttering for about three years at the time of treatment and was most likely beyond the window of appreciable spontaneous recovery. Child C, in the lower left graph, also shows an appreciable decrease in stuttering, after twelve sessions. However, note that Child C had only been stuttering for about three months at the time of treatment. Hence, Child C, it is fair to say, may have been the beneficiary of spontaneous recovery facilitated by intervention! Of course, at this point, we don't know that, and given the child's relatively severe problem at time of diagnosis, 20 to 25 percent stuttering, we probably would do the same thing again, given the child's severity level and parents' clearly and deeply expressed concerns at the time of initial diagnosis. However, when we do so, we must be honest with ourselves and realize that some of the "benefit" of our treatment for these children may be as much spontaneous recovery as it is intervention! Child B (upper right) and Child D (lower right) present an entirely different picture. Both apparently received little or no benefit from the intervention, although there is always—and I want to emphasize this, particularly with children growing, learning and developing at different rates—the possibility that a longer period of treatment might be effective and/or necessary for these type of children. Be that as it may, it is this writer's opinion, that Child D (lower right), particularly given the child's long TSO, probably needs some other form of treatment, be it individual and/or direct, stuttering modification, fluency shaping, or an integration of both. While Child D was initially

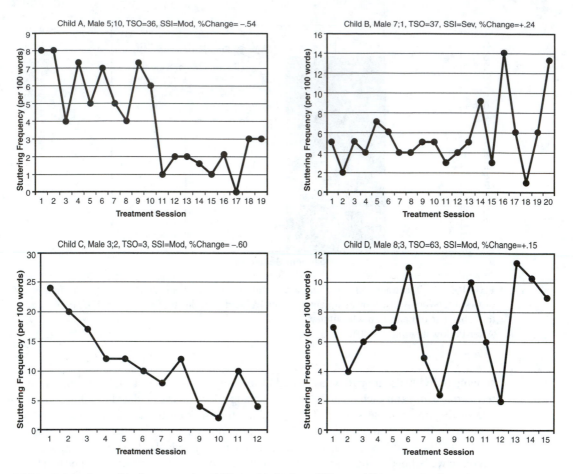

FIGURE 3.4 Stuttering frequency (per 100 words) for four different children (A, B, C, and D) who participated in twelve to twenty weeks of parent–child (indirect) group therapy, with two children (A and C) exhibiting successful outcomes and two (B and D) nonsuccessful outcomes. See text for details. After Pellowski et al. (2000).

brought into the parent/child group because the home communication environment was far less than ideal (e.g., parent and child, more often than not, simultaneously talking), it seems apparent that this child needs a more direct, individualized approach because his stuttering problem was too entrenched, or habituated, for an indirect, group approach to significantly modify. Child C (upper right), on the other hand is, in our opinion, another story. Note that Child C's TSO is about the same as child A, the latter child being an apparently successful client while Child C seems far from it. Why then didn't Child C appear to benefit from treatment? In our opinion, Child C's stuttering frequency was starting to stabilize during treatment weeks 8–12, when, shortly after in rapid succession, his father lost his job, the father was in the home during the day, the mother had to work more and be away from the child more, and the family moved. All were appreciable changes in the child's routine. Further, we had earlier documented, through the Carey Temperament Scale and by repeated parental reports, that this child was very sensitive to any type of change of variation in his routine, schedule, or environment. Any reader who has worked with children who stutter, particularly preschool children, of sensitive, slow-to-warm-up, or behaviorally expressive temperaments, will recognize the reality of this situation and the apparently strong influence changes in routine, schedule, and environment can have on the stuttering of a child. This is particularly true for a child whose temperament is initially reactive to change and continues to remain so, long after the change has occurred (see Hill, 1999, Table 12.1, where she presents a scale attempting to document and rate "specific life changes that may affect children," p. 154).

In summary, for the group of 26 children who stutter, we see evidence that indirect treatment can bring about a significant decrease in stuttering frequency; however, we can also see that spontaneous recovery can confound the degree of certainty we have in such conclusions as well as recognize that this treatment might not work with all children, at least initially. Children who receive minimal or no benefit from this or any form of therapy may need (1) different forms of intervention; (2) longer periods of the same treatment; or (3) in those situations where appreciable life changes have occurred for the child/child's family, help for the parents, as rapidly as possible, to stabilize the home environment and the reactions to same, especially if child's temperament is such it reacts and continues to react to such variations and breaks in routine. Again, it is recognized that this is preliminary data, limited in scope in terms of sampling several different speaking situation as well as insights into maintenance, but the longest journey starts with a single step, something Pellowski and colleagues (2000) have done. To paraphrase Robert Frost, we realize we have many miles to go before we can ever rest: We still have to settle whether this therapy works, for whom, how long, and under what conditions.

Children with Some Stutterings Whose Parents Are Also Concerned

Children in this category can certainly be initially placed in the P/C group and, if they are not successful, after say two or three ten- to twelve-week therapy blocks, individual therapy may be necessary. Some other children, for scheduling or other reasons, may need to begin with individual therapy, without ever receiving group therapy. Even with this latter group, some involvement with the parents, particularly in the beginning to keep them informed as to the type and progress of the child's therapy, is strongly recommended. Some of these children can still be helped with an indirect approach, as discussed above, while others will need a "combined" indirect/direct approach, and still others need mainly a direct approach. Truly, one size therapy will not fit all in this category.

Getting Therapy Started

Much of the first individual session with a young child who stutters is spent getting to know the child, setting down rules of the road for the therapy sessions (and for the parents, if they are involved), and trying to develop some procedure for the first and subsequent therapy sessions whereby the SLP can assess whether the child's speech disfluencies warrant therapy. This last task—developing a strategy to assess progress or lack thereof—is oftentimes overlooked. All too frequently, SLPs will assume that the fluency achieved in the clinic is also manifest outside the clinic, without either asking the client or the client's parents or doing their own testing. Many times it seems that therapy begins without much thought given to when the SLP will know that therapy should be terminated. We have already discussed the fact that speech fluency in the clinic does not necessarily equal speech fluency in the home does not necessarily equal speech fluency in school. At the least, then, the clinician should routinely ask the parent how the child's speech at home and school is progressing, and not be surprised if the parent says that there is little change in the home or school even though the child's behavior in the clinic suggests otherwise!

Encouraging Parents to Interact (Play and/or Read) with Their Child Outside of Treatment.   As with the P/C group, if at all possible, we like to have and think it instructive for parents to observe us playing and talking with their children. An ideal number of observations would be once every other session but even once every ten sessions would be better than none. Although parents frequently say, "I simply don't have the time to spend playing with Mario like you do," or "We don't have *all those nice toys at home*," or "I don't like to play with children," we try to emphasize to the parents the *quality*, rather than the *quantity*, of our play interactions with the child. Although the wise SLP would never say this directly to a parent who complains about not enough time, the issue is not really the *amount* of time but the parents' willingness to *take* whatever time they have to interact with the child ("it's boring to play with him"). Simply put, some parents find it boring to play with children; others find it not particularly intellectually stimulating, and still others simply don't know how and when to play and/or read with their children. We are not talking about hours and hours of playing with or reading to the child each day, but 10 to 30 minutes a day. We can't state this strongly enough: It's not a matter of amount of time spent by parents with their child but parent priorities for the spending of what time is available. Certainly, parents clearly need and should be encouraged to take the time to relax and unwind themselves on a daily basis. However, they are, like it or not, a parent also and must be helped to see, in firm but gentle ways, that some daily time spent interacting with their child should receive a reasonably high priority. No one ever said that being a parent was easy.

We also try to quickly point out that it is not the toys themselves that determine what they child gets out of playing as much as it is how the child and parent actually play with the toys. A cardboard box can, and very often is, a more attractive toy to a young child than the latest Death-Ray-Stun-for-Fun-Dream-Laser-Beam toy gun. We try to point out to and demonstrate for the parents such things as: a clinician's unconditional, positive regard for the child, the clinician's attempts to listen to the content of the child's utterances, the clinician's clear but firm setting down of rules for communication as well as general behaving, and the clinician's showing as well as telling the child how to do a particular task. We find, all too often, that parents will *tell* Chantra to do something like make her bed and think their mere telling her is sufficient, even though they have never really spent time instructing and *showing* Chantra how to actually go about making a bed (see Bettleheim, 1985).

Introducing the Concept of Hard and Easy Speech

Although these preschool and school-age children may be relatively inconsistent in the production of their stutterings, if the situation strongly suggests that there will be continued negative development (i.e., greater numbers and varieties of stuttering), we may and do become fairly direct in our approach. Elaborating upon Williams' (1971) concept of *hard* (i.e., physically tense and relatively rapid) versus *easy* (i.e., physically relaxed and relatively slow) speech, we start by having the child identify "hard" and "easy" speech in our speech. We then progress to having the child listen to audiotape recordings of others, to listening to tape recordings of him- or herself, and finally to the stutterings in his or her own speech *as* he or she is actually producing them. We prefer to begin with audio rather than videotapes because it allows the child, clinician, and parents, if they are involved, to focus on speech behavior rather than being distracted by any associated, inappropriate nonspeech behavior and/or how the child looks or acts on the television monitor.

The terms *hard* and *easy* speech are nice, simple terms with minimal negative connotations associated with them (Williams, 1971). These terms may be used by the SLP to help children (if this seems appropriate) *identify* instances of hard and easy speech as well as describe speech targets that the child can aim towards. The *initial* goal with hard versus easy speech, contrary to what some think, *is not* reduction in the *frequency* but reduction in the *duration* (length) and *manner* (tensing, pushing, avoiding) of stuttering. Eventually, of course, as the duration shortens, and the manner becomes more physically relaxed and forward flowing, reduction in frequency will come naturally as well as be encouraged and taught by the clinician. But in the beginning, the client learns to change the manner in which he or she stutters, to make it shorter, less physically tense, and more normal sounding and looking. As the child demonstrates increased ability to quickly and accurately identify hard and easy speech, we then help the child learn strategies to facilitate (1) increased production of easy speech and (2) the ability to change from hard to easy as needed. In essence, as will be seen, this sequence—*identification* preceding but being overlapped with *modification*—provides the foundation for all of our therapy procedures with children, teenagers, and adults. And, of course, the (3) *transfer/maintenance* stage is overlapped with and eventually follows (2) modification.

Parents' Role in Hard/Easy Speech. One caution, however, is that some parents, once they hear and understand the terms *hard* and *easy* speech, *rewrite* or *rephrase* these terms into their own vocabulary and usage, employing these terms in statements like, "Stop that hard speech!" (we have a similar problem with some parents in the P/C group with the terms *rabbit* and *turtle* speech). We never cease to be amazed at how some parents can continually and consistently selectively attend to mainly the negative aspects of their children's behavior. Ironically, these same parents will ask us whether they should or can say to their child in nice, positive tones, "That's it, that's good easy speech" while never once asking us whether they should say "Stop that hard speech this instant!" While we certainly don't want to continually make a big deal out of the child's fluency and thus indirectly highlight the "terribleness" of the child's stuttering, we tell the parents that a little praise now and then, anything that builds their child's positive self-image and confidence, must be correct and should be good for them to do and for their child to hear. Likewise, we tell the parents that a little support ("talking to the child's feelings") for when the child is obviously frustrated or discouraged about the difficulties of talking is always appropriate. For example, the parent might say to the child, after watching a child struggle, get frustrated and/or discouraged while trying to say his name, begin a story about something that happened at school, or ask the parent a question, something like, "Yeah, sometimes it's hard to do things the way we want to do them . . . we try but just can't do it the way we want . . . like just the other day I was trying to bake some bread and I just couldn't get it to turn out the way I wanted it to . . . you know that old door I've been trying to fix? I get so frustrated when I just can't make it close right." Recognizing the feeling and then sharing similar feelings under similar situations helps the child recognize the parents' and thus the child's humanness.

As we've said before, parents want to do the right thing, it's just that their methods are not always the most effective means to achieve the ends they seek. Likewise, parents are anxious to help their children, and such help is typically viewed by parents to be an active, hands-on, direct involvement with their children. They want to *DO* something to help. Such parents find it quite difficult to accept the fact that sometimes the best thing they can *DO* to help their children is *NOT TO DO* anything more than being a loving, attentive, non-interrupting listener. Surely, they'll ask, there must be something I can DO or say to help my child? (As mentioned before, we are always reminded, in this situation, of the phrase from Thomas & others [1972] record album, "There is some kinda help which is the kinda help we can all do without.").

Unfortunately, no matter what we say, some parents can and do sometimes take matters into their own hands. In some cases, this is a well-intended but misguided attempt to get the child to "slow down" or "speed up" or "take a deep breathe before you begin to talk" or have the child "sing" through his or her stutterings or have the child rapidly and correctly name single-word picture cards, apparently in the belief that fluent production of single words will automatically generalize to conversational speech. These overt, direct procedures are generally easy to spot (if the clinician is watching for them) and relatively easy to get the parents to curtail. What is not as easy to observe, however, and what might be even more insidious and detrimental to the child's fluency, as mentioned above, is those parents who simply substitute the word *"hard"* for the word *"stuttering."* These parents then proceed to reprimand, correct, nag, or badger the child regarding the continuing production of "hard" speech (or the reciprocal instruction "use your easy speech now, like you were taught"). As should be obvious, such usage, on the part of the parents, defeats the purpose of the term and the effective use of this term with the child in treatment. This misapplication of a fundamentally helpful procedure is a good example of the child's parent doing something he or she thinks will help the child but which is clearly not helping. That is, the parent's advice to the child becomes part of, rather than solution for, the problem. Parents must be assisted to understand that such active helping on their part may have to wait until both they and their child have progressed to a more advanced state of therapy. For now, we want parents to *teach by model not by instruction*, to show not tell their children what to do.

Nature of Communicative Interaction Between Clinician and Client

Van Riper (1973) and others have discussed the benefits of engaging the young people who stutter in low-level types of verbal conversation. We are particularly receptive to Stocker's (1976) notion of level of demand in which she has developed five categories of questions that require different levels of linguistic and cognitive formulation (see Conture & Caruso,

1978 and Martin, Parlour, & Haroldson, 1990 for critical reviews of Stocker's procedure). Surely, future work will refine these levels of demand and probably expand on their number and quality; however, for the present, the idea of relatively systematically controlling the child's utterance by the nature of the questions one asks has intuitive appeal. This is very similar to the notion (that we discussed in Chapter 1) that the "demands" of people who stutter exceed their "capacities," an idea that appears to have received its first theoretical elaboration by Andrews and his colleagues (Andrews & Neilson, 1981; Andrews et al., 1983; Neilson & Neilson, 1987) and then by Adams (1990) and Starkweather and Gottwald (1990), who have amplified upon this concept and discussed its clinical application.

Of course, one would not want to restrict an entire therapy session to questions of only one type, for example, "Is the ball big or little? blue or red? hard or soft?" Instead, we would vary the nature of our questions of and comments to the child so as to positively control, influence, and shape the child's fluency as well as reinstitute fluency after a period when the child has become disfluent and/or to elicit speech from the child once the child is talking. By experimenting with each individual child, the SLP may even be able to find types of questions that routinely elicit, for that child, fluency or disfluency and instruct parents in the use or avoidance of such questions, as the case may be. Knowledge of how the length and complexity of utterances and questions (e.g., Logan & Conture, 1997; Melnick & Conture, 2000; Silverman & Bernstein Ratner, 1997; Weiss & Zebrowski, 1992) influence stuttering in children gives the clinician a tool with which to regulate the amount of stuttering exhibited by the child.

The Child's Communicative Interaction ("Pragmatic" or Usage) Abilities

While we first and foremost want to modify the child's disfluency, positive changes in fluency are often impeded by difficulties the child appears to have with verbal expression or communicative interaction abilities. Technically, this relates to the pragmatics or use of language, but for our purposes we will stay with the term "verbal expression" because this communicates a bit better to our clients. *Verbal expression*, for lack of a better term, is here used to describe such things as the amount of time spent talking, selecting the appropriate place or point in time to begin talking, logically organizing thoughts into language, knowing when it is a good time to interrupt people who are talking, knowing how to take the listener's perspective into account in order to most effectively communicate ideas whose content is outside the immediate environs, and knowing how to appropriately achieve listener attention. While some of these issues were previously discussed in our coverage of the P/C fluency group, these subtleties of verbal expression (see, e.g., Bates, 1976 and Rees, 1980 for an overview of the pragmatic aspects of language) need to be further discussed in this space since they are seemingly difficult for some young children who are beginning to stutter.

Some of these children may:

1. Monologue rather than dialogue at the dinner table (to everybody's discomfort and utter boredom)
2. Seem to "put the cart before the horse" in many of their verbal expressions

3. Not wait their turn—instead they will repeat sounds, syllables, words, and phrases in seeming attempts to gain listener attention or to hold the floor during a conversation or interrupt an already ongoing conversation (and yet seem to expect no one to interrupt them after they have begun to talk)
4. Use long, relatively complex utterances in situations that really require shorter, less cognitively or linguistically involved replies
5. Begin and continue a conversation while others are talking that has little or nothing to do with the present topic of conversation.

Now, before the reader begins to say "Where are the data?" let me reiterate that I said *some* and not all children who stutter exhibit such verbal interactions; further, these are clinical observations and require empirical, objective investigations in order to refine, refute or support their veracity (e.g., investigations like the series conducted by Weiss & Zebrowski, whereby they assessed parental conversational behavior in relation to stuttering/fluency [Weiss & Zebrowski, 1991], influence/relationship of questions to childhood stuttering [Weiss & Zebrowski, 1992], and conversational/narrative abilities of children who stutter [Weiss & Zebrowski, 1994]).

Now, it needs to be pointed out that many other children who do not stutter also do these things, but at this point we are not sure what the frequency and consistency of these behaviors are in the population of children who do not stutter. Further, in terms of parental reactions to their child's undesirable verbal expressions, we are sure that some parents have a shorter fuse than others. Likewise, siblings who are also trying to gain the speaking floor and their parents' attention may not be too tolerant of a brother or sister who takes up more than his or her fair share of "talking time." These same brothers and sisters may not appreciate a sibling who takes what *they* think is too long a time to begin speaking or to get to the point of their speaking (this can sometimes lead to criticism, mocking, or teasing on the part of brothers and sisters, an issue that will be discussed in a following section). Sometimes these siblings cause problems for the young child who stutters because the siblings themselves exhibit the following concerns: use more than their fair share of talking time, take too long to get to the point of their communication, inappropriately correct the child who stutters, and/or inappropriately interrupt the speaker who has the floor. In more than a few cases, the parents have seemingly given up trying to socialize their children and/or play linguistic traffic cops and merely let the children verbally slug it out for communication supremacy. Suffice it to say, this is a battle that a child who has difficulties with speech fluency will seldom win. (We have also observed situations where a live-in relative—e.g., a grandmother—continues to routinely interrupt and talk for a child who stutters long after both parents have ceased doing so.)

If at all possible, the SLP should try to address and try to change inappropriate means of verbal expression, particularly those exhibited by the child who stutters and the child's parents. At the very least, the parent should be encouraged to examine the home situation to see if these problems exist and if they do, how the various members of the family may be reacting. The problems some children who stutter have in this area lead, in my mind, to one of the many Catch-22s of stuttering. For example, the child who takes too long to get to the point of his or her topic (or the child who tends to monologue once he or she does get the speaking floor) becomes the child that other children, parents, and adults find less and less enjoyable to verbally interact with. However, if this child is continually told to be quiet, "slow down," "hurry it up, I don't have all day" or to "shut up," the child will get less and less opportunity to practice verbal expression. Thus, with lessened opportunities, the child's skills in this area have less chance of being exercised, which results in the fact that the child remains less than fully undeveloped in these areas. In the end, all of this may mean that the child still gets called on less frequently to speak! Such vicious cycles, with which the problem of stuttering seemingly abounds, should be identified at an early age. Through early identification and modification, these concerns can be mitigated, to the degree possible, before they develop into consistent, undermining problems possibly contributing to the maintenance and perpetuation of stuttering.

Parents' Reading to Their Children

In General   In general, we believe that parents of children who stutter should be encouraged to talk and read more with their children. However, as Van Riper (1973) notes, particularly with parents reading to their child, there are some cautions. Before we get into these cautions, let me say that it is my experience that with patience, persistence, and support on the part of the SLP, most parents can learn, and even come to enjoy, reading to their children. Reading to a child can become a family ritual or tradition that closes out the day in a relatively relaxed, mutually satisfying way. The parent gets a chance to talk to the child, and the child has an opportunity to listen to and ask questions of the parent. It is a wonderful way to provide the child with a chance to attend to the spoken word (something the child will need to do repeatedly in school) and should stimulate the child's vocabulary development and interest in reading as well as inform the child about the world outside the home.

Problems in this area, as Van Riper suggested, do exist, and the SLP needs to and should be familiar with these problems if this reading at home is to have a positive or facilitative influence on the child and the child's fluency. First of all, too much of a good thing is bad. The child can be verbally interacted at and with to the point of fatigue, satiation, and unnecessary stimulation. The child, like all of us, needs quiet times, time to think, daydream, or just plain rest. Second, attempting to read to a child when that child is obviously more interested in playing with toys or coloring in a coloring book is going to be a frustrating experience for everybody involved. Thus, not only the *amount* of time the child is read or talked to must be monitored but the *timing* of when to talk and read to the child must be assessed. Clearly, in our experience, some parents will need help assessing the amount as well as timing of their reading and talking. Parents' reading and talking with their children should be an enjoyment rather than a regimen. Third, the parents should be helped to select books and stories that the child can understand, relate to, and enjoy. At the risk of greatly simplifying the situation, books for preschool/early elementary school children can be categorized into four groupings:

1. *Prereading books*: Books that make noises, can be scratched and sniffed, made of material the child can put in his or her mouth, all of which may have only pictures or at the most, one word per picture/page.

2. *One-word, one-picture per page books*: Books that have one word per page per picture that with repeated readings the child can memorize and say along with, just after the parent.

3. *One to three short phrases/short sentences per picture per page*: Like the one-word per page books, a child can, after repeated readings, memorize, and say along with or just after the parent.

4. *One to three short to long paragraphs per page*: These books contain more story-like or actual stories like Pinocchio or Cinderella. These are books the parent can read to the child for content, entertainment, and vocabulary development, but probably with minimal expectation that most preschoolers can actually read with or just after the parent.

Reading for Content Versus Reading for Development of Oral Reading Skills   Given the various distinctions in reading materials available for parents of preschool children, it is important, in this writer's opinion, that parents be helped to understand that besides companionship and parent–child sharing, reading has at least two other, related but different functions: (1) It provides the child with cognitive, language, and vocabulary enrichment and stimulation; and (2) it provides the child with a model of speech-language production that he or she can use when starting to read orally or read aloud themselves. Unfortunately, many parents opt for what I call the "Fairy Tales from the Old Country" type of book. These books are usually long on intellectual content, moral messages, and imagination. However, these books typically present a model of oral reading well beyond what the typical preschooler could be reasonably expected to follow, at least in terms of "reading" memorized or sight vocabulary words from the page. Instead, the parents should be encouraged to mix, blend, or interchange their reading material. That is, sometimes the parents should "read for content," for example, reading from the Babar the elephant series, and other times reading to provide for the child an obtainable oral reading model, for example, reading such books as "Go Dog Go" or "Left Foot, Right Foot." Both types of books—those high on content versus those providing an obtainable model of oral reading—have a place.

The speech–language pathologist can help parents understand that one type of book is not better than the other. Instead, the two sources of reading material just have different functions. Both functions, it should be pointed out to parents, are important in helping their child learn to love reading as well as love to learn how to read. Likewise, parents need to be helped to understand that it really does little good to read or talk if nobody is listening. One mother of a 5-year-old stutterer we remediated could not understand why her son seemed bored with her reading of a *National Geographic* article on the Apollo space mission! Such parents need help in learning what kinds of stories, print, and pictures a child of their child's age might understand and enjoy. Dodson (1970) presents a very comprehensive listing of books and stories appropriate for various ages of children. And, as obvious as this may be, try not to give parents the impression that they must buy *all* these books (or books on tape) themselves; encourage them to visit local libraries and bring their child with them. Be patient and supportive, and tell them that with time and experience their child will select books independently; but that in the beginning the parent will have to do much of the selecting. Indeed, parents can put themselves "on tape" (audio and/or video) reading the child's favorite stories (a wonderful procedure for a mom or dad who must travel a lot for business purposes).

Also try to help the parents determine which parent, mother or father, has the most patience for and interest in reading *aloud* to the child (the parent who has fewer skills in this area can and should be encouraged to help their child in other ways). The athletic, relatively frenetic father or the extremely quiet, but impatient-with-mistakes mother may not be your best bet. Try to figure out who would be the best (but not perfectionistic) out-loud reader and who would have the most interest in and patience for same. It also helps if the SLP helps parents learn that when they read to their child that they should do so in as calm, relatively physically relaxed and unhurried fashion as possible. These parents should be told to expect, even encourage, the child to interrupt and ask questions or make comments. Indeed, if the parent simply cannot tolerate the child's interruptions for questions and/or the child's comment about text and pictures, that parent is a poor risk for a reader. Again, with such a parent, other types of opportunities for parent–child verbal interactions should be sought and encouraged—for example, the simple-to-minimal verbal chatter that accompanies throwing or kicking a ball back and forth. Most of the time, however, we have been able, by employing patience and persistence (no one ever said this was going to be easy!), to help parents like this learn how to modify their behavior in this area so that they can become good, or at least, adequate oral readers—and try to minimize their guilt when they are unable to easily read to their child for whatever reason. That is, while we encourage parents to read every day to their children, we should also try to make it clear to them that it certainly is all right to skip a day or two when they or their child is just not in the mood.

We have found parental reading to children to be an excellent vehicle for parent–child sharing; for providing the child with an obtainable adult model of relatively physically relaxed, unhurried speech production; and for giving the child practice in listening to an adult speaking to them for a period of time (the very thing they experience in school classrooms every day). We think that it is clear that such reading is also a stimulant for the child's vocabulary development, and that it also helps the child to learn that reading can be enjoyable and entertaining. If we can believe what we read about television's being a less-than-positive influence on our children (Winn, 1977), then the more reading we expose our children to and that they do themselves, the better.

Deciding When a More Direct Approach Is Warranted

The above is mostly suited for the child who is producing, albeit quite frequently, relatively physically relaxed ("easy") sound/syllable repetitions, appropriate eye contact with listeners, and appears essentially unaware of his or her speech problem. As always, of course, there will be children who fall in the cracks, children for whom the above approach will not be specific or direct enough to achieve improvement in speech fluency but for whom more direct approaches seem somewhat inappropriate. It is not always easy to identify these children prior to therapy, and many times their needs only become apparent after three to twelve months of seemingly appropriate but relatively ineffective remediation. And, unfortunately, some of the reasons some of these children haven't received benefit from therapy is that their parents could not or would not make a number of simple changes in the home communication environment—for example, they continue to speak for their child "because its hard for him," routinely correct him for disfluencies and/or misarticulations, and the like.

To repeat, we have developed through experience several behavioral guidelines that we have found helpful in deciding whether a particular child needs a more direct approach:

1. Sound prolongations comprise 30 percent or more of all their stutterings (e.g., Yaruss, LaSalle, & Conture, 1998).
2. There is more than occasional presence of stuttering-stuttering clusters in the child's speech (LaSalle & Conture, 1995).
3. Stutterings comprise 70 percent or more of their total speech disfluencies (Yairi, 1997a).
4. Less than 50 percent of the time, the child makes eye contact with his or her listener.
5. The child makes frequent reference to his or her speech and problems with it (e.g., "Mommy, why can't I talk right?" or "Daddy, I didn't stutter at all today" or "Mommy, I can't talk").
6. Delays and/or deviant speech and language development are present—for example, a child who exhibits a score on the Goldman–Fristoe Articulation Test of 20 percent or below or who exhibits delayed and/or unusual phonological development.

It is fair to say, however, that children exhibiting several of variables (1–6) mentioned above will generally be "picked up" at the time of initial evaluation and more direct therapeutic regimens recommended. A far more challenging situation is the child who weakly exhibits only one or two of these variables (e.g., 15-20 percent sound prolongations + reduced but not seriously diminished eye contact) along with occasional indicators of that the child may be aware that speech is difficult, a concern or different. It is difficult, with these "in-between" children (i.e., on the cusp between needing indirect versus direct treatment), to be sure which way they are going to progress and whether indirect approaches are sufficient or whether direct methods will need to be instituted.

What is desperately needed is empirical investigations to assess which speech and related variables predict positive, negative, and minimal change in speech disfluencies. Recently, Hancock, Craig, McCready, McCaul, Costello, Campbell, and Gilmore (1998), studying 9- to 14-year-old children who stutter, found that pretreatment stuttering frequency and trait anxiety posttreatment significantly predicted stuttering frequency one year posttreatment. That is, those children exhibiting the most severe stuttering pretreatment and least anxiety immediately posttreatment were those who were most susceptible to frequent stuttering long term. Whether these findings hold true for preschool and early elementary school children is unclear, but such data is very much needed for us to improve our treatment of people who stutter.

In essence, why implement direct therapy regimens when with time and positive parental intervention some of the children initially evaluated, who are just beginning to stutter, will become more fluent? Conversely, why implement indirect therapy regimens and significantly involve parents when the child needs specific and direct modification of inappropriate speech and related behaviors? Unfortunately, at present, we are still missing the empirical evidence that would allow us to make such decisions based on a more solid foundation.

Children with Some to a Great Deal of Stuttering Whose Parents Are Reasonably to Somewhat Concerned

These children are frequently and routinely producing within-word disfluencies (probably well in excess of 10 stutterings per 100 words spoken), and adults (most likely, but not necessarily, the parents) explicitly notice and report these disruptions. Interestingly, parents appear most concerned about (1) the child's sound/syllable repetitions and (2) associated nonspeech behavior, particular facial gestures. Facial grimaces and bodily movements many times seem to be the final straw that breaks the camel's back! Associated nonspeech behavior (variously called secondary behavior ["secondaries"], physical concomitants, accessory behavior) seems for many parents to be the *sine qua non* of stuttering, the essential condition that defines the presence of a problem. Observing these behaviors, parents (and other professionals) call and set up an evaluation for their children. Furthermore, some parents seem to breathe a sigh of relief when their child begins to prolong more than repeat, particular if the prolongations are silent and the child's mouth is closed or nearly so. Such parental acceptance is in opposition to our clinical intuition and experience, which suggests that when a child begins to prolong more (i.e., changes from reiterative or oscillatory speech gestures to more fixed or stabilized gestures) that the child's stuttering problem is worsening. Indeed, Pellowski and Conture (2000) provide preliminary empirical support for the preceding clinical observation with their finding (based on a sample of 40 CWS) that as children who stutter get older, specifically after age 5, sound prolongations become a larger percentage of total stuttered disfluencies while sound/syllable repetitions become a smaller percentage. While further empirical investigation of this topic is clearly warranted, we believe that these findings lend support to the notion that as stuttering persists in a child, the child tends to "shift" his or her predominant disfluency type from one of a reiterative to cessation (or fixed) form of speech production. It probably goes without saying, but it is a waste of both the parents' and clinician's time to try to convince or persuade the parents to be less accepting of physically tense sound prolongations and more tolerant of physically easy sound/syllable repetitions. It may have to be explained to some of these parents in a clear, gentle, but firm manner that as the child becomes more fluent, he or she may resume repeating, at least for a while, sounds and syllables; but this is expected and not to be concerned about.

Unfortunately, some professionals without enough experience, knowledge, or interest in stuttering will use up precious time in the early stages of the development of the child's stuttering problem. Such professionals only seem to refer to a more qualified professional when the child is showing very obvious signs of a worsening and generally more habituated speaking problem. Or, sometimes, when the child begins to frequently exhibit facial grimaces, some clinicians may stop trying to remediate the fundamental problem—the child's speech disfluencies—and instead focus on changing the child's facial grimaces and eye contact. This is most unfortunate, since these problems will remain, albeit in different forms, until the child becomes more fluent. However, our observations of these sorts of problems are not meant to nor will they cure these or other worldly woes. Their inclusion in this space merely serves as a comment on their all too frequent occurrence and a hope for a better tomorrow for children who stutter and their families. Hopefully, the future will witness more publications such as Guitar and Conture (1991), addressed to professionals like pediatricians, that help increase more timely referrals for childhood stuttering by those without primary education, training, or interest in stuttering.

Try Not to Bug the Children Just Like Their Parents Do

At the outset, we want to reiterate that the following treatment suggestions *assume* that the child is frequently stuttering, to the point where direct, individualized therapeutic intervention is necessary. While indirect methods may still be useful and necessary (e.g., teaching parents not to unduly interrupt their child), in this section, we are more and more dealing with direct methods. Likewise, simply because we move from a more indirect to a direct approach, we must not forget about the child's emotional/social needs. Indeed, a child with a frequent, nonresolving-by-indirect-means problem is a child who needs as supporting and encouraging a therapy environment as possible.

First of all, we cannot emphasize this point enough: The SLP should not bother, pester, cajole, nag, or otherwise harass the child the same way as the parents and other individuals may be! All too often we tend to communicate with children who stutter in an "old wine in new bottles" vocabulary that does little more than change the name while the game remains the same: *Stop that stuttering!*

Many youngsters who stutter are not particularly eager to hear, see, or feel what they are doing when they stutter; some of them may be afraid to closely examine their stuttering or may be denying the fact that they speak differently from their friends. Whatever the case, more than a few of these children appear to want to avoid all mention of and confrontation with their speech behavior as if they are ostriches with their heads in the sand. These youngsters' reluctance to examine their stuttering on any level is, of course, a frustrating situation for both clinician and parent alike. Getting them to objectively examine and identify their stuttering, for the purposes of subsequently changing it, will take patience, time, and encouragement.

These children, because they are human, would ideally like some passive procedure, technique, cure, or device that they could use, wear, or ingest that would take their stuttering away from them (or in the words of the old pharmaceutical advertisement, "Relief is just a swallow away"). In the beginning of therapy, the child and parents are particularly receptive to any and everything that promises to lift the burden of stuttering off their backs. It is the role of the SLP to gently but firmly disabuse the parents and child alike of such get-fixed-quick notions.

Helping the Child Accept a More Active Role in the Changing of Stuttering

The SLP can help the child accept a more active or doing role in changing his or her stuttering by helping the child, right from the beginning of therapy, to understand that there are different ways we can begin and continue to speak and that there are various ways to produce speech that make it sound, look, and feel better than others (it is quite helpful, with some of these children, to use the "talking about talking" procedures described by Williams in the earlier part of this chapter). We like to use analogies with our clients—children, teenagers, and adults alike—in attempts to take the complex task of speaking and break it down into terms and objects that make sense to the client. We like to explain the child's problem on a level he or she can relate to so that they can begin to understand and *do* something about their own behavior. Not only do analogies help children understand their role in their problem, but they take some of the fear and mystery out of the situation and treat their speech in a more matter-of-fact or objective manner. Speech-language production is such a complex act, often involving behaviors hidden from view and changes in muscular tensions and structural movements that quickly move through time and space. It takes years for even the speech scientist to gain some familiarity with the many activities and functions of speech. Therefore, the SLP should not be surprised that the lay client, particularly the child, has difficult grasping what he or she is *doing* to interfere with normally fluent speech production.

Helping Parents Understand That Many Aspects of Speaking Are out of Sight and Therefore out of Mind

The first analogy, which involves the activity of the heart, is really more for the benefit of the SLP and the parent. Its purpose is to make the SLP and parent understand that (1) most people take speech-language production for granted and (2) that the location of the speech musculature deep within the vocal tract obfuscates the nature of its structure and function. Basically, we are trying to help the parents and/or child understand that the speech-language production behavior we are trying to change is unknown to them because of (1) and (2). Of course, we don't expect the child and the child's parent to understand speech anatomy and function like a speech-language pathologist, but we want them to have sufficient appreciation for the process of speech production to be able to identify and change inappropriate behavior.

This analogy (see Figure 3.5) is particularly useful in explaining to parents why their child seems unable to identify and/or modify clearly inappropriate behavior. We believe it also helps the SLP to better understand why the child is having such difficulty doing what clearly needs to be done. The SLP might start by asking her- or himself or the parent: "What is your heart doing right now?" To which most people say, "I don't know." Hammering the point in a bit further, we might ask "Where is your heart, exactly? What does it look like? Is it contracting or expanding right now?" and so forth and so on.

Most people have little or no clear idea regarding the color, shape, structure, or function of their hearts, nor should they. I mean, after all, why should they know about something that is always there when they need it? Why should they be concerned with something that takes care of itself? Why should they worry about fixing something that is not broken? Clearly, there is no need to know about the heart, since it is taking care of itself for the most part just fine (obviously, we are not advocating diets or lifestyles that abuse or increase the risk of heart disease, we are simply commenting on the fact that few if any of us consider the size, shape, and workings of our internal organs, as a routine matter of course).

But what of the child's speech-language production system? Perhaps it is not performing as it should but everyone still treats it like the heart: out of sight and out of mind. The parent is helped to understand that some rudimentary understanding of speech pro-

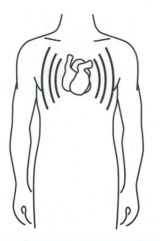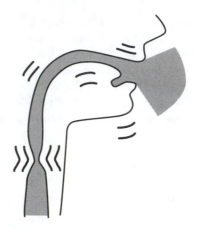

Heart beating/movements   Speech structural movements
deep within chest cavity   deep within vocal tract

FIGURE 3.5.   Out of sight, out of mind analogy. The heart's shape, size, and function are "out of sight" and thus "out of mind" for most people. Likewise, the shape, size, and function of the person's vocal tract is out of sight, thus out of mind for most people. While most people need not concern themselves with cardiac structure and function, the stutterer with a problem that requires direct intervention must gain some rudimentary understanding of vocal tract structural movements in order to effectively change inappropriate to more appropriate speaking strategies.

duction may be useful for the child to make a lasting change in his or her stuttering. However, given the fact that neither the child nor parent have much understanding of the nature and function of the speech production mechanism, such understanding will not come easily. While speech behavior, just like cardiac function, may be taken for granted that doesn't mean that the child has to relinquish his or her ability to change behavior. The child may not be able to change the size or shape of the speech production mechanism but he or she can influence its behavior even though very little of its actual movement can be seen. This ability to change will not come overnight, but it can and will develop, especially with the guidance of an SLP and the emotional support of the child's parents.

Helping Parents Understand What It Feels Like to Stutter

To an individual who is normally fluent, the act of "being stuck," of being unable to move on to the next sound even though you know what you want to say, is relatively foreign. And probably there are no words or analogies that can adequately or completely describe the frustration, embarrassment, and fear associated with the act of stuttering. However, we believe an attempt should be made, if the normally fluent parent of a young child who is stuttering is to gain some degree of reasonable empathy for the child's problem.

The feelings of stuttering involve a number of levels of experience and certainly when talking with parents it is not necessary to go into all these levels, especially for the parents of a younger child who stutters. It is not to be assumed, for instance, that *all* of these children are fearful and/or embarrassed by the way they talk. They are more likely to be frustrated, but even that is not a given. Therefore, with the parents, at least to begin, rather than concentrate on the child's possible feelings of frustration, embarrassment, and fear, we focus on the feelings of "unexpectedness," "suddenness," and "startle." The two analogies we use are jumping into a swimming pool and touching a hot burner. Both analogies, we think, help parents better appreciate what the act of stuttering sometimes feels like to their children.

Jumping into a Swimming Pool (see Analogy 1, Figure 3.6). We tell the parent to imagine jumping feet first into a swimming pool that he or she thought was warm or at least room temperature. As the stomach and chest hit the water, however, he or she discovers that the water is like a liquid ice cube—that is, real cold. The person is shocked at the *unexpectedness* of the water's temperature, and the *suddenness* of the experience is even a bit scary, especially as the head sinks below the water as the body descends into the water. The unexpected, startling nature of the experience may even "take the breath away," to which the person may respond with a forced inspiration.

This unexpected, suddenly occurring, startling, and maybe even scary experience leads most people to respond with a quick, forced inspiration and try to make every effort to get out of the water. The unexpectedness, the startling quality of the experience, the forced inspiration, and attempts to "leave the scene of the crime" are somewhat akin to their

Air Temperture 85°

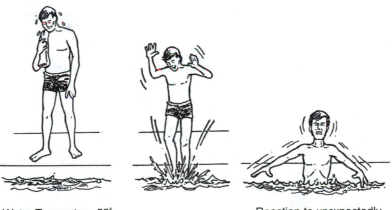

Water Temperture 58°

Reaction to unexpectedly
cold water

FIGURE 3.6. Bodily/physical reaction to unexpected circumstances. Analogy 1: On a hot day in early summer a swimmer might forget that the water is still quite chilly and be surprised (if not shocked) when hitting the cold water. Sudden gasping, inhalations, and /or muscle tensing might all be exhibited by the surprised swimmer, much like the sudden gasping, inhalation, or muscle tensing exhibited by a stutterer when attempting to produce a sound, syllable, or word he or she suddenly and/or unexpectedly finds difficult to produce.

child's feelings during the act of stuttering. The child's unexpected feelings, forced inspirations, and feelings of wanting to escape when he or she feels unable to move forward are no more "willful" than the parents' reaction to the ice-cold pool water. The child may be observed to physically tense various aspects of his or her throat, jaw, lip, and tongue muscles, in apparent effort to "blast" the sound, syllable, or word out (see Figure 3.11). Something, to the child, seems "stuck." Now, at this point, we must remember that most preschool or early elementary school children are not typically known for rationality, reflectiveness, reason, and reservation in their responses! Indeed, rather than wait for the feeling of "stuckness" to pass and/or the word to become available to produce, the child physically tenses, pushes, and strains in apparent attempts to "dynamite" a fluency logjam out of his or her mouth!

Touching a Hot Stove Burner (see Analogy 2, Figure 3.7).   With this analogy, we ask the parent to imagine a stovetop with four electric burners. We then ask the parent to imagine running his or her hand across the top of the stove looking for some utensil, all the while assuming that all burners are turned off. To their surprise and shock, one of the burners has been left on. Recoiling in fear of being burned, the parent may take a sudden, forced inspiration. Here, we explain to the parent that the recoil, the pulling back or backing away from something feared while taking a sudden, forced inspiration, is similar to some of their child's instances of stuttering. While the intensity of the fear or depth of inspiration might not be as great nor identical to what their child experiences in each and every stuttering, there is some degree of similarity in the two situations.

In general, with such analogies, we are trying to help the parents develop a greater sense of empathy with what their child experiences when he or she stutters. In specific, we

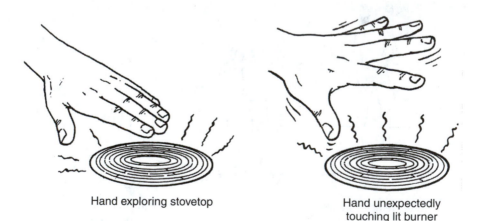

Hand exploring stovetop   Hand unexpectedly
                                           touching lit burner

FIGURE 3.7.   Bodily/physical reaction to unexpected circumstances. Analogy 2: A person exploring a stovetop with his hand unexpectedly touches a lit burner. The person reacts by *physically pulling* the hand *away* and perhaps by gasping, suddenly inhaling, and tensing muscles up in the hand, arm, and elsewhere in the body. Likewise, a person who stutters may react to the sudden, unexpected inability to say a sound, syllable, or word by *physically pulling back* the tongue, jaw, head, neck, or shoulders while simultaneously gasping or inhaling.

use these analogies to help the parent understand the suddenness, the unexpectedness, the fear, and out-of-control feelings of stuttering. We want to help the parents better appreciate their child's startlike need to take a deep breath and/or escape the situation by whatever means necessary. In this way the parents are helped to better empathize with what their child maybe experiencing and helps them to realize that what at times may appear inappropriately purposeful on the child's part is many times a normal reaction to an abnormal situation. These analogies should *never* be used to admonish or scare parents for their apparent lack of understanding or concern regarding their child or their child's behavior. Rather, we use these analogies as a way to increase the parents' appreciation of the challenge their child faces. We use these analogies to provide a better basis for our communication with the parents about their child and things the parents can do to help. Analogies should not be used or taken to be an explanation of a behavior, person, or process but as a vehicle to better help someone—in this case, a parent—better appreciate, deal with and understanding a seemingly complex situation.

The Garden Hose Analogy

The Basic Concept. One analogy we like to use with children (and, given the proper approach, teenagers and adults) is what we call the garden hose analogy (see Figures 3.8

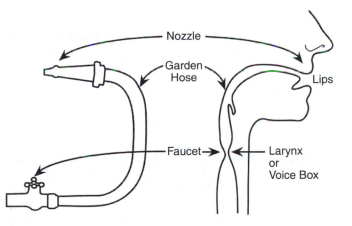

FIGURE 3.8. Garden hose analogy: The parts. A lateral view of the supraglottal and glottal structures with their analogous parts to a garden hose–nozzle–faucet is presented. The lips are equated with the nozzle of the hose in that both can be constricted to stop or modify airflow (lips) or water stream (nozzle). The vocal tract is analogized with the flexible, bendable garden hose in that both can be manipulated in such a way (the garden hose can be kinked or bent, and the vocal tract can have the tongue partially or completely occlude airway) as to impede or modify the airflow or water stream. Finally, the larynx or vocal folds (housed in voice box) are equated with the faucet in that both can be constricted or adjusted to stop or modify airflow or water stream. This analogy helps the young child identify the nature and function of each part of the vocal mechanism and the means by which his or her strategies to interfere with speech take place.

and 3.9). Most children have played with and used a garden hose with a nozzle at one end and a faucet at the other, and thus the analogy generally works. I explain the three parts of interest: the *faucet* on the side of the house, the flexible or bendable *garden hose* itself attached to the faucet, and the *nozzle* on the end of the hose. We begin by describing the garden hose and its parts and how the parts work separately as well as together as a unit to (1) permit the water to flow out of the hose (2) minimize the amount of water that flows or (3) completely stop the water from flowing out of the hose. Technically speaking, of course, something like the air hose and pump used to inflate bicycle or automobile tires might be more appropriate, given that air and not water is used to speak. However, most children are

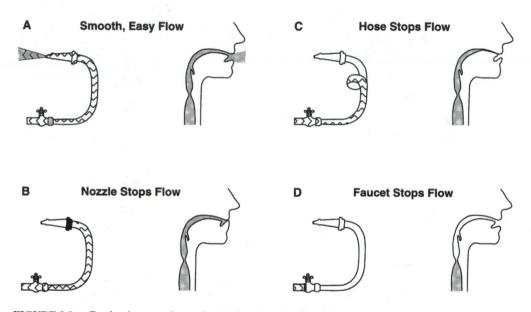

FIGURE 3.9.   Garden hose analogy: the mechanism. The four aspects of this figure (A, B, C, and D) depict the nature and function of the vocal tract during fluent and stuttered speech. The smooth, easy flow of air (A) for fluent speech strategies also shows how water flows through a garden hose in such a procedure. Naturally, during normal speech, the state of affairs depicted in A would be continually changing, but the idea of smooth, sequential movement from one speech posture to the next to produce a continuous flow of speech would still be apparent. In the first interfering situation (B), the client contacts long and with too much pressure on the lips and stops the airflow in much the same way as the nozzle on the hose when tightened would stop water flowing from the hose. In the next interfering strategy (C), the person is seen contacting the hard palate with too much tension for too long, which stops airflow in an analogous way to a kink in a garden hose blocking water from flowing. Finally, the vocal folds can be constricted (D) in such a way to impede airflow, much like turning a faucet off will impede water from flowing from the vocal tract. What is not easy to analogize is the inappropriate laryngeal strategy of opening the vocal folds (see Conture, McCall, & Brewer, 1977; Conture, Schwartz, & Brewer, 1985). It is also possible for the three inappropriate strategies (B, C, D) to be combined in a variety of ways to interfere with speaking. In fact, such combinations of strategies are probably closer to the reality of the situation than the present examples, which were independently presented for the purposes of clear explication to the reader and client.

not as familiar with air hoses and pumps as they are garden hoses, and the parts of an air hose and pump don't quite lend themselves, by analogy, to the vocal tract like a water faucet, garden hose, and nozzle.

To begin, we explain to the child that we could shut the water off completely or slow down its flow by turning the faucet at the house, bending the hose, or turning or twisting the nozzle. After the child seems to understand how a faucet, garden hose, and nozzle arrangement works (while using a real nozzle attached to a short length of real, flexible hose makes this more alive, some youngsters may become overly attentive to the actual object, the hose—this calls for clinical judgment), we begin to discuss the similarities between the garden hose and our speech production mechanism. Our larynx (voice box) becomes the faucet, our throat and tongue the garden hose, and our lips the nozzle. We then practice— first us and then the child—"closing off the water (air)" with our *voice box (faucet), tongue (garden hose),* or *lips (nozzle).* Some have come to call these "air stoppers" and others "speech helpers." Use whatever terms seem appropriate and communicate the basic point: *We,* the speaker, *have control* over our speech and can influence it in a variety of ways!

As we mentioned above, to the lay person, especially a child, much of the speech production mechanism is out of sight and out of mind, particularly the voice box. Thus, it is hard for them to visualize or realize or feel exactly what they are doing with the parts as well as whole of their vocal tract when they stutter. We have found, however, that children can come to some appreciation for the way they (mis)use their larynx by having them take a deep breath and then hold it with their mouths open (Figure 3.10a). This gives them the idea of how they can use their "faucets" to stop air from flowing. Conversely, having the child take a deep breath and then hold it with lips closed and cheeks puffed out gives him or her the idea of how to use their "nozzles" to stop air from flowing (Figure 3.10b). Having the child hold the /s/ and then gradually stop air flowing through the constriction created by raising the tongue close to the alveolar ridge/hard palate and then finally totally occluding airflow by touching the hard palate with the tongue gives the child the idea how the "hose" can slow down and then completely stop flow (the child can, although it is harder at first, do the same thing with /z/, only gradually closing the vocal folds to minimize and then completely stop voicing/air flowing). We play with these various air or water *flowers* or *stoppers* or *helpers* until we think that the child has the idea or has had all the fun that he or she can stand!

Air Stoppers.   We then introduce the idea of *air stoppers* in the child's actual speech by having the child observe us slow, restrict, or stop the airflow through the vocal tract through the use of the nozzle, hose, or faucet. We encourage the child, at this point, to do the same as we are doing on selected words, sounds, or syllables. For example, the word-initial /b/ in the word *ball* could be used to demonstrate air stoppage at the level of the nozzle (lips); the word-initial /k/ in the word *key,* for the level of the hose (tongue against palate); and a word-initial vowel like /i/ in the word *eat,* or a sound like /h/ as in the word *hot,* for the level of the faucet (larynx).

As mentioned above, of the three levels—lips, mouth, or larynx—laryngeal constriction or its converse, abduction, is a most difficult concept to get across to children (or adults, for that matter). Again, as shown in Figure 3.10, one helpful way to reinforce or explain the idea of air stopping at the larynx is to have the children hold their breath, after

(a)   (b)

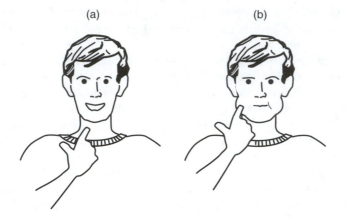

FIGURE 3.10.   Informal determination of laryngeal involvement during typical stutterings. (a) Person holding his breath, mouth opened, larynx (vocal folds) closed. He is pointing to the place on the body, that is, on the neck, at or slightly below the larynx, where he feels/perceives resulting physical tension and/or aerodynamic back pressures from the column of air "pushing up" from the respiratory system onto the laryngeal/voice box area. (b) Person holding his breath, mouth/lips closed, larynx (vocal folds) opened. The person is pointing to the place on his body, that is, lips, cheeks of the face, where he feels/perceives resulting physical tension and/or aerodynamic back pressures from the column of air "pushing up" from the respiratory system into the oral/mouth region, puffing up the sides of the face, and pushing against the closed lips.

taking a deep inhalation, with the mouth open (another way is with a blown-up balloon, an analogy we'll cover in greater depth below). It must be emphasized that the laryngeal area is not particularly rich in sensation that would allow the speaker, particularly, a child speaker, to visualize or sense its activity. Furthermore, much of the activity of the larynx is invisible to the naked eye, and children have no real good picture or mental image of what the larynx or vocal folds look or act like. All this vagueness makes this task all the more challenging. Unfortunately, for some children whose stuttering is a real problem and concern, laryngeal involvement can be a major aspect of the peripheral manifestations of their stuttering. Indeed, the careful observer will note that some of these children, in the interim between the listener's questions and the child's response, seem to take a quick, deep inhalation and hold it with the larynx (the mouth may or may not be open) as if to prepare themselves for the task of speaking. This seems to be a bit like when you take in a deep breath and hold it in order to prepare yourself for the task of lifting or moving a heavy piece of furniture. To these children, the sensation in their throat will feel like being "stuck." For many of these youngsters, therefore, the resultant and/or associated oral and nonoral movements observed during the stuttering seem to be their attempts, albeit inappropriate, to "free" themselves or "release" or "work through" or "break through" the "block" they sense occurring in their throat. Like dynamiting a log or ice jam in a river (Figure 3.11) to get the river flowing smoothly again and release the pressure of the backed up water. While this reaction, to push or force through or "dynamite" out the feeling of "being stuck," is very understandable, it is also a solution that becomes part of the problem! Indeed, this rapid, initial response—to "break through the block"—must be mitigated if the child is to have a chance for significant improvement.

"Tightness" Due to Air Pressure Versus Muscle Tension.   Laryngeal, vocal tract, or lip closure during speech can lead to some degree of aerodynamic back pressure (Netsell, 1973), as well as normal feelings of muscle tension-tonus. Obviously, when these constrictors or complete closures within the vocal tract are held for too long or too tightly, associated aerodynamic back pressures and muscle tensions will be noticed and felt to be inappropriate. It is important that the SLP be clear on the difference between aerodynamic back pressure and muscle tension since (1) most lay people who stutter confuse the two and (2) changes in one—*muscle tension and movement*—many times must precede the other—*aerodynamic back pressures*—before positive changes in fluency are achieved. In a very real sense, the "tension" felt in the vocal tract, as shown in Figures 3.10 and 3.11, is very much related to aerodynamic back pressures.

  We speculate that the "feelings of pressure . . . tension . . . tightness in the chest" that children and adults who stutter many times report result from these unusually high levels of back pressures of air below the point of vocal tract constriction or occlusion (e.g., the air pressure felt behind or below the back of the tongue during the stop phase of "k" in the word "kite"). Not only must we help our clients separate out these aerodynamic events from muscle movements and tensions, but they must be distinguished from those *autonomic events* associated with sympathetic nervous system discharge, for example, heart palpitation, lightness or heaviness feeling in the stomach, flushed feelings, and sweating palms (see Brutten & Shoemaker, 1967; Guyton, 1971; Turner, 1969).

Feelings of Tension Versus Feelings of Fear.   The reason we try to help the child understand the nature of these feelings of pressure (besides helping to take away some of the mystery of the problem) is so the child can come to realize that these feelings result from something he or she is *doing*. To *change* speech disfluencies, we need to change the length, amount, and kind of physical tension the child is using prior to and during the stuttering. Conversely, the feelings of heart palpitation, butterflies in the stomach, and so on, associated with autonomic arousal, while necessarily kept within normal limits, will probably always be with the child, teenager, or adult. Feelings of frustration that a listener wasn't paying attention to us, feelings of fear about telling the truth about who broke the window with the baseball, and so forth—these feelings and others like them will always be with the person who stutters (as well as people who do not). Again, it will important for the person to have such feelings of a nature and level that fall roughly within normal limits, but it will not be appropriate for any clinician to remove these feelings—they are part and parcel of the human condition. What IS important, however, is to help the person who stutters learn to physically feel (identify) and change inappropriate amounts and durations of physical movement and tension within the vocal tract WHILE in the midst of normal, although less than pleasant feelings—for example, the feeling of uncertainty and dread at being wrong in front of everyone when answering a question in class when not really sure of the answer.

  We revert back to the garden hose analogy and say that a quick, overly tight closure of the nozzle makes the garden hose stiffen and even jump in our hands. This stiffening or

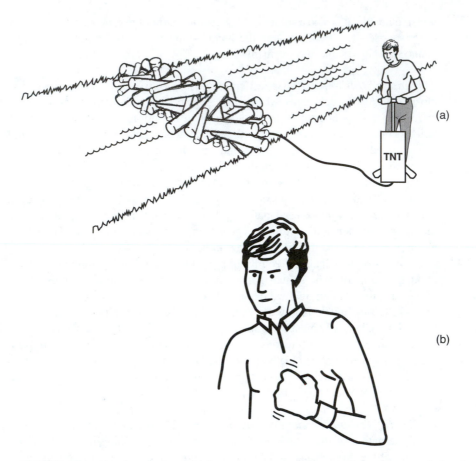

FIGURE 3.11.   Log jam analogy. (a) Just as a person might try to dynamite or explode a log jam to release water dammed up in a stream, (b) so too might a person who stutters push and physically tense the fist as well as the mouth (in this case, the lips), lower the head, and tense facial, neck, or chest muscles in attempt to "force" or "blast out" the seemingly stuck sound, syllable, or word. What is "stuck," of course, is not the literal sound, syllable, or word, but the person's articulatory posture, one that he or she may actually make firmer, tenser, and/or hold for an inappropriately long time, in order to "blast out" or "push out" the element of speech that they perceive to be "lodged," "stuck," or "caught" somewhere in their speaking mechanism.

movement results from water pressure or the fact that the flow of water is suddenly stopped and has nowhere to go so it pushes out the sides of the flexible garden hose. We explain to the child, if this seems appropriate, that the water in the hose behaves in much the same way as the air flowing up from the lungs that can suddenly be dammed up or closed off by the child using the "faucet," "hose," or "nozzle." This "dammed" volume of air below the larynx, mouth, or lips exerts some degree of pressure within the respiratory and vocal tract and can cause feelings of tightness, tension, or constriction. The child can learn to sense these physical feelings and understand them sufficiently to change them during conversational speech.

Blown-up Balloon Analogy: "It's Stuck down Here." One excellent way to help the child understand tightness resulting from aerodynamic back pressure is through the use of a blown-up balloon, using the thumb and index of finger of one hand on the balloon's neck to stop the flow of air out of the balloon (Figure 3.12). As shown in Figure 3.12, you can blow up the balloon and have the child feel the taut or tense sides of the balloon. Then explain that this is a bit like the tension created by air pressure in the lungs and vocal tract. Have the child gently squeeze the side of the balloon and feel the changes in pressure on the sides of the balloon. Have the child hold the neck of the balloon him- or herself and feel the pressure against the "laryngeal-fingers" as you squeeze the sides of the balloon. Have the child figure out the best way to let the pressure out of the balloon, for example, by (1) push-

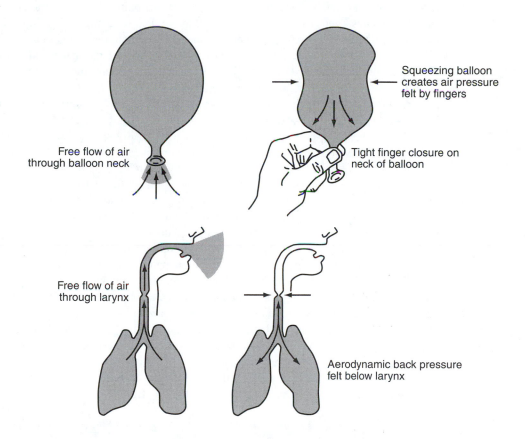

FIGURE 3.12. Balloon analogy to the tight closure at laryngeal or vocal fold level. Since it is difficult for most clients to visualize and understand vocal fold structure and function, some "real-world" analogies are needed. Here a blown-up balloon is squeezed and the aerodynamic "back pressures" are felt by the fingers holding the balloon neck. Likewise, tight vocal fold closure can create aerodynamic back pressure felt at, below, or within the larynx, trachea, and chest. Some of the "tension" that stutterers frequently mention in their neck and chest is undoubtedly due to these aerodynamic back pressures resulting from laryngeal and, at times, supraglottal constriction.

ing hard on the sides of the balloon (2) squeezing the thumb and index finger together or (3) slowly releasing the air through slightly separated fingers and thumb. With some imagination, this analogy can help the child see the various reasons why he or she feels physically tight and constricted in various places within the vocal tract and how these feelings of physical tension can be changed by doing different things.

Lily Pad/Barrel Bridge Analogy: Changing and Moving Forward.   If the child seems to get the general gist of what he or she does that interferes with speaking, seems to be able to describe and identify his or her interfering behavior, and appears willing to make at least some of the necessary changes, we move on to the next stage. Here, too, we use some analogies to help the child (and parents, if necessary) understand what the child must do to increase speech fluency. Two analogies we use at this point operate on the same theme: Speech involves a movement from one sound to the next (one might also, if a sidewalk is nearby, use the child's skipping, jumping game of hopscotch to make similar points).

The first analogy (Figure 3.13) involves pretending a frog or the child is jumping from one lily pad to the next to cross a stream (an analogy perhaps more useful for younger children). We pretend that each pad is a letter of a short word like *baby* and that we must hop from the bank to the first pad, then to the next pad, and so on until we reach the other bank. We explain that we will get wet, go the bottom of the creek, have to climb out and start all over again if we stand too long on any particular lily pad or if we jump on the pad hard with both feet (i.e., if we prolong the sound) or have trouble smoothly and easily getting across the stream, or easily say the word. Likewise, if we hop up and down for too long or several times on the lily pad (i.e., repeat the sound) rather than moving on to the next pad, we will also get wet, possibly go to the bottom of the creek and have to climb out and start all over again. In other words, we'll have trouble smoothly and easily getting across the stream, or saying the word. In either case, we explain to the child, we won't be able to *easily*, *smoothly*, and *quickly* get across the stream if we land on one lily pad and stay there too long or repeatedly jump up and down on the same pad.

Essentially, the same idea is conveyed by another analogy (Figure 3.14), a floating barrel bridge. Here, the bridge is created by having each barrel tied to the other with rope and is used to cross a stream (an analogy perhaps more useful for an older child). Again, a barrel that is jumped on too hard and stood on (Figure 3.14c) *or* repeatedly jumped up and down on (Figure 3.14 b) will keep us from getting across the stream or from producing the phrase "an apple." Again, the use of the child's game of hopscotch, whereby the child must sequentially jump from one square to the next, might actually be used to help the child understand "lightly landing on" and then "moving on" from one point to another.

For Older Children: Thumb and Opposing Fingers Analogy.   For older children, teenagers, and adults, who would naturally scorn or feel patronized by the perceived juvenile nature of the lily pad or barrel bridge analogies, we use one of our thumbs and its opposing four fingers in much the same way (Figure 3.15). Here each finger is a letter or sound of a short word and our opposing thumb, the tongue, or speech system, is used to "produce" each letter or sound. Fluent speech, we tell the client (and his or her associates, if necessary), is something like having the thumb move smoothly, sequentially, and easily from one finger to the next. Conversely, we explain, stuttered speech is much like pressing

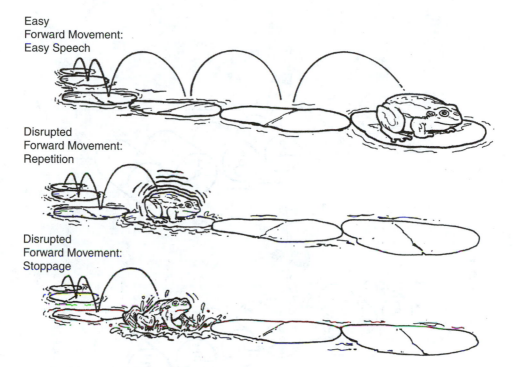

Easy
Forward Movement:
Easy Speech

Disrupted
Forward Movement:
Repetition

Disrupted
Forward Movement:
Stoppage

FIGURE 3.13. Lilipad/frog analogy of forward versus disrupted sequencing of movement (for younger children). For a frog to hop across a pond or stream on lily pads, it would have to smoothly, easily, and sequentially hop from one pad to another. However, if it landed on one and repeatedly hopped up and down (repetition) or landed on one in a physically tense, fixed manner (stoppage), it would disrupt forward movement across the pond. Likewise, speech requires physically easy, smooth, sequential behavior to make forward movement from beginning to the end of a sound, syllable, or word.

for too long with too much force between a person's thumb and any one of its opposing fingers (i.e., a fixed articulatory posture or audible or inaudible sound prolongation) or repeatedly contacting the thumb and one particular finger (i.e., a reiterative speech posture or sound/syllable repetition). And, at the risk of redundancy, with cautions already made: These analogies will, I believe it obvious, not help anyone get fluent in and of themselves. Rather, they serve as concrete examples of abstract concepts, as a common ground of understanding between client and clinician. They provide essential insight for the young client into what he or she *does* that interferes with speech and what is necessary for them to change in order to speak more fluently.

Closed-Fist-To-Relaxed-Hand Analogy. One last analogy that is often used by experienced clinicians involves nothing more than one's hand. Sometimes called the "fist" or "clenched fist" analogy, it can be seen nicely demonstrated by Barry Guitar, while treating a child who stutters, in the Stuttering Foundation of America video (#79), *The School-Age*

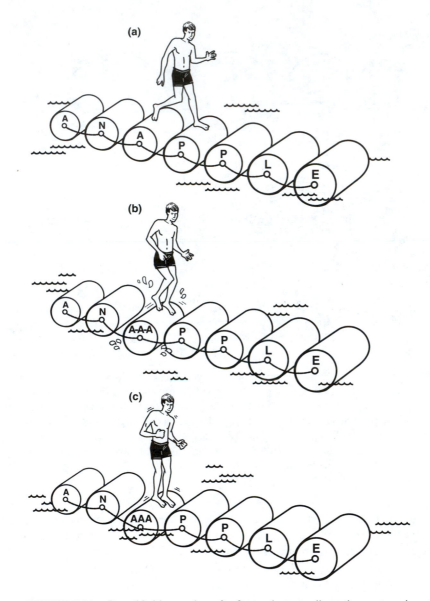

FIGURE 3.14. Barrel bridge analogy for forward versus disruptive sequencing of movement (for older children). In (a), the man is walking across a floating barrel bridge, neither too fast nor slow, neither too physically tense nor loose. He "touches" each barrel, representing a sound in the phrase "an apple," just long enough and strong enough to move between barrels. In (b), the man jumps up and down, on the first "a" barrel in "apple," not going forward, repeating his position (and the sound). In (c), the man comes to the "a" barrel in "apple" and just pushes down, with physical force/tension, not going forward, which prolongs his position (and the sound).

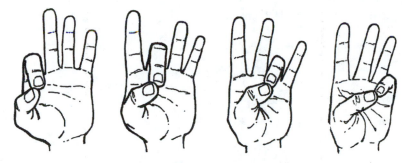

Smooth, easy forward movement

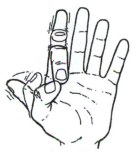

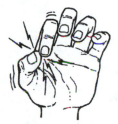

Disrupted forward movement:
Repetition

Disrupted forward movement:
Stoppage

FIGURE 3.15. Sequential finger-to-thumb analogy for forward versus disrupted sequence of movement (for older children/teenagers): Sequential touching of fingers to thumb. To successfully touch each of the four fingers to the thumb, the person must smoothly, easily, and not hurriedly move each finger to thumb in proper sequence. If thumb-to-one-finger contact is made repeatedly (repetition) or prolonged (stoppage), sequential, easy forward thumb to finger movement is disrupted. Likewise, with speech "forward" movement of vocal tract structures through the sound, syllable, or word requires physically easy, smooth, and sequential movement. Repetitions or cessation of vocal tract structural movement will disrupt forward movement through utterance.

Child Who Stutters. Guitar parallels this analogy with relatively physically tense speech behavior, but in the beginning it can also be used by itself to teach the child (as well as the teenager) how *time* can be used to relax *physical tension*. Once the child appears to grasp the concept—and this doesn't take long with most clients (something the child can demonstrate by copying the clinician's behavior)—the clinician may, as Guitar demonstrates, parallel fist/hand behavior with stuttered speech behavior. A graphic version of the fist-to-relaxed-hand analogy employed by Guitar (but without accompanying speech) can be seen in Figure 3.16 below.

With this analogy, which can also be used effectively with older clients, the clinician is essentially teaching the client *to use time to release physical tension*. In essence, analogizing an instance of stuttering to a closed fist, the clinician gradually, over several seconds, releases or lets the physical tension out of his or her hand. As the hand relaxes, it moves

Time   **Physical Tension**

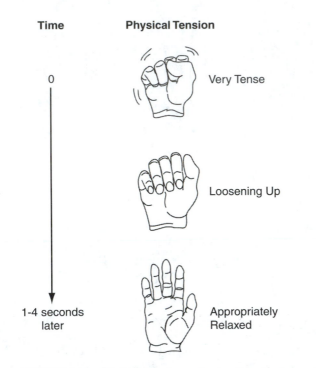

0   Very Tense

                                           Loosening Up

1-4 seconds   Appropriately
later   Relaxed

FIGURE 3.16.   Tight fist analogy of using time to change tension. Here, the clinician uses *time* to help the client *gradually* release/change physical *tension* during speech. This analogy can be used with or without accompanying speech postures, for example, a fixed articulatory contact on /b/. By tensing the fist, and then gradually releasing it, the client can be helped to understand how time can be used to gradually reduce physical tension. Note: The clinician *does not* want the client to learn to speak in association with or by clenching and then relaxing the fist. This is an analogy only, not a substitute for the client's being able to gradually move, with lessening tension, a speech posture that is being stuttered onto the subsequent speaking posture of position.

from a fist to open palm. Through repeated demonstrations, with or without accompanying speech, the child comes to understand that time can be used to change tension. Praise of the child by the clinician for gradual, smooth release of tension in the hand, especially if it parallels similar gestures in speaking structures, is appropriate. Again, what is being taught here is the interface of time and tension, and how one aspect of this interface (time) can be used to appropriately change the other in the direction of physically easy, nonrushed speech production. (In light of the above analogy, it is interesting to note Bloodstein's [1975, p. 81] observation, when trying to help the person who stutters understand that he or she is must learn to identify and hence change his or her own behavior, that the person who stutters ". . . must learn to unclench his tongue as he unclenches his fist.")

Again we caution: Some clients may get the notion that they should be unclenching their fists *throughout* conversational speech, whenever they are stuttering, in attempts to "ease out" of the stuttering. They seem to believe that the fist unclenching, through some magic we are still unaware of, will release their tongue, lips, and so on. While a little of this in the therapy room, to teach the idea, is okay, its routine use outside of therapy when speaking should be discouraged. We are NOT trying to teach them more tricks to "get out of stuttering." We are merely trying to help them learn that tension can be changed by time, whether in their hands or mouth. The final emphasis, as always, is with the person's speaking behavior, not hand gestures. The final goal here is to focus on means to facilitate reasonably fluent speech, not developing creative ways to time speaking with fist clenching and unclenching.

Helping the Child See, Hear, and Feel Stuttering

One of the fundamental problems with assisting young children to do more and more things that normally fluent speakers do when they speak (Williams, 1971) is that the child cannot really see much of what he or she is doing that facilitates or inhibits fluent speech. Furthermore, although the child can *hear* what he or she did that interfered with or facilitated speech, audition is, by and large, an *after-the-fact* type of feedback. That is, although the child may have heard the stuttering, the speech behavior of interest has already taken place by the time the youngsters has heard it! What we need to be seeking, if we are to change behavior *during* its actual production, is feedback that indicates inappropriate behavior is about to be produced or is being produced!

Learning about speech and how to change it is different, therefore, than when the child is learning to hold a crayon or pencil for writing. When learning to write, the child can readily visualize—as these events or behaviors are actually happening—most of the correct hand postures, positions, and to some extent the necessary movements and coordinations of fingers, thumb, hand, wrist, and arm needed for writing. Likewise, most sports that the child can learn can be readily visualized and thus practiced and compared to the visual model (even though, of course, such visualization slows down actual production). On the other hand, many aspects of speech production, as mentioned above, are, for all intents and purposes, invisible to the naked eye. Thus, you really cannot watch and, therefore, easily visualize (or draw a mental picture) the necessary movements of the tongue, soft palate, pharyngeal and laryngeal musculature and structures needed for speech production as you can, say the hand and arm movements used for tennis, soccer, or baseball.

Again, our young clients are as baffled by the how and why of speech production and movement as we are probably by the how and why our heart behaves the way it does. While we know the heart pumps blood and that it beats, few of us could really describe the physical movements, contractions, and configurations of our heart at work. (To get some idea of how naive most of us are regarding our heart, ask a few of your acquaintances to point to the location of their heart; many will point to the upper left side of their chest when in actuality the heart is located more centrally behind the sternum!) For most of us, speech and cardiac behavior are automatic events that we give little thought to: We simply speak, and our heart simply beats. For children who stutter, however, some knowledge of how they speak and how they interfere with speaking is crucial in order for them to improve their speech fluency.

To counteract these difficulties, we have found that acoustic and videotape recordings are an excellent means towards the end of helping the child see, visualize, and thus change the interfering (with fluency) speech behavior. Mirrors and clinician modeling or imitation are also useful in this regard, and have long been used. Likewise, the "speech helper" diagram of a person, demonstrated by Dr. Peter Ramig on the Stuttering Foundation of America's video (#79, *Stuttering and the School-Age Child*), helps the child identify places within the vocal tract where the he or she may interfere with speaking. However, all such work must be done with caution and with a sensitivity toward the particular child's needs.

Some Children React Strongly to Audio and/or Audio-Video Recordings of Their Own Speech and Language Behavior.   We have observed that some children are excellent at discussing and demonstrating speech behavior and disfluency in the abstract but become very emotional, resist, or refuse to cooperate when their own actual speech behavior is touched, or visualized, or heard. For example, we recently had a 7-year-old child (with a mild/moderate stuttering problem) repeatedly ask us, during a diagnostic session, if he could see the video of our diagnostic session with him, during which he mainly conversed with his mother, the examining SLP, or responded to (in)formal tests. We agreed, and at the end of the session, we had he and his mother watch a brief section where he was talking to a clinician. As I was watch the television and adjusting the contrast and sound, I heard a sound behind me coming from the 7-year-old child, who was standing behind and to my left. I looked back, and the child was recoiling from his image on the television, much like someone might watch a pet dog being run over, with horror, fear, and throwing his arms up over his eyes. He slowly backed out of the room, went rigid, and refused to watch further. Only when I turned the VCR off and the image went blank on the television screen would he put his arms down. Were these extreme reactions on the part of the child? Of course, but slightly less extreme reactions of fear, discomfort, and dislike can and are observed with people who stutter (indeed, with many people who do not stutter), when hearing or viewing themselves and behavior for the first time. These children need time and patience on the part of the clinician because they are not going to get over these feelings of fear, avoidance, and denial in a hurry. (We have also observed, in the P/C stuttering group, that children can, with clinician support and experience, readily identify their *own* speech behavior; however, we have also observed that inappropriate competitiveness and criticism *between* children starts to emerge if we require them identify *each other's* speech behavior. Thus, experience has shown us, tasks that require a speaker's identification of his or her own behavior are very useful, but we have learned to be cautious when using tasks that require child speaker A to identify child speaker B's speaking behavior. Such is a bit more possible, with appropriate support and guidance, with teenagers who stutter.)

Sometimes actually showing older, more science-oriented children who stutter a model of the vocal tract or the larynx and allowing them to explore and ask questions about the model is helpful. They should be encouraged to ask questions about their own speech behavior and structures. Using any appropriate, reasonable means available to mitigate the mystery and vagaries surrounding the child's speech behavior and the structures that produce it is desirable. Of course, any approach with children must be done with an eye towards the child's level of understanding, experience, and ability to remember and assess complex concepts. And while there is a danger of being too intellectual with a young child who stutters, clinicians—particularly younger clinicians who have minimal experience with youngsters—must also guard against the opposite: oversimplification. Clinicians and teachers quickly come to realize that an 8-year-old child in the third grade is not exactly receptive to approaches that would be used with a preschool child who stutters. Not making assessment and intervention procedures (not their underlying principles) age-appropriate is one of the most common mistakes made by beginning clinicians. We should make every effort to interact with children at the level they present, rather than the level we think they should present or that they sometimes present. Furthermore—and this is very important—if parents are to be a part of the solution, as they should be, we have to help the parents realize that as we fine-tune our procedures to match the child's actual not hoped-for level of development, mistakes will be made, on the part of the child and the clinician. For example, we might believe that a 3-year-6-month-old child understands the vocabulary that normative tests suggests he should be able to understand; however, for whatever reason, the child doesn't readily respond to that level and thus the clinician may have to present words at say a 3-year-old level, at least until the child is more comfortable with the clinician and the clinical situation.

Explaining to Parents That Children Make Mistakes. And while we are in the neighborhood, it is a very wise policy, if you are having a parent watch his or her child's response on a standardized test like the *Peabody Picture Vocabulary Test (PPVT)*, to explain to the child's parents that mistakes on the part of the child are expected. Some parents, for whatever reasons, appear to believe that their child's responses to a clinical test or procedure must be essentially flawless or there is something wrong, their child is "not right," or even "slow." Indeed, you must explain to the parents that with most such tests that you will start slightly below or at the child's expected level of development and go well beyond that to find out the child's absolute best performance. Parents unsophisticated in the ways of standardized or even non-standardized testing will become quite concerned (and think something wrong with their child) when their child is failing unless you tell them that the test is designed to do just that: achieve the child's highest level of performance as denoted by a string of incorrect responses. Likewise, the parent is to be assured that a mistake here or there along the way is normal for all children, that the child doesn't have to get EVERYTHING right to be well within if not well above normal limits. Beginning clinicians, in particular, will be surprised how much more relaxed the parents will be once these facts are explained to them and they can rest assured that some mistakes during testing are acceptable and that the child's best performance is signally by a series of incorrect responses.

Helping the Child Understand "Forward Movement" in Speech (Changing Arresting and Releasing Gestures)

In our opinion, direct modification of the speaking behavior of youngsters who stutter (as with adults but using different methods) should focus on three factors: (1) the child's psychological and physiological reaction *just before* he or she speaks (i.e., what the child does and how he or she gets ready to initiate speech); (2) the child's speech production strategy used to *enter* or *go into* the production of the initial sound of the word, syllable, phrase, or sentence (the child's arresting gesture [McDonald, 1964]); and (3) the child's speech production strategy used to *release from* or *move away* from this sound and onto to the next sound. The concept in the area of phonetics/phonology of "arresting" and "releasing" has salience here, but in broader sense. Like a stack of blocks, these three factors support and relate to one another, and, for example, the child's apparent difficulties with *releasing* from a particular sound and moving on to the next is probably an end-product of a be-havioral chain that originated prior to the child's beginning to speak. We hasten to add: The child should not be given the impression that the sound is like some sort of tar baby that once touched, he or she can never let go of; instead, we want to emphasize that it is the child's *behavior* that needs modification and not the *sound*. Because if the problem is within the sound rather than within the speaker, then one logical conclusion is to avoid the sound, an approach that would be as inhibitory to fluency as it is impractical to do.

Therapy procedures like Van Riper's (1973) "pullout" or Williams' (1971) instruc-tion to "move on" or our suggestion to "change" or "change and move forward" are among the many ways of assisting the child to make the necessary and appropriate arresting, releasing, and transitional gestures onto the next sound. When helping the child learn to *change* speech production behavior for the sound(s) of interest and move forward, we want to make sure that we don't (1) simply have the child prolong the end of the stuttered sound or the sound after the stuttered sound or (2) engage the child in long, didactic lectures about speech sound transitions and arresting/releasing gestures. As always, with young clients, your demonstrations or examples of the model or target behavior are worth a thou-sand words. *Show* the child what you want him or her to do and try to minimize the *telling*. When it comes to helping the child learn to change his or her speech behavior: *Model* for rather than *instruct* the child. Closely observe the child's more common behaviors during stuttering, and with appropriate support and guidance, help the child to identify, in your own speech, behavior that closely resembles the child. This form of modeling is *only* done *after* the SLP has spent time helping the child identify speech disfluencies, first from recordings of other people who stutter, then recordings of the clinicians and then recordings of the child him- or herself. *Do not* engage in overt modeling of the child's stuttering until you are reasonably confident that the child can readily and quickly identify, with no unto-ward or inappropriate emotionality or concern, his or her own behavior during recorded samples of speaking. Even when this is apparent, be explicit with the child: "I (here, the clinician is talking) am not making fun or mocking or anything like that . . . I am merely showing you what you are doing, what it sounds and looks like, so you can begin to iden-tify and change it in your own speech."

Cursive Writing as an Analogy to "Forward Movement" in Speech

If the child has even a vague idea of what cursive writing looks like (as opposed to printed writing), the clinician can use the transitional gestures between cursive written symbols as an analogy to transitions between speech movements. For example, in Figure 3.17 the curved elements between "a" and "p" and "p" and "p" in the word "apple" are what we are referring to (in Figure 3.16, the thumb-to-finger analogy, it would be the movements *between* successive finger-to-thumb contacts). That is, the child can be shown that the con-necting lines, curves, and so on between cursive written letters are something like the tran-sitional gestures known to occur during speech production. These connecting lines, the child is shown, need to be made in a smooth, easy, and continuously forward-moving fash-ion for the writer's cursive writing to appear "fluent." Carrying the analogy further, we ask the child to guess what would happen if the writer refused, was reluctant, afraid, or embar-rassed to, or could not make the necessary curved elements or transitional lines between let-

(a)

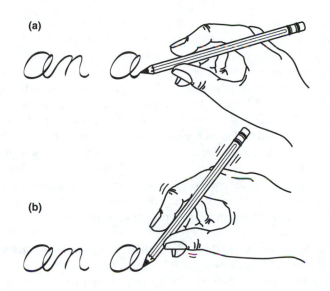

(b)

(c)

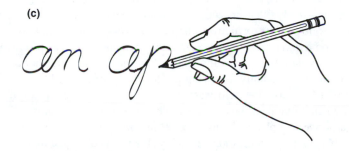

FIGURE 3.17.   Cursive writing analogy. The person in each panel (a-c) is trying to write, cursively, the phrase "an apple." In the top panel (a), *smooth, easy writing*, the person is quickly and physically easily moving the pencil from one letter to the next, in smooth, fluid, cursive writing fashion; in the next panel (b), *physically pushing with tension*, the person is physically pushing down with the fingers/hand on the pencil, at the transition point between "a" and "p" in the word "apple." In the last panel (c), the person has released the tension exhibited in (b) and moved on into and through the "p" that the person was "stuck on" in (b).

ters. We help the child understand that the writer would probably get stuck on or go back and repeat the initial letter of the word. We use this analogy to help the child learn to appreciate and more readily produce a more appropriate rate and level of physical tension when (1) initiating speech and (2) when moving between speech sounds.

Sometimes having the child slowly and easily say his or her name in synchrony with the writing of same may help the child develop the idea of forward-flowing sound production and, in particular, the speech production gestures needed to move between sounds, to move from one sound to the next. Similarly, attempting to produce the word-initial sound too rapidly with too much physical force or tension will throw everything off. This too can be analogized through the use of writing. Indeed, the child can practice "hard" versus "easy" writing (with and without accompanying speech production) to help the child get the message that he or she must enter the word-initial sound with appropriate force and tension (neither too much nor too little, perhaps like Baby Bear's porridge!) and then concentrate on smooth, easy release and transition into the next speech sound. This approach helps the child learn what forward movement in a seriated motor task like speech is all about. Most importantly, it can help the child understand what he or she is *doing* that interferes with smooth, forward movement. As mentioned above, we emphasize strategies, plans, programs, or rules rather than concentrate or focus on the child's so-called "problem" sounds, syllables, or words. We believe that the child needs help in understanding that he or she can use the same principle for many different sounds or sound combinations rather than a sound-specific means of "getting through" the sound, syllable, or word.

Sound-Specific Versus Speech-General Rules For Achieving Reasonably Fluent Speech.
Indeed, we want to help the child, as best we possibly can, to learn rules of speech-language production (both those that apply to initiation of speech as well as movement between sounds) that can apply to *all* sounds rather than learning one rule for /s/ and than another for /t/. Bluntly, the child just isn't going to expend the energy to learn *sound-specific* rules for achieving reasonably fluent speech. Rather, we want to teach one or two *speech-general* rules for achieving reasonably fluent speech. Technically speaking, a salient speech-general rule can be stated as follows: *Use an appropriate rate and level of physical tension to begin or initiate speech production as well as move from the first sound into the following sound.* Obviously, we don't explain this rule to the child using these words; furthermore, stating this rule is much easier than actually following it! However, for the child to become more fluent, he or she will have to have help learning to change the time/tension domains of speech, particular when initiating as well as moving between speech gestures, to initiate and continue speech at a rate and physical tension level that maximizes his or her chances for producing reasonably fluent speech. And reasonably fluent speech is just that—speech that is essentially full of fluency with some disfluencies permitted and accepted. As we have said elsewhere (Conture & Melnick, 1999), to strive for zero disfluencies, to have zero tolerance for speech disfluencies, is neither reasonable nor realistic. Of course, there is little doubt that all of this will require concentration and work (once again, we never said any of this would be easy). Simply put, lasting behavioral change takes time and effort! It is our job, however, to encourage the child to expend the necessary time and effort without becoming overwhelmed and discouraged with the task. Indeed, as we were motivated to learn and grow by those teachers, parents, mentors, and the like, so must we be motivators for our clients, particularly when they are at their lowest ebb of confidence, energy, and interest!

Trying Not to Turn off Child and Parents to Speech Therapy

Sometimes, our sincere desire to help, our zeal for "improving" the child as fast as possible, overcomes our abilities to consider long-term consequences. Again, there is some kinda help which is the kinda help these clients and their associates can do without. We really must try not to turn the child or his parents off to speech therapy. Sometimes waiting until a child's and his or her parents schedule is more conducive to therapy is preferable to forcing everybody to begin therapy when it requires the juggling skills of a circus clown just to get their feet in the clinic door. Granted, a child can be *too* organized with tuba lessons on Monday, soccer on Tuesday, Boy Scouts on Wednesday, choir practice on Thursday, and so on. However, this frenetic schedule is the reality that the child and his or her parents live with, and it is the wise clinician who doesn't insist that each and every one of these activities take a second or third priority to beginning speech therapy. Instead, the SLP should use gentle but firm terms to make it clear that the child needs therapy and that as soon as it can be done, some room in the child's busy schedule should be made to accommodate weekly therapy sessions. This "schedule adjustment" might take as much as three to six months to effect. Indeed, the SLP is often brought into conversations by parents, to help them prioritize their child's schedule. No problem, but an SLP's opinion in these matters is not the same as an SLP's decision about schedule. In the end, the child is the parent's responsibility and the parent needs to be explicitly reminded of that (e.g., "Here are my thoughts on the matter, Mrs. MacDonald, but remember, Angus is your child, in the end, you can and must do what you think is best for him"). Once this has been completed, however, on the initiative of the parent and child and not as a command performance because of clinician demands, this particular horse is going to be a lot more inclined to drink when brought to the water.

Change Sometimes Occurs After Difficult Sessions   Maintaining a child's interest in therapy does not mean, however, that all therapy sessions have to be a rollicking good time or that children and their parents will not have to work hard during as well as outside of therapy. In fact, this writer has often observed, that intervention improves *after* difficult, contentious, or seemingly failed sessions. Sometimes both clinician and client must do poorly for one or both to realize that they must adjust, change, and/or work harder/smarter for progress to be made. And, if all else fails, we are simply trying to maintain, as much as possible, the child's enthusiasm for change in speech behavior and a belief that such change is possible. Maybe not right now, but in the future, such change can and will take place. Speech-language pathologists can do harm by providing the child with such an aversive, non-rewarding experience at an early age that it may take many years before the child can forget this experience and be willing to resume therapy.

Giving the Child a Break by Creating a Break from Therapy.   Speech-language pathologist should be willing to give a child a break from therapy when he or she or the child appears to become stale or bored with the process. However, the clinician should also, at the time of the break, let the child, parents, classroom teachers, and other important adults in the child's environment know of the break and provide some explanation for why the clinician is instituting the break. Moreover, it is helpful to let the child and related adults know the exact time and date when therapy will be resumed. Three to six weeks is a good break period, but individual clients' needs dictate the exact length and nature of such a break. Homework, if any, given during the break should be minimal; leave the children alone, give them some time to think about and reflect on whether they are interested and willing to make the necessary changes in their speech. It helps to explicitly tell the parents that they may call you any time they want during the break. It also helps to emphasize that they should not revert back to older, less appropriate ways of correcting the child's speech during the period of the break from therapy. When the child and parent(s) return after the break, try to greet them in as positive a tone as possible, let them know that you are glad to see them once again and that you both can now get down to the business of helping the child speak more fluently. Of course, such breaks are different from changes in therapy that need to take place if a child's learning disorder, attention deficit, hyperactivity, excessively perfectionistic, obsessive/compulsive tendencies, extreme competitiveness, emotional fragility, or intellectual difficulties prove to be significantly getting in the way of speech-language therapy. In these cases, clear explanations to the parents of what is observed, similarly clear explanations to an appropriate referral source, and then discontinuation of SLP services is probably most appropriate (more on such referrals below).

Motivating the Child to "Think I Can."   The power of suggestion is tremendous, as Van Riper (1973) aptly points out and the field of medicine has long understood (Benson & McCallie, 1979). In my opinion, the speech and language clinician should use it appropriately to help children (and their parents) believe in themselves, their ability to change, and their ability to work to the goal of improved fluency. Like the little train engine, the young child can be helped to believe, "I think I can"; conversely, the clinician certainly does not want to add to the young stutterer's all too common "I think I can't" philosophy. Undoubtedly, the speech-language pathologist is, as Starbuck (1974) and Prins (1974) discuss and as this writer mentioned above, a motivator as well as changer of behavior.

The clinician must routinely assess the child's degree of motivation and try to adjust clinician strategy to accommodate the natural rises and falls of client motivation. The SLP must not assume that the child's recognition of a problem is sufficient motivation to change, because if mere recognition of a problem was all that was needed to improve, then people who knew they were heavy would easily lose weight and people who knew they smoked would easily quit. No, recognition of a problem may be necessary for motivation to change, but it is clearly not sufficient.

Referrals to Other Professionals

It has been said that the trouble with education is that everybody has a little of it. Unfortunately, SLPs suffer from a similar problem: Everybody uses speech and language, and therefore everybody understands it, right? Wrong! Many readers of these pages devote their professional lives to an understanding of normal and disordered processes of speech, hearing, and language and yet still may think that they have an inadequate understanding of these processes. This does not imply that our profession corners the market on information or knowledge regarding speech and language behavior, but it does imply that our professional education, training, and experience puts us in a very good situation to assess and manage the myriad of communication problems that people present.

While it is important to know what we know, it is just as important, if not more so, to know what we don't know. And, we hasten to add, that this such lack of self-knowledge is not only a problem for SLPs but for other professionals as well. We need to realize that

certain clients have problems and concerns that go beyond our scope of training and juris-
diction, or practice. Likewise, other clients may have concomitant problems besides stuttering, problems and concerns that warrant attention from other professionals. With
children, such professionals are most apt to be classroom teachers, special education teachers, reading specialists, family physicians, pediatricians, child psychologists (and psychiatrists), social workers, audiologists, and otolaryngologists. Academic and related matters
are often detected *prior* to your entrance into the child's life; however, it is not uncommon
for certain behaviors such as reading problems, difficulties with neuromotor development,
psychosocial adjustment, and so forth to be detected for the first time by the SLP during an
initial speech and language evaluation. The parents should be told, in as nonalarming tones
as possible, when such problems are apparent and that you will (with their permission) pass
this information on to the appropriate school authorities.

Certain other problems—for example, a child who fails a hearing screening; appears
to have abnormal reflexes; has difficulties learning; or is extremely hyperactive, inattentive
or distractible, impulsive, hyperperfectionistic, or fearful of any normal changes in the
environment—may require the SLP to consult with nonschool professionals. Once again,
the SLP should try to explain to the parent, in as clear and nonalarming tones as possible,
his or her observations and recommendation that the child receive a *routine* or *standard*
screening test or evaluation by the family physician, pediatrician (whichever the parents use
and prefer), or child psychologist to assess whether your observations warrant concern.
Referrals, of course, are a two-way street. We are not physicians, nor are we psychologists
or classroom teachers. Neither, we hasten to add, are these professionals speech and language pathologists! Thus, while we refer to other professionals when needed, we also need
to be prepared to receive referrals from other professionals. While a psychologist might
observe and describe what to him or her is a speech problem, it is our purview as well as
professional responsibility, after having the case referred to us by the psychologist, to
administer a diagnostic evaluation and make, if needed, therapy recommendations regarding the child's speech and language function. When receiving such referrals, it is hoped the
decisions we make and report regarding the child will be based on as well as give the
appearance of resulting from a careful mixture of clinical intuition and objective data and
avoid the appearance of being arbitrary and capricious.

Again, and speaking in general terms, when making a referral, it is most appropriate
to tell the parents of your observations and allow them to decide if they want further consultation with appropriate personnel. Certainly, you want to strongly encourage such referrals, particularly in those cases where you believe a referral is essential, but in the final
analysis the decision to pursue the matter further rests in the hands of the parents. In a few
cases, with parents of limited understanding, you may have to be more insistent and actually make some phone calls yourself, especially if the nature and degree of the problem
(e.g., a child who is physically acting out against other children, small animals, who routinely talks about fires, knives, and guns, and/or one who has threatened to harm him- or
herself or take his or her own life) require thorough and immediate attention from a professional other than a nonspeech and language pathologist. It is our routine policy to tell the
parents (after they have signed the appropriate parental consent and release form) that we
will send to their family physician or pediatrician, or any other professional of their choosing, a copy of our report, findings, and recommendations, unless, of course, they would

rather we did not. Although the SLP runs the risk of another professional's misinterpreting, misunderstanding, or ignoring the written report, it our belief and experience that more factual information is better than less and so we continue to routinely forward reports to the family's other attending professionals.

In the relatively few situations where the child has a psychosocial rather than stuttering problem, a referral to appropriate psychological or psychiatric agencies is in order. Many times, however, the parents and/or the child may resist such referral and insist that there is nothing wrong with the child besides speech. If, on the other hand, you firmly believe, based on your clinical insights and objective data, that speech disfluency is not a significant problem or that it is secondary or even tertiary to some more chronic or serious psychosocial adjustment concern (our experience indicates that this is the case for appropriately 5 to 10 percent of the children, teenagers, and adults who stutter that we encounter), then the parents should be told. And if push comes to shove and the parents disregard your recommendation, then you may have to decline speech therapy for the child (of course, providing the parents with the names of other SLPs who might be willing and able to handle the child). Simply put, we believe it inappropriate to administer speech therapy for a child whose real concerns lie elsewhere. Obviously, it is in your and your clients' best interest for you to develop and cultivate professional interactions with psychologists who work with children and their families. Such professionals can enter into such tough counseling situations and assist the parents in seeing that psychological services are warranted and most appropriate.

Concluding Remarks

At the risk of stating the obvious, let me do so: The child is not a small adult! Large amounts of information about child development make that clear: The child is progressing or developing toward adulthood, and in many ways, the child has a long way to go behaviorally, emotionally, physically, psychologically, and socially. Thus, while our principles about what stuttering is and/or what might cause it remain the same, regardless of age, our assessment and treatment of children *must* be geared to the skills and ability and level of development of the child. We either maneuver according to the circumstances the child presents or the circumstances the child presents will maneuver us!

Parents' Gift of Independence to Their Child.   Given those remarks, we have tried to view the remediation of stuttering in children in the context of dealing with the child's skills and abilities as well as the child's environment. Neither aspect—the child's abilities or environment—appears to be sufficient to cause stuttering, but both appear to be necessary for the problem to develop. Hence, the two aspects appear to complexly interact in such a way as to make the whole greater than the sum of the parts. For the clinician, of course, working with both the child and the child's environment provides a sizable challenge, but it is a challenge that can be met with rewards for so doing that far outweigh any initial trepidations. Alluded to in Chapter 2, this author likes to say that the greatest gift a parent can give his or her child is the gift of independence—an independence to readily and effectively deal with the slings and arrows of outrageous fortune that we all experience as children, teenagers, and adults. And while the burgeoning independence of children cannot be divorced from their overall dependence on their parents, helping the child who stutters learn to speak more fluently and appropriately cope with any instances of disfluency that remain contributes to the child's growing forays into the land of independence, while still allowing the child to dart back under the protective wing of appropriate parental dependence. For the parent, no greater challenge exists than appropriately letting the child learn by doing, trial and error, and thus developing the internal resources to handle future challenges rather than doing for the child to help the child avoid the pain and discomfort of making mistakes, but also stripping the child of the ability to develop internal resources for adjusting and adapting to an ever-changing world.

Segue into the Land of Teens Who Stutter

As we move from the young child to the older child (although don't let any teenager hear you call him or her a child!), we are presented with a different sort of challenge. Here the environment provided by the parents becomes less and less significant while the environment provided by peers takes on increased importance. More than anything else, the teenager does not want to appear different from his or her peers, for example, by having to leave the classroom to go to speech-language therapy! The teenager finds him- or herself betwixt and between the role of the child that he or she so willingly seems to discard and the brass ring of the adult role model he or she so eagerly seems to be reaching for. Like a snake half in and half out of its shed skin, the teenager clamors for the independent privileges of the adult but is quite content to revert to the dependent ways of a child if the less-than-pleasant responsibilities of adulthood are thrust upon him or her. Onto this sea of adolescence physical, mental, social, psychological, and emotional disequilibruim, we must sail if we are to effectively deal with stuttering in the teenager. Indeed, much more is going on than merely stuttering in teenagers who stutter (a point clearly made by Guitar & Conture, 1996, in a video entitled: "Do You Stutter? A Video for Teens Who Stutter").

While calm winds may be relaxing, they don't fill our sails and we can't make headway when becalmed. Likewise, while hurricane-force winds may fill our sails, they also may rip them asunder and leave us at the mercy of the elements (simply ask the sailing crews in the 1998 Sydney to Darwin racing disaster!). Instead, it is the moderate-to-strong winds that test our sailing mettle, teach us how to sail, and make progress toward our destination. Between the relative calm of childhood and the hopefully steady tradewinds of adulthood arise the unpredictably strong winds of adolescence that wax and wane and test the mettle of teenager and parent alike. Hopefully, in the end, however, experience with these turbulences help develop independent sailors who no longer need parents or a skipper, navigator, or crew. Parents may not like the fact that their crew has taken to skippering another boat, but perhaps they can take some comfort in the fact that even though the young skipper may be sailing to other unknown ports, he or she now also has the means to return home when he or she so desires without the constant supervision of parents.

Summary

This chapter started by establishing the widely held notion that stuttering is a disorder of childhood, in that the vast majority of those people who stutter, begin to so by 7 years of age, with a few more continuing to onset until 12 years of age. This so-called "developmental" stuttering was contrasted with "acquired" stuttering, the latter typically beginning in adulthood, usually after disease, trauma, stroke, and/or psychosocial difficulties. It was also made clear that childhood stuttering is quite variable with more than a few children resolving without formal treatment; however, while strides have been made, we are still a long way from accurately predicting which children will become chronic, persistent people who stutter. Furthermore, while the precise relationship between chronological age and presence or absence of a stuttering problem is less than clear, it does seem to be the case that the child's chronological age significantly influences the exact procedures used to treat the child's stuttering, regardless of its level of development or severity.

This chapter also made apparent that strides have been made in the treatment of stuttering, with more and more workers in this field advocating intervention as soon as possible, or at least as soon as it becomes clear that a problem exists and that there is less likelihood that recovery without treatment will occur. For the clinician, therefore, it was pointed out that they had to be aware of the growing literature for professionals in terms of treating childhood stuttering (e.g., Onslow & Packman, 1999) as well as the growing literature oriented toward public information (e.g., Conture, Guitar, & Fraser, 1997). A strong case was made for the involvement of parents in the treatment of childhood stuttering (e.g., Conture & Melnick, 1999), and part of this approach involves helping parents understand that their influence, if any, on their children's speech (dis)fluency is most likely to be one of exacerbation and maintenance rather than causation.

Subsequent to that, and before treatment *per se* was covered, the present chapter discussed a variety of general "treatment process" issues, concerns that all clinicians must deal with when treating stuttering—for example, when to begin treatment, how often, how long, and so forth. Likewise, there was discussion of selection criteria for who should and should not enter treatment. This was followed by description of three variables (i.e., "using the 's' word," "talking about talking," and the influence of chronological age on treatment) that clinicians typically deal with when remediating stuttering. Subsequently, issues pertaining to *direct* versus *indirect* versus *combined* approaches were presented.

This chapter then spent considerable space describing the characteristics and treatment approaches for four groups of children typically assessed and treated for childhood stuttering, running the gamut from children with no apparent problem with stuttering to children very involved with stuttering. Qualifying each of these four groups was their parents' relative concern or lack thereof with their child and their child's stuttering. Woven through much of this was the role and impact of other problems—for example, phonological problems and the quantity and quality of intervention services the child would receive. Considerable space was devoted to the author's parent–child stuttering group approach (e.g., Conture & Melnick, 1999). The chapter then spent considerable space discussing and presenting a variety of analogies to use with parents and/or their child to better help the child understand the complexities of stuttering, the child's role in same, and what can be done about it. This chapter ended with discussion of the rationale behind as well as general procedures for referring children who stutter who exhibit other problems—for example, psychosocial adjustment—that are either more of a concern than stuttering and/or appear to be confounding the treatment of stuttering. Last, the difficulties all parents experience helping their children develop independence, its role in therapy, and for appropriately setting the stage for becoming an older child or teenager were discussed.

4 Remediation: Older Children and Teenagers Who Stutter

Older Children Are Not Just Older, They Are Different as Well

As we have said before, young children are not small adults! Likewise, older children (those of about 9 years and older) and teenagers who stutter are not just larger preschoolers. Older children and teenagers differ in more ways than just age from those who are younger. To begin, older children and teenagers many times have had some form of prior therapy experience. Although some older children have had little formal therapy and thus, at least in theory, are eager for help, many others have several months to years of relatively unsuccessful formal speech therapy and are not as motivated and interested to receive more. Second, besides stuttering, these older children present the typical preteen and adolescent concerns unique to their age group. Put another way, these youngsters are not only older but exhibit concerns that differ somewhat from those of the preschool, early elementary school child.

For example, the third- to fourth-grade child, who in the first and second grades readily left class for speech therapy, now begins to resist. In fact, the leaving of classmates, for some third to fourth graders, may be of far more concern than their stuttering! Another example might involve a 14-year-old girl who stutters, even one who noticeably and severely stutters, who may balk at receiving help for her problem. Again, being different from her peers becomes of paramount concern. The 14-year-old girl may complain that she does not want to seem different from her friends, leave school at unusual hours, or attend special classes not attended by her normally fluent peers. She may even tell you (as these young people have sometimes told this author) that she feels like a "retard" by coming to your speech therapy sessions. Indeed, the author just did a preliminary assessment of a 19-year-old male, a sophomore in college, whose main concern, besides the stuttering, was that his college peers/fraternity brothers might think he was "different" if they knew he was receiving speech therapy. Thus, one of the main driving forces of these older children and teenagers is to "fit in," to avoid being different from their peers at all costs, to be like their friend but, of course, different from their parents!

Third, and segueing from the above discussion, is the developing importance and influence of peers for older children and adults. And conversely, the diminishing importance and influence of their parents. While the influence of parents cannot be denied (indeed, some clinicians, [e.g., Mastrud, 1988], actively and extensively involve parents in the remediation of stuttering in teenagers), neither can the tremendous influence of peers on the likes, dislikes, motivations, and so forth of the older child. To manage the older child *without* understanding the influence of his or her peers on the child's behavior is to manage the child from a relatively incomplete perspective. Indeed, understanding the unique concerns of the older child and teenager who stutter are crucial for successful remediation. For example, about three months ago, we removed a teenager from our teenage therapy group and placed him into individual therapy. Why? He enjoyed the group immensely, was cooperative and socializing well with his peers, but was making absolutely no progress in terms of changing his stuttering. It became clear that he needed the quantity and quality of attention, focus, and amount of instruction afforded by an individual session. However, when asked which treatment format he liked best, he quickly replied, "the group." When further queried about his success in the group, he admitted that he had made little progress and that individual treatment was what he needed. After all that, however, he still stated his intense desire to be in the group rather than individual therapy, to skip individual therapy, even though he knew individual treatment was what he needed. Attempts on the reader's part to use logic and rational thought to understand the above is relatively fruitless; the emotional magnet of peer camaraderie, influence, and support attracts the emotional iron filings of most teenagers, regardless of what their own (or their parents') logic and rationality may tell them.

Paralysis Through Analysis

The present author agrees with individuals with considerable experience, like Guitar (1997), Rustin, Cook, and Spence (1995), and Schwartz (1999), that more than a few older children and teenagers who continue to stutter have and/or are continuing to develop strong emotional reactions, negative attitudes toward their speech, their abilities as speakers, and communication. For example, a teenager who stutters may feel "different" because of his speech, a feeling in direct contradiction to his strong desire to look, act, and be like other teenagers, to conform, to fit in with his peers. Likewise, an older child who stutters may have developed so much fear and dread about stuttering, an "emotional whiteout" during instances of stuttering that is so strong, that no amount of well-intentioned attempts to modify stuttering may be able overcome this fear without attending to these strong reactions. Interestingly, in this writer's opinion, some of these teenagers' own attitudes about themselves as speakers appear far more negative than any feedback they seem to have received from their peers. (Teens, of course, are not the only people who may continually seek the cloud rather than the silver lining in themselves. Some adults who do and who do not stutter may have a low self-esteem and a negative opinion of themselves, regardless of environmental reactions to the contrary.) While it is appropriate in a society as complex as ours to care about what others think of us, it is not conducive to our mental stability and self-esteem to be chronically, deeply, and persistently concerned about how others assess our every waking act. However, such continual concerns are exactly what some teenagers who stutter experience, and this can lead to a "paralysis by analysis" whereby people, places, and things are avoided. Indeed, some teenagers seem to feel that it is better not to act at all than to risk ridicule by their peers for their actions. This is a bit similar, perhaps, to the old adage, "Better to be silent and thought a fool than to open one's mouth and remove all doubt." Again, none of us can have a total "sense of freedom" from what others "think of us," but when our first and foremost concern is what others and not ourselves think of us, our ability to easily function on a daily basis can be compromised. This issue—of always looking "outward" to see if our "inward" self is appropriate, correct, and acceptable—is something we will discuss in some depth later in this chapter.

Understanding the Parents of the Older Child and Teenager Who Stutter

Continuing with our preceding remarks regarding the treatment of older children and teenagers who stutter, Schwartz (1999) makes an important point, "When some clinicians begin to work with older children and adolescents, they fail to recognize the continuing need to involve family members in therapy" (p.113). For example, parents of teens, as well as young children, cannot expect their children to pay attention to their advice to speak with a normal rate of speech but ignore the parent's own examples of talking at 300 words a minute! Parents of these children also have special concerns. First, some of these parents may have been trying for several years to get appropriate assistance for their child but have met with little success. Naturally, therefore, they may be somewhat frustrated by the time an SLP, who has the training and experience necessary to significantly help them, meets them for the first time. Second, some of these parents may have observed their child receive numerous hours of therapy and related services without much appreciable progress. These parents, therefore, may be quite skeptical or uncertain that yet another SLP can actually help their child. Third, another group of parents—some of the ones we discussed in the previous chapter who were unconcerned about their child's problem—may have consciously decided to keep their child out of therapy. Perhaps they were previously denying the problem or hoping against hope that the child would "outgrow" the stuttering. Whatever; now, when their child is a teenager, they seek services but probably do so with a great deal of guilt or concern for the fact that their child should have previously received therapy. These same parents may now feel that their child's continued stuttering is their fault.

Fourth, and perhaps most important of all, many of these parents are also having the typical concerns with their rapidly maturing youngster that all other parents of children of similar age experience: (1) concerns with schoolwork, homework, and academic achievement; (2) responsibility for carrying out household chores; (3) respect for adults and/or parents; (4) willingness to listen and respond to parental requests and rules; (5) dating and relations with the opposite sex; (6) ability to get along with peers inside and outside of school; (7) (mis)use of drugs and alcohol; and (8) concerns about education beyond high school and future employment possibilities. Yes, no one ever said that parenting was an easy job! However, the job of being a parent to a teenager is not made any easier by professionals who fail to recognize the tremendous number of variables these parents must deal with, on a daily basis, to properly raise and interact with their older children/teenagers. To effectively treat stuttering in teenagers is to try to come to grips with the period called "adolescence," a period of time where most of us have one foot planted in childhood and the other in adulthood, and hoping back and forth between the two, as the spirit, convenience, and circumstances dictate.

We have mentioned before that the child who stutters and the parent of that child are children and parents first and only secondarily involved with stuttering. Our belief that stuttering relates to a complex interaction between the person who stutters and his or her environment suggests that stuttering neither develops nor operates in a hermetically sealed container but is interwoven with the fiber of human existence. We would encourage SLPs to gain understanding of the general human background against which the stuttering foreground exists.

Based on our understanding of this background, we have come to the belief that when managing the older child who stutters, we become less and less able to separate out our own feelings of how things should be done because the child gets closer to our own age. I feel that this dilemma (a concern also apparent when we try to treat adults who stutter) arises because we begin to observe with these children and their parents, more clearly than with younger children and their parents, problems that we ourselves have not successfully coped with in our own personal lives. These clients act as mirrors that reflect some of our own inadequacies. This is not something that makes us comfortable, but it is something we should clearly understand. Indeed, a basic understanding that it is the teen's *duty* to break the ties of childhood, to overthrow the shackles of childhood dependence, and forge new liaisons with a world that has little to do with his or her parents. As we mentioned in Chapter 3, the greatest gift a parent can give his or her child is the gift of independence! This is true no matter how hard it is for the parents to see their little Johnny or Susie sailing away from them and into a realm where the young person not the parents set the rules, agenda, and the means to get there.

How Older Children Differ in General from Younger Children

It goes without saying that older children relate to adults in different ways than they did when they were younger. Whereas 5-year-olds generally do what the clinician tells them to do because the SLP is an adult, the clinician finds that with the older child, explicit rationale may have to be given for each and every request of the child. Paradoxically, older children and teens may want explanations for adult requests of them but be very much put off if the explanation is too detailed or stated in language they cannot understand! The SLP, to be successful with these "children," must recognize the older child's growing independence (or need for same) as well as appropriate assertiveness (not to be confused with inappropriate aggressiveness; for an excellent discussion of the distinctions between aggression, assertion, and nonassertion see Lange & Jakubowski, 1976, pp. 7–53). In essence, the SLP must be prepared to interact with these children as they present themselves rather than as we might ideally like to see them behave.

Likewise, it is important to discuss with the older child's parents, school personnel, and others familiar with the child whether the child seems to be socially, emotionally, psychologically, physically, and academically developing on course. A child who is afraid to speak, has very few or no friends, is reluctant to use verbal expression during social and academic situations is a child who may nonverbally act out to seek peer and adult attention, recognition, or approval. The SLP must be sensitive to these signs and try to get parents and appropriate personnel to intervene to insure that the child's acting out and other inappropriate behavior, inside and outside the classroom, does not become the child's standard operating procedure as he or she develops into his or her teen years. We have observed situations where stuttering becomes the least of a child's problems when that child keeps the classroom in a state of mild uproar, and the police routinely visit the house because they suspect the child of the latest piece of neighborhood vandalism. (Conversely, we also deal with the child who is not "causing trouble" in the neighborhood, and who may actually be a good student, but whose hyperperfectionism, inability to make and tolerate a mistake, hyper-competitiveness, and/or obsessive-compulsive rituals make it nearly impossible for him or her to benefit from speech–language therapy.) The SLP and other professionals should be sensitive to the child who, because he or she can't master the academic information and social rules of the typical classroom, tries to "master" his or her classmates by acts of physical and verbal aggression and interference. In our opinion, these children are crying out for help and should receive it as early as possible in the form of family or individual counseling, individualized academic instruction, and the like.

With the older child who stutters, but who exhibits minimal awareness, we like to continue the emphasis on parent–child activities. Any event that brings the family together is one that can potentially foster opportunities for positive emotional, intellectual, and communication sharing. Allowing the older child to spend week in and week out with minimal adult–child communication besides, "Clean up your room," "Don't talk that way to your mother," "Use your easy speech," or "Be quiet, can't you see I'm talking" is counterproductive to successful remediation of the child's fluency problem. For example, a father who enjoys working with tools around the house could be encouraged to explain their use to his son; a mother who enjoys reading could explain her books to the child, in terms the child would understand; a father who collects coins could involve his son; a mother who likes to garden could involve her child in some of the less physically demanding aspects of gardening. An opposite tack, but one that works as well, is to focus on what the child wants to talk about and listen and learn while the child talks. Indeed, some of my toughest cases have been "cracked" when I requested at home and in the clinic that conversations be increasingly child-oriented, allowing the child to take the lead and talk about what he or she wants to talk about.

Verbal sharing (which is to be differentiated from verbal lecturing) or quiet interactions between child and parent, regardless of what is discussed or the specific nature of the shared activity, should be encouraged by the SLP. Every opportunity can and should be used to encourage the child to keep talking, to praise him or her for his attempts to converse; that is, the child should not be allowed to become reluctant and afraid to verbally converse with his or her parents, other adults, and peers. Simply put, a child cannot practice speaking, cannot attempt to modify inappropriate speaking behavior, if he or she does *not* talk except during therapy sessions! A child who essentially holes him- or herself up in his or her room playing computer games or watching television has no real reason or incentive to talk and hence no opportunity to modify speech. You can't modify something you never do!

How Stuttering Problems of Older Children Who Stutter Differ from Those of Young People Who Stutter

As mentioned above, it is fairly obvious that stuttering in a child of 9, who has been stuttering since he or she was 4, will be different from that of a child who is 4 who has been stuttering since he or she was 3.5 years of age. Exactly how stuttering changes over time, for the group of people who stutter or any one individual, is still less than clear (although, with advancing age, stuttering does appear to become increasing more apt to contain *cessation* [e.g., prolongations] rather than *reiterative* [e.g., repetitions] disfluencies [Pellowski & Conture, 1999]). However, it is far less than clear what these differences might be. In Chapter 1 we discussed some differences that might be observed as the problem develops. Similarly, Bloodstein (1995, pp. 52–56) discusses the "four phases in the development of stuttering," which are based on his assessment of the clinical case histories of 418 children who stutter ranging in age from 2 to 16 years. Bloodstein provides broad ranges of age limits for each of these stages, suggesting, he appears to believe, as do we, that chronological age is loosely related to routinely observed behavioral characteristics of stuttering.

What is needed is empirical research that investigates whether the older child and teenager who stutter are different, on dimensions other than frequency, duration, and severity of stuttering, from those children who, at an earlier age, with or without therapy, become normally fluent. If we had this information, we might be better able to predict, at earlier ages, which children will more or less likely to recover and plan frequency and type of therapy accordingly. As mentioned in Chapter 2, Riley's (1981) *Stuttering Prediction Instrument* (SPI) represents an attempt to make such prediction; however, independent investigators need to empirically assess the SLP's ability to do what it is designed to do: predict chronicity of stuttering in young children who stutter. Yaruss and Conture (1993), examining select acoustic aspects of the fluent speech of children who stutter, used the SPI to distinguish between those children at low versus high risk for stuttering. While one of the acoustic measures (transition duration) did appear to differentiate between the two groups, we are still a long way from having reliable indexes of chronicity in early childhood stuttering.

Furthermore, we need to know whether the older child and teenager who continues to stutter presents different or more complex problems than does the young child who stutters who becomes fluent. Do older children who stutter exhibit more concomitant problems in speech and language, for example, delays in phonological development, than do younger children who stutter? Did these older children, for example, take longer to develop reading skills or fine motor control over speech musculature? Are there subtle differences in the home life of these older children that contributed to and perpetuated stuttering? Why are people who stutter, between the ages of 12 to 14 years, sometimes so challenging in terms of achieving successful remediation? These questions and others must await empirical investigation for answers. For the present, however, we must rely on insights and knowledge gained from clinical practice managing older children and teenagers who stutter, which, we hope, has some general applicability to these clients in other clinical settings and locales.

The Age of the Client Is a Guide Not an Imperative

Earlier we mentioned that the age of the client may be useful with the logistics and planning of therapy strategies but that it is our experience that chronological age tells us little about the nature of the child's stuttering problem (although Pellowski & Conture, 1999, suggest that increases in age are associated with increases in cessation-type speech disfluencies; see Au-Yeung et al., 1999, for related speculation). What we were and are trying to point out is how important it is to consider each child in terms of his or her present situation rather than be locked in or blindly follow some a priori rule that such and such an age child should be dealt with in such and such a fashion. Unfortunately, the problem with taking this approach—that age is more important for therapy planning than determining the nature of the problem—is that it does not readily lend itself to the confines of an organized book! Thus, for the sake of discussion, we have partitioned our clients who stutter into three age groups and assigned them each their own chapter: Chapter 3, children who stutter; Chapter 4, older children and teenagers who stutter; and Chapter 5, adults who stutter. This partitioning into separate chapters is not completely arbitrary since each age group does appear to have unique aspects and concerns; however, this does not mean that each and every client in a particular age group will present with similar problems or be treated in exactly the same way. Ranging around the central tendency for any of these groups is tremendous individual variation. What we are trying to emphasize here is that there are some common themes among older children and teenagers who stutter, but that each of these clients presents his or her own unique variation on these themes. Our job, as SLPs, is to learn to recognize common themes but to be simultaneously cognizant of and prepared to deal with their numerous variations. It is a bit like understanding that the mean has a range of scores around it and thus it is silly to expect, for example, everybody to have an IQ of 100 just because that is what the mean for the population might be. Again, a tolerance for ambiguity is necessary for being a successful clinician, if not human being.

Variations Among Older Children and Teenagers Who Stutter

Keeping in mind the above, we assume that older children and teenagers who stutter will vary a great deal among themselves. To make some sense of these variations, as well as to present a more organized chapter, we have divided these children in to three different groups: (1) older children with little or no awareness of stuttering; (2) older children with definite awareness of stuttering; and (3) teenagers with definite awareness of stuttering. This writer has observed some teenagers who stutter with minimal emotional and/or intellectual awareness of their stuttering but he believes that these are probably the exception rather than the rule. Further, we have observed a handful of individuals who began their stuttering in their teenage years (and even into adulthood), but this group is also probably the exception and not the rule. For the most part, in this chapter we will be discussing older children and teenagers who have been stuttering for some time (two or more years at the least), and the onset or origins of their problems are generally reported to occur during preschool or early elementary school years. While some of these youngsters will have received previous therapy, some will have had little or no contact with SLPs, some of them seemingly only realizing they have a problem when they are in the latter stages of elementary school. To begin, therefore, let us consider older children with apparently little or no awareness of stuttering.

Older Children with Minimal or Little Awareness of Stuttering

The book by Rustin, Cook, and Spence (1995); Kully and Langevin's (1999) chapter; the video, co-produced by Guitar and Conture (1996); and the Stuttering Foundation of America booklet (No. 21), edited by Fraser and Perkins (1987) are among the handful, to our knowledge, of modern-day materials specifically addressed to stuttering in teenagers (although Guitar [1998], Ham [1999], Schwartz [1999], and Shapiro [1999] devote some attention to teenagers who stutter as part of the overall coverage of stuttering in their treatment-oriented textbooks.) Another type of publication (Ginott, 1969) deals with the unique relations between parents and their teenage children. These stuttering-by-teens and psychosocial-emotional-life-of-teens publications deserve, in our opinion, consideration by any SLP required to or interested in managing stuttering in older children and teenagers. Just as children are not little adults, teenagers are not big children but individuals with unique needs and concerns that should be understood, at least to some degree, by individuals who must professionally interact with them.

Awareness of Stuttering: What It Is, What It Means, and How to Deal with It Therapeutically

One of the first issues that SLPs encounter with the older child or teenager that is generally different from that observed in younger children is the level and type of "awareness" of stuttering. Awareness is a topic frequently discussed in clinical circles but one whose external manifestations and internal motivations are minimally understood, at best. In our opinion, awareness of an event takes at least two different forms: general or specific. The former is predominantly, for the sake of this discussion, an emotional-feeling level of awareness while the latter is a cognitive-intellectual (perhaps rational) level of awareness. Dichotomizing awareness in this manner is somewhat artificial because most of our awareness of ourselves, our actions, and interactions with the world around us involve both emotional and intellectual processes. That is, our intellectual (relatively objective) and emotional (relatively subjective) selves are inextricably related to one another. However, for the purposes of this discussion, differences between the two can be discussed, since although the two are related, they do differ.

We have found, in the clinic, that it is useful to treat and discuss our clients' awareness of their behavior in terms of objective and subjective components. Many clients in the age group presently being discussed will tell you, sometimes in a very emotional manner, that they stutter because they are people who stutter (an interesting tautology) but when asked to show or describe what they do that they call stuttering, they will say, "I stutter" (this harkens back to the classic "Point of View About Stuttering," by Dean Williams [1957], whereby Williams suggests that much of the malaise of people who stutter relates to the manner in which they think and talk about themselves and their speaking, to themselves as well as their listeners). Teenagers who stutter (and adults, for that matter) use the word "stutter" or "stuttering" as if that is all the listener needs to know to understand what they *do* when they produce, as Young (1984) termed it, a "fluency departure." Along these same lines, Wingate (1976) has remarked (about people who stutter), that ". . . it is surprising how poorly most people who stutter are acquainted with their own difficulty." We hasten to add, and with some certainty on our part based on our clinical experience, that this acquaintance is not as poor on the emotional (or more subjective) level at it is on the intellectual or behavioral level.

When we say that a person who stutters is "unaware" or "lacks awareness" of his or her stuttering, we seem to be actually saying that the person is not concerned about or bothered by his or her speech. Such "unawareness" is, we believe, not really possible, at least at all levels—intellectual as well as emotional. In our opinion, even a young child, who is reasonably emotionally intact and has any degree of intellectual ability, must be aware, on some level, of the fact that he or she talks differently from his or her parents, siblings, relatives, schoolmates, or friends.

Awareness of a Difference Versus a Disorder.   Now, for the young child, this awareness may be nothing more than "Susie has freckles . . . Johnny can't ride a bike as well as I . . . Mario wears glasses . . . and sometimes its not easy for me to talk straight." Young children seem aware of a *difference* not a *disorder*. Conversely, a parent's "awareness" that his or her child has a "problem . . . he may have trouble in school, socially, finding friends and a job . . . ," can be a red herring for the SLP. The SLP, if she is not careful, can get swept up in the parent's emotionality about "disorder," when, at the most in young children, all that many of them sense is a "difference." But such sense of difference is quite common. For if in the beginning the child is not aware of the difference in his or her speaking behavior, we can be reasonably sure that some other, less sensitive youngster will unsubtly remind him or her of the child's differences and difficulties when talking. (For a fascinating, although horrifying, account of how individuals deal with and seem compelled to ostracize, ridicule, shun, and condemn that which is *different* from themselves, read Kosinski's [1966] novel *The Painted Bird*.)

Perhaps, then, what we are saying when we say that a child is *unaware* is that the child shows no *overt* indications of being concerned or worried, in any fashion, about his or her abilities to speak or speaking behavior. We submit, however, that not being concerned and not being aware are related but different issues. Intuitively and ideally, we would like to see the child's speaking difficulties diminish prior to the child's becoming concerned about them, but we really cannot assume that the child does not recognize differences in his or her speaking abilities and behaviors.

It's Type Not Mere Presence of Awareness That Matters.   Certainly, as speech-language clinicians, we try to do nothing to increase children's concern, worry, anxiety, or bother about themselves or their speaking abilities or behavior. Thus, for example, we would not hammer away at the occasional articulation errors of a young person who stutters, teaching him how hard or difficult these sounds are to produce, to be ever on guard for even the slightest mistake, and how much physical effort he or she must use to try and correctly produce them. Such an approach has, in effect, the real potential for making the child inappropriately aware as well as fearful of producing his or her "problem" or "error" sounds. In our opinion, it is not just awareness of a problem that is a problem but the *type* of awareness and whether the type of awareness experienced by the people who stutter increases or generates concern on the part of people who stutter (and his or her friends, relatives, and family), which inhibits fluent speech production. Awareness based in shame, guilt, and fear will do little to foster improvement and everything to exacerbate or maintain stuttering. Conversely, awareness based on acceptance, the notion that things are different not disordered and trying to physically feel what is being done so that it can be physically changed, can significantly aid the therapy process.

Matter-of-Fact, Objective Approach Helps Counteract Negative Aspects of Awareness

Some older children and teenagers who stutter can be quite concerned and aware, in an emotional, fairly negative way (e.g., highly ashamed and feeling fearful about stuttering), regarding their speaking abilities and behavior. If this is case, then it helps (indeed, it is probably necessary) that the SLP maintains an accepting, nonjudgmental, objective, matter-of-fact approach to the young client and his or her speaking problems. This does not mean, of course, that the SLP becomes overly philosophical or intellectual or totally ignores the child's obvious fear, anxiety, and worry about him- or herself. However, neither should the SLP excessively dwell or focus on these concerns, spending considerable therapy time with wringing of hands, crying woe is me, and the like. What the SLP should do is accept and recognize the reality of these concerns, and clearly acknowledge how these concerns may make the client feel when he or she experiences them—and, of course, ideally try to help the teen that stutters minimize the further development of such concerns. Essentially, the SLP wants to arrest or stop the future growth in the number and strength of these concerns. This is, of course, harder than it sounds, and not all clients will react similarly to the SLP's attempts to do so.

We have observed children with little apparent emotionality associated with their speech behavior refuse to listen to themselves on an audio tape recorder or watch themselves in a mirror as they speak. These children are obviously concerned, at some relatively unobservable level, about their speech, and these concerns or fears need to be dealt with if long-term improvement is to take place. We have also observed children with apparently high levels of emotionality associated with their speech appear to react reasonably objectively and positively to the clinician's description of their speaking problem. Thus, the "awareness" of someone who stutters need not be observable to an external observer to interfere with the therapy process. Paradoxically, the client can externally exhibit "awareness" of his or her speaking difficulties but as long as this "awareness" neither engenders nor stems from dread, embarrassment, fear, guilt, and shame, the client is probably going to have some degree of readiness and willingness to examine his or her own speech behavior. Whatever the case, the type and level of awareness is difficult to judge in advance of therapy, and it is this difficulty that makes the thoughtful SLP hesitant to rush headlong into making assumptions about the child until further experience and testing of the child has taken place.

"Everybody Makes Mistakes" as Another Means for Counteracting the Negative Aspects of Awareness

Older children and teenagers who present physically effortless repetitions are probably aware, on some level, of their speech disfluencies, of the fact that they may sometimes sound or look different than their peers when they talk. These children can often be helped through parental counseling, support, and encouragement to continue and enjoy talking. Their classroom teachers can also be enlisted to assist the child to learn that talking can be pleasurable and contain some naturally occurring errors but still be usable for all normal purposes. At the least, the classroom teacher can be encouraged to ask the child to talk on those days when the child seems particularly fluent and, conversely, call on the child far less on those days when he or she is particularly disfluent. These youngsters, we have found, can gain a great deal of perspective on their problem by considering their speech disfluencies as mistakes, mistakes that are not unlike those observed in other activities they are familiar with, for example, sports, walking, riding a bicycle, schoolwork, and so forth.

Williams' (1971) *hard* and *easy* speech concept may be used when discussing "mistakes," depending on the degree to which the client appears to be moving in the direction of producing more and more speech disfluencies. Particularly for the beginning or less experienced clinician, fostering awareness of "mistakes," as in subsequently discussed procedures where we will be actually increasing the child's awareness of speaking behaviors, should generally begin by focussing on those events "far away" from the client. In other words, the clinician should begin helping the child develop appropriate awareness by employing events that do not directly influence or are not produced by the child.

Worry About "Mistaking" Overshadows the True Purpose of Speaking: Communicating.
Starting with events and people a bit removed from the child, we might begin with a talk about how other people make mistakes when they are learning to print the alphabet, read aloud, write their name, or ride a bicycle or how we, the SLP, are having trouble learning how to ski or use a computer. Many young clients, as long as the stories aren't overly long or moralizing in nature, appreciate hearing stories about the trials and tribulations of their SLP trying to learn or develop X, Y, or Z ability and skill. And it's important in these stories to show the young client that the SLP can fall down, flat on his or her face, but get back up again, learning from the mistake, and try again. We suggest that the clinician begin by using audio- or videotapes of *other* people making mistakes when they talk or walk or do anything. We try to help the child begin to understand the concept that learning is not a smooth, error-free progression to mastery of a skill but a process that is filled with mistakes, errors, and picking oneself up and trying again. Above all, we try to get the child to focus on *communicating*, not *mistaking*, to understand that talking is about sharing our thoughts, feelings, and opinions with others, not about fluency. We try to help the child develop an understanding for the gradualness of learning, so that he or she can develop an awareness of his or her own behavior based on reality, not some unattainable ideal of totally or

completely fluent speech. The awareness we are trying to help the child develop is objective, as nonemotional as possible and specific to speech behavior and disruptions in same. The SLP tries to foster this awareness by his or her words and demeanor, by being as nonjudgmental, objective, and rational as possible in his or her examination of the child's and other peoples' speech and related behaviors.

The SLP's noncritical but analytical assessment of the child's speech disfluencies will go a long way toward helping the child appreciate and come to deal with these behaviors in objective ways. One caution: The SLP, like the parents of children who stutter, can convey concern, fear, anxiety, and worry through nonverbal as well as verbal means. In fact, as we discussed in the previous chapter, it is entirely possible that children, older ones and teenagers as well, may actually pay more attention to and learn more from your facial gestures and prosody of speaking than any of the specific words you say and use. Our clinical observations suggest to us that many listeners, when they listen to a child, teen, or adult who stutters, tend to hold their breath, move their eyeballs to the left or right, close or blink their eyelids, turn their head, or immobilize their facial expression. Older as well as younger children, we believe, can pick up on and react to these nonverbal gestures. We believe it highly instructive to the SLP to have a mirror behind the client so that the SLP can study his or her own nonverbal behaviors during the client's stutterings in order to learn how to identify and eventually change any untoward behaviors.

Use of "Awareness" as a Positive Influence on Changing Behavior

The above discussion of awareness calls attention to the ambiguities and uncertainties of dealing with awareness of stuttering, particularly with the older child or teenager. Objective awareness would appear to be a positive force for identifying and changing unwanted or inappropriate speech and related behavior. Subjective awareness, with its often attendant negative emotionality and feelings of fear, frustration, embarrassment, shame, and the like, is not viewed as a positive force and can contribute to a child's negative reaction to speech. The SLP should strive to understand the difference between the two types of awareness— objective and subjective—and how to change both if the need arises.

Desensitization

One procedure that we find of assistance with this type of child (and the younger child who clearly stutters) is a desensitization approach (e.g., Gregory & Hill, 1980; Hall, 1966; Van Riper, 1973). With this approach, the clinician attempts to assist the child/teenager develop more tolerance for events and stimuli that are associated with or seem to precipitate his or her stuttering. In essence, the SLP, when attempting to *desensitize* the young client, tries to raise the youngster's tolerance level for those *fluency disrupters* for which the child seems to have a low threshold for reaction. Children are systematically presented with stimuli that they have indicated have greater or lesser abilities to negatively influence or disrupt their speech fluency. Because the clinician never actually deals with changing or modifying speech and language behavior or concerns, desensitization is particularly useful when applied to children whose subjective awareness and concern regarding stuttering appears minimal. That is, the clinician can create and control the communication situation in such a way that the child's involvement is that of a spontaneous speaker rather than someone who is trying to be overly focused on modifying his or her own speech behavior.

Beginning to "Desensitize" the Young Client

To begin, the SLP tries to create a communication-emotional situation that is as free as possible from any criticisms, corrections, pressures, or frustrations (fluency disrupters) believed to precipitate the child is disfluency. The following is a partial listing of potential fluency disrupters: being an inattentive listener, talking at a rapid rate, interrupting the child, talking for the child, using very short or no turn-switching pauses, continually questioning the child, continually correcting the child's speech/language productions, always setting the conversational agenda and seldom letting the child talk about what he or she wants to talk about, and so forth. Modifying the communication situation, for example, using a slow-normal rate of utterance when talking with the child, requires the SLP to practice these modifications and be willing and able to discontinue them and use another approach if the child's behavior dictates. In essence, with this approach—and nearly everything we do with our clients—the SLP gauges the success of this situational modification or control by monitoring the child's speech. When the child's speech is essentially fluent, when the child has reached what has been termed a *basal fluency* level (Hall, 1966), the clinician assumes that he or she has been able to minimize important fluency disrupters. The child's speech at this point should be normally disfluent, not perfectly or abnormally fluent, and the child should appear to communicate with a reasonable degree of freedom and apparent comfort.

Although apparent to those familiar with stuttering, it is nonetheless true as Yaruss (1997a) notes in his study of situational variability in stuttering, that "variability is one of the hallmarks of stuttering" (p. 187). Thus, the SLP must observe, if at all possible, the child's stuttering across several situations (or at least receive reports from reliable sources about the child's speaking behavior). The clinician should carefully observe—audio and/or video recording help with retrospective study—the number and nature of salient aspects of the situations in which the child exhibits basal fluency (again, this raises the issue of situational influences on stuttering, something frequently mentioned, but seldom studied empirically, noting such exceptions as Yaruss, 1997a). This is because during therapy the child may have to be repeatedly brought back to basal fluency and the clinician needs to clearly understand what variables are most highly related to the child's basal fluency.

Once basal fluency can be reliably and predictably obtained and maintained for appropriate periods of time relative to the child's severity of problem and stage of therapy, the SLP can begin to introduce fluency disrupters or *barbs* or *probes*. It should be pointed out that for a child with a moderate to severe stuttering problem, basal fluency will look and sound considerably different than it might for a child with a mild stuttering problem. Basal fluency does not mean totally fluent speech, a feat that few if any of us can achieve! Furthermore, before we proceed any further, let us make it clear that this form of therapy, as with many other forms, relies heavily on the SLP's ability to accurately and quickly "read" or discern those stimuli and events that are facilitatory versus those that are inhibitory to the client's speech fluency. The clinician's observational skills are every bit as important as his or her manipulation of environmental events to the success of desensitization. Once again, the SLP should observe and manipulate the fluency disrupters that *actually* seem to influence the child rather than those the SLP *assumes* to be of influence or is familiar dealing with. Again, try, as much as possible, to follow the lead of the child's behavior rather than preconceived notions of how the child should or should not behave. In our experience, many therapies achieve little success in the clinic, not because they are fundamentally unsound forms of remediation but because the therapies are poorly applied or understood relative to the child's *actual* behaviors.

In all fairness, of course, some therapies are poorly conceived as well as stated and thus lead to less than ideal results when put into practice. With desensitization, the SLP must spend some time assessing and testing out which events are fluency inhibitors and which are fluency facilitators for which children, and when. This continual assessment and experimentation, at least in the initial stages of therapy, is no small task and is just another reason for considering remediation as ongoing diagnosis.

Introducing "Barbs" or Fluency Inhibitors

The barbs or fluency inhibitors introduced into the speaking situation are used to toughen or strengthen the child's resistance to fluency-disrupting influences. Barbs should be selected from those events the child is likely to encounter in the daily, outside-the-clinic environment and should be based, as much as possible, on clinician observation of the child speaking while in the presence of these events. As mentioned above, we have used the following events as barbs:

- Answering children's questions with questions
- Asking questions that involve rather large, abstract responses from children; changing the topic of conversation with children
- Looking away while children talk; interrupting children while they talk
- Asking children to repeat themselves
- Asking children to hurry up their responses
- Asking the child a question and then answering our own question without giving the child a chance to respond
- Talking very rapidly ourselves
- Providing minimal or no turn-switching pause between the end of the child's response and the beginning of our reply

This is, of course, only a partial listing and is presented solely for the purpose of providing the reader with some examples of fluency inhibitors or barbs. The list is not meant to be all-inclusive and in no way should it inhibit or preclude readers from adding or developing their own "barbs" as they so desire. At first glance, the reader may think that the listed fluency disrupters are "cruel and unusual punishment," but under the right circumstances, done in the right manner (mildly stressing the child's resistance to fluency disrupters without ever provoking the child's stuttering), they can be used to positively influence the child's fluency and strengthen the child's tolerance for or desensitize the child to such unfortunately all-too-often-occurring fluency disrupters. At no time should these barbs be used by the SLP or other interlocutors to correct, chastise, punish, or ridicule the child or to show SLP disapproval for client behavior judged to be inappropriate or undesirable by the SLP.

It is quite safe to assume that many children experience fluency disrupters in their everyday communication situations. Therefore, it seems both commonsensical and prudent to help these children learn how to effectively deal with these disrupters if they are demonstrating that dealing with these disrupters makes it difficult for them to speak fluently. Each disrupter, or barb, is presented into the speaking situation only *until* the child shows that he or she may is about to become disfluent. The SLP removes the disrupter(s) *before* the child begins to stutter, not *after*. An analogy would be the process used by the medical specialist (allergist) the current writer has visited and who treated him for allergies. The allergen dosage—for example, ragweed pollen contained in a serum or liquid form—used in the desensitization injections I received would be slowly increased but leveled off if I exhibited any signs that the desensitization shot was precipitating an allergic reaction (sneezing, wheezing, itching, or watery eyes). If need be, the allergist may even back down the level of our allergen dosage, say from 0.3 cc to 0.2 cc, if the higher level caused too many problems. Likewise, the SLP is not trying to elicit or precipitate stuttering but to slowly and systematically increase the child's ability to *react* fluently to communicative situations that that the child apparently finds increasingly stressful.

Inattentive Listeners: A Potent but Difficult to Discern Fluency Disrupter

One relatively subtle but potent fluency disrupter that some parents and other listeners unwittingly expose their child to is ignoring the child when he or she talks to them. I am convinced that some of the yelling and shouting of children that some parents of children who stutter report to me results from the frustration a child may experience talking to a zoned, tuned-out, or checked-out parent, a parent whose mind is elsewhere and stays there all too often. For example, this may be seen when the parent and another adult are conversing, and the parent's child *continually* tries to interrupt to ask the parent something or to get the parent's attention. The child may repeat ten to fifteen times (I've actually counted!), "Daddy" before the father will respond to the child; sometimes the father may never respond but continue to converse with the other adult, seemingly oblivious to the child's presence or attempts to communicate with his or her parent. Instead of momentarily stopping the adult conversation and explaining to the child that it is impolite or inappropriate to butt in or telling the child to wait his turn, the parent essentially ignores the child.

To my mind, the only thing worse than continually and destructively criticizing someone is not paying any attention at all to that person—ignoring the person. When children are *frequently* ignored by their parents, some youngsters seem to figure that any attention is better than none at all and do things that their parents simply can't ignore—for example, throw a match into the paper in the kitchen wastebasket, punch out or verbally abuse or tease the younger brother or sister, draw on the walls with crayons, and so forth. Children who must constantly repeat and lobby for their parent's attention experience far more than their fair share of fluency disrupters (besides desensitizing the child to these disrupters, we should also try to mitigate their excessive occurrence).

Being a parent is very rewarding, but like any other endeavor, these rewards are earned through a lot of hard work. Perhaps it is fair to say that a parent's work is never done and dealing with young, many times demanding children, especially after a long day of work (either inside or outside the home), can be exasperating. Particularly at these times, the parent needs to make some effort to let the child know that he or she was heard, but that mommy or daddy is busy and tired right now and after such and such is done, the child will be listened to, talked, interacted, or played with. Another example of this type of situation is the mother who is busily preparing dinner when her child comes up behind her and starts excitedly explaining how he just scored the winning goal in a neighborhood soccer game. The mother, as she slices the carrots and scurries around the kitchen looking for the cookbook containing the recipe for tonight's main course, says such things as, "Hmmm" or "Oh yeah" or "That's nice" while the child rattles on about this most recent example of his athletic prowess (perhaps, she thinks, her youngster's soliloquy is only too similar to her husband's reminiscences about the halcyon days when he was a star high school basketball player!). Sometimes the mother may not even say anything to the child but silently nods her head and silently prepares dinner. Meanwhile, the child may begin to feel that he or she is losing his or her listening audience (if there ever really was one) and gets frustrated, nervous, and upset over the parent's apparent lack of interest or willingness to communicate. This frustration may cause the child to talk more rapidly because he or she is losing his or her audience and perhaps begins to repeat sounds, syllables, or whole words. Interestingly, *now*, with the emergence of disfluencies, the mother turns and reacts either overtly or covertly to this new form of the child's verbal expression. Perhaps the message the child is getting is: When you begin to lose your audience, when your audience pays you little or no attention, when your audience seems unwilling to communicate, start speaking rapidly, repeat and prolong—it gets their attention every time! The mother's disregard for the content of the child's communication but attention to its manner acts as a differential reinforcement that may actually lead to more of the very speech behavior on the part of the child that she actually doesn't like (see Ryan, 1974; Shames & Sherrick, 1963).

Helping parents recognize (and reduce) and the child resist such fluency disrupters is one of the tasks of the speech-language pathologist. While this desensitization procedure has been used with younger children who stutter (Hall, 1966), its use with older children is quite appropriate. This approach is very similar to Schwartz's (1999) description of systematically increasing communicative demands to "toughen up fluency" skills beyond the therapy room (pp. 94–96). One cannot claim that the child will successfully deal with all fluency disrupters and frustrations as a result of this form of therapy or that parents will cease and desist each and every instance of fluency disrupters. However, this approach is a good beginning , a good way to, as Van Riper (1973) suggests, "toughen up" the child.

Evaluating Successfulness of Desensitization Approach

In truth, there are no firm guidelines that the SLP can follow to evaluate the success of desensitization approaches with children who stutter. Success with this procedure will be relative to the nature of the individual child and the type and severity of stuttering that the individual child presents. As mentioned previously, "fluency" during the introduction of fluency disrupters or barbs for one child may contain as much as 5 percent disfluency whereas for another child it may contain 1 percent or less. The clinician is using this procedure in an attempt to help the child successfully deal with as well as resist the types of fluency disrupters that he or she will encounter during everyday speaking situations.

Desensitization may or may not be employed when the SLP is *directly* helping the child learn to identify and modify specific instances of disfluency (its use being determined by the clinician's judgment regarding its compatibility with these procedures). The emphasis with this desensitization or increasing communicative demands or "toughening up fluency" procedure is on the situations that evoke disfluency and the child's ability to respond or react to these situations in a reasonably fluent manner. With desensitization, it is the child's *tolerance level for fluency disrupters* and *not the disfluencies themselves* that the SLP is directly trying to influence. In this case, the disfluencies are used by the clinician to determine the relative success with which the child is coping with communicative pressures and demands. It is also helpful, when employing desensitization, to meet with the child's parents and discuss some of the fluency disrupters they may knowingly or unknowingly be exposing their child to (e.g., "When your child is stuttering a great deal, what is typically going on in the home? What are you typically talking about or doing?" and so forth). Along these lines, Zwitman (1978) explicitly describes some parental reactions to the child's speech that *do* (e.g., pay attention to *what* the child says) and *do not* (e.g., appear angry or impatient) facilitate fluency. The key to uncovering fluency disrupters that seem highly related to the child's stuttering is the frequency and consistency of their occurrence. Why? At the risk of redundancy, it should be pointed out that all parents—indeed all listeners—exhibit fluency disrupters when they are talking with other people and so the occasional occurrence of these disrupters should not be surprising.

Encouraging the Child to (Non)verbally Interact with Peers

We like to spend some time discussing with and encouraging parents to see what hobbies, sports, or extracurricular activities their child might like to become involved in or would benefit from participating in. It is not uncommon for these older children to come home every day after school go in their rooms by themselves, play with their computers, or turn on the television after dinner. Again, occasional isolation is no problem, even a desirable means of unwinding, but when isolation, detachment, and noninteraction is routine, the child needs to be encouraged to break out of such habits of nonengagement with peers and adults. Certainly these children, like all children, need some time to themselves, but *routine* isolation from peer interaction makes it difficult to develop interpersonal skills (and, after all, it is their peers not their parents that these children will be spending their school years and later life with). Indeed, while we concern ourselves with parent-influence-on-child, we seldom consider child-influence-on-child—and the latter is quite germane to normal social maturation. Further, watching television three or more hours *every* afternoon provides the child with little opportunity to communicate verbally with others (Winn [1977] likens the experience of watching television to that of staring into a fireplace relative to the amount of intellectual stimulation that takes place!).

Children who stutter, like all children, should be encouraged to develop friendships with other children their age. Perhaps this will mean, initially, inviting other children over to their house to play (it is certainly okay to have some friends markedly younger or older than themselves; but when this is the rule, then gentle, parental encouragement to form friendships with their age peers should take place). Alternatively, an organized team sport like baseball, soccer, basketball, or football or more individualized activities or sports like chess, karate, tennis, archery, fencing, wrestling, bowling, swimming, gymnastics, golf, or track might be good ways for the child to develop friends and learn appropriate verbal and social interactions. Perhaps lessons at a local school or community center in how to play the guitar, take photographs, raise tropical fish, learn how to juggle, obedience train the family dog, learn more about computers than blowing up aliens, magic tricks, crochet, painting with oil colors, first aid, or using woodworking tools may help the child get out of the house and interact with new and different people. Needless to say, if mom or dad gets involved in these extra activities, the greater the likelihood that parent and child will socially and communicatively share with one another common experiences or skills to be learned or, once learned, mutually enjoyed. If these children learn some skill, sport, or special information (e.g., knowing detailed information about Civil War battlesites or United States stamps since World War II) in which they can take pride and gain the respect of others, so much the better. These skills, sports, hobbies, or expertise can only serve to build the children's positive regard for themselves. Further, there is no better place for a parent to see how typical his or her child is then by regularly watching the child perform, play, or interact with other children of the same age.

The Gradual Process of Learning or Learning About Learning

One caution: Some parents, like their children, do not understand the gradual process of learning, in general, and the gradual process of learning to change behavior, in specific. That is, these parents give the impression that all one must have to master a particular skill, event, activity or sport is will power and positive thinking ("all is mind"). They seem quite reluctant to accept the fact that complex skills—for example, catching baseballs, reading, riding a bicycle, using a hammer and nails—take months and years to develop and that the first time you sit down at the piano you do not play like Chopin! This attitude, on the part of some parents, is most unfortunate because their children, by their immaturity, are already impatient with learning! Thus, instead of helping the child learn patience, reflectiveness, nonimpulsivity, and how to concentrate on small signs of positive improvement, some parents become impatient, discouraged, "shop around" for "quicker cures," or push their child to use skills he or she is simply not ready for or has had insufficient opportunity to develop. Once again, time urgency, this time on the part of the parents, or the inappropriate attempt to "speed things up," interferes with the therapy process.

In these cases, the SLP must be patient and continually encourage the parents to accentuate the positive in their child; the SLP should try to support the parents' positive intervention in their child's development and help them change or mitigate their more negative forms of intervention. Our experience suggests that *parental* impatience with or intolerance for their child's overall development is one of the main reasons that they express impatience with their child's progress in speech therapy. Recognizing the existence of such impatience leads the SLP to be as clear as possible regarding the short- and long-term goals of therapy and how long, in weeks, or years, the SLP plans active speech therapy. If a period of "maintenance" therapy or a "transfer" period is to follow active speech therapy, the parents should be so instructed with the timeline explicated as clear as possible. Parents need and want such timelines and, while it may not decrease their impatience for the relatively slow process of human change, it certainly makes things less ambiguous for them.

Older Children with Definite (Cognitive/Emotional) Awareness of Stuttering

It is difficult to provide a precise age range for these individuals. They could be as young as 7 or 8 but are probably at least 9 or 10, with a ceiling somewhere around 12 years of age. Once the child gets much beyond 12, adolescent concerns begin to enter the picture and considerably change the course of remediation and prognosis for improvement. Older children with cognitive and/or emotional awareness of stuttering are probably producing both sound prolongations and sound/syllable repetitions, and glottal fry and breathy voice quality may be associated with both disfluency types. They are increasingly more likely during their stutterings to move their eyeballs laterally and/or blink their eyelids. Indications of physical tension may be associated with these youngsters' stutterings, particularly on the cessation-type of speech disfluency. As a result of lateral eyeball movement and/or eyelid blinking, eye contact with listeners, as mentioned in Ainsworth and Fraser (1988), may be poor, particularly during instances of the child's speech disfluencies. The child may give verbal as well as nonverbal indications that he or she is psychologically and physically tense prior to or during speaking. Many people, even casual observers, in the child's environment will recognize that this child is stuttering, and the parents and the school system will often express a good deal of concern. The child may increasingly try to avoid or escape situations requiring speech, for example, Sunday school recitations, oral book reports in class, using the telephone, and so forth.

Within the context of his description of the four phases in the development of stuttering, Bloodstein's (1960a, 1960b, 1961), would probably characterize these children as phase three people who stutter (i.e., chronic; certain situations, words, and sounds more apt to be associated with stuttering; word substitutions and/or circumlocutions; and little or no clear evidence of fear, embarrassment, or avoidance of speaking, and like situations). While, as Bloodstein (1995) notes, these phases represent an attempt to describe the typical (or "average") people who stutter of a particular age-development level, they may inadequately describe any one individual people who stutter (just like the mean IQ hardly describes the IQ of one typical individual).

It is important to note that any attempt to use categorical "phases" to describe what appears to be a continuous process (i.e., the development of stuttering) is problematic. This is due to the fact that the variables being categorized are dynamic and ever-changing and are resistant to being "pigeonholed" into static or relatively fixed slots or groupings (see Smith, 1999, for further discussion of stuttering as a "dynamic" disorder). While the use of such categorical schemas (e.g., mild, moderate, and severe stuttering) certainly provides one reasonable means to organize and more clearly discuss the multidimensional nature of stuttering, such categorical labels and terminology should be taken as conventions for the improvement of thinking and communication about stuttering rather than inviolate laws of nature.

The emotional concern exhibited by these children is clearly unclear. It may be, as Bloodstein suggests, *irritation*, but it can be concern, which is more aptly described as *emotional discomfort*. On the whole, with these children (and of course there are exceptions here), we don't think that their emotional concern has yet developed to the point where terms like *anxiety* or *fear* could be applied, at least not in the sense that these relative strong concerns are chronic. Once again, we are talking about the rule rather than the exception, the group rather than a specific individual. And, as mentioned above, it is always difficult to place categorical labels onto behavior and events that our continuous as well as multidimensional in nature. We can say, however, that it is apparent that these youngsters "know" and are "concerned," at some level, that they stutter, although the nature and degree of their knowledge and concern is probably dissimilar from that of older teenagers and adults who stutter.

Motivation

One of the first, most important but probably most challenging things to ascertain when remediating any client, and these clients in particular, is the nature and depth of motivation for seeking therapeutic services. The essence of this investigation can be summarized in the following modified analogy: Is the horse being led or is he coming of his own free will and desire to water? Obviously, not too many 10-year-olds will actively seek help (e.g., pick up a telephone and call a professional agency), but many of them will at least tell their parents (or some other adult they trust) that they are concerned about their speech ("Mommy, I can't talk," "I can't talk right," or "Why can't I talk right, Daddy?") or that they wish their parents would take them to someone who can help them with their speech. Another group of children will say nothing as direct but indicate indirectly that they are concerned, irritated, or frustrated regarding their speech. Still yet another group will express very little, either explicitly or implicitly, that indicates concern. Parents may be the motivating force behind this latter group coming in for therapy services; sometimes it is a concerned physician, social worker, or teacher who makes the referral.

Unfortunately, no matter how severe, frequent, or noticeable the stuttering, children with a passive or blase attitude towards their own speech will be children whom the SLP will find difficult to help. The child has to care somewhat about changing his or her speech. No matter how badly the parents or teacher desire fluency for the child, if he or she is minimally desirous of expending the necessary effort to change behavior, then prognosis for change is poor (Van Riper, 1973). Starbuck (1974) and Prins (1974) discuss these problems and make a number of suggestions for dealing with them. I might add that one asset (acceptance of the child and his or her behavior by other children) can be a liability. While we absolutely don't want the child's peers to belittle, demean, mock, ridicule, or in any way tease the child because of the way the child speaks, it is nonetheless true that if all the child's friends are completely tolerant and accepting, this is minimal encouragement, it would seem, for the child to change in the presence of his or her peers. Again, we often think of the influence of adults on children, but there is ample evidence that children influence children and their acceptance of the child and the child's problems may lead the child to feel, in essence, "why fix what ain't broken."

Identification

Although situations impact these children's stuttering, other than the aforementioned sensitization procedures, we do not generally attempt to modify the association between situation and stuttering. For more complete description of situations associated with stuttering, developing situational hierarchies, and systematic desensitization, one may read Brutten and Shoemaker (1967). Brutten and Shoemaker present rationale and therapy for dealing with situational fears and concerns that may be negatively impacting a person's speech fluency. Instead, when possible, we have the child's parents provide us with a general situational hierarchy—from those situations where the client exhibits the most to the least number of speech disfluencies—in order to gain some perspective on those events and stimuli associated with the child's stuttering.

Working on Problem Sounds.   Again, we want to mention, at this point, the notion of "problem sounds." The concept of "difficult . . . problem sounds" is seemingly borrowed or at least consistent with treatment of articulation/phonological disorders. The notion, simply put, is that the person who stutters has more or only "problems" being fluent on certain sounds, sound combinations.

We submit, however, that concentrating on a child's "problem" sounds, syllables, or words is therapy time misspent. In our experience, this procedure all too often leads the child to develop more, rather than fewer, concerns, fears, and avoidances regarding specific sounds, syllabless or words. It is almost like telling someone driving a car to be extra special careful and on guard anytime he or she crosses a bridge. If the instructor gives these instructions persistently enough and the driver listens and takes them to heart, it would not be surprising to see this same driver quite physically and mentally tense when driving over bridges. We might also see the driver go out of his or her way to avoid bridges or get someone else to do all the "bridge driving." Instead, we like to have children and teenagers (and adults for that matter) deal with their speech behavior and disruptions in same by using a more general, problem-solving approach where the emphasis is on changes in their *overall* communicative strategies to initiate and continue speech rather than to watch for and modify their behavior when *specific* speech "hurdles" must be jumped. Our emphasis during treatment is on the client and the way the client acts when speaking (an active approach) rather than on the way various sounds, syllables, and words act upon them (a passive approach). The "problem" is not in the sound, syllable, or word but in the means and ways the person attempts to initiate and move through these sounds, syllables, and words.

The Use of Analogies.   To begin, we use the previously mentioned garden hose analogy and others like it to help these older children learn something about their speech mechanism and the various ways they can *use* it. This approach helps them come to grips with what they do that is *facilitating* versus *inhibiting* their speech fluency; however, it does this in a rather down-to-earth, understandable fashion (one that these youngsters can relate to). Once again, rather than concentrate on certain sounds or words, we concentrate on *strategies* the child appears to use to interfere with the smooth, fluid flow of ongoing speech (e.g., "stopping the air from flowing at the nozzle" or "making sounds hard with the faucet").

We believe it extremely important to get these older children to *physically feel* what they do when they produce speech, both the disfluent and fluent aspects. Hearing and seeing what takes place during stuttering is nice and supports the changes in client speech behavior that must take place; however, audition and vision are generally *after*, rather than *before* or even *during*, the act of stuttering. Many times, by the time the client hears and sees the stuttering it has already begun. While we want the client to change once he or she has begun, we also want the client to change prior to or at the very beginning of speech production. To do this, the client must *physically feel* what they are *doing*. This age client can come to *physically feel* and recognize what he or she does that interferes with speech and contrast this with what he or she does that facilitates speech, that is, what he or she does to produce fluency. Identifying and recognizing inappropriate strategies used to produce speech are crucial, in our opinion, for the child to learn how to modify speech. Once such modification is learned, the client can recognize those situations where he or she is reverting back to inappropriate behavior or strategies so that change can be made. Long-term recovery, we think, requires these clients to understand that if they can physically feel and closely imitate these inappropriate strategies and that these strategies can be changed in ways that they can physically feel, this will facilitate their fluent speech production.

Imitation Is Not the Same as Mocking.   One problem with identifying and recognizing speech disfluencies is the amount and ability of clinician's imitation of the child's disfluencies. Demonstration or imitation, in and of itself, is not inherently bad, but some clinicians may do it, albeit unconsciously, in such a fashion that the child may feel mocked or "put down." I want to emphasize that this is *not* a common problem, and many times it is the child's hypersensitivity toward imitation, rather than the clinician's imitation, that engenders a problem. However, the sensitive as well as sensible clinician should be aware of such events and head them off before they happen (in some cases, the child will have to be specifically desensitized to observing his or her own stuttering before any imitated stutterings are presented to the child). The clinician should realize that even for children, there may be relatively strong fears associated with stuttering (see Guitar, 1997, for excellent, thoughtful suggestions for how to deal with these concerns, therapeutically) and that showing the child, no matter how innocuous, what his or her stuttering sounds or looks like may be a fairly unpleasant experience, at least at first, for some of these children.

Unnecessary Emphasis on Nonspeech Behavior During Imitated Disfluencies.   Another problem with imitating the youngster's disfluencies, and one that seems more common in our experience, is the clinician's inappropriate, unnecessary emphasis of nonspeech behavior during imitated disfluencies. Here, for example, a clinician may be showing a child a sound prolongation on the /b/ in the word *boy* by pursuing her lips and then quickly and tensely jerking her head forward as she releases the /b/ and moves through the word. Make no mistake: At least in the beginning, the child will notice and copy the gross, the visual nonspeech behavior rather than the subtle, auditory/physical behavior of speaking. In essence, this clinician is teaching more than just the nature and feel of the speech disfluency and its locus within the speech production mechanism. She is also teaching the child inappropriate nonspeech behavior. These more molar or "grosser" nonspeech behaviors are readily perceived and picked up by the child and can easily come to be part of the child's disfluency. Clinicians should try to avoid producing such unnecessary head and body movements and only imitate what is necessary to produce the actual speech disfluency. If the clinician feels the need for emphasis, large magnifying glasses, small high-intensity lamps and the like can help the child focus in on the area of the lips, tongue, mouth, and so on and speech behavior of import.

The Older Child's Desire for a "Passive" Cure.   Of course, these children, not unlike many of us, wish and hope that a pill or some passive device was available that would take away their stuttering. This wish is only natural since humans, like electricity; tend to take the path of least resistance (this doesn't mean that we are inherently lazy, it means that we are just human). As difficult as this can be, especially with a child with strong fears, the SLP needs to help children use their minds and sensing powers to intercede between the communication environment and their speech reaction in the presence of that environment.

Such intercession obviously takes some work ("we never said this would be easy") and patience on the part of the child and the SLP. Change, long-term change, can only come about if the young client takes some degree of an active role in the process of changing his or her behavior. Some clients and their associates seem to hope against hope for divine intervention, a miracle drug or device, passive, osmotic assimilation of the SLP's admonishments to change! These very-human hopes of finding the "silver bullet" to eradicate the problem is about as productive as staying up all night in an attempt to catch the tooth fairy. What a shock when we realize that the magical appearance of money under our pillow comes from good old mom and dad. Likewise, it is an equal shock to learn that any seemingly magical change in our speech must come from our own acts, thoughts, and efforts. To hope for and believe in tooth fairies and miracle cures may be human, but it also reflects an earlier stage of development as well as an inability or unwillingness to face reality as we now know it.

Getting off the Identification Dime.   We, as SLPs, sometimes make the process of change unnecessarily difficult for our clients when we get so involved with identifying and recognizing the child's behavior that we fail to make the adjustments necessary to move into the next phase: modification. That is, the SLP carries on the identification phase of therapy long after it has achieved its desired goals. Once a client has reached 75 percent or better identification of stutterings during conversational speech, modification should definitely be co-occurring with identification. Once identification during conversational speech has reached 90 percent or better, the treatment sessions should mainly be modification. At the risk of putting too fine a point on things, identification is a means not an end. It sets the stage for modification—it, by itself, is not the ultimate goal of treatment.

Indeed, moving toward modification is something the SLP must be doing, in at least small steps, from the initial evaluation onward. Nothing is as motivating as change, even it is slight and temporary; it signals to the client that things can get better. Indeed, the clinician must constantly assess the client's ability and willingness to change as well as demonstrate to the client that change is possible, that there is hope for the future.

Modification

Modifying a child's speech assumes that the SLP knows what changes in speech signify movement in the right direction, in the direction of " . . . doing more and more things like normally fluent speakers do" (Williams, 1978). That is, the SLP must be able to recognize and reward small positive changes in the child's speech if they are to appropriately reinforce and shape (cf. Shames & Egolf, 1976) that child's speech. It is not too difficult to recognize that a decrease in the frequency of a particular within-word disfluency is indicative of positive change. Likewise, it is fairly easy to see that diminution of inappropriate facial gestures or bodily movements during stuttering indicates positive change. However, in the beginning of therapy, when changes are less noticeable, more subtle in nature, what can we use to indicate to our clients (and ourselves) that they are changing? That is, before the client produces noticeable changes, what can we use to indicate improvement?

We Can Count Behavior, but Do We Know What Behavior to Count?   In the beginning of therapy, before dramatic change takes place, what changes indicate that positive change is occurring? Here, unfortunately, we come up against a blank wall. In the past twenty to twenty-five years, our rush to be clinically quantitative, to count and assess behavior within this or that behavioral theory framework, has, to some degree, led us to lose sight of the *content* of our client's behavior. While we can easily design charts to depict behavior change over time, we cannot as easily explain to ourselves and others *what* behavior *needs* to be charted! Fortunately, information has accumulated (e.g., Caruso et al., 1988; Conture & Kelly, 1991a; Conture, McCall, & Brewer, 1977; Conture, Schwartz, & Brewer, 1985; Denny & Smith, 1992; Freeman & Ushijima, 1978; Guitar, 1975; Hutchinson, 1974; Kelly & Conture, 1988; Shapiro, 1980; Yaruss & Conture, 1993; Zimmerman, 1980b) that objectively describes those speech production behaviors associated with those speech behaviors we perceptually evaluate as stuttering. These studies make it abundantly clear that the number and nature of these speech production behaviors vary as much as the labels—for example, broken words, sound prolongations, and so forth—we use to describe our percept of them. And, as Howell, Hamilton, and Kryiacoupoulos (1984) and Howell, Sackin, and Glenn (1997a, 1997b) have shown with their attempts to identify stutterings automatically through the use of computer algorithms, no single algorithm can probably capture or identify all instances of stuttering. Therefore, as much as we find the counting of behavior attractive and understandable, it may not adequately circumscribe all aspects of stuttering. Indeed, it may overlook very salient behaviors.

Typical Improvements Observed in the Beginning of Therapy: Changes in Duration and Number of Sound Prolongations and Physical Tension.   Our clinical observations indicate that during the beginning of therapy, three of the first things that signify positive change in stuttering are: (1) decreases in the duration of stuttering; (2) a change in the ratio of sound prolongations ("cessation" type of disfluencies) to sound/syllable repetitions ("reiteration" type of disfluencies)—fewer sound prolongations and more sound/syllable repetitions; and (3) subjective listener impressions that instances of stuttering are being produced with less physical tension (they sound more physically "easy" or "relaxed"). These changes may occur even while the child continues to stutter at about the same frequency during treatment. In essence, we need to look beyond the frequency count of behavior and examine more closely the time course and relative predominance of certain other behaviors, some of which may be less quantifiable than frequency of stuttering (see interchange between Cooper & DeNil, 1999).

For example, it has been our observation that duration of instances of stuttering will start to change as children become more and more objectively aware of where, when, and how, within the speech utterance, they are or are beginning to stutter. As they learn more and more about the *where* as well as *when* of their own behavior, they seem to begin to learn more and more about the *what* that they *do* that interferes with speech. This level of objective awareness appears to help many children and adults shorten or truncate the duration of their speech disfluencies. It is my hunch that when compared to shorter disfluencies (under one second), longer disfluencies (over one second) are associated with higher levels of muscle activity or physical tension (particular if they are the cessation kind of speech disfluency earlier mentioned, e.g., blocks or sound prolongations). It is my experience, therefore, that objective awareness of these longer, more apparent disfluencies assists children, in the early stages of therapy, to begin decreasing the amount or level of physical tension associated with their speech disfluencies. In essence, to help the child begin to identify and subsequently to change instances of stuttering, it is a reasonable policy to begin identifying and then change the longer, more physically tense and apparent instances of stuttering.

Helping Children Change Physical Tension Levels. Helping children *directly* decrease the duration of their disfluencies is hard but not impossible. First, the child needs to understand something about the difference between physically tense versus relaxed muscles *and* the gradations of physical tension in between these two states of muscle tonus. This is, of course, a difficult concept for even older children to grasp because the vocabulary used to describe gradations in the temporal, physical tension aspects of speaking is generally beyond the comprehension of most youngsters. Besides, even adults, in our experience, have trouble sensing physical tension in their muscles (perhaps, biofeedback may be of some assistance in this regard; for a critical review of the use of biofeedback with school-age children, see Guitar, Adams, & Conture [1979]; for examples of the use of biofeedback to assist people who stutter in achieving more appropriate levels of muscle tension, breathing, airflow, etc. patterns during speech, see Guitar [1975]; Dembrowski & Watson [1991]). Readers of these pages may get some perspective on the difficulty of recognizing amount and sites of bodily tension by trying to figure out, without palpitating or touching with fingers/hands, whether the muscles of their forearms and shoulders/neck region are physically tense and, if they both are, which one is the most tense!

We try to help children understand, at a level they can relate to, the concept of physical tension by using the Scarecrow and Tinwoodsman in the *Wizard of Oz* (see Figure 4.3) as analogies with the cartoon or stick figure of Gumby as midway point between the excessive floppiness of the Scarecrow and the excessive tension or stiffness of the Tinwoodsman. Most children have seen or read the *Wizard of Oz* (and seen or heard about Gumby) and can readily identify and imitate the floppy, relaxed scarecrow and the creaky, stiff Tinwoodsman. It is, however, very instructive to see them imitate how Gumby might talk, walk, or run, since this gives the clinician some idea how they view the more in-between, necessary for speech production, state of physical tension. We explain through word and deed that speech takes some degree of muscle tension, but not as much as the Tinwoodsman or as little as the Scarecrow but more like Gumby. We have children throw balls, walk, skip, run, sing, write, or clap their hands with Tinwoodsman, Scarecrow, or Gumby-like muscles or movements. In these ways the idea of (in)appropriate degrees of muscle tonus is imparted, to a greater or lesser extent, to the children.

Changing Tension During Speech Production "When They Need to."   Assuming that the child understands muscle tension in terms that are clear, that the child can relate to us and show us by example, we show the child how to apply these ideas to his or her own speech. In essence, we want the child to understand that *he* or *she* can decrease as well as increase muscle tension throughout the vocal tract, that it is well within the child's power to make changes in muscle tension during speech production, *when he or she needs to.*

The latter phrase, "when he or she needs to," is key. Giving our young and/or older clients the notion that they must *continually, constantly,* and *pervasively be vigilant and scrutinize their speech* is really no way to run a railroad! Speech, communication, is supposed to be an enjoyable, relatively effortful experience, not an experience where we continually fear that the wrath of the Fluency Police will come crashing down on our heads if we relax for a minute and mess up! We want to instruct people who stutters to develop strategies that can be used when they need to use them. We should not, either consciously or unconsciously, consign people who stutter to a life of hypervigilance regarding their speech behavior. We do not want to encourage them to continually look for stuttering breakdowns as they drive their conversational vehicles from one speaking situation to the next. Rather, we want to teach them effective strategies that they can use as need be. Above all, we want to teach them flexibility, not fanaticism, in the application of what they learn with us. Helping them adjust and maneuver their speaking behavior according the circumstances they find themselves in is, in my opinion, one of the highest goals we should aspire to in our attempts to help people who stutter and their families.

We also find it helpful to employ the garden hose analogy (Figure 3.9) to assist the child to more readily identify and sense the various locations within the vocal tract where physical tension can be felt and changed. With mirrorwork and face-to-face observation, the clinician makes speech production physically tense ("hard") at the level of the faucet (larynx) or nozzle (lips) and then has the child do the same. Using magnifying glasses and small high-intensity lamps helps emphasize the areas that the clinician wants the child to attend to. We repeatedly demonstrate to children through both word and deed that they have the ability to tense and relax various aspects of their speech mechanism and that these states of muscle tension are within their control, that they can govern the tension level of their muscles. The child is then given practice in tensing on sounds and relaxing on the same sounds. In the beginning, the use of bilabial sounds like /b,p,m/ helps the child more readily visualize what is going on. Again, however, it is not the specific sounds that are of import. What is of important is the child's recognition and sensing the difference between muscles that are physically tense versus relaxed versus the states in between. Here we are not talking about an understanding of the level of a speech physiologist or scientist but an objective awareness that is sufficient to serve the child as a basis for subsequent modification.

Changes in Time and Tension: The Essence of Modification of Stuttering. At this point, other therapy procedures may be employed—for example, Van Riper's (1973) well-known cancellation, pull-out, and preparatory set sequence, Webster's (1978) precision fluency shaping, or Williams' (1971) "hard"/"easy" speaking approach. Although the names of various therapies change and philosophies differ in whole or in part, one common element seems to stand out: The modification of stuttering involves, to greater or lesser degrees, changes in the *time and tension* domains of speech-language production. Whether, as with precision fluency shaping, it involves a systematic change in the initiation of vocal sound pressure level ("vocal loudness" or "volume") over time (neither too gradual nor too sudden a change) or, as with the pull-out procedure, a gradual stretching or elongation in time of the sound following the word-initial stuttering or, as with the hard/easy procedure, starting or "going into" the sound in an "easy" (less physically tense) manner, all modification procedures for stuttering appear to involve, in one way or another, manipulation of the *time* and *tension* factors of speech production. In essence, the person who stutters is encouraged to begin and continue speaking in a less rushed, more physically relaxed fashion—a goal that is easier said than done but is the essence of *all* stuttering therapies. Again, the means to achieve this end—more appropriate use of time and tension during speech production—may differ, with some means being more effective than others, but at the base, all such treatments attempt to change time and tension elements of speech, when trying to help the person who stutters become more fluent.

It is appropriate that therapies focus on changes in the time/tension domain of speech production, since an instance of stuttering takes more time per sound or syllable than it ordinarily should and probably is produced with inappropriate levels of muscle tension with the speech and related musculature. Therefore, even if not described, the unspoken goal of therapy is to help people who stutter normalize the time course and physical tension level of those sounds/syllables/words they stutter on or at least bring the temporal/tension aspects closer to typical values for producing these speech events. Interestingly, some stuttering therapies appear to change the stutterings of people who stutter by *lengthening* the duration of their sounds and syllables (see Metz, Onufrak, & Ogburn, 1979; Metz, Samar, & Sacco, 1983). It is my hunch that there is an unspoken reason why some therapies require people who stutter to *volitionally* increase the duration or length of sounds and syllables in order to bring about a change in stuttering. In essence, I believe that these approaches change stuttering, when and if they do, by bringing about a *decrease* in physical tension levels when compared to instances of stuttering. Elongating the time domain of a sound provides the person a great chance to physically feel and *gradually* change and decrease the level of physical tension.

Time and tension are different but related aspects of speech production, and it is by no means clear which of these two aspects of speech production should be "worked on" first in therapy. It is our guess, however, that therapies that concentrate first on tension and then time result in speech that contains more disfluencies but sound more natural, whereas therapies that concentrate first on time and then tension result in speech that contains fewer disfluencies but sounds less natural. These are, of course, empirical issues that must await careful, objective therapy evaluation research studies.

Personally, with children who stutter, we are partial to Williams' (1971) hard/easy approach to try to help them learn to quickly recognize what they are doing—in terms of temporal as well as tension disruptions—to interfere with their speech fluency and then learn how to modify such interfering behavior. At this point in therapy we continually instruct the child to: "move on to the next sound," "move on," "change" (reduce the physical tension level associated with speech production and move on to the next sound), "make the sound easy" or "easy." Such instructions must obviously be repeated, and praise should be offered for *small* as well as *large* changes in the child's demonstrated ability to successfully follow such instructions and make appropriate change. Indeed, praise, positive reinforcement, and support for the small change, the successive approximations to more normally disfluent speech, are crucial paving stones to lay down on the child's road to increasing more fluent speech.

Once again, we hasten to add that these instructions SHOULD NOT become an old-wine-in-new-bottles situation: changing the name ("stuttering" changed to "hard") but keeping the game the same (instead of criticizing for "stuttering" the listener now merely criticizes for "hard" speech or even tells the child to "stop that hard speech!"). If the child appears discouraged or confused, or is having a great deal of trouble, the therapy task should be changed, and this direct work discontinued until later in the session or the next session. My experience suggests that with some clients, long-term change requires long-term therapy! We may have to prolong this challenging stage of therapy for some time until the child demonstrates that he or she is ready to consistently make these changes.

Older Children Who Stutter May Do Almost Anything to "Get Unstuck."   As I write these words, I am in receipt of correspondence from a grown adult who works in a professional field, who tells me that when he is on the telephone and starts to speak " . . . words just don't come out . . . and . . . I try, even with force, like banging my feet to the ground, even then nothing comes out." Similar to our discussion in Chapter 3 of "dynamiting" the sound, syllable, or word out of the mouth, the notion or feeling here, I guess, is that like hitting a piggy bank to pop loose a coin that is stuck, banging your feet on the ground will jar loose an apparently jammed up word!

Why do I mention this adult? Well, if a supposedly more mature, sophisticated, and learned adult feels the way the above person feels apparently, that jarring his body will free words up, what might a younger, less mature, and less educated individual thing or feel! Without a doubt, not being able to move on from one speech posture to another, feeling stuck on a particular sound, syllable or word and being unable to move forward, is a frustrating, frightening feeling for a young or even more mature speaker. It is indeed a sense of helplessness (in the last chapter we will discuss the concept of "learned helplessness"), of being out of control or being unable to control one's acts. For some older children, some of the time, the feelings surrounding these events can be strong enough to create a temporary *white-out* from reality or tuning out of one's surrounds and behavior. Physical pressures are felt in the chest, neck, vocal tract, and stomach regions (we've had a few adults who stutter also tell us that they felt that their head was "under pressure" or "about to explode"). During these sensations, the child who stutters is solely occupied with getting the sound, syllable, or word *out*, and, if sufficiently panicked and afraid, he or she will use *any* means at his or her disposal to do so. If you will, the ends (getting the word out) justify the means (any strategies that seemingly complete the word or "shake the word loose," like banging your feet on the ground).

Coming to Grips with the Whiteout of Stuttering.   As discussed before, it is unfortunate that at the very moment when change is most important for children to make, they are the least aware or objective regarding what they are doing that interferes with talking. This is particularly true for a child who is afraid of his or her stuttering, who is ashamed of it. Like a hot stove, the child approaches with caution, if at all. Perhaps we can equate these feelings of unclarity to those we have if we almost fall off a high ledge but in the nick of time pull ourselves back from the edge. We feel momentarily panicked, frightened, and try to do something, anything that we can, to keep from falling. If I then ask you, "Describe for me what you did when you almost fell off the ledge," it is almost certain that you will have some difficulty. Even some time later, when trying to recall the events surrounding your near fall, you may become emotionally uncomfortable and draw a blank or be very hazy on details. Indeed, you'll probably remember the emotion far better than the specific acts involved in righting yourself. You will probably be even less clear if I say, "What did you do to get yourself in such a situation in the first place?" The antecedents to, as well as the events of, the near fall are most likely lost in a haze of emotion.

The point of this analogy is often we try to have youngsters try to make changes in their speech fluency by quickly and objectively attending to specific physical aspects of their speech production *at the very moment in time* when they are the least objective regarding their own behavior (see Williams [1978] for elaboration on this point). Thus, the emotionality associated with the child's instances of stuttering must be brought within some reasonable limits if children are to make the necessary changes (as mentioned previously, Guitar, 1997, discusses this concern and how to deal with it in children who have strong emotional reactions and feelings about their stuttering). The good news is that we find that success with making changes in speech—no matter how small the change—many times leads to increased willingness to make further changes and lessen of emotionality.

Once children have demonstrated an ability to make the type of change necessary (physically moving their speech structures to the next posture from the posture they were holding or repeating), you may then engage them in spontaneous conversation. Again, beginning with the more noticeable, longer instances of stuttering, the clinician instructs the child—near the beginning or at least in the middle of the stuttering—to change what he or she is doing (not necessarily what he or she is feeling). We often do this by saying gently but clearly to the child "Change," "Now," or "Easy," or "Move on" in association with a slight head nod or motioning or gentle pointing to the child. We clearly and emphatically reward ("Good!") the child's attempts at changing speech behavior, whether a partial or clearly apparent change. We believe that our verbal instruction, hand gesture, and/or head nod help the child focus on the specific behaviors needed to make the change and, we think, help break through the white-out of emotionality associated with the instance of stuttering. As we will subsequently note, the SLP can also demonstrate for the child, with his or her own speech, what changes are desired in the child's speech (some children is our clinic call these "change-outs").

Handling a Child's Inability to Make Change.   If the child does not seem to make an attempt at changing upon our instructions, we immediately back up and halt the forward flow of our own therapy! Does the child know or understand what we mean by change? Is the level of the child's emotionality surrounding his or her instances of stuttering still so high as to preclude objective appraisal and change of behavior? Can the child *show* you an easy change on an isolated syllable or word? Can the child imitate an instance of stuttering and then, with your help, change it? We clearly do not want the child to spend the entire session, or large portions thereof, being frustrated, discouraged, and embarrassed by his or her inability to make change. We try to assess right then why change is not taking place. (Schwartz [1999, p. 114] suggests, based on his experience, that older children or teenagers who continue to stutter despite treatment have two general characteristics: speech motor skills that are slow to develop and at the lower end of normal limits and strong emotional reactions to his or her speech and environment.) With clients who are not changing, we cannot overemphasize the clinician's sensitivity to the client's behaviors and feelings. The effective clinician is the sensitive individual who constantly monitors his or her client's activities and makes changes in procedures, on the spot, as the client's behaviors dictate. Let the data (i.e., child's behavior) talk to you!

Model the Type of Change You Want the Child to Produce.   Have the child mimic your model. Then have the child shadow your modeled change immediately after you. The perceptual reality of the change—moving forward to the next speech posture—is that it sounds a bit like a fluent pull-out. That is, the child is moving from the physical cessation of forward speech flow (i.e., the stuttering that is typified by a fixation or reiteration of speech postures) on a sound by making more appropriate speech production gestures, movements, or transitions for the next sound. At first, these transitions might appear longer and more gradual in nature than they would ordinarily, but as the child more quickly and precisely recognizes and changes the original nonmoving-on posture, he or she will shorten these articulatory transitions. We do not, repeat do not, want the child to end up with speech that sounds like the ends and beginnings of adjacent sounds were elongated like so much stretched taffy. This results in nonnatural speech, speech that is hardly "suitable" (see Franken, van Bezooijen, & Boves, 1997, for discussion of communicative "suitability" relative to stuttering). Rather, our goal is to help the client produce speech that sounds reasonably fluent and natural. Of course, on a particular day, in a particular speaking situation for a specific sound or word, a deliberately longer moving-on posture might be appropriate because it handles, in the best way possible, a particularly difficult-to-change disfluent production. In the main, however, the child will, with time, learn to make more and more of the movements that are necessary to produce the sound within a reasonable timeframe and within reasonable limits of physical tension. Make no mistake: Speech that sounds and looks unnatural, is less than suitable for work, school, social situations, no matter how fluent, is speech that just isn't going to fly! The person who stutters feels and probably is better off continuing to stutter rather than accept some win-the-battle-and-lose-the-war type of speech modification, one that creates a manner of talking that is unnatural and not suitable for many forms of communication.

Changing Rather Than Pushing or Pulling on Speech Postures.   We try to emphasize to the child that pushing or pulling on the speech posture of the sound they are stuttering on is only causing them to hesitate or stutter even more. For emphasis, we might tell the child that it is as if he or she was some other silly cartoon or comic figure they know who keeps running into a closed door, each time with a little more force and with a longer start. Instead, we say, open the door and move on to the next room (or speech posture)!

As Figure 4.1b shows, "Opening and moving on or through" is one more relatively graphic way we have of explaining to children what they do when they fail to move on to the next posture and exhibit inappropriate levels of physical tension. We tell them they can repeatedly kick at the door, each time with a harder and harder kick, or they can push on it with their shoulder with all their physical might, but they will not go on to the next speech posture (or into the next room) until they smoothly turn the handle, open up (the door), and move on. Most children seem to comprehend such descriptions and act, to greater or lesser degrees, on these recommendations. Another good analogy to help the child understand the differences between "pushing" versus "letting go" and "moving on," involves the clinician sticking his or her foot between the door and doorframe (be sure you use the hard soles of your shoes and not sandals, sneakers, or your actual toes or foot!) to keep the door from closing. To close the door, the clinician can push and push on the door, but to no avail. The door will *only* close once the foot is removed from between the door and doorframe. This is another way of helping the child understand that "letting go" rather than "pushing" achieves the desired goal.

Children Must Speak Before They Can Change Their Speech. Children who stutter must be encouraged to and supported in their efforts to communicate. We firmly believe

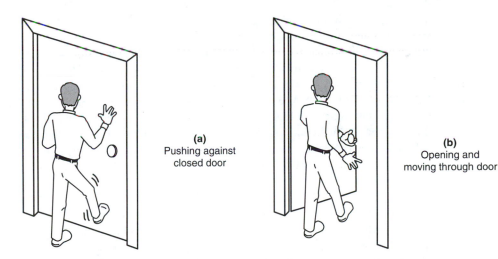

(a)
Pushing against
closed door

(b)
Opening and
moving through door

FIGURE 4.1 Pushing versus opening the door analogy. In both (a) and (b), the person is trying to go through the door, move from one room to the next. In (a), however, the door is closed and rather than smoothly grasp the doorknob, twist and turn it and open the unlatched door, the person is pushing on the closed door with his hand and foot. This is similar to "pushing," with muscle force and/or air pressure, against lips that are tightly closed, in attempts to "push or blow the sound out of the mouth." In (b), the person grasps the doorknob, twists and turns it and smoothly moves from one room to the next. This is similar to releasing the articulatory contact for the sound being stuttered on and moving on to the next sound or syllable.

that an important adjunct to therapy with this age group—indeed, any age group—is to keep the client talking, to foster his or her attempts to communicate (cf. Johnson, 1961). Talking should be encouraged and fostered at home, at school, at play, in therapy, and in any situation where verbal communication is appropriate. One of the real tragedies of stuttering, when the problem goes unchanged and worsens, is that the people who stutter begin to talk less and less, and society begins to lose their potentially beneficial, worthwhile, and interesting contributions. In our parent–child groups, we have seen more than a few children who stutter, during the first few therapy sessions, who only produce 50 words during a 50-minute group treatment session! Indeed, one of the goals with such children is to increase the amount that they talk. Simply put, talking is required to learn how to change talking!

The well-known clinical practice of having people who stutter accompany their clinicians on visits to stores and shops has, as one of its goals, the maintenance and reinforcement of talking. It seems logical to assume that if the child only talks and practices changing his or her talking during the therapy session, the child has less than a favorable prognosis for improvement in speech fluency. For example, one of our current clients, a 15-year-old boy, only wants to talk about sports. Small talk, "flow" (Czikszentmihalyi, 1975), is seemingly out of the question for this teenager, and his progress in therapy suffers because of that. It is much like practicing to drive only in the driver education class and in the school parking lot. (Conversely, we shouldn't only practice during the Indianapolis 500 race!) Classroom or in-therapy practice is important, but nothing can take the place of actually using the skilled behavior in the forum or situation in which it must be displayed. "Learning by doing" is as at least as important to remediation of stuttering as all of our skillful and supportive in-clinic therapy procedures.

One suggestion to encourage talking in older children who stutter was made by Johnson (1961). He encouraged children to read aloud, at first to themselves, then to their mother, father, or friend. His suggestion, which I sometimes use with this age group, helps the child practice talking. The parents, after instruction, are encouraged to listen to the child and be uncritical of the child's speech fluency during the reading. The parents are to attend to the content of the child's reading; children are encouraged to read something they find interesting that can be read in three- to five-page blocks. This activity is not to take a half-hour of the parent's or child's time but more like five to ten minutes every day, or at least every other day.

What the clinician, parent, teacher, and so forth want to encourage is the act of talking aloud, the physical feel of speaking, the joy of conveying a message to attentive listeners. Fully realizing the relative intolerance of some adults for listening to oral reading, this activity is not to be undertaken by every child and his or her parents. When it is used, the clinician needs to clearly, and sometimes repeatedly, describe the purpose and procedure of this task and to maintain weekly monitoring of its progress. The clinician should not be hesitant to discontinue such an assignment if it appears to be more of a hindrance than a help.

Practice.   Related to talking and using what is learned in treatment outside of treatment is the notion of practice. Getting children to practice outside of therapy what they demonstrate they can do during therapy is a major task for the SLP. First, the SLP must make the practice exercise or assignment something that can be done within a short period of time each day between therapy sessions. Second, the child must be helped to see or understand some reason why the homework assignment is given—busywork will seldom get done. Some time should be spent with the child helping him or her figure out a time, each day, outside of therapy that is convenient for them to practice—on the school bus in the morning, during dinner at night, on the playground, and the like. Leaving this open-ended (i.e., practice everyday when you think about it) generally means the practice is open to not being done! Setting up specific times during each day when practice is to occur is a "treatment process" facet of therapy (much like setting the day, time, length, and number of treatment sessions), and one of the more crucial "treatment process" to ultimate transfer of change into the everyday, nontherapy world of the child. Third, we should explain to parents the nature of the practice exercise and its rationale. As mentioned above, parents need to be given positive ways of responding to changes they notice in their child's speech. Fourth, partial or totally *uncompleted* practice assignments need to be dealt with as they occur and not allowed to become a routine occurrence. Why wasn't the assignment done? Was it too hard? easy? silly? unclear? irrelevant? Again, did the child have a particular place, listener, and time each day to practice? Is the child sufficiently motivated to change? Are you a sufficient motivator (a necessary if challenging role for the SLP)? We want to make clear that allowing "homework" assignments to go undone from week to week is poor therapy and sets a poor precedent (better, almost, to give no "homework" than to assign exercises that never get completed, handed in, or checked up on). Make it clear to the child and parents that change in speech will come but not without time and effort on their part *outside* the confines of the therapy session.

I Forgot to Practice.   One of the big problems with practice assignments is that they are handed in, so to speak, at the beginning of each therapy session. What more discouraging way—at least for the clinician—to start a therapy session than with the child's report, in deed or in words, that he or she forgot, was not interested in, or did want to do the assignment? Your post hoc scolding generally accomplishes very little. Conversely, neither will ignoring the situation accomplish much. Some sort of talk is in order, where you ask questions and listen to the child's answers. Try to impress on the child the need for practice and with its importance to you and the child's success in the therapy program. Show that you care about the assignments getting done but that you aren't disappointed in the child as a person. Request the child's help in carrying out the assignment. Many times, with an older child or teenager, having him or her write down the assignment in a notebook to treatment can be a big help. Let the child know you trust him or her to do the right thing, and encourage the child to ask questions and raise concerns if he or she feels your homework assignments are unclear, unfair, too hard, or simply meaningless to them.

Show the child: Actually demonstrate the assignment for the client before he or she leaves. Tell the child that the assignment requires so many minutes each and every day. Again, we want to state our opinion that a brief period *every* day is, in our opinion, worth much more than a long period that gets done only one day per week. In some cases, helping the child to develop a chart that can be hung up at home allows him or her to check off the days and times when homework was done. Praise the child for successfully completed practice assignments; try not to just accept the assignments as if it is a "you-understood" that they get completed.

When the assignment has been accomplished, clearly show the child you are pleased with his or her completion. Let the child know you are proud of him or her and that it is important to you that he or she has done the assignment successfully and on time. We really shouldn't expect sudden or dramatic change with such a complex human problem as stuttering; however, we should make every attempt to reward for successive approximations to the final goal: regular successful completion of reasonable practice assignments.

Parents' Role in Modification with Older Children.   Sometimes, when parents observe you directly trying to modify or change their child's speech, they may ask what they can do at home to help. This is not a situation to be feared, but it is one to be dealt with in a thoughtful manner. Once again, some kinds of help are the kind of help these kids can clearly do without! For example, parents may observe our *neutral tone* suggestion to their child to change speech behavior but only attend to the word "change" and ignore the neutral affect of our voice. Later, when irritated or concerned that the child is not "doing what he or she was told in therapy," the frustrated parents may use the word "change" with their child in a manner that is nothing more than "stop that stuttering." If the same word is said by the parents (or us!) with the wrong inflection or as a means to "get at" or "pick at" the child for unwanted behavior, then the use of that word is counterproductive to long-term success in treatment.

What Parents Should and Probably Should Not Do to Help.   For these reasons, we routinely caution against parents using the same instructions we use, at least in the beginning of therapy, because we have so little control over how some of the parents will use these instructions. Our tentativeness in this area reflects the fact that our treatment has sometimes been hampered by parents who inappropriately use our instructions, outside of the clinic, to the point that when we employ them in therapy, they negatively influence the child. Instead, what we like to encourage parents to do is to keep their child talking. We routinely encourage the parents to try to listen to the content of the child's speech and not to overly request speech from the child on a day when the child is obviously disfluent. We don't want them to make such a big deal about the child's attempts to change speech that the child feels bad when he or she doesn't change or when he or she stutters. We do want to encourage parents to parents to appropriately reinforce any and all positive *changes* they observe their child making in his or her speech. Further, we try to help parents learn to develop the discipline NOT to talk for their child or fill in the word but to let the child do this for him- or herself. I might add that one of my suggestions—reinforcing changes in the child's speech—is difficult for parents to implement because it requires them to be able to detect changes, just like you, the SLP. This, of course, means training the parents to be more observant of their child's behavior, which, of course, means more work on the part of parent and clinician. Very importantly, this also means that parents must learn *what differences* in their child's speech and related behaviors *make a difference* in terms of long-term recovery from the problem. For example, in the beginning of therapy, this may mean helping parents observe that even though their child's frequency of stuttering remains the same, the duration of each instance of stuttering is shortening, suggesting that the child is beginning to make progress toward becoming more normally disfluent. Helping parents learn to appreciate positive changes in the "typography" of stuttering (e.g., short duration stutterings, stutterings with less physical tension, "change-outs," etc.) helps them understand and relax about their child's progress and not be so overly concerned that the frequency of the stuttering has not yet changed appreciably.

Collaborative Efforts Between Public Schools and Clinics.   In a public school situation, of course, parental involvement is often very difficult because of facilities, time factors, and school policy, but in a clinic, involvement of parents is not as problematic. Perhaps this suggests that schools and local clinics could cooperate in such a fashion that in the beginning, when parent concerns, information sharing, and the like are most acute, the child could be managed by the clinic. However, as the child progresses and parents become more facilatory and less of an issue, the public school SLP could take over management of the child. In our opinion such collaborative efforts are feasible—we have often implemented them ourselves, and many times in the child's best long-term interests.

The Engaged Parent Is the Helpful Parent.   In our opinion, some engagement in the treatment process on the part of the parent is necessary to the long-term success of the child. The disengaged parent is often, in our experience, the parent who fails to understand the purpose and procedure of treatment and who continually does things in the home that are at odds with what we are trying to do in treatment (e.g., providing words for the child when the child is "stuttering"). As a matter of course in our clinic, *all* parents of children who stutter must be present and observe during a proportion of their child's therapy sessions (this is particularly true for our P/C groups, as previously discussed). Parents, unless there is an extremely pressing reason, cannot routinely drop off their child at the clinic—like a pair of pants at the dry cleaners—go shopping and then come back in an hour.

We explain this policy kindly, clearly, but emphatically to parents *prior* to the beginning of therapy. If they decline to become so involved, we give them names, addresses, and phone numbers of other agencies that they can consider. We are very desirous of having the parents know what is going on, and we want the parents to be a part of their child's remediation program. We show the parent what we mean by change in their child's speech; we have them observe the child in therapy and point out to them changes their child makes. We tell the parent that spontaneous examples of these changes at home or elsewhere outside the clinic should be praised by the parent: "Boy, Melissa that was a nice change you made there." Not in an outlandish or overly effusive manner, but in manner that conveys support and pride for a job well done.

How to Handle Parental Observation of Therapy.   It should be noted that parental observation of therapy, not unlike student clinician observation of therapy, must be *guided* to be of any real value. If the clinician does not guide the parents' observation, tell them what behaviors and events to attend to and why, the parents may gain little real understanding from the observations other than fatigue! This procedure may require two clinicians, one managing the child and the other with the parent, pointing out therapy's strategy, procedure, and rationale; changes in clinician behavior that appear to influence changes in child behavior and progress (or lack thereof). Two SLPs are obviously not a luxury every clinic or school system can afford. One way around this, if the parent can observe without the child being aware, is for the SLP to arrange in advance with parent certain nonverbal signals or verbal cues or codes that the parent is to listen and watch for and then attend to this or that aspect of the child's behavior. Another simple solution is for the clinician to audio or videotape the session and then go over salient parts of the session with the parent, explaining and stopping the recording to allow for discussion and questions. Furthermore, at least in the beginning, the parent should not discuss with the child what the parent has observed in therapy. In fact, in the beginning, the parent should probably not tell the child that he or she is observing therapy. This can be too distracting to the child, especially for the child who is distractible to begin with, whose threshold for reaction to extraneous stimuli is low, and whose reaction to events is typically intense, regardless of their nature. If the child directly asks the parents if they are watching therapy, they can say that the clinician discusses what is going on in therapy with them. With time and positive change on the part of the child, the child will probably come to realize that mom and/or dad occasionally watches therapy; but this will concern the child less and less. In fact, we have noticed that this lack of concern seems to closely parallel the child's positive change in his or her speaking difficulties.

(Dis)continuing Therapy.   When children do not change their speaking behavior, no matter how hard the clinician works, several things must be considered: (1) Do the individual children really understand how they are interfering or disturbing their speech production and how, when, and where they can change these interfering behaviors? (2) Is the environment counterproductive to the child's making significant (or any) change in his or her speech disfluencies? We have had parents complain, once a child becomes significantly more fluent, that the child is talking too much and they do not like this! Some of these children may revert back to their earlier forms and frequencies of stuttering. (3) Does the child practice outside the clinic, to a sufficient degree, what you and the child do during the therapy sessions? (4) Is the child and his or her family ready, willing, and able to put in the time, effort, and energy to make the necessary changes that will facilitate the child's speech fluency? and (5) Have you adequately assessed the child's problem and sufficiently geared your therapy to the child's particular needs? These and many more questions arise when change does not occur or when change plateaus and levels off. Again, we should also consider Schwartz's (1999) observation that strong emotional reactions and/or less than well-developed speech and language abilities are associated with children who do not change in therapy. Perhaps the strong emotional reactions must be dealt with (see Guitar, 1997) and/or the concomitant speech and language problems dealt with—for example, a child with a very depressed vocabulary, especially relative to syntactic skills—is a child who is going to take more time retrieving and encoding words, a situation that can and does contribute to hesitating, pausing, stopping, and so on while trying to produce speech. Perhaps such a child needs to be helped with vocabulary enrichment before treatment for fluency can be effective.

Lack of change may also signal that it is time for a break from therapy with all the precautions previously mentioned in Chapter 3 duly taken into consideration. It may also be the time for you to reassess the client's intellectual and social skills; perhaps you have been overestimating his or her ability to quickly and clearly follow your therapy plan. It is also possible that the child's social maturity is still not at a level where he or she can independently carry out assignments at home. Perhaps these children understand the idea of change in the abstract, but when applied to their own behavior during an instance of stuttering, when many things are happening rapidly and they are the least objective, they cannot apply what they actually know, feel, and can do. Perhaps, they know those behaviors that will facilitate their speech fluency but will not do them because they feel, "It won't sound like me" or "It doesn't sound or feel right." Sometimes lack of change simply comes down to the fact that it takes too much work too often for the child to maintain or increase his or her speech fluency. For more than a few of the clients we have worked with who are less than successful, we are convinced that their inability to communicate simultaneously with changing the motoric aspects of their speech is their main impediment. They can do one, for example, relate a story, but not two together, for example, relate a story *and* modify their stutterings while relating the story. In effect, the child finds it easier to stutter and/or that the costs of improved fluency outweigh the benefits. As much as we want to and try to help, we must recognize that in order for anyone to be helped he or she must be helpable.

Appropriate Use of Placebo Effect. Sometimes in our rush to be absolutely truthful, to provide complete "truth in advertising" with our clients, we fail to encourage their attempts even when those attempts are less than successful. This is a most challenging situation for the clinician, reinforcing the good faith efforts of our clients even when these efforts do not result in successful change. With such clients, while being reasonably honest about their present status, we also try to continue to encourage and support those children. We have already mentioned the *placebo effect* in therapy; however, rather than reject this out of hand, I think that we should recognize a powerful therapeutic adjunct when we see one. Better, in my opinion, that we recognize its presence and use it for our clients' benefit than deny its existence like a ostrich with our collective clinical heads in the sand.

Nothing is to be gained from being reluctant to tell parents and children that they are doing a good job, that you see signs of positive progress, or that this was a good session, even when things are not exactly ideal, when the child or parent is progressing as fast or as far as we had hoped or expected. We realize that unwarranted touting and praising of a particular therapy approach has given the placebo effect a bad name (and deservedly so), but we also recognize that every clinician, either consciously or unconsciously, is involved with the components of the placebo effect in his or her therapy: (1) the beliefs and expectations of the client; (2) the beliefs and expectations of the clinician; and (3) the client and clinician relation (Beecher, 1955; Benson & Epstein, 1975; Benson & McCallie, 1979; Shapiro, 1964).

We can reinforce and raise children's expectations for change by encouraging and supporting them. Likewise, the parents' feelings that change has taken place can be reinforced and supported; this in turn should help the parents try even harder to change and maintain change in themselves and their child. Nothing succeeds like success, and we can gain much by telling our clients and their parents in positive tones when they are making change, when their efforts appear to be paying off in improved performance. We don't want to be so quick to report each and every client misstep that we throw the positive baby out with the negative bath.

Teenagers with Definite Awareness of Stuttering

Twelve- to Fourteen-Year-Old People Who Stutter: Turning the Corner into Adolescence

Along the road to becoming a reasonably organized, stable adult, we all go through a period of relative disorganization and instability called adolescence. This period of personal development begins for some by 11 to 12 years of age and for most, by 14 years of age. During this period of time, young people begin to find themselves in the throes of physical, social, emotional, and psychological forces and changes over which they have little control. Emotions are readily expressed and keenly felt. The strong urge to be like and to be liked by their peers many times replaces their better judgment. Indeed, as Gladwell (1998) describes, some professionals believe that teenagers are not trying to be like adults, they are trying to contrast themselves with adults! Teens (and young children as well) are powerfully attracted to their peer group. The here and now become paramount. Parents discuss the future—for example, plans for college—while the farthest into the future the teenager is thinking about is this weekend and whether the girl in third-period math will go with him to a party.

Sometimes one of the last things members of this age group may want to hear and attend to is speech therapy! Things such as speech-language therapy is the concern of parents, and teens are trying to be good at being teenagers, not parents! Without a doubt, the mood swings of this period make speech therapy less than a steady course of action. The young person's struggle with independence from parents reminds one of the approach–avoidance conflict previously discussed by Miller (1944) and Sheehan (1958, 1975). One minute teenagers want freedom and disassociation from parents, and the next they are asking for parental advice and support. While they clamor for the privileges of adulthood—for example, staying out late, driving a car, drinking alcohol—they may simultaneously refuse adult responsibilities—for example, taking out the trash, saving for the future, cutting the grass, or taking care of their rooms and their health.

Into this whirlpool of human change and disequilibrium enters the speech-language pathologist trying to help teenagers become more fluent. These clients present us with a unique challenge in terms of remediation. To start to begin understanding this age group, one might want to read Ginott's (1969) common sense approach to interactions between teenagers and adults. Ginott covers many of the feelings, actions, and issues involved with being a teenager, and for this reason alone his book is worth reading. I am a firm believer that we, as SLPs, must be well grounded in the totality of the children and adults we remediate. Shames and Egolf (1976, p. 14) put it better when they said, "Stuttering neither develops nor exists in a vacuum. Stuttering is a behavioral response of a living, feeling, reacting individual who is operating in some form of socially interactive system with other people." With teenagers, young teens in particular, it is crucial that the speech and language pathologist knows the general bounds of that system so that he or she can successively navigate through its pathways. Such knowledge can also be enhanced by the video produced by Guitar and Conture (1996) or the therapy-oriented text of Rustin, Cook, and Spence (1995). The video, especially directed to the teenager who stutters, contains material that the teenager who stutters, his or her parents, and the SLP can benefit from reading.

Teenagers' Interest in and Cooperation with Therapy

It will come as no surprise, given the above remarks, that we have sometimes observed that adolescents do not appear particularly interested in speech therapy! One fundamental reason for this disinterest, in our opinion and experience, is that speech-language therapy "brands" the teen as *different* from his or her peers. And given their strong desire to fit in and be like other teens and not like their parents, they resist anything that they perceive to set them apart from their peers. I just did an informal evaluation of a 18-year-old college freshman who readily admitted that his friends know he stutters and that he probably needs help with his stuttering, but that he doesn't want to receive help because "my friends would think I'm weird." Translated, getting such assistance would mark him as someone different from his teen peers and this, above all else, must be avoided like the plague!

Paradoxically, this disinterest in therapy can also relate to the fact that teenagers are becoming acutely aware of their stuttering and themselves as speakers, and this awareness is beginning to become increasingly emotional in nature (which is completely in keeping with teenagers' general modus operandi). While some develop such fears and emotional reactions, sometimes a person who stutters becomes a teenager before he or she starts to develop real fear and avoidance of speech and speaking. This person's speaking may be making an already challenging age period even more so because he or she may be reluctant to be outgoing and speak in view of the embarrassment that speaking causes. Just when the teenager might want to become one of the gang and impress friends (particularly those of the opposite sex), he or she may become shy, withdrawn, and reticent to talk because of fears and concerns regarding his or her speech.

Once again, paradoxically, the last thing this person may want to do is touch, see, feel, and discuss (with an SLP, or anyone else for that matter) what is bothering the person the most: his or her speech. Of course, this is exactly what the speech and language pathologist wants them to do: touch, feel, see, hear, and confront the very thing (speech) that the teenage people who stutter fear the most, their speech behavior. Some of these clients give the impression that they'll change the problem as long as: (1) none of their friends know they are receiving speech therapy, and (2) the therapy process involves them as passive recipients of the clinician's administrations! Along with these concerns goes the fact that so many things are changing for adolescents. They must attend to so many different things that they may feel they have little time left over for attending to or changing their speech behavior. Perhaps teenagers may be likened to a beginning juggler with too many clubs to juggle—some of them are going to get dropped and only picked up later on when the juggler becomes more proficient at balancing many things at once. One teen told us last week that he wasn't sure he could come to treatment this week on Thursday, because on Friday he was having an exam! This would not be so unusual except that this same client has repeatedly told us that he didn't know how X or Y teen, in the same treatment group with him, could practice changing his or her speech outside of clinic. He said he figured that they just weren't as busy as he, that he had too much schoolwork to really think about changing his speech outside the clinic!

Obviously, when the speech-language pathologist is confronted with such rationalization as the above, patience is a watchword. Teenagers need adults who will be patient with them and provide them with support; yet, as adults we often feel inclined to direct, instruct, and scold teenagers. (As an example of how our patience can be tested by teens, a teen, when asked to practice "stuttering" and then "changing" on the word "pop," refused to do it on the grounds that the word "pop" is a Yankee word! Resisting the urge to chastise him for an obvious attempt to thwart appropriate attempts to change his speech, we replied that we didn't care what kind of stop-plosive he used, as long as it came out something like Consonant +"op." He won his little victory of resistance, and I won my little victory that he try to attempt to make the changes he had been learning.) We find it too easy to lose our patience with teenagers' apparently flip dismissal of what we consider well-thought-out therapy plans or suggestions for change. Sometimes the best course of action when we face the challenge of remediating adolescents is a break from therapy where client and clinician can separate, regroup forces, and wait for a more advantageous time to resume therapy. The SLP must make it clear to the teenager, however, that therapy will resume after a period of time when more time, effort, and thought on their part can be applied.

Of course, discontinuation of treatment does not mean disregard of all that has been learned during treatment. That is, the SLP's discontinuation of therapy should not be taken by the teen to mean that the SLP is disregarding the teen's speech problem but that the SLP is calling time out from formal active, weekly therapeutic intervention. The SLP's decision to discontinue therapy may not be agreed to by the client and his or her parents, but periods of plateauing or stabilization or lack of forward progress in behavioral change and/or relative uncooperativeness in therapy dictate that something should be done. It is neither fair to the teen nor is it good therapy practice to prolong the agony of unsuccessful treatment when a break would be a better long-range solution even though the short-term security of weekly therapy ("At least I'm doing something about my speech") is missing. Some parents will be quite insistent that the child "toe the line," and continue to go to therapy long after it is apparent that the child is merely "marking time," with the only "line" in sight, apparently, being the one he or she crossed over from enthusiasm to apathy.

Using Other People to Assist with the Teenager's Therapy Program

Specific procedures for speech modification used with this age group are not unlike those used with clients slightly younger or older; however, with the 12- to 14-year-old client, we must apply procedure in somewhat different ways. We need to enlist, if we can, people in the client's environment that the client can relate to—for example, a friendly school guidance counselor, a kindly piano teacher, or a supportive mother or father. We don't want these individuals to become unpaid, unlicensed, pseudo-SLPs—as I recently explained to a well-intended music teacher who wanted to provide a 16-year-old boy who stutters "lessons" to become more fluent. Rather, these people, whom the teen routinely contacts outside of the clinic, can be asked by the SLP to reinforce change outside the confines of therapy, to praise the client's increased amount of talking and so on. When sufficiently informed regarding the client's problem and therapy plan, individuals outside the clinic can help monitor the client's outside-of-clinic progress.

It is important to remember that the SLP should also consult with the teenager client (and his or her parents) regarding whether the SLP may discuss with the outside person the client's speech problem, therapy plan, and progress. We have found that the client's discussion and responses in these matters are very instructive regarding the client's desires to avoid, conceal, cover up, or hide his or her problem from friends and relations (for discussion of the *interiorizing* of stuttering see Douglas & Quarrington, 1952). Such responses give us insights into the degree to which he or she is willing to share personal information with friends, and the degree to which discussing stuttering with anyone is a fearful, shameful, or embarrassing topic. Some teenage clients may balk at your suggestions and others will readily agree; however, it is prudent, as well as good therapy, to obey your client's desires concerning the discussion of personal matters with outside-of-clinic friends. Besides, given some time to think about it as well as the SLP's encouragement and support, many of these clients eventually come around to the point where they will accept the involvement of outside-of-clinic friends, particularly as they become more fluent and begin to receive the spontaneous praise of their friends and adults for their improved speaking abilities. Indeed, it is not uncommon for the praise of those outside the clinic to be more valuable than that from inside the clinic!

Differences Between Young Teenagers and the Younger Child Who Stutters

A 12- to 14-year-old person who has been stuttering since, say, 4 or 5 years of age probably has a more *habituated* speech problem than the 6-year-old who has only been stuttering for six to twelve months. This habituation plus the young teen's fundamental flux in development can make it a challenge to change speech behavior. Lasting change, I believe, is predicated on engaging more of the client's intellectual cooperation than his or her emotions in the change process (this is a relative increase in cognition since teenagers' emotions are something that even they find hard to dampen). Interestingly, as Ginott (1969) points out, this comes about by talking to the teenage client in a manner that conveys your understanding of some of the emotional changes and concerns the client has and is going through.

Effective communications and interactions with teenagers do not mean that the SLP becomes a psychoanalyst or psychotherapist; however, as a professional, the SLP should have and be developing sufficient sensitivity to recognize the adolescent client's particular needs and concerns. While the SLP is not directly involved in influencing the teenager's psychosocial-emotional behavior, the SLP should make it clear to the client that he or she appreciates the client's feelings. Perhaps it is obvious, but understanding the young teen's feelings provides the SLP with a broader perspective from which to view his or her stuttering problem. Further, the SLP must search, largely through trial and error and the use of common-sense, for a "middle-ground of expression." Such a "middle ground" means that, on the one hand, the teenager does not feel patronized by the apparent immaturity or childlike manner of the clinician's expression or, on the other hand, overwhelmed and confused by high-level, sophisticated, and adultlike vocabulary and manner of clinician expression.

Some "Demographics" Re: Teenagers Who Stutter

Interestingly, little published information exists regarding the specific nature of the speech and related problems of teenagers who stutter (for more clinically germane information

TABLE 4.1   Descriptive Information Regarding a Sample of Older Children and Teenagers Who Stutter (*N*=15)

Stuttering per 100 words spoken
  Mean 16.5
  Range 1.0–43.0

Stuttering Severity Level
  Mean 3.5
  Range 1.0–6.0

Disfluency Type
  Most frequently produced by most clients: Part-word repetitions (8 of 15 clients)
  Least frequently produced by most clients: Part-word repetitions (7 of 15 clients)

Child's Age at Time of Initial Evaluation
  Mean 13.6 years
  Range 12.2 to 14.8 years

Sex of Child
  Male 14
  Female 1

Child's Position in Family
  First 7/15
  Second 3/15
  Third 3/15
  Fourth 2/15

Presence of Speech Articulation Disorder
    10/15

Significantly Consistent Stuttering
    10/15

Source: Iowa Scale for Rating Severity of Stuttering (Johnson et al., 1963).

Descriptive information regarding a sample of older children and teenagers who stutter (*N*=15). Clients were selected because of their representativeness of this age group of people who stutter whom the current author has evaluated and remediated. Significantly consistent stuttering determinations were based on the Iowa Measure of Stuttering Consistency (Johnson et al., 1963). Presence of speech articulatory/phonological disorder resulted from either reported histories of three or more sounds in error or actual observation by the present writer of such a disorder. Note: Data pertaining to the teen's former/present articulatory problems are to be considered preliminary and in need of further, more refined, and controlled analysis; however, if one can consider teens who stutter as "persistent," which seems reasonable, these findings are consistent with those of Paden, Yairi, and Ambrose (1999) suggesting that children who stutter who persist with their problem are more apt, than those who recover, to exhibit difficulties with phonology.

about teens who stutter, see Rustin et al., 1995, particularly Appendixes XIV, XV, and XVI). Therefore, we decided to remedy this in part by selecting a small but representative group from our clinical population and studying its characteristics. Table 4.1 presents information for fifteen people who stutters in the 12- to 14-year-old age range (as usual, most of these clients are boys). Approximately two-thirds of these clients report or have clinically demonstrated speech sound articulation/phonological difficulties. A similar proportion were significantly consistent (values of 1.0 or greater; cf. Johnson, Darley, & Spriestersbach, 1963, pp. 272–276, 292) in the loci of their instances of stuttering, which suggests that there is a fairly well established relation between certain speech-related stimuli and their instances of stuttering. Eight out of the fifteen clients produced sound/syllable repetitions as their most frequent disfluency type. We might add, in the time since this data was developed, we would add that some teens who stutter also seem to have a tendency to monologue, in a rambling, less than coherent, organized manner. Once started, they monopolize the speaking floor and seemingly have little sense of whether their listener understands and/or is listening to them. If the topic of their conversation is outside the immediate environment of the listener or outside the listener's understanding, some of these teens who stutter seemingly ignore providing referents and context (e.g., rather than start out by saying "I'd like to tell you about my gerbil, his name is Ralph. Gerbils are small, about the size of a chipmunk, light brown rodents that make neat pets for inside the house" they might typically begin by saying, "Gerbils like to hide things. Ralph hid one of my bottletops. He saw the bottletop when he was spinning"). They don't seem to understand that the listener needs this information to better understand what the person is talking about, so the listener won't and doesn't keep stopping the person to ask "What?" or "I don't understand" or "Could you please repeat it? I didn't catch what you are talking about."

While these facts suggest that persons who are still stuttering at ages 12 to 14 are in some ways similar to those who resolve their stuttering, with or without therapy, before 12, these facts also suggest that their stuttering has become more consistent and that more of these teenage clients appear to have had (or still have) concomitant speech/language problems than younger people who stutter. At the least, these observations suggest that the entirety, not merely fluency-controlling aspects, of speech and language production are less than fully developed for these children. As Louko, Conture, and Edwards (1999) point out in their review of the phonological characteristics of children who stutter, evidence mounts that phonology plays some role (though unclear) in stuttering. Its role, however, is not necessarily that children who stutter exhibit a phonological "disorder," but that they are, as a group, within the lower ends of normal limits in terms of articulation/phonology (for supporting data, see Pellowski, Conture, & Anderson, 2000), being less than efficient, rapid, and precise in terms of phonological encoding rather than being disordered. Perhaps such inefficiencies are of no consequence when the child is not attempting nor being encouraged to attempt, rapid, precise, adult-like oral communication. However, the child's speech tends to break down when routinely attempting to do so. Such speculation must await future research, but for now provides intriguing food for thought. Whether our rather small sample ($N = 15$) is representative of teenagers who stutter as a whole remains a question that must await subsequent study. For the present, however, we need to keep these facts in mind as we plan our remediation programs and realize that teenagers who stutter may not be representative of all younger children who stutter but originate from a select strata of children who stutter, a strata whose overall speech and language development may be different from both children who do not stutter and those children, with or without therapy, who recover from stuttering during preschool or schoolage-years.

Planning Therapy: Factors to Consider

Assess the Entirety of Speech and Language, Not Merely Stuttering. First, as the data in Table 4.1 suggest, the SLP should try to determine whether concomitant language, articulation, cognition, or social concerns are evidenced by the teenager. Far too often significant problems in other areas are overlooked or overshadowed by an SLP's overly focusing on the client's stuttering (we'll give an actual example of this in Chapter 6). Significant problems in any of these related areas may dictate that the concomitant problem, and not stuttering, should be evaluated in greater detail and, if appropriate, remediated initially.

Assess the Teen Client's Track Record: To Be Helped, You Have to Be Helpable. Second, the SLP should make every attempt to assess the teenage client's past track record in terms of speech therapy. For example, did he or she already receive three years of public school therapy to no apparent avail? Why does the teenager think or feel that this therapy was of little help? Why do you think previous therapy was unsuccessful? Likewise, has this person received two years of therapy for speech sound misarticulations/disordered phonology only now to be referred to you for a "stuttering problem"? What was the nature of this former articulation therapy? Are the "problem sounds" (i.e., sounds in error) that were concentrated on in the articulation therapy now the sounds the teenager stutters upon? What role did the parents have in changing clinicians or therapy agencies? Do the client and/or parents blame previous therapy and therapists for the client's lack of progress?

In our opinion, nothing is more predictive of the present and future than the past. If the client failed to regularly attend treatment, complete homework assignments, practice outside of therapy, and so on with previous treatment, then chances are he or she will do the same with us. However, SLPs typically start by looking elsewhere. They will often think that a client's past failure or relative failure was due to poor therapy elsewhere or a misevaluated case. However, many times these failures are just as much due to the client, his or her particular problem, relatives and/or associates, or some combination of all three.

Any client of this age group who is referred to you for evaluation and assistance should be carefully assessed by *you* (see Rustin et al., 1995, for excellent suggestions regarding assessment of teens who stutter), and all such background questions should be asked ("look before you leap"). If the child was in treatment before he or she came to you, try to find out all you can about the time course, scope, and nature of that treatment. If the client's attendance record was poor and you know this for a fact, you should discuss it directly with the client and his or her parents *before* you begin therapy. At the risk of redundancy, we cannot help repeating (and slightly changing) Santanya's famous remark that those who ignore history (or a client's history of therapeutic progress) are destined to repeat it themselves (see Van Riper, 1970 and Rieber, 1977 for an overview of historical perspectives on stuttering therapy).

Attempt to Discern Typical from Atypical Problems. It will help if you try to decide whether the teenager's presenting problems—for example, withdrawal from social events, reluctance to use the phone, meet new friends—are more related to teenagers' typical "disorganization" or to the client's stuttering. Realistically, we seldom can make such fine distinctions, but by trying to do so we are encouraged to give the client every benefit of the doubt so that we are less eager and willing to label each and every one of his or her problems as those *typical* of people who stutter. Simply put, some of the problems of teenage people who stutter will have little to do with stuttering but everything to do with his or her unique personal characteristics as well as being a teenager. If the teen or the SLP or the parent think that all the teen's problems will be "fixed" if the teen becomes more fluent, I suggest they dial 1-800-GETREAL! The shoulders of stuttering are simply not broad enough to carry all those problems! A reserved, cautious individual is going to be reserved and cautious after becoming more fluent. Becoming more fluent may significantly facilitate communicative, social, vocational, and academic interactions, but there is little evidence it will significantly change basic, inherent temperamental characteristics like a cautious approach to novel stimuli, flexibility in dealing with stimuli, level or threshold of stimuli necessary to evoke a response on the part of the person, and so forth.

Our knowledge of typical teenage mood and personality swings and quirks also should help us explain the client to his or her parents (conversely, the SLP's knowledge of parent–child interaction should help in translating "parentese" to the teenager)! Particularly nowadays, when grandmothers and grandfathers do not live at home and do not routinely provide parents with perspective, parents tend to think that they and their child are the *only* ones with these problems (of course, grandparents living in the home are not always helpful with children, as we noted in Chapter 3, if they are *routinely* communicating in ways that interfere with the teen's speech fluency). You can help with all of this if you strive to deepen your understanding of typical teen concerns so that you can begin to explain them to parents, if the need arises. Obviously, we do not want to overly generalize and ascribe all problems to being a teen or temperamental characteristics; instead, we will want to identify any real problems that relate to the teen's stuttering or related matters and that need our attention.

Teens Need Adult Support Not Adults Posing as Peers. Fourth, try not to fall into the trap of becoming a buddy, compatriot, groovy or cool friend, or the like; teenagers need and want *adult* guidance, help, and counsel. Just because teens are striving to become like their friends doesn't mean you have to try to join them! Indeed, teens learn as much from your model as from all your words. This, as in most things, requires moderation. While you do not want to be overly authoritative and become like a Marine Corps drill instructor who coldly and loudly barks out orders and assignments, neither do you want to be overly chummy and essentially deny your adult experience, dignity, and maturity as well as professional training in a mad rush to relate like a teenager to the teenager who stutters. The latter posture—that of a chum or teenage-like buddy—is easier for older, more experienced clinicians to avoid than for those in their twenties who more vividly remember their teens; however, it is not unusual to see 40-year-olds act like teenagers themselves in order to better relate to their teenage clients. Again, understanding where your teenage clients are coming from is not the same thing as trying to come from the same place yourself!

The SLP Does the Guiding, the Client Does the Walking. Fifth, finally, and most importantly, make it as apparent and as clear as you can to the teenager that you are the *guide* and he or she is the person who must do the *walking* (that is, work). Promising quick cures and fantastic, overnight changes are what everybody, particularly the uncertain teen, appears to want to hear, but nothing, in the long run is more debilitating to the client than the subsequent reality that indicates that they were misled. We all seek the quick, the easy, the passive, the no-brainer solution but no one said any of this, that is, long-term changing speech, was going to be easy.

If the Public Does Not Pay, the Charlatans Cannot Play.   Related to the paragraph immediately above, I'd like to stand up on a soapbox and pontificate a bit. People who stutter and their families are not going to like what I have to say. I am sorry for that, but the truth, as I see it, is that people who stutter and their families have a definite role in fostering therapies that claim quick cures. While the charlatan may know in advance that his or her fast fluency therapies only produce temporary, albeit dramatic, changes in stuttering, the lay public seems only too eager to believe and shell out their hard-earned money and patronize such charlatans. Obviously, these charlatans, these mountebanks, are telling the public what the public wants to hear, because if they weren't, these charlatans would quickly go out of business. In essence, I am suggesting that charlatans won't be able to purvey bad therapies if no one enrolls in them. Their legerdemain approach to treatment, their hocus-pocus of now-you-see-stuttering-now-you-don't simply would not exist if the public did not patronize them. The bogus, fast-fluency trade of the charlatans, mountebanks, and all the others who leech off the unsuspecting, all-too-gullible, suffering elements of the public would dry up overnight.

Professional groups should certainly be taking a leadership role in eradicating the therapies of these quacks; however, I submit that professional organizations cannot do this *all by themselves*. As long as the public continues to flock to and patronize these therapies in hopes of receiving fast fluency, the silver bullet to "cure" their stuttering without any real or active attempts on their part to make long-term changes in behavior, these sleight-of-hand therapies will be encouraged to develop and multiply. Our only hope here is developing a more educated, knowledgeable, and sophisticated public—a public who will, *before beginning therapy*, ask themselves questions, as well as question the so-called authority about his or her claims. This same public needs to particularly scrutinize claims that the changes resulting from fast fluency therapies will last longer than a week or two. The irony in all this is that the public, who will comparison shop to buy a toaster, a car tire, getting someone to paint their house, will throw all such caution to the wind when seeking health care for problems like stuttering.

Encouraging an Active Rather Than Passive Role in Therapy.   Contrary to the fast fluency, silver-bullet forms of therapy, we try to help the teenager understand his or her *active* role in changing his or her own speech. We try to explain to our teenager (and adult clients) and their parents that we are a bit like a person guiding a tour on which the client and their parents are about to embark. We say that we will facilitate their trip and point out salient aspects for their consideration along the tour, but they are the ones who must do the considering, they are the ones who must do the walking and touring. It is they who must pay attention to the landmarks we point out and think about what they mean to them and how to use them, if need be. We tell them that we cannot and will not carry them on our backs but will, on occasion, let them lean on us for support. If they refuse to go down trails we think are of importance, we cannot (and will not) force them. We are guides not magicians: We point out ways and means for them to change, but we cannot make their problems disappear into thin air. This involves perspiration not presto-chango your stuttering is gone!

Is the Cost of Effort Worth the Benefit of Fluency? Obviously, the concept of us being a guide versus magician is not one that makes all clients and parents particularly comfortable, because it will undoubtedly mean more work on their part. However, it is said, on our part, in as honest and straightforward fashion as we can muster. I think that it is this honest and directness that convinces and motivates people to try to help themselves. We try to show that we believe that the teen, with sufficient guidance, can and will change and that we trust him or her to put out the necessary effort, to spend the needed time, to make these changes. Indeed, we have to trust the teen because if he or she is not going to make these changes, who will?

When to Begin and When Not to Begin Therapy

As we mentioned in Chapter 3, knowing when to begin therapy is a skill that takes a long time to develop. Sure, any clinician can begin treatment when a problem is apparent, when the child's parents are insistent, but this does not mean that treatment *should* begin at that time. This reminds me of British sportscasters who sometimes say, while describing soccer games, that a soccer player "will only get one bite of the cherry, and he missed it when he had the chance," meaning: He had a chance to score a goal, and he blew it! In other words, we only have so many times we can "begin" therapy with a particular client (before they lose interest, become discouraged, give up), so we had better make sure that when we do we are starting at a time in the person's life when there is an optimal chance for success and client cooperation and motivation.

We think it best to begin speech therapy with young (as well as older) teens when they begin to show signs of wanting to actively participate in therapy and have reached some degree of emotional, psychological, and social stability. It is probably the case that every day that these clients continue to stutter makes their stuttering behavior that much more difficult to change, that much more habituated. However, initiating therapy when a teen is clearly not ready to attend and cooperate or is minimally motivated is courting clinical failure and frustration. We would prefer that a client actually says to his or her parents, "Dad, I'd like to get some help with my speech," rather than the SLP and parents deciding *for* (rather than with) the client that now is the time, regardless of whether the teen is willing and able to begin remediation.

With teens (and most clients for that matter) we need to be patient and exhibit trust in the client's ability to recognize when he or she is ready for speech therapy. However, this is not to say that some friendly, gentle but firm coaxing and persuading might not be of benefit for a teenager who is a bit uncertain or hesitant to begin therapy. Friendly, gentle persuasion, however, is not the same as threatening and browbeating ("If you don't go to therapy and get help with your speech, you can't drive the car") a teen into resuming or initiating therapy. Speech therapy that begins when a teenage client is not ready (or is diametrically opposed to) may leave an indelible mark that subsequent clinicians may be unable to remove regardless of the strength of their therapeutic cleanser. While such therapy may not "make them worse," it may turn them off so badly to the therapeutic process that they want little to do with it, even though they may still need it. We have had parents of teens insist, over the loud protestations of the teen, that treatment begin and, in our nonwisdom, we agreed with the parents, only to have the teen sabotage therapy through poor attendance, poor motivation to work or change, lack of cooperation, reluctance to do homework assignments, and the like.

Objectively Changing Speech Behavior

With teenagers who are or appear ready to receive speech therapy, it is important to positively indicate from the beginning that you know that with time and effort on *their* part change is possible. It is helpful to demonstrate to clients in the first therapy session or two that they are capable of changing their speech, if only temporarily. It also helps if you can make some of your therapy procedures objective and make some of the abstract concepts regarding speech production and change in same a bit more tangible.

Making Speech "Visible": The Basic Concept.   An audio tape recorder or even a video tape recorder with a needle deflector or bar graph indicator VU meter can be used for a variety of clinical purposes. First, you can record the teenager exhibiting both stuttered and fluent speech while speaking or reading and then play back the recorded tape. The VU meter—whether the needle or bar kind—can be used to show the client the objective difference in vocal level or intensity between his or her stuttered and fluent utterances. You should probably practice this a few times by yourself with a previously recorded sample of stuttered speech so that you can readily and quickly discern instances of stuttering and how changes in the VU meter correlate to instances of stuttering and comparable instances of fluency. A even better way of doing this is with devices such as Visi-Pitch or Computer Speech Lab (CSL; KayElemetrics, NJ). However, few clinicians, particularly in school systems, have the necessary time and/or technology to implement such procedures. These computer-based devices allow the SLP to quickly and easily digitally record and play back to the client his or her speech utterance. The CSL, for example, can be used as a digital oscilloscope or 3-D display, showing in real-time (i.e., as it is happening) changes in the client's formant frequencies, vocal level, intensity or loudness, and pausing over time. This provides immediate feedback to the client that his or her speech is different during a stuttered versus fluent utterance.

The Characteristics of Speech During Stuttering, as Viewed on a VU Meter.   As a general rule, *during* a sound that is stuttered (whether prolonged or repeated), the VU meter indicates a *lower* than usual or minimal vocal intensity level. This may tell us one of a number of things, but our earlier research (Conture, McCall, & Brewer, 1977; Conture, Schwartz, & Brewer, 1985) suggests two types of laryngeal behavior associated with this low level meter reading: (1) very closely approximated or adducted vocal folds; or (2) widely separated or abducted vocal folds. At the *end* of the stuttered sound or as the people who stutter makes the transition into the following *fluent* sound, you may notice either a temporary surge of relatively high level (the VU meter going beyond or above 0 into the "red zone") speech reading and/or erratic, normal to relatively high level (louder) speech.

In other words, *during* the stuttering itself the VU meter will often give a *low* reading but at the *end* of the stuttering, as the person who stutters makes the laryngeal/articulatory adjustments to move into the following fluent sound, the VU meter will sudden and sometimes erratically "redline" as the person who stutters apparently uses more vocal level (becomes louder) in attempts "to get it out."

Depending on the level of understanding of the particular teen, you can decide how much, if any, detail to provide them regarding the specific nature of their laryngeal and/or articulatory speaking behaviors. With most of them, though, you can discuss the fact that they may actually become softer during their stuttering as viewed on the VU meter. Teenagers can be shown and understand the difference between the relatively soft levels associated with stuttering and the more normal (below or around "0" on the VU meter) as well as louder (above "0" or in the redline area of the VU meter) levels associated with normally fluent speech.

What is important here is that the teenager comes to realize that it is *his* or *her* behavior that is *making* or causing the needle deflector (or bar graph indicator) to move up and down, to go into the redline area, stay near the bottom, or hover around 0. In other words, the client can be helped to understand that it is *he* or *she* who is stopping the forward movement of speech production, in one way or another, when he or she stutters. The VU meter is not going up and down by magic, this is something being done by the person. This is something the teenager *does*; if the person *does it*, he or she can learn to *undo it* or at least do it in an easier, briefer more acceptable fashion.

Making Speech "Visible": Learning How to Change. The needle deflector or bar graph VU meter on an audio or videotape recorder can be used to help the client understand the idea of *moving on* to the next sound. Indeed, the lack of *moving on* when speaking is one of the hallmarks of stutterings. The arresting, freezing, or cessation of forward movement is what instances of stuttering are all about. Even repetitions represent a lack of forward movement in speech production, although they appear less "stuck" than prolongations or "blocks" (at least with repetitions of sounds or syllables, movement is taking place, albeit repetitive movement of the same speech gesture).

With regard to changing these behaviors, clinicians can be instructed to guide their clients to maintain, for example, a tight constriction of their lips during the isolated production of /b/ in the word "bee" while watching the VU meter. The VU meter in this case would probably indicate a very soft or low level of vocal intensity. The client would then be gently told to "open up" (to "change") and "move on" to the next sound, say /i/, while still watching the VU meter. As the client opens his or her lips and articulatorily moves on, the needle will quickly move from the left to the right or the bottom to the top (the green or similar color light on the bar graph indicator quickly moves up into the orange or red area), which indicates a sudden rise in vocal intensity, produced by the client's making the appropriate adjustments in speech production behavior.

Rock star Michael Jackson sang about looking at the man in the mirror, musing if he could change his ways. So to it is with therapy. What we are trying to do with these teens, through the use of the VU meter, is to help them see that *they* influence the way they speak and that *they* can change the way they speak with the appropriate amount and kind of attention and effort on their part. (Remember during these types of activities to try to insure that the client keeps a relatively constant mouth-to-microphone distance. Otherwise, unpredictable changes in mouth-to-microphone distance will cause changes in the VU meter rather than the client's behavior! A relatively inexpensive tie tack [that can be purchased at places like Radio Shack] or lavalier microphone clipped onto the client's shirt collar or thereabouts will minimize this problem).

Magic Is in the Man or Woman, Not the Machine.   One major caution in all of this: Instruct teenagers (and adults) that the tape recorder is *only a means* to an end and that it is *not the end*. That is, you are using the VU meter only as a vehicle, an instrument, a means to help them visualize what is going on when they speak, when they change their speech behavior, or when they work on using more appropriate means of initiating and maintaining speech production. The VU meter is a means to help them *focus on the physical feelings* associated with their speech behavior. In the end, it is the *physical feelings* of fluent and disfluent speech (and changes between the two) that they need to attend to. The VU meter and any other device like that is an in-between step, a bridge from where they are now (largely *unaware* of the physical feelings associated with their stutterings) to where they must go (considerably *aware* of the physical feeling associated with their stutterings and changes in their stutterings). We like to tell them that by watching a visual representation of their acoustic speech output, they can more quickly and accurately attend to and focus on these physical feelings within their vocal tract. If clients are not given these sorts of cautions and instructions, they may come to be overly dependent upon the tape recorder or any device used to objectify or feedback what they are doing when they speak. Periodically, turn the tape recorder off or block their view of the VU meter and observe whether they can do as well without it.

Phasing out the Use of Instrumentation.   Weaning clients, right from the start, off their need to rely on such instrumental assistance is *very* important in establishing the all-important transition between in- *and* outside-of-clinic changes in behavior. This "weaning" is necessary to the development of sufficient carryover of clinical changes to everyday conversation outside the clinic, where, obviously, VU meters are seldom seen! In other words, the young and older client must be clear that you realize that he won't have the VU meter handy when he gives an book report to his English class or asks a girl out for a date! Instead, the client must be told by you and come to realize that the VU meter is a means to help him concentrate on his speech and the physical feelings associated with fluent and disfluent aspects of same. (Several years ago, we mentioned some examples of "biofeedback" approaches with people who stutter; one good example of this is Guitar, 1975; for discussion of pros and cons of biofeedback with young people who stutters see Adams, Guitar, & Conture, 1979.)

Making Speech "Visible": Learning Easier Onsets.   The VU meter can be used with teenagers to show them how to make appropriate vocal initiations and transitions. We begin with clients watching the VU meter while we demonstrate a very gradual or "easier" (slower with less physical tension) onset of voicing on a vowel like /i/ or /a/. We point out to the client the relative slowness of onset and the gradualness of initiation. We are here trying to help the client unlearn what appears to be a problem for many people who stutter: getting going! While some claim that people who stutter begin speaking too fast and with too much physical tension, there is little data to support or refute this contention (indeed, research into the speech reaction time of people who stutter suggests, if anything, that they are slower not faster when they initiate speech [see Bloodstein, 1995, Table 15]). Paradoxically, we believe—although we don't have data to support our contention, only clinical observations—that people who stutter rush the planning of their speech-language production. Overly rapid planning, we believe, is one of the reasons that the various facets of speech/language production—syntactic, semantic, phonologic, motor execution—do not synchronize well, leading to hesitations, stoppages, and errors in production (see our discussion of "mismatches" in Chapter 1).

Helping the Teen Distinguish Between Categorical and Continuous Forms of Speech Production. With some teens who stutter, we must help them understand that fluent speech involves physically easy, neither overly fast nor slow movements from one vocal target to another. Instead of this "gliding" from vocal target to vocal target, they seem to want to move from one vocal posture to another like going from black to white, night to day, without any shades of gray or twilight or dawn. As the skier (writing) versus pogo sticking (printing) analogy suggests (Figure 4.2), they appear to approach speech like print-

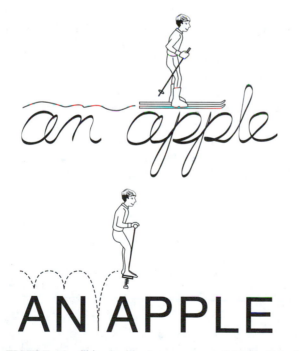

FIGURE 4.2 Skier (writing) versus pogo sticker (printing). In (a), the skier, like the talker, glides from one sound to the next whereas in (b) the pogo-sticker hops, jumps, or attacks each sound, syllable, or word, with little or no attempt to transition or glide smoothly between sounds. Breaking speech down into discrete units, rather than an integrated whole, tends to lead to hesitations, slowness, disruptions, and disfluencies in speech.

ing or the Morse code or stringing discrete beads on a chain rather than like cursive writing. They appear to want to hop from sound to sound rather than smoothly make the necessary articulatory transition (the in-between "sound") from one sound to the next sound (many years ago, Bloodstein [1975, p. 6] made similar observations in his discussion of how people who stutter "fragment" their speech, breaking "its natural transition into the next sound"; see simular observations by Van Riper, 1954, p. 249). To approach speech in a categorical rather than continuous way—to eliminate rather than use transitions between sounds, syllables, or words—would be like typing or keyboarding by, after striking a key, lifting each finger all the way up then pressing all the way down on another key rather than quickly sliding or transitioning the fingers laterally from one key to the next, just gently touching each sufficiently to make contact!

In my opinion, the apparent tendency, of at least some people who stutter, toward abrupt, almost categorical (discrete state to discrete state), rather than continuous (discrete state–transition–discrete state), forms of speech-language production is particularly noted during their initiation of speech (a problem that may be driven, as we suggested above, by rushed, incomplete, or inappropriate planning for the utterance they are about to produce). It appears that any place in the utterance where change must be made, whether silence to speaking, voiceless to voiced, voiced to voiceless, between-phrase pausing, and so forth, has potential, for some people who stutter, to move from one state to another *without* the necessary transition (this is a bit like a frog that attempts to hop from lily pad to lily pad without going through the air). It is unclear whether these transitions between sounds are inherently difficult for the people who stutter to produce or whether the people who stutter have learned, for whatever reasons, to exhibit such difficulties. Whatever the case, the inappropriateness or lack of these transitions need to be emphasized to the client. Figure 3.13, showing the successive movement of the thumb from one finger to the next, points out the transition (thumb moving between fingers) versus target (thumb touching a finger).

Through whatever means possible, we have to help the client learn how to employ different speech production strategies. One such strategy involves helping the people who stutter understand that a word-initial sound can be initiated *without* abrupt, physically tense onsets of respiratory, laryngeal, and supraglottal activity. No matter what the real or perceived time pressures in the communicative situation, people who stutter can initiate speaking with an appropriate gesture that moves them from the silence of being a listener to the vocalization of a speaker. And sometimes pausing a bit longer (a second or so) before beginning to talk or respond to a listener, helps the speaker get the various facets of formulation (i.e., syntax, semantics, and phonology) properly aligned before the beginning of execution of or overt speech production. Again, through analogy (Figure 4.3), behavioral demonstration, and other techniques, the teen must be helped to understand that *time* and *physical tension* are the two elements that can and must be adjusted to become more fluent—adjustments that the teen can learn to make, perhaps not overnight, to achieve more normally fluent speech.

Transitions between sounds can be shown on the tape recorder in such a fashion that teenagers can understand that they must open and move on to become more fluent. Again, the use of cursive writing helps them get the idea that whether they are continuing (prolonging) or reiterating (repeating) a speech posture, they must make movement transitions between letters (or sounds) for their writing (or speech) to look (or sound) smooth. On the

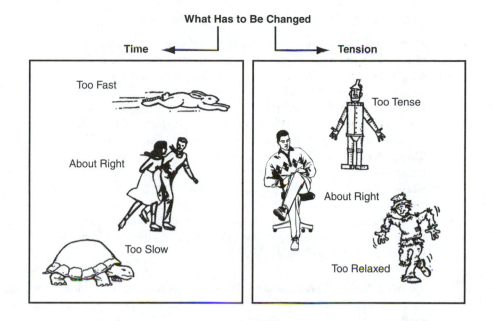

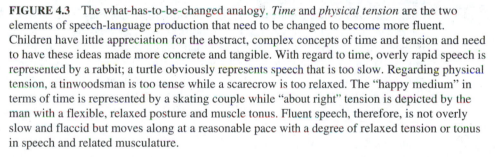

FIGURE 4.3   The what-has-to-be-changed analogy. *Time* and *physical tension* are the two elements of speech-language production that need to be changed to become more fluent. Children have little appreciation for the abstract, complex concepts of time and tension and need to have these ideas made more concrete and tangible. With regard to time, overly rapid speech is represented by a rabbit; a turtle obviously represents speech that is too slow. Regarding physical tension, a tinwoodsman is too tense while a scarecrow is too relaxed. The "happy medium" in terms of time is represented by a skating couple while "about right" tension is depicted by the man with a flexible, relaxed posture and muscle tonus. Fluent speech, therefore, is not overly slow and flaccid but moves along at a reasonable pace with a degree of relaxed tension or tonus in speech and related musculature.

tape recorder, the VU meter will probably be a low level and look stationary during a sound prolongation and then make a rapid change up or down as the client moves into the next sound. The needle will stay relatively still for the prolonged sound but make a quick movement up or down during the transition between the prolonged sound and the subsequent sound. With the development of various physiological sensing devices, for example, the electroglottograph (see Childers & Krishnamurthy, 1984; Colton & Conture, 1990 for review; see Adams, Freeman, & Conture, 1984; Conture, Rothenberg, & Molitor, 1986; Rothenberg, 1981; Rothenberg & Mahshie, 1988 for examples of application to people who stutter as well as procedural/analytical considerations), it is already becoming possible for the SLP to more quickly and accurately show the client his or her speech behavior than with an audio tape recorder. For the present, however, the audio or videotape recorder can be used for a variety of purposes besides recording and playing back of speech. The SLP should be continually evaluating the rapidly developing technology in this area, which promises to influence many of our current and future clinical practices.

Motivating Client to Make Speech Changes

Emphasize Activity and Not the Actor.   Perhaps nothing is more challenging, with some clients, than to motivate them to change! Indeed, one of the main roles of the SLP (professor, coach, etc.) is to motivate clients, to help them come to believe they can do what they have to do, to expend the time and energy necessary to do the work inside and outside the clinic to change. While beginning clinicians, in particular, believe that their main job is to help clients make the preceding changes in their speech, they must realize that without their encouragement, motivation, and support, their client is unlikely to make these changes. This is done, at least in part, by praising, positively reinforcing, rewarding, and congratulating, and supporting them for their attempts at changing their behavior and by demonstrating that you, the SLP, believe the person can and will do what is necessary to become more fluent. At selective points in treatment, particularly with a teen who feels discouraged, frustrated, and disheartened about progress and the work ahead, I'll smile, gently point a finger at him or her and say, "Amanda, you can do this . . . I know you can . . . it won't be easy or quick, but you can do this!"

Praising Activity Not the Actor.   From another perspective, Ginott (1969) suggested that it is important with teenagers to emphasize events rather than personalities. If the teen makes a nice change in his speech, let him know, "That was a nice change, Dwayne," rather than "You've become a good talker." Ginott suggested that you emphasize *activity* and not the *actor*. In truth, I think you need to do both, sometimes praising activity and sometimes praising the actor! Whatever you praise, make it clear and emphatic (this does not mean yelling or jumping up and down, just very apparent). Be demonstrative in your praise (but not ridiculously so) and use positive emotional tones in your speech, "That was a *good* change, Harry." Harry may not do much but look at you when you say this, but emphatically stated praise for his acts will help him develop the confidence and willingness to work at as well as make change in his speech. The praise not only *informs* the teen what is the goal/target is but *confirms* that he did it correctly. The teenaged client should, hopefully, come to value your descriptions of his behavior and appreciate your praise. When in doubt, however, keep your descriptions and praise *focused*, as much as you can, on his or her *behavior* and try, as best you can, to avoid evaluating and critiquing him or her as a *person*.

Sometimes Even Your Best May Not Be Good Enough.   If, after several sessions, a teenaged client does not make change or does not seem to be moving in a positive direction, reevaluate your therapy procedure and whether the client's parents are being sufficiently supportive. Parents can make or break a SLP's best laid plans, and you should assess whether your client's parents have a contributing role in the client's lack of therapy progress. Sometimes these teenager–parent problems are so pervasive and complex that family counseling or individual psychotherapy is the only alternative. It is, however, just as important to avoid a rush to judgment. The teenage years can be normally difficult for many of us. Just because there is friction, fighting, and disagreements at home does not necessarily mean that the teen and his or her family need psychotherapy.

Psychosocial Issues.   It behooves the SLP to recognize psychosocial problems in the teenager who stutters that he or she remediates and to make appropriate referrals. For example, *frequent* reports by the client or her parents that she stays up all night, is chronically fatigued, finds little joy in things that used to bring her joy, cannot sleep, or does not seem to be at all interested in food should be thoroughly investigated. Referring the client for psychological services may be warranted if these problems seem frequent and consistent. Such referrals, we hasten to add, will many times be rejected by the client and parents. It is therefore important that you only make such referrals *after* careful study of the case and the facts. We all get blue and out of sorts sporadically, but when the above behaviors are more *present* than *absent*, more *chronic* than *sporadic*, referral is warranted. Above all, don't confuse *your* (or that of the parents) discomfort dealing with a typically taciturn teenager (Parent: "Where have you been?" Teen: "Outside." Parent: "What did you do." Teen: "Nothing.") and behaviors that are typical (e.g., angst, emotionality, and apparent lack of concern) for teenagers. In specific, we need to learn to distinguish between our sometime discomfort dealing with teens, the typical concerns of teens, and behaviors that are atypical of adolescence (e.g., demonstrated or expressed interest in hurting small animals, continual discussion of setting fires, use of knives and guns, inability to sleep night after night).

Practice and/or Carryover of Change

Once clients exhibit an ability to make change on isolated sounds, syllables, or words, you should begin to test their ability to make these changes in more *realistic*, everyday-speaking situations. As any clinician can tell you, however, finding such realistic situations is very difficult (and now with liability laws being what they are, transporting or taking clients to off-site places like shopping malls and stores is quite problematic). Traditionally, clinicians have taken their clients around to other individuals in the building where therapy takes place or into nearby stores or shops. We hasten to point out that these activities, if not closely monitored, can degenerate into a series of coffee breaks where the client and clinician come to relate to one another in a most cordial, but therapeutically nonproductive manner (once in a while this is fine, if not very important, but as a routine event it is a waste of precious therapy time, and given the current realities of managed healthy care, therapy time is precious!). Phone calls may also be used to help the client practice changes, but this, too, becomes difficult if the clinician shares a phone with others or does not even have a phone and must borrow that of others.

Advance Planning for "Road Trips."   One secret to the realistic speaking situation is advanced planning. Before taking clients any place outside the therapy room, we should plan which places to visit, whether anything needs to be purchased or requested or inquired about, and to whom the client may be talking. It is a wise policy to call or discuss, in advance, if you are visiting people inside or outside your building, what you want to do and when and what you will be doing. People are generally willing to help as long as it does not take too much of their time and does not interfere with the routine running of their business, establishment, or office. Prepare them for the client and his or her problem and insure that the client asks a simple question like, "When do you close?" or "How much does this cost?" Be sure to thank them for their cooperation (make it clear to them how much of a help they have been) and you will likely be welcomed back again with other clients. People generally want to do the right thing if only they know what is expected of them and get a little encouragement and praise for their efforts.

Conducting and Evaluating Outside Assignments.   Besides advance planning, it is wise to make these activities reasonably short and to the point. Instead of ten phone calls, three may do, especially if they are well prepared for and each one is immediately assessed in terms of accuracy and correctness of desired activity or behavior. Explain to the client why you think he or she hesitated on the phrase-initial sound of the phrase, "What time do you close?" For example, specifically tell him or her that "You went back to your old way of talking when you began. You first took a deep breath and then held it with your tongue pressed hard against the roof of your mouth (or you held your vocal cords tightly together, or your two lips were pressed together, or some combination of two or three of these events)." Explain and then *show* the client ("show don't tell") what is necessary for them to smoothly initiate that sound and to smoothly make the transition between sounds. Again, show and not tell the teen what you expect!

Praise the teen for his or her effort and encourage the client to try again. Obviously, this much a priori planning and post hoc assessment takes time, but it is time well spent. Try not to let the client just go through the motions of talking to strangers over the phone, in your building or in stores, but explain to the client when and why he or she was (or was not) successful during a particular outside activity. Sometimes it is very instructive to the teen (and adult client) to role-play the situation, several times, before it actually occurs outside the clinic.

Once again, when interacting with a teenager, try to concentrate on the event, the behavior, the activity, and not the personality of the client. For the stranger's (e.g., a store employee) sake, try to keep your client's verbal interactions with the client to a minimum. Simple statements that can be answered with either a yes or no response or a short one- to three-word phrase are best. Further, these rather simple, brief statements give the client more control over the speaking situation and minimize elaborate discussions on the part of the client and listener. The emphasis here is on the *quality*, rather than the *quantity*, of the client's talking. Physically *easy*, somewhat *slower* initiations of the word-initial sound are generally, but not exclusively, the item of main import. Try not to allow the client to be continually unsuccessful with the exercise; back up and reevaluate: Is this task too advanced and have we prepared the client sufficiently? Have I demonstrated what I want in a clear, concrete fashion? Have I adequately confirmed and informed the client about behavior when he or she did or did not "hit" the target behavior. Don't be reluctant to *repeatedly demonstrate* for the client what you want done and then encourage him or her once more to do it.

The Use of the Phone in Outside Assignments.   Personally, we prefer the use of the phone as an "outside assignment," since it can be done in the school, home, or clinic and allows the client to experience brief but realistic communicative situations. Teens readily understand that the phone is an "outside" activity. That is because it is one of the means they have at home of "escaping" parental supervision! That is, parents of most teenagers are familiar with the frequent as well as long phone conversations their teenagers conduct when they are at home. These conversations, in essence, allow the teen to be "outside" the home and away from parental supervision while at the same time placating parents by not physically leaving the house.

Establishing Low-Cost, Local-Call Phone Systems, One Person's Dream.   Unfortunately, not every SLP has access to a phone, and using the phone costs money. I would like to see our professional organization lobby for the use or availability of a reduced-rate, limited-to-local calls phone as part of our professional apparatus, something set up nationwide that SLPs or their employers could rent at minimal costs. I would think it good business, and public relations for phone companies to develop special, low-budget, local-call phone services for SLPs that would allow unlimited local phone calls and that provided outlets for the recording of these calls for future study by the client and his or her SLP. The latter (recording of calls) might be impossible since it could be construed as an invasion of privacy, but the former (low cost), could be easily developed and designed for the exclusive use of SLPs working with teenage and adult people who stutter. Making our therapy procedures as similar as possible to that of the outside world makes our chances for successful carryover and transfer to everyday conversation that much greater. In the next chapter we further discuss the use of phones with adults who stutter and how procedures like the Relaxation Response (Benson, 1976) in conjunction with our change-of- speech procedure can be used effectively to help the adult people who stutter more successfully use the phone when they want to do so.

Assessing Changes in Speech Outside of Therapy

Carryover or transfer of inside-clinic change to the everyday world can often be difficult to assess. Which outside-of-clinic situations do we assess? Which are the most important for the person who stutters? What people and places are the most and least important for the particular person who stutters to exhibit fluency with? Obviously, answers to these questions are answered on a case-by-case basis, but it can be said that there are, for a teenager, at least four "settings" of relevance: (1) the clinical setting; (2) the school setting; (3) the home setting; and (4) the social setting, with peers. (Adults, of course, can add a fifth [work] and possibly sixth [a significant other] setting.)

In essence, we cannot be sure that the significant increase in fluency we observe in the clinic is similar to that produced outside the clinic because the two speaking situations are so different. This difficulty is in part the reason for the previously mentioned store and restaurant visits; however, even these visits are a bit artificial because the SLP tags along with the clients when they go into the store or sits next to them when they use the phone. These are good, sometimes excellent approximations to reality but they aren't quite the reality of "going it alone." Simply put, they provide some insight, but they are still less than a complete means for assessing the teenage client's ability to use changes during everyday communicative stress.

Fluency "Stress Test."   This problem is a bit like the one experienced by doctors when they listen to and measure (electrocardiographically) the activity of the heart while the person quietly sits or rests (same could be said about blood pressure, which varies continuously throughout the day). These tests may indicate a normally functioning heart, whereas the same procedures used while the patient is undergoing physical stress may indicate cardiac difficulties. We need the stuttering equivalent of a physician's cardiovascular stress test: How does the speech of the person who stutters hold up under conditions similar to those the person finds himself or herself speaking in? This is not quite the same, but related, to the question of how "functional" the person's speech is in everyday situation. In a sense, the study by Franken and colleagues (1997), with its attempt to measure when the fluency resulting from treatment is "suitable" across a variety of speaking situations, moves in the direction of the functionality of the person's speech. Likewise, despite some of its shortcomings (see Martin, Parlour, & Haroldson, 1990), the *Stocker Probe* test (Stocker, 1976) is a step in the right direction of assessing the speech of children who stutter under speaking conditions that approximate everyday speaking situations. The well-known *Job Task/Home Town* procedure (Johnson et al., 1963) is another attempt to obtain speech similar to that used outside the clinic, and Thompson's (1983) "surveying" parents' and teachers' observations of outside-of-clinic assessments of the child was developed for similar reasons. Yaruss's (1997a) data pertaining to situational variability in stuttering is quite helpful in terms of documenting this issue; however, the problem still remains: having a clinically feasible, meaningful way to assess the client's everyday communication (for a highly germane discussion of variability of speaking situations, see Ingham & Cordes, 1997, pp. 423–427, for a description of a "three-factor model for stuttering treatment outcome evaluation"). Truly, in this writer's opinion, this is an issue that deserves serious attention and one that will continue to make our therapy carryover procedures difficult to assess until we resolve this concern.

Related Concerns: Academics, Social Life, and Employment

What May Be True for the Group Is Not True for the Individual.   There are numerous references to indicate that for all intents and purposes, people who stutter are essentially the same as normally fluent speakers in terms of a variety of emotional, social, psychological, and physiological parameters (see Bloodstein 1987, 1995; Perkins, 1970; Sheehan, 1970b; Van Riper, 1971). The SLP should remember, however, that these findings pertain to people who stutter as a whole. That is, they hold true for people who stutter as a group, but for any one individual person who stutters (perhaps the very one the SLP is currently servicing!), they may be invalid. Thus, we can expect to observe older children and teenagers who may have *significant* problems with speech and language development, attention deficit disorders, schoolwork, socializing, psychosocial adjustment, and so forth. Conversely, we should not assume that other problems exist for most people who stutter; however, we should be aware of the possibility of other problems so that if they manifest themselves and/or impede our progress in helping someone become more fluent, we need to act and plan accordingly.

Hierarchical arrangements may need to be made whereby concentrated attention to school problems takes priority over speech therapy for stuttering. Parents and their children should not be expected to attend, on a weekly basis, six different professional settings (talk about being run ragged!). Unfortunately, all too often we are less than knowledgeable about these other areas of concern and professional services as well as extracurricular activities. It is not uncommon for SLPs in school settings, for example, to find themselves less than adequately prepared to understand concerns that their student–clients may have with reading and academic subjects.

Sometimes, of course, people familiar with the child, including yourself, will decide that the child's stuttering is central to other problems and that with remediation of his or her stuttering, the other problems will improve. This is fine and we have seen it happen; however, it is up to you, the SLP, to see to it that business does not go on as usual with all other professional activities as well as extracurricular ones—especially if these other professional services all require that the client take an *active* role in changing behavior or learning new skills.

How many balls do we think the teenager can successfully juggle? The client and parents can only do and be expected to do so much. We need to allow the client some free time to think, daydream, and rest. None of us would try to simultaneously learn golf, tennis, squash, sailing, and plumbing; and yet we seem to expect similar types of multitasking abilities from teens who simultaneously receive speech therapy, reading remediation, special physical education classes, tutoring with math in addition to regular schoolwork, baseball practices/games, Boy Scouts, and tuba lessons! Such "multitasking" is particularly problematic for individuals who find it difficult to do more than one thing at a time, and such individuals *do* and, ironically, seem to be the very people who gravitate to multitasking situations to place themselves under incredible stress.

The Concerns of a Teenager Who Stutters Regarding Future Employment Shouldn't Mean That the SLP Must Become an Employment Counselor. Present and future employment concerns with the teenage people who stutter and parents are many times very serious and need consideration. Indeed, the social, vocational, academic, and so on *handicap* of stuttering is real; some teens and their families are well aware, perhaps too much so, of the possible handicap stuttering may have on vocational choices and opportunities. The two best sources for such services are school guidance counselors or local rehabilitative counselors. Of course, we can't reasonably question whether 14-year-olds are concerned with employment. However, they are somewhat concerned with college and life after high school, so why not vocations?

Generally speaking, concerns about employment center on future, rather than present, employment. The SLP can provide such professionals—for example, the guidance counselor—with the status and prognosis of the teen's speech problem, and he or she in turn can provide you with information regarding the client's (and parents') employment aspirations. Ideally, you may receive information regarding the client's abilities to do those things he or she professes to want to do for a future job. You must realize that your input into these matters may influence other professionals in their decisions, and thus you need to *carefully* consider the firmness and accuracy of the data/observations from which you will draw you conclusions. Whatever the case, avoid getting into heavy-duty employment counseling with the parents and the teen. Remain as general as possible regarding such issues, especially when you are talking with a 12– to 15-year-old teen for whom the future workworld is still way off. Refer, as much as possible, to appropriate counsel in these matters and keep in touch with that counsel and offer information, copies of reports, and the like (obviously, only if you have the permission of the teen and/or his or her family). Your job is to diagnosise as well as remediate speech and language and to be cognizant of those events that pertain to these activities—you are not to try to help the client determine and find employment best suited for him or her. As SLPs, we need to be clear that stuttering can and does handicap academically, vocationally, socially, and so on, but also need to be clear when our clients and their families ask us to make decisions in areas that are outside of our professional purview.

In extreme cases, however, there may be a need for SLP counseling to handle the teen's and parents' reasonable employment aspirations; this counseling may even have to take place prior to speech therapy. Of course, when employment aspirations are in line with the client's skills, and these aspirations seem to be a prime motivator for the client's coming in for speech therapy, it may be appropriate to occasionally mention these aspirations. This should help maintain therapy interest through discussion of how speech change will make these employment goals more or less possible. Under no circumstances, however, should the SLP say in effect (no matter how tempting it will be to do so), "You can't expect to become a lawyer (clinical psychologist, politician, etc.) if you aren't going to work any harder than that at changing your speech." Besides being against the spirit and letter of the American Disabilities Act, this also is an obvious negative evaluation of the teen's personality and/or aspirations. Equally important, this is also probably harassing the client in the same way that his or her parents do. When in doubt, don't!

Teenage People Who Stutter with Apparent Psychosocial Concerns.   Sometimes the teen who stutters appears to, or is reported to, have psychosocial concerns (once again, listeners should not confuse the typical angst of teenagers, particularly teenagers who stutter, with their own level of emotional discomfort or uneasiness felt while listening to the teen people who stutter). For example, one 13-year-old we managed began to act out in class as well as against his parents. He stuttered quite severely, and it seemed that the only way he could get people to listen to him and pay him some attention (using the axiom that any attention is better than no attention at all!), was to misbehave. His stuttering was changed little in therapy, and psychological services were recommended to the parents. They declined such services, insisting his only problem was stuttering. (They were partially right, stuttering was a problem, but it clearly was neither his only nor most important one.) They changed their minds, however, when he set fire to his sister's bedroom! Obviously, not all cases are this dramatic or clear-cut, but we need to be aware of their occurrences and should be prepared to deal with them. At the risk of being redundant, the emotional discomfort exhibited by the teenager who stutters when stuttering and that of his listeners should not be misconstrued, and the SLP should avoid making a rush to judgment regarding the teen's level of psychosocial (mal)adjustment. Most of these reactions on the part of the teen are normal reactions to an abnormal situation, that is, being unable to move forward during speech production.

Teasing/Mocking of Teens Who Stutter.   Sometimes, as Robinson (1964) discussed, all these children may need is the companionship and attention of a significant adult; for some this is an older male, and for others an older female, while for others the sex of the adult is not as important as the personality and warmth of the adult. Other times we may need to spend considerable time discussing the mocking and ridiculing these children receive from their peers. It is not uncommon for parents to report, during an initial diagnostic, their concern regarding " . . . other children's reactions to his speech behavior . . . these other children's reactions to his stuttering may have a negative influence on him." These concerns should be dealt with and discussed by the SLP because they are one major reason these children have come to avoid talking to others, avoid situations where they may have to talk with others, and in general withdraw from social interactions. While these avoidances and withdrawals may be normal reactions to abnormal situations, they nevertheless interfere with these youngsters' development. Telling the teen and his or her parents to simply ignore these taunts, jeers, and wisecracks is about as effective as telling you to disregard the negative comments you get from friends and relatives when you have just gotten a new hair style!

Instead of ignoring the comments of other children and adults, the child and parents need to: (1) understand why certain people make such comments (the other people actually have a problem, not the person who stutters), and (2) learn how to say something, perhaps slightly humorous, that will defuse the situation and stop the ridicule—for example, "Sometimes my talking will be interrupted due to technical difficulties!" Furthermore, some children/teens "tease" because they actually think that the person who stutters doesn't realize he or she is doing this, that by bringing it to their attention they could stop doing it! And of course this assumption, explicitly or implicitly conveyed to the teen who stutters, makes him or her all the more upset because the teen knows that he or she really can't stop stuttering, at least not unassisted.

Dealing with such concerns, which are the everyday stock and trade of the SLP who remediates people who stutter, needs to be differentiated from the psychosocial concerns stemming from psychosocial adjustment problems. To paraphrase an old saying, we need to understand those things we can help with (and change), those things we cannot, and, hopefully, be able to recognize the difference between the two.

Other Concerns Exhibited by Teenagers Who Stutter. Again, as mentioned above, and in other places within this book, reading concerns, language delays, hyperactivity, attention deficits, and learning disabilities also occur in this population (people who stutter have just as much right to have these other problems as you and I). The latter—learning disabilities— is an area where, admittedly, controversy still exists but much is becoming known. In Chapter 2 we mentioned ADHD/Attention Deficit Disorder (ADD) in children—a problem frequently associated with learning disabilities—but it is quite possible that this problem could also occur with older children and teens who stutter. Whatever, the learning disability (LD) specialist and yourself, if you both treat the same child, must come to terms with the significant problems of the child (and his or her family) and try to decide which needs the most immediate attention. Further, you may have to do much in-service training in this area, discussing what is known and unknown about stuttering with the LD specialist. Obviously, a child with a learning disability who is finding school a difficult place to succeed and who also stutters is a child with a complex problem, but that may be the reality of the child's situation.

Whatever the case, as an SLP you should try to say nothing to the child and parents that either raises false hopes regarding cures for stuttering or gives an overly pessimistic, hopeless, or inaccurate picture regarding the problem and its origins. Communication between professions is particular crucial for both the client and the involved professionals, especially if the child has a several co-occurring problems. Such communication can result in a better understanding of each other's profession as well as mutual respect between professions. Once again, other concerns, like syntax, vocabulary, phonology, or reading, may also need more immediate attention than stuttering, and it is important for the SLP to understand this and set priorities for remediation accordingly. The severity and nature of these problems will dictate, to a large degree, whether they can be treated simultaneously with stuttering or whether one will need to be dealt with before the other.

Maintaining Contact with the Family Physician.   The older child's or teen's family doctor or pediatrician should, if the parents so decide, at least receive a copy of your initial evaluation, findings, and recommendations. If reevaluations and therapy are planned, it is also wise policy to inform the physician. Although there is always a risk that other professionals may misread (or not read), misinterpret, or poorly understand our communications, they can generally tell when another professional knows what he or she is about and is proceeding in a reasonable, prudent, and cautious manner. Nothing ventured is nothing gained in these matters, and it is a good clinical policy to let the family's main health professional, the doctor, know of your findings and plans for remediation. This is particularly important when you have decided that speech therapy is contraindicated and/or some other professional services seem more appropriate. Furthermore, if the referral comes from the doctor, you are ethically bound to send him or her information regarding your findings (unless, of course, the parents refuse permission).

Maintaining Contact with School Personnel.   While perhaps obvious, school personnel are another group of professionals who need to be considered. Far, far too often SLPs in clinics fail to communicate with school personnel regarding individual clients and vice versa. The excuse that both groups are "too busy" to communicate is no excuse. While it may take longer than usual because of the differing time schedules of clinics and schools and large caseloads of both, the SLP must take the time to confer with school personnel about individual clients. Our experience with these interactions is that the client typically benefits and our therapy is more effective when *all* interested parties know what is going on and what they can do to help.

Many times school personnel see the child almost as much as the parents do and certainly more than an SLP in private practice or in a clinic. An experienced schoolteacher, administrator, guidance counselor, or nurse can often provide you with information and insights that the child and his or her parents cannot. Conversely, some of these personnel may have what this author calls *long ears* and hear problems when none exist. We have had situations where every year a particular nursery school or public school teacher sends us a child who stutters. This would not mean much except when you realize that the teacher may only have one class of 25 students every year! Highly coincidental we might say, but experience indicates that these individuals—be they teachers, principals, or other school personnel—probably knew or were related to a person who stuttered when they were younger or that they have extraordinarily high standards for fluent, articulate verbal expression (and aren't afraid to let children know of their standards). Phone calls, letters, and memos to them explaining the problem of stuttering and what a classroom teacher can do to help should be of assistance. We generally do not send literature until we feel the classroom teacher, principal, and so on seem to have some basic understanding of the problem. This is because I believe that observations and readings in new areas of information should be a priori guided to be of maximum benefit and the individual should demonstrate *a priori* some willingness to read and learn. Teachers can become very powerful allies to the SLP in his or her remediation of a older child's or teen's stuttering problem; however, allies, like anything that should grow with time, must be cultivated and developed through continued interactions. We never said any of this was going to be easy.

Some Parting Thoughts

Clinician as Guide Not Curer

This chapter tried to show that older children and teenagers who stutter present us with a variety of issues to consider in planning and carrying out therapy.

In general, with this age group, we must start from a base of understanding of teenageland. This is a country that everyone enters without a passport and leaves without the possibility of return but is immensely changed by the visit. A country where the residents strive to be like each other and unlike the residents of adultland and childland. People who live in teenageland do visit other lands; indeed, shortly after they enter teenageland they frequently revisit childland (much to their parents' dismay), and after they have been in teenland for a while they make forays into adultland, with each foray lasting a bit longer and visiting a wider number of sites. Teachers, parents, and speech-language pathologists, to name a few, are often allowed day passes and visas to enter teenageland, but unless these visitors understand the rules and regulations of teenageland, they will not enjoy their stay.

More specific to stuttering, the issue of objective versus subjective awareness of stuttering must be dealt with and appreciated for successful remediation to take place. We have seen with this age group that it is particularly important for SLPs to realize that they not only *help* and *guide* people in the changing of their own behavior but that the SLP also must *motivate* them to want to change that behavior. We have discussed impressing client and parents with our role as guide rather than curer (or magician or wondrous healer), but that this must be done by the SLP in a positive manner, one that explicits conveys that the client is capable of changing and that the clinician can help in this process.

Objective Awareness Before Speech Objectively Changes

We have also seen that change in speech behavior involves an objective awareness of (ability to identify) the specific things, behaviors, acts, or events the client *does* that interferes with as well as facilitate fluency. I believe it was my mentor, Dean Williams, who said something to the effect that "stuttering is what you do that interferes with normal speech." It is one of the SLP's biggest challenges to helping the teen accept the reality and full implications of the simple verb "to do," relative to his or her stuttering and changing same. This objective awareness is followed by discussion and demonstration (hopefully more of the latter than former) as well as practice at physically feeling the behaviors associated with stuttering, staying with those behaviors long enough to truly sense them, opening up, moving on, and changing at or on the word-initial sound or transition between sounds. We have tried to show ways to objectify these changes—for example, audio and video tape recorders—and some of the problems we have when we test these changes inside and outside of the clinic.

Sometimes Some Kinda Help Is the Kinda Help People Who Stutter Can Do Without

Most importantly, we have tried to show that it is very helpful to know when to let go; that is, it is professionally correct to terminate therapy when it is obviously going nowhere. Likewise, it is professionally correct not to begin therapy for stuttering with a teen when all the cards are stacked against successful remediation. It is also professionally correct to prioritize the client's problems and decide that other speech and related issues need attention *prior* to stuttering either because of their severity, pervasiveness, or seeming causal relation to stuttering.

Finally, we discussed related concerns—for example, ADHD, reading problems— and knowing when and when not to refer to other professionals. We discussed the fact that receiving referrals means making referrals and a cultivation and development of a circle of professionals the SLP can consult with and turn to when the need arises. Hopefully, some of these thoughts will help you help others at a point where the problem of stuttering has lingered too long but has not quite settled in for the duration. Anything we can do for these older children and teens to reverse as Van Riper (1971) put it, the "morbid growth" of stuttering, is a step in the right direction for them and their families.

Summary

This chapter, in essence, presented the classic stuttering–modification treatment sequence (identification, modification, and transfer), as we will see again in the next (Chapter 5). Adapting this approach to the teen requires us to help the teenager see that it is behavior, not personality that we seek to change ("Sure, you may stutter, but that doesn't make you a bad person"). The clinician, with the teen who stutters, should attempt to concentrate on helping the teen change behavior and related attitudes while minimizing evaluations and lectures regarding emotions, feelings, and so forth. The clinician can do this, to the extent possible, by engaging the teen's intellectual skills for reasonably objective, nonjudgmental analysis of behaviors, feelings, attitudes, and beliefs. Again, we want to emphasize what the teen is *doing* and how he or she can *change* same, and avoid, as much as possible, lectures, instructions, diatribes, and the like regarding those feelings, thoughts, or evaluations of thoughts or feelings that we find problematic.

Woven in around our discussion of treatment procedure, in this chapter, we also tried to stress the fact that teenagers who stutter are people first, and people who stutter second. Hence, assessing, diagnosing, and treating stuttering in teens who stutter requires the clinician to know something about adolescence as well as stuttering. The teenager, whether he or she stutters or not, is neither fish nor fowl, neither child nor adult. Thus, many teens who stutter exhibit elements of the child they were and the adult they are becoming. The period of adolescent disorganization that we all pass through on our way to becoming, we all hope, more organized adults is no less a period of disequilibrium for teens who stutter than for their nonstuttering peers.

We tried to explicate, in this chapter, that one of the great challenges to any clinician who attempts to treat a teenager who stutters, regardless of approach, is to adjust treatment to the teen's level of intellectual, social, and psychological development. While the teen will make it clear that he or she does not want the clinician to talk to or treat them like "a baby" or "a kid" (something that happens when the clinician uses age-inappropriate language and treatment procedures), neither will the teen appreciate it if the clinician talks to and expects them to be adult-like. These concerns are particular acute with the 12- to 14-year-old person who stutters, an individual seeming, more often than not, half in and half out of his or her skin, going on 37 with touches of 4 and 5 thrown in! Analogies suitable for teens are still very useful to help them grasp the details of the behaviors they must physically feel and/or exhibit to become more fluent. For treatment can fail, not merely because it is poorly planned or inappropriate, but because the individual is not ready, willing, or able to respond to it. Despite the best intentions of the clinician, a teen client's level of motivation, ability to grasp concepts, attend to the clinician, attend treatment, and so forth are all client-dependent variables that must be dealt with for any treatment to be effective. We discussed in this chapter a myriad of extraclinical issues (and means for dealing with them) that cannot be expunged from the realities of dealing with teenagers, no matter how much we would like these issues to go away—for example, *chronic* failure to make appointments or make them on time; *chronic* absenteeism or tardiness at school; difficulties with schoolwork; difficulties meeting members of the opposite sex, worries about "being popular"; lack of opportunities to verbally communicate at school, at home, and with friends; chronic obsessions with not being different, with acting, looking, thinking, and talking *exactly* like peers and so forth.

An additional challenge, implied throughout the chapter, is those (clients, clinicians, or the client's family) who believe that becoming more fluent, in and of itself, will *completely* remove the various interpersonal and intrapersonal concerns described above. Such individuals appear to have a stuttering-centric view of reality; that is, they appear to believe that all bad things exhibited and experienced by the person who stutters begin with and are exacerbated by stuttering. Simply put, the shoulders of stuttering are neither strong nor broad enough to carry the weight of so much human misery, discontent, and suffering! And this point must be made clear to both the teen and his or her family—for example, a slow-to-warm-up teen, one who takes his or her time to meet and greet people, appropriately respond to novelty—is not going to suddenly become gregarious and extroverted merely because he or she becomes more fluent. Yes, becoming more fluent should not hurt the situation, but will increasing someone's fluency cure or solve problematic temperament characteristics? I don't think so.

Finally, the chapter suggests that the teens' parents be brought into the arena when treating teens that stutter. Parents of teens, in our opinion and experience, still may have a role in encouraging, discouraging, facilitating, or interfering with treatment. After all, in most cases, the teen still lives with the parent and much of the child element, noted above, exhibited by the teen is still very much an issue between parent and child. Of course, as with younger children, parental involvement with the treatment of teens who stutter may be minimal, moderate, or considerable, depending on the teenage client's individual circumstances. No one size fits all here, but what we are saying is to give strong consideration, for every teen who stutters, to how the parents *may* or can facilitate or interfere with the teen's progress in treatment. For example, a mother and/or father, who routinely look on (even if they say explicitly say nothing to the teen) in apparent sadness, shock, horror, or worry when their child "is having trouble" speaking, is a parent who needs the clinician's help to minimize such behaviors. For as long as the child clearly feels that he or she is disappointing, upsetting, worrying, or shocking the parents with his or her stuttering, he or she will continue to physically tense, struggle, push, and so on to "try not to stutter," exacerbating at the least and perpetuating at the worst the problem. Parents can and do still have an influence on the teen who stutters. However, it is fair to say that the amount and nature of parents' influence on teens who stutter is probably different than it is with children who stutter. And while the challenge of assessing and treating teens who stutter may be somewhat greater than it is with children, there is no question that it is just as satisfying to the teen and the clinician alike and can be, as I said in the second edition of this book, an effort that makes a significant difference in the teenager's life.

5

Remediation: Adults Who Stutter

The General Lay of the Land

The Past Many Times Influences the Present

Individuals who still stutter in the latter years of high school and beyond qualify as *adult people who stutter*. While some will have received no formal therapy of any kind, most will have previously received partially to completely unsuccessful speech and language therapy in addition to a wide variety of other forms of remediation, for example, hypnotherapy, transcendental meditation, primal scream therapy, traditional forms of psychotherapy or psychoanalysis, pharmaceuticals, or specialized academic or vocational counseling. On rare occasions, you may be the *first* professional who evaluates and remediates an adult who stutters, but these adults are the exception rather than the rule. Naturally, a history of past therapy in the presence of continued stuttering means that the adult who stutters may have legitimate reasons for doubting your (or any other clinician's) ability to help him or her at this point in their life. These doubts, whether explicitly or implicitly expressed, may threaten the SLP, especially when many such professionals have their own self-doubts regarding their ability to help adults who stutter. Clearly, SLPs who attempt to remediate adults who stutter have their work cut out for them; however, it is just as clear that adults who stutter can be helped—they can be assisted in learning how to speak more fluently and leading lives that are more enjoyable, comfortable, and productive on both personal and professional levels.

Habitual Inappropriate Behavior May Feel More "Normal" Than Novel, Appropriate Behavior (Subtitle: Better to Deal with a Known Devil Than an Unknown Angel)

In addition to the doubts are the client's relatively *habituated* attitudes, speech behaviors, and beliefs relating to stuttering in specific and speech in general. Indeed, the adult who stutters may know that his or her stuttering is inappropriate, a major handicap, a personal and professional hindrance, or the like but for them, the atypical (stuttering) has become, over the years, typical. Thus, dealing with the devil that is known is often more attractive than risk dealing with an unknown angel. Better to stick with what one knows and is albeit grudgingly familiar with than to risk the uncertainty of trusting in unknown pie in the sky. These are not beliefs unique to adults who stutter but are part of the human condition; since these adults are human, one can expect them to feel the same.

The habituation that adult people who stutter often exhibit implies that their stuttering and related concerns will be fairly resistant to change. This is because adults who stutter, like all adults, spend many years developing their own personal behavior (neither Rome nor an adult's personal behavioral repertoire was built in a day). They are, like you and I, most comfortable with their present behavior—the maladaptive as well as adaptive elements—because it is what they *know* best and routinely perform. It *feels* like them, and any change in their behavior "doesn't feel right," doesn't feel like them. Whether an adult who stutters exhibits speech behavior that is appropriate or not, it is the behavior that the adult who stutters *routinely* produces, it is this behavior that feels, looks, and sounds most like him or her. This is the behavior that seems most natural since it is most typically produced even though it is atypical of what others produce! Perhaps the naturalness of and familiarity with his or her own behavior is why the adult who stutterers presents the SLP with something of a Catch-22 situation: Clients may ask the clinician to stop their stuttering but they do not as readily request that the SLP help change their means of speaking, reacting, feeling, or thinking! And, of course, to do one (i.e., "stop my stuttering") without the other (i.e., "change my speaking, reacting, feeling, or thinking behavior") is a bit like trying to stop smoking without giving up cigarettes!

Levels of Emotionality

A client's possible *doubts* in *therapeutic effectiveness* as well as *resistance to change* may also be coupled with rather high levels of emotionality concerning the problem. Indeed, for many listeners, it is the apparent *emotionality* of the adult who stutters—the apparent nervousness, uneasiness, lack of self-confidence, excessive cautioness, unsure-of-oneself or self-deprecating quality—that is the hallmark of adults who stutter (see Woods & Williams, 1971). We all should, from time to time, engage in periods of self-assessment and self-scrutiny in attempts to change inappropriate facets of our behavior. However, such self-assessment should not be confused with continual, chronic bouts of self-deprecation where we become not our own best friend but our own worst enemy.

We cannot count the number of times we have been told by well-intended (non)professionals outside (as well as inside) the field of communication disorders that such and such an adult who stutters "just needs to get more self-confidence (or be less nervous or more relaxed) and then he or she won't stutter." While there may be some truth in this advice for some adults who stutter, it is obviously an overly simplistic solution to an extremely complex problem. Besides, if such suggestions worked, there would be far fewer adults who stutter than there are. Further, if lack of confidence caused stuttering, the prevalence of stuttering would be far greater than the 1 percent we typically observe! We believe that the emotionality of the adult who stutters is something that should be dealt with by the SLP; however, too many times this dealing is either nonexistent, misdirected, superficial or too far beyond the bounds of the SLP's training and experience, or simply not relevant to the problem(s) of the adult who stutters.

The SLP May Have to Encourage Those Who Are Discouraged.   Finally, after the doubts, relative resistance to change, and related emotional concerns, the SLP may also find that the adult person who stutters is someone who, on one level or another, is *discouraged*. Adults who stutter (and who could blame them?) may be discouraged that they do not talk like others, that speech is not as automatic for them as for others, that they may never talk like they see other people do. They may also be discouraged that they have thoughts they'll never be able to contribute to conversations because of their stuttering or that their stuttering makes them unacceptably different from their friends and associates. Like their doubts regarding your ability to help, their discouragement with themselves and their behavior must be addressed by the SLP and somehow mitigated if therapy if is to stand a chance of being successful.

Cautious Optimism Is Not the Same as Pessimism

Thus, we approach the adult who stutters with caution but with optimism as well. We believe that the SLP can appreciably help adults who stutter, but we also know that this is no easy task where success will come quickly. The therapy will require continued review on our part and an ever-watchful eye on those aspects of therapy we should modify, terminate, or introduce. If we can begin therapy with adults who stutter knowing what we know as well as what we don't know, we have a better likelihood of helping the adult who stutters change in the long term. We realize, of course, that the adult problem with stuttering differs in both degree and kind from that presented by younger people who stutter. And we also know that these differences in the problem create differences in our procedure because the clinical problem generally dictates the clinical procedure.

Problem Dictates Procedure

Late Onset

In Chapter 2 we discussed the diagnosis and evaluation of people who stutter and stutterings and do not intend to reiterate this discussion in this space. However, there are a few nuances to the evaluation of adults who stutter that should be mentioned prior to the description of remediation. It will be recalled that stuttering has been described as a disorder of childhood (e.g., Beech & Fransella, 1968; Bloodstein, 1995); that is, it has its origins in the developing child. Thus, adults who tell the SLP that their stuttering just began last year when they were a senior in high school or just after they got married and so forth, are adults who do not have what we would consider a run-of-the-mill stuttering problem. Earlier in this book we described adults who have a relatively late onset of stuttering as having *acquired* rather than *developmental* stuttering. Adult "stutterers" who report such late onset of stuttering need careful assessment, a second opinion from another qualified SLP, and perhaps a routine medical or psychological evaluation (oftentimes acquired stuttering follows neurological, physical, or psychosocial trauma). We have sometimes been the fools who have rushed into places where angels or at least wiser heads feared to tread, but fortunately we have learned some things from these "rushes to judgment." One of the things we have learned is to be cautious, careful and reasonably deliberate with regard to remediating adults who stutter when their stutterings began in late adolescence or adulthood.

Similarities to Other Problems

A similar but different issue relates to the overlap in the adult population between stuttering, organic-neurological, and psychosocial problems. That is, some stutterings or stuttering-like behavior have organic-neurological or psychosocial origins and do not fall into the category of problem (stuttering) that this book is attempting to deal with. For instance, some adults with certain types of apraxic disorders (e.g., Messert, Collins, & Wertz, 1978; Rosenbek, 1978), organic brain damage (e.g., Ackermann et al., 1996; Helm-Estabrooks, 1999), or psychosocial adjustment problems (Baumgartner, 1999) have stuttering-like behavior, but this does not mean that they are similar to people who begin to stutter in childhood. Conversely, a person who actually stutters may get referred to a physician, particularly a neurologist, because his or her excessive eye blinking and facial grimaces are thought to be indicative of Tourette's syndrome. Some of these adults who stutter may even exhibit nonverbal behavior when *not* speaking, but careful observation suggests that when this happens (nonverbal gestures without overt speech), they may be either silently rehearsing what they are about to say or "talking to themselves" about things that have previously happened.

Likewise, some individuals have deep-seated psychoemotional problems that appear to relate to their speech hesitations. Dealing with these two classes of individuals—adults who stutter with either psychoemotional or organic-neurological etiology—as if they are typical people who stutter does not appear to be a good policy. Indeed, the ability to know when and how to refer these individuals to appropriate agencies or professionals is a skill worthy of development.

Referrals from Employers

Last, some adults who stutter may be referred to us by their employers. For example, an up-and-coming young salesperson who stutters may be told by the employer indirectly or directly, that advancement (or raises) will be determined by improvement in the salesperson's speech fluency. After discussing this situation with the adult client and directly asking the client if we can discuss this situation with the employer, we may ask the client to have the employer get in contact with us. When we make contact with the employer, we discuss the employer's perception of the client and the client's problem(s). During this conversation we try to impart to the employer basic information regarding stuttering and see how receptive he or she is to such information. We promise no rose gardens, but we do tell the employer that we are positively supportive of clients in their attempts to assist themselves. We try to determine how realistic (e.g., expected length of treatment program), supportive, and understanding the employer is with regard to the client, the client's feelings, and the client's problems.

In some cases, we have referred the client elsewhere or declined services because we thought that the situation was untenable in terms of successful therapeutic outcome (e.g., the employer was putting unreasonable demands on the client and wanted them fulfilled in a very brief period of time). Obviously, the door to our clinic swings both ways and our services remain open to this client, but I explain that given present conditions, therapy else-where or at a later date would seem most appropriate. Once again, some kinda help is the kinda help adults who stutter can do without. In essence, we, as SLPs, have to continually see to it that we become part of the solution rather than part of the problem. We may be ready and willing to help but if the client isn't presently helpable, for whatever the reason, then declining or waiting on services or referral elsewhere may be the best as well as only approach. However, before we delve further into the specifics of treatment for stuttering, to get some overview of the situation, we should, briefly examine the ABCs of stuttering and one clinician's attempt to simultaneously deal with them.

A (Affect), B (Behavior), C's (Cognition) of Stuttering

In the clinical literature in the area of stuttering, one can find, increasing discussion (e.g., Kully & Langevin, 1999) of the interplay or interaction between A (Affect), B (Behavior), and C (Cognition) (see Figure 5.1, adapted from Yaruss, 1998a, where the author nicely shows relation between etiology, impairment, ABC reaction, disability, and handicap of stuttering). Likewise, as Neilson (1999) points out, many modern-day treatments for adults who stutter involve attending to cognitive processes as well as behavioral change. While some therapies for stuttering emphasize one aspect of the ABC trilogy (e.g., behavior), sev-eral emphasize an integrated approach (e.g., Ramig & Bennett, 1997). In particular, in this writer's opinion, the treatment approach of Jan Bouwen (1999), an SLP who works mainly with teenagers and adults who stutter in at the University of Rotterdam (The Netherlands), nicely exemplifies the melding of the ABCs of stuttering. Whether Bouwen's treatment is more or less effective than other forms of treatment is *not* the point here. Rather, Bouwen's approach is described because it is a good exemplar of treatments that take all three aspects (A, B, and C) into consideration.

Bouwen describes his treatment goals, with older people who stutter, as a five-step progress:

1. May stutter (*mental* permission to stutter)
2. Dare to stutter (*emotional* acceptance that stuttering will occur)
3. I may use the technique (*mental* permission to use *behavioral* change)
4. I dare to use the technique (*emotional* acceptance that technique will be used)
5. I want to and can use the technique to speak as normally as possible (*mental* permission to make *behavioral* change).

Bouwen reportedly achieves these goals through individual as well as group treat-ment and appears to believe that the three parts—affect, behavior, and cognition—are each important but interdependent, requiring change within each part to achieve lasting change in the whole. He appears to believe that as long as the person who stutters is afraid of his or her stuttering, the person may have minimal confidence in the behavioral technique. As long as adults who stutter remain afraid, Bouwen suggests, they will "panic" when the stut-tering "returns," as it often does with adults, and their panic will undermine their ability to resume using the technique(s) they have learned. Bouwen appears to believe that by mak-ing the behavior and as a result of this emotion "opvallend" (obvious, striking or conspic-

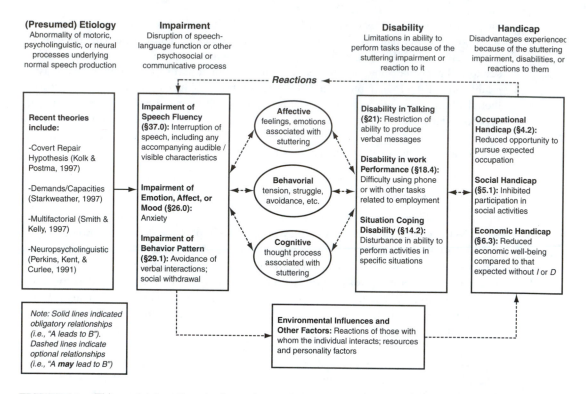

(Presumed) Etiology	Impairment	Disability	Handicap
Abnormality of motoric, psycholinguistic, or neural processes underlying normal speech production	Disruption of speech-language function or other psychosocial or communicative process	Limitations in ability to perform tasks because of the stuttering impairment or reaction to it	Disadvantages experienced because of the stuttering impairment, disabilities, or reactions to them

FIGURE 5.1. This model describes the "experience of the stuttering disorder" in reference to 1980 World Health Organization guidelines. For our purposes, this graphic is primarily displayed to show some of the possible ABC (affect, behavior, cognition) relationships that may exist with stuttering, and their relationship to the "impairment" (actual speech disruption) and "disability" (limitations in abilities to perform some tasks). After Yaruss (1998a, Figure 1, p. 254), with permission.

uous) in the most difficult speaking situation, he can help the person who stutters gain control over his or her feelings and control in a wider variety of speaking situations.

Clearly, without appropriately conducted, collected, and analyzed treatment efficacy research/data, no one knows whether Bouwen's (or any other clinician's) sequence of goals and/or the goals themselves are salient to long-term improvement in stuttering in adults. However, on the surface, Bouwen's approach does make apparent how feelings, thoughts, and behavior *might* interact. Clearly, the role of cognition in human emotions is quite well appreciated in the area of psychology (e.g., Burns, 1980), and we see no reason to believe that people who stutter don't similarly use cognition in ways that influence their emotions. Neilson (1999) discusses what she calls a "rapprochement" between behaviorally oriented and cognitively oriented treatments for stuttering (see Guitar, 1998, for excellent attempts and discussion of melding behavioral with traditional, more cognitively oriented treatments). We can only hope that the future will mean that cognitive-behavioral intervention for teens and adults who stutter will become an increasing reality for more and more people who stutter.

Humans feel, humans think, and humans behave. This is the reality of the human condition. And if we make the reasonable assumption that people who stutter share the same human condition that everybody else does and that interactions may occur between these events—affect, behavior, and cognition—for people who do not stutter, we must also assume, I would think, that such interactions are possible for people who stutter. Indeed, it would seem that the burden of proof is on those who view these three events as independent of one another, as isolates rather than as interdependent, overlapping circles in a Venn diagram or ballentine, freely interacting and influencing one or another, sometimes in ways that facilitate and sometimes in ways that interfere.

Group Therapy for Adults Who Stutter

Modern-day emphasis on behavioral modification, structured individual therapy, individual instructional plans, and "bottom-line" mentality (i.e., exactly how long will it take for the client to get cured and how much will it cost), has led to a movement away from group therapy with adults who stutter. Unfortunately, this emphasis on getting results as quickly as possible means that long-term change is somewhat an afterthought. We believe that this is unfortunate, because group therapy for adults who stutter can be a positive experience and one that significantly contributes to long-term change as well as supports adults' continued efforts to maintain change once it has been established.

Adult Fluency Groups

In these groups, adults who stutter can share past as well as present experiences, feelings, attitudes, and beliefs with others who share the same concerns, that is, adults who stutter. The group provides a nonjudgmental, sheltering atmosphere whereby the adult who stutters can say what he or she wants to do about his or her problems and feelings toward same and others will at least listen, even if they do not always agree! Through a group, adults who stutter come to learn that they are not alone in the world with this problem, that others share their troubles and feel much the same way they do. Groups provide speaking opportunities for people who might otherwise go literally for days or weeks without verbally communicating to other nonprofessionals.

Client Reluctance to Participate in Group Therapy

Conducting group therapy for adults who stutter is, however, no easy task. First and foremost, the disorder itself interferes with the very medium the clinician needs to use in group therapy: talking! If it were easy to talk for people who stutter, they would not be coming to you for therapy in the first place. Thus, for you, the leader of the group, there are periods of discouragement when it appears no one wants to talk or contribute to group discussions. However, with patience, time, and support on your part, even the most reluctant to speak can be encouraged to talk and contribute to the group. Second, based on our experience recruiting adults who stutter to group therapy, I think I can safely say that group therapy, to the average adults who stutter, appears to be something of an anathema. For sure, they may want therapy but only the individual kind. Coming together with a group of people who also stutter seems far less than what they want. They appear reluctant to even see or hear another person who stutters; the reasons for this reluctance seemingly varying with each client. The following is but a *partial* listing of reasons: (1) some have strong fears about their stuttering, fears that they may be reluctant to deal with, explore, and expose in a group setting; (2) some seem reticent to see themselves in others; that is, they realize that the stuttering problems of others may mirror their own problems, and they resist having to face this reality; (3) some may deny or avoid facing the reality that their feelings, beliefs, and attitudes may be contributing to their problem, a reality clearly illuminated in a group setting but one that may be deemphasized in an individual setting where modification of speech is primary; (4) some seem to believe that by hearing and seeing others who stutter that they will get worse or stutter more or regress; and (5) some appear to believe that by seeing and hearing others stutter that the stuttering "may rub off" on them, that they may catch or pick up more stuttering. Actually, (5) is just another way that clients state (4).

Logistics of Group Therapy

We have reached a point in our experience whereby, if at all possible, we request that all adults who stutter attend weekly group sessions (exceptions: the adult person who stutters who speaks English as a second language, has receptive language problems, or a significant enough hearing problem to make the group situation an extremely difficult one for him or her to understand). Attendance in our group permits us to monitor the progress in individual therapy of adult people who stutter and the specific nature of their speech and related problems. We have found through experience that the ideal group size is about seven people, but we have had as many as twelve or thirteen and as few as two or three. We try to keep the day of the week and time of the day fixed throughout the year; generally, a late afternoon or early evening time works out best. We have also found that an odd block of time, say one hour and fifteen minutes, allows people to arrive late and leave early but still get in about 30 to 45 minutes of group therapy; however, sometimes one-hour sessions are all that can be arranged. With one-hour sessions, however, the SLP must learn to adjust to the fact that many clients will come and go in 30 minutes or less. Whatever the case, the SLP must keep on keeping on because, particularly in the beginning stages of establishment of a group, attendance may be erratic; it is the SLP's weekly presence and support that will be the foundation around which the superstructure of the treatment group will be built.

Composition of Group Members

If at all possible, groups of adults who stutter should be composed of a mix of individuals, for example, college students, laborers, executives, secretaries, and so forth. By forming such "mixed" groups both you and your clients learn how stuttering cuts across all walks of life and how it influences different people in different as well as similar ways. Such variety also insures that student clinicians, if you work in such a setting, get experience observing and managing individuals from different backgrounds. This is a much more realistic experience and good preparation for their professional careers after graduation. Thus, the

SLP working within the confines of a university clinic is going to have to make many different "outreaches," at many different times, to various agencies in his or her area to encourage the type of referrals that will lead to such diversity of clientele.

Group Therapy by Itself

It is possible for an adult who stutters to receive group therapy and nothing else. This is particularly true for the marginally disfluent adult who stutters whose level of concern regarding his or her speech does not seem warranted by either the nature, severity, or frequency of presenting speech problem. Through exposure to other members in a group, these individuals quickly realize that the frequency, nature, and severity of their speech problems are quite different and considerably less than that of others. Sometimes even the most patient, clear presentation of a SLP cannot help them come to this realization as quickly and as surely as an hour spent interacting with three or four adults who stutter with moderate-to-severe stuttering! Thus, minimally disfluent clients also benefit from learning that some of their communication concerns are shared by others but that objectively they have less reason for concern. Also subtle, as well as not so subtle, group pressures ("Why are you in the group? You don't stutter.") influence minimally disfluent speakers to reconsider the level and nature of their concern, to think about their problems in light of external reality. And, after all, getting our clients to think and change behavior and related issues is what our therapy is all about.

The SLP as Group Leader

None of the preceding, however, should be taken to mean that group therapy with adults who stutter is a panacea—it will not make a silk purse out of a sow's ear. This becomes obvious immediately because the same problems with tardiness, attendance, and failure to do homework assignments that plague individual therapy bedevil group therapy. The SLP who leads a therapy group must wear many hats and at times be a little bit of all things to most all people. Now a motivator, now an organizer, now a talker, now a listener. At times this SLP group leader must be rather authoritative in manner, at others very much laissez-faire, and at still other times turn the leadership of the group, albeit temporarily, to a member of the group. As mentioned above, the group leader is the common thread that runs from one year of the group to the next, the person who provides the anchor for and continuity of the group as individual clients fade in and out. The SLP group leader must be sufficiently structured to get and keep each group going but be prepared to backtrack and discard all such structured plans if group behavior so dictates. The classic opening line of public speakers that they have prepared the talk but after meeting the audience or viewing the situation have thrown away their notes is true when running a group for adults who stutter. Be prepared, but also prepare to do things you haven't prepared for!

Mechanics of Versus Feelings About Speech

During the group, the group leader must tread a thin line between dealing with what clients call *the mechanics of speech* and *feelings about speech*. When there is too much group discussion about attitudes, beliefs, and feelings about speech, some clients—whether they should or not—seem to lose interest and feel that the group is becoming too esoteric, non-substantive, and of minimal relevance to *their* specific problem(s). On the other hand, when there is too much discussion of this or that client's or of all clients' specific speech *mechanics* or behaviors, some clients may feel that we are slighting *their* specific problem(s) or their personal beliefs, feelings, or attitudes. Indeed, besides the mechanics-versus-feelings dichotomy, there is also the general-versus-specific dichotomy that must be addressed by the SLP. The SLP must address specific individual concerns but continually relate them to general group issues; conversely, the SLP must try to help all group members see general or common themes but continually try to relate them specific individual concerns. Perhaps a treatment group can best be defined as a collection of individuals whose understanding of common concerns must be translated through their own individual needs.

As many adults who stutter have told me, in one way or another, "I'm more than just a mouth and larynx . . . I'm more than just speech, I'm also a person who feels and thinks." Thus, the group leader is constantly shifting within as well as between group sessions from discussions of *attitudes* to discussions of *speech behavior* and back again. The SLP continually shifts from discussions of how a particular individual's concerns relate to general or common concerns among the group members to talking about a particular individual's specific problem and how it can be best addressed by that person. It is no place for those who have a low tolerance for ambiguity. Group therapy, therefore, is no place for the faint of heart; it is no situation for the professional who finds it difficult to juggle more than two balls at once! We are convinced, however, based on our experience with adults who stutter, that such groups are beneficial to the client and clinician and should be given serious consideration in the development of a therapy program for adults who stutter.

Individual Therapy for Adults Who Stutter: Starting Up

First Impressions

We previously mentioned the impact that first impressions have on young children and parents we deal with in therapy (as an old ad stated, "you never get a second chance to make a first impression"). First impressions also impact adults who stutter, but the means by which these impressions are made differ with the older client. We hope that it is obvious that our attempts to convey positive first impressions to the adult should not be a show, a forced procedure or performance or a hype of the wonders of ourselves and our approach. Most adults can easily detect a show of insincerity or a "sales pitch." Rather, most adults who stutter seek a SLP that demonstrates: (1) an understanding of the problem, (2) a willingness to listen, (3) an ability to help, and (4) the integrity and confidence to be honest. It is important to the adult who stutters that the SLP make apparent, right from the beginning, his or her *understanding* of stuttering in general, and the adult's problem in specific. Reasonable, clear, and cautious answers to the clients' questions about cause, symptoms, and the like help establish the SLP's credentials (ethos) in this area. It is also important to the adult client that we *listen* to his or her individual story, concerns, beliefs, and feelings (such listening does not imply agreement with all of the client's beliefs but it does imply acceptance of same). You may have heard similar stories before, but you haven't heard this person's particular version and it behooves you not to give the impression that you have. It is also important to the adult client that we make explicit our willingness and ability to *help* (without overly exaggerating this ability).

While the client wants the SLP to give signs of support as well as indications that therapy will be of some help, it is important to the client that the SLP be *honest* with him or her. We should make it clear to the client if we are guarded in our belief concerning the client's prognosis for positive change in speaking and related attitudes, beliefs, and feelings. Some clients will need more. Some clients will need some specific concrete, tangible, up-front "proof," no matter how temporary, that things can get better, that they can improve their speech. Demonstrating to the adult client that his or her speech can be changed, even through an artificial means, for example, metronome, choral reading, or whispering, can be used to show that: (1) the adult client's speech disfluency is malleable, it's not a fixed, never-changing property etched in stone for all time; (2) that speech fluency, given certain circumstances is obtainable; and (3) that you, as a professional SLP can assist him or her in the modification of speech. However, it should be noted that giving early, concrete examples to an adult who stutters that change is possible in his or her speech is not without its problems, and these need to be discussed.

We Are Guides, Not Magicians. As mentioned before, when remediating stuttering we use the orientation of *helping with* rather than *curing* the speaking problems of the person who stutters. We want to clearly and emphatically convey to the adult that our role is one of a guide rather than a magician. Furthermore, while we are not Merlin, neither is whispering, for example, the silver bullet the average adult who stutters seeks. Part of being honest with the client is repeatedly and clearly explaining to him or her that quick changes in fluency are generally followed by equally quick relapses, and that such procedures as the metronome and the like will not be the principal means by which we will assist him or her to change speech and related behavior. We try to make it clear that "our technique" begins and ends with *their* involvement, engagement, and effort. We emphasize to the adult who stutters that procedures like the metronome, if we use them, are used *merely* as a means to show that change is possible. Leading the adult client—or any client for that matter—to dream the impossible dream that we can quickly cure him or her of stuttering (while the adult who stutters passively stands around and watches and hopes to absorb "the cure" through osmosis) is, in my mind, the ultimate cruelty, because time will show that such a dream cannot be realized. In a nutshell, therapy helps those who help themselves!

The short-term gain of wowing the client with clinical legerdemain is counterbalanced by the long-term pain of reality. The quick cure is the domain of the clinical mountebanks and represents procedure that the SLP of integrity and sincerity will want to avoid like the plague. Quick cures for long-standing, human behavior disorders are not compatible with the present state of the human condition. In short, we want to provide the client from the very first meeting—usually a diagnostic evaluation—with as positive a therapy atmosphere as possible. We want to convey an attitude that change appears possible and desirable rather than deceiving the client that we are able to change lead into gold! Our field needs competent guides willing to stay the course not glib alchemists who fold their tent and move on before the inevitable relapse occurs.

How Many Times per Week?

Assuming the client agrees and we think it appropriate, the client begins therapy. And, as discussed before, the first question we ask is: How often and how long? This is, of course, no easy question to answer but hopefully we have told the client in the initial evaluation (see Chapter 2) the approximate time line of the therapy. We must then square the ideal with the real: Therapy every day may be best, at least for rapid behavioral change, but our clinical program and the demands on our time may only permit one hour per week. We recognize that the intensity and/or frequency of speech therapy (see Gregory, 1978) may be of primary positive significance to our client's improvement; however, while the jury is still out regarding the relative merits of *intensive* (e.g., once or twice per day for three weeks) versus *extensive* (e.g., once a week for twelve months) therapy, our experience indicates that *lasting*, *long-term* change of stuttering and related matters may take much longer than we or our clients would like. This is especially true, in our opinion, for adults who stutter. As we said earlier, our observations tell us that *intensive* therapy provides quicker changes in speech behavior but insufficient time for meaningful change in associated attitudes, beliefs, and feelings which, if left unchanged, may impede long-term recovery. Conversely, our observations suggest to us that *extensive* therapy takes longer to achieve changes in speech behavior but provides the needed time to change associated attitudes, beliefs, and feelings that, if when changed, may facilitate long-term recovery. These are empirical issues, however, and must await the sort of careful, meticulous therapy evaluation procedures advocated by individuals like Ingham (1984, pp. 433-464). Whatever the case, given the time and space considerations of most clinician's clinical realities, adults who stutter are probably most apt to be remediated on a once- or twice-a-week basis (generally one group and one individual session per week), and the usual timeframe (start to end) runs from three to twelve months.

Trial Therapy

Before we begin any therapy regimen, particularly one that looks like it may be protracted, we inform our clients that we plan to initiate what we call *trial therapy*. With adults this trial period usually lasts from three to six weeks. We inform the client of the beginning and end of this trial and that a judgment will be made somewhere between the middle and end of this period regarding the continuation of therapy as well as the nature of same. We emphasize, several times, that the client does not have to produce total change for continuation, but it must be apparent that change seems possible or that the client is moving in the right direction. We stress the positive but inform clients that before they or we get involved in an extensive therapy program, it must be apparent that the situation warrants the necessary time and effort. It is not unusual in these situations for clients to want to hurry up and get therapy whether they are ready and willing to expend the necessary time and effort. For some adults who stutter there is little connection between their *goal* (more fluent speech) and the *means* (time, effort, and work) by which this must be accomplished. It is up to the SLP to explain this connection. For these reasons, and more, the author wants to emphasize: *The SLP should not be stampeded into untenable therapy situations.* Explain to the adult client that his or her talk about change is necessary (and appreciated) but not sufficient. The client needs to understand you'll be much more impressed by his or her behavior, doing something, and actions than all the verbal expressions of good intentions (actions do speak louder than words). Conversely, the SLP should try to recognize a client's sincere and honest desire to commit the necessary personal resources to obtain the type of desired therapy outcome. Simply put, it takes effort, time, and thought to change behavior, and you must make it clear to the adult client that you recognize this difficulty and will support him or her in his attempts. Although it is not easy to spot the difference between sincere motivation to change and "talk is cheap" forms of motivation, it is an ability the SLP needs to work at developing.

Bringing this discussion to a close, if we find that the client is able to make the necessary effort and commitment and we believe we can assist him or her in modification of stuttering, we begin in earnest. The first step, not unlike what we do with direct treatment of older children and teenagers, is to assist the client in quickly and accurately identifying instances of stuttering and related behavior. The emphasis here, as elsewhere, is on the inappropriate *strategies* and *behavior* the client employs to interfere with fluent speech. For the most part, the problem lies in the strategies the client employs and not in the sounds and syllables the client produces.

Individual Therapy for Adults Who Stutter: Identification Phase

Identifying and Physically Feeling (In)appropriate Behavior

We firmly believe two things about achieving *lasting* change in stuttering: (1) people who stutter need to be able to quickly, correctly, and objectively identify when and what they do when they stutter; and (2) that most of this ability to identify must relate to the physical *feelings* (not emotions) of speech movements and muscular tensions. Unless they can do these two interrelated things—quickly and correctly identify the appropriateness of their behavior and physically feel it—we think it is difficult for adults who stutter to *lastingly* change their stuttering. That is, how can individuals change stuttering when they cannot identify when and how they stutter and what it feels like? As we'll see, hearing and seeing these behaviors are important adjuncts to identification; but in the final analysis *physically feeling* these behaviors is key since, as we've said before, by the time the person who stutters sees or hears the inappropriate behavior, it has already happened. Those who stutter need a sensory modality—conscious proprioception, kinesthesia, and so forth—that is associated with the antecedents or least the concurrent speech-language production *processes* of their behavior and not the *outcome* of those processes, that is, acoustics.

Many adults who stutter attempt to improve their fluency without ever becoming aware of what *they do* that interferes with their speaking, but the *long-term* success of these attempts is not overwhelming. Indeed, one of the first things we find out in the previously mentioned trial therapy period is whether the client is ready, willing, and able to quickly and correctly identify the physical feelings associated with his or her instances of stuttering. While, as we'll see, identification—just like modification—requires the adult who stutters to simultaneously monitor the *manner* as well as *content* of speech, the SLP can structure the speaking tasks, at least in the beginning, to make this simultaneous monitoring easier to do.

"Devices" Used with Identification

While physical feelings of stuttering are our ultimate goal, we still must, at this stage of therapy, use devices that give the client auditory or visual information: audio tape recorder, an audio-videotape recorder (with associated television monitor), computer software that converts the microphone signal to a image on computer monitor, magnifying glass, mirrors, language-master-type tape recorder and/or player, oscilloscopes (signal generated by microphone fed to scope), flashlight with pushbutton on-off switch, clicker (like those used by children around Halloween), or any other device that quickly and clearly provides a visual or auditory stimulus for the client's observation. Technology, however, is very rapidly developing in this area as witnessed by the development of interactive computer software and "biofeedback devices." Unfortunately, most computer applications—for example, Visi-Pitch (Kay Elemetrics) or Speech Viewer (IBM)—while quite useful, are based on the microphone signal and not on directly related to physical behavior or feelings. Conversely, devices such as the electroglottograph (EGG) and surface eletromyography are much closer to the actual movements and tensions of speech muscles and would, therefore, seem to have a great deal of potential for quickly and accurately informing the client regarding the physical aspects of speech behavior. However, EGG and EMG technology is still not at a level readily available to the average SLP. Perhaps, where available, devices that portray acoustic information about speech production could be initially used with the person who stutters. Then, once the client gets more comfortable and capable of identifying acoustic aspects of speech, he or she could move to such devices as the EGG that more directly measure or monitor speech production activity.

Adults' Reactions to Identification

Whatever the nature of these devices, they can be used in a variety of ways. For example, the client and clinician can each employ flashlights or penlights, with on-off pushbuttons, with the object or goal begin to see who—the client or clinician—can push the button first when an instance of stuttering occurs. In the beginning, this procedure works best if the SLP decides only to identify more obvious instances of stuttering, which generally are those that are longer and are repetitive in nature, for example, longer sound/syllable repetition and monosyllabic whole-word repetitions. One word of caution: It is not always easy, however, to get individuals who stutter, particularly adults with a long history of the problem, to listen and view themselves on tape. This is no small concern and must be, with some adults, approached with sensitivity, thoughtfulness, and concern for the client's feelings. On the other hand, no one ever said any of this process was going to be easy for the client (or clinician), and at times some degree of emotionality and self-recrimination must take place in order for therapy to move forward.

Likewise, some adult clients do not react favorably to clickers, flashlights, or other indicators used to "highlight" or make more apparent or conspicuous their instances of stuttering (see Siegel, 1970 for further discussion of "highlighting"). Adults who stutter may say that this procedure makes them nervous, self-conscious, feel hurried, or other statements to the effect that they are reacting to this aspect of identification with feelings of discomfort. These feelings—which may be much more central to the person who stutters than his or her recognition of instances of stuttering—should be discussed with the client, and the SLP should try to make explicit his or her understanding of these feelings and reactions. That is, the SLP should neither ignore nor downplay these feelings and reactions, but discuss their nature and their possible causes. The SLP should explain his or her appreciation for the unpleasantness of such emotions. ("I know that hearing this clicker every time you stutter is unpleasant and frustrating, but this is one way I have of helping you help yourself identify behaviors you produce that get in the way of fluent speech.")

Amount of Time Spent on Identification per Session

In the beginning do not use these identification procedures for extended periods of time (fifteen to twenty minutes at a stretch); instead, break them up into smaller blocks of say three to five minutes with a few minutes' rest in between to discuss possible reasons for success or failure. You can gradually increase the time spent in identifying stuttering and related behavior as clients get more and more adept at recognizing instances of stuttering, as they begin to get better than you or beat you at identifying quickly and accurately their instances of stuttering. Likewise, more and more time can be spent on identification as the client consistently identifies the stuttering during the middle or toward the beginning of its occurrence.

By no means, however, devote an entire session to identification or week in and week out to identification. Mix it up with, for example, with discussion of group therapy events. Or, if group therapy is not part of your adult client's regimen, then mention success or lack thereof outside the therapy room, identifying situations that are becoming easier to speak in or still remain difficult. Ask the client if friends, relatives, or associates are commenting on or reacting to any changes in the client's speech or the client's therapy progress (more on this in a moment). Whatever, mix up the content of this therapy hour to avoid boredom and also because identification of instances of stuttering is hard, intense work requiring focused attention, concentration, and effort. Extensive immersion (i.e., all session every session) in this procedure is, in the long run, counterproductive to a successful remediation program.

Three Early Signs of Improvement

We firmly believe that long-term recovery, particularly for adults, requires a *gradual* change in speech and related behavior. As we mentioned earlier in this chapter, sudden improvement is too often followed by sudden relapse. Thus, improvement will not be dramatic, but there are some early signs that are true indicators that improvement is taking place: (1) shortening of the duration of instances of stuttering even though there is little or no change in stuttering frequency—this may or may not be associated with changes in physical tension during speech; (2) individuals in the clients' environment are starting to report to the client and/or the SLP or others that they are noticing an improvement in the clients' speech and related behavior; and (3) relatively consistent identification at the beginning and/or middle of stutterings that may or may not be associated with the client's sometimes spontaneously changing his or her stuttering behavior (this is related to (1)—shortening of the stuttering—but can also lead to changes in the type and frequency of stuttering). When the SLP notices these early signs of improvement, he or she should tell the client. Make it quite apparent to the client—don't let him or her guess—that improvement is apparent and that progress is being made. Don't assume the client sees the improvement you see—explicitly tell the client.

Continuing with Identification

We begin identification in earnest once the client demonstrates a willingness to see, hear, and feel (emphasizing the latter) his or her instances of stuttering (this demonstration need not be one of absolute but of relative willingness). It should be stressed that it is not only important that you know *why* you employ identification but that your adult client also realizes its importance and rationale. Obviously, identifying something is not the same as changing that thing; however, changing something presupposes that the person changing can identify what they want to change (similar to the famous educator/psychologist E. Thorndike's "specificity doctrine"—for example "in order to do something about anything you have to know specifically what you are about," Hilgard & Bower, 1966, p. 45). The accuracy and speed with which such identification is made is also important. Once again, the *mode* of identification (vision versus audition versus physical feeling of physical tensions and movements) needs to be considered. Steps used when employing identification with a client are, therefore, as follows: (1) introduction to the concept; (2) helping the client become more objective and less subjective when identifying his or her instances of stuttering; (3) increasing the client's accuracy with identifying instances of stuttering; and (4) helping the client concentrate on the mode of identification that is most crucial for long-term change in stuttering, that is, feelings of physical tensions, movements, and positions of speech structures.

Accuracy of identification of instances of stuttering has been covered in other sources (for example, Van Riper, 1973, 1974). Basically, identification with adults who stutter involves giving them an opportunity to observe themselves during speech and then asking them to label through voice or gesture each and every time they perceive a target behavior, for example, all sound/syllable repetitions or all sound prolongations that are 1 second or longer in duration. These opportunities, as mentioned above, can be made available through audio or audio-video recordings of the client's speech productions (*off-line* analysis) or during real-time or the actual speech production itself (*on-line* analysis). Off-line analysis, although initial reactions of people who stutter may be negative, is the preferred and generally easiest place to *begin* using identification with adults. Once accuracy of identification during off-line analysis is 80 percent or greater, the SLP can proceed to on-line identification (which we assume has more generalizability to everyday speaking situations). However, as mentioned above, most adult clients have difficulty, at least in the beginning, accurately, objectively, and quickly monitoring their speech productions simultaneously with carrying on a lucid conversation. We might add that clinicians have the same difficulty simultaneously identifying instances of stuttering in the client's speech while at the same time trying to maintain normal conversation with the client. This parallel processing (simultaneously monitoring speech production and maintaining thoughts so that a cogent communication can take place) is a necessary skill the clinician must develop as well as to try to help his or her clients develop.

Off-Line Identification

Off-line analysis is best employed when the SLP has a priori knowledge of all instances of stuttering contained within an audio or an audio-video recording. Several rules apply: (1) Start "away" from the client, (2) begin with audio recordings then video recording of the client, and (3) progress from more obvious or longer, more physical tense stutterings to shorter, less physically tense and less apparent stutterings.

Start "away" from the Client.   First, it is best to start off-line identification "away" from the client; that is, start identifying the stutterings of some other client, preferably an adult. In this way both client and clinician can be objective and say pretty much what they want about the anonymous adult who stutters and his or her stuttering. While the client's objectivity is enhanced by this procedure, he or she also gains experience being a constructively critical listener and observer. To facilitate matters even further, the SLP can analyze this recording in advance and even type up a transcript of the recording (this transcript/recording can be used for several adults who stutter at this stage of therapy). The typed manuscript permits client and SLP to easily compare notes and go back into the taped conversation at precise points. If an on-screen tape counter is not available, tape counter numbers should be tabulated every ten words or so on the manuscript to enhance the clinician's ability to readily go back and forth through the tape recording, instead of wasting time guessing where a particular section of the recording lies on the tape. Most importantly, however, the SLP's a priori listening, analyzing, and tabulating the number and type of stutterings contained on the recording allows the SLP to more fully devote his or her time and attention to the present client's ability to accurately and quickly identify and label instances of stuttering. All too often, the SLP spends precious time in these initial therapy sessions off-line assessing and/or identifying instances of stuttering and thus cannot pay as much attention as needed to the client's difficulties with this task.

Progress from Audio to Audio-Video.   Second, begin by having the client identify his own stutterings on audio rather than audio-video recordings. If audio-video recordings are all that are available, somehow black out or turn off the video portion and only listen to the audio segment. We recommend *beginning* with audio for two basic reasons: (1) A video recording can be a rather confrontational medium, that is, it directly and rather starkly portrays the client's behavior, and some clients, at least in the beginning, simply aren't ready for this sort of reality. They will be, given time and patience on the part of the SLP; however, in the beginning, we recommend sticking with audio recordings alone. This procedure increases the chances that the client will be far less defensive and more objective when listening to him- or herself, at least in the beginning. (2) Visually apparent behavior such as eyeball movement, eyelids blinking, head movement, and facial gestures are more apt to be attended to, in the beginning, by the naive client than auditorily apparent behavior such as sound/syllable repetitions. In essence, until the client becomes more used to observing him- or herself, the auditory medium will take precedence over the visual. While this procedure will not speed up therapy, it will support the SLP's desire that the client become adept at quickly and accurately attending to disfluent speech behavior.

Progress from Obvious to Less Obvious Stutterings.   Third, the SLP should begin identification with longer, more physical tense and auditorily apparent stutterings (these are generally, but not necessarily, sound/syllable repetitions). In essence, this makes the client's task easier in the beginning. Success begets success. As the client quickly and accurately identifies longer, tenser, and more obvious stutterings in his or her speech and the speech of others, the SLP can change the behavior to be identified to those stutterings that are shorter, less tense, and less obvious. It is best to start where success is maximized—this not only helps the client more quickly learn the task but facilitates motivation as well.

While it is important that the client recognize the same *number* or close to the same number of stutterings recognized by the SLP, it is also important that the client recognize the same *type* of stuttering (for example, sound prolongation versus sound/syllable repetition). Perhaps the difference in number of stutterings recognized by client and SLP relates to the fact that the client easily and quickly identifies all sound-syllable repetitions but seemingly misses most sound prolongations. Or perhaps the difference in numbers results from the fact that the client can readily and quickly identify stutterings of 1.0 seconds and longer but misses the shorter stutterings, say 0.5 to 1.0 seconds (it should be noted that stutterings shorter than 0.5 seconds *definitely* exist; but the beginning client, as well as beginning student–clinician, cannot be expected to readily identify such brief stutterings without some experience and/or guided observations). Such problems need to be discussed with the client as well as the reason(s) for such successes and failures and exactly what the client calls stuttering in him- or herself and others. In essence, the SLP needs to be clear regarding the client's relative skill as an identifier of stutterings before embarking on more complex identification. These sorts of conversation between client and SLP—where the client's definition of stuttering and basis for identifying same—can provide the SLP with fascinating insights. It is not uncommon for the client to identify behaviors the SLP "misses," particularly behaviors that are self-produced, because while the SLP's judgment can only be based on audition and vision, the client can also employ physical feelings (e.g., kinesthesia), and these physically feelings may "indicate" stuttering in the absence of any auditory or visually apparent behavior.

Once again, it is very important that the client is clear on the purpose of these procedures; here, as elsewhere, redundancy of instruction will be necessary. It is not bad policy to continue to discuss with the client "What are we doing here?" and "Why do you think we are doing it?" You may be surprised at the response! Obviously, your long-range goals are other than merely getting the client to make quick, accurate identification of stutterings, but does the client realize this? And if the client doesn't understand the ultimate reason for identification, you will have to make this fact explicit. All clients need to be told and periodically reminded that there are short-, medium-, and long-range goals. The client also needs to be clear on the fact—and you need to explicitly tell him or her—that learning is a *gradual* process and the identification step is but one point along the gradual learning curve that leads the client from stuttering to becoming a more normally fluent speaker.

Bridge Between Off-Line and On-Line Identification

It is time to move beyond off-line identification when the client demonstrates relatively accurate off-line identification (e.g., 80% or greater) of most medium-to-long instances of stuttering from a tape-recorded sample of his or her own speech. The client is ready to proceed to the bridge between off-line and on-line analysis. This *bridge* involves using an audio tape recorder or an audio-video cassette recorder that has a pause or instantaneous stop switch, lever, or button on it.

The object of this bridge is the *speed* of identification, which, of course, presupposes accurate identification. Clients are now required to listen to the same audio recordings of their own speech that they accurately identified and to quickly stop the forward movement of the tape or cassette as soon as they perceive the stuttering. Another way this may be done, when the tape recorder lacks a pause button or switch, is to use two flashlights or penlights that have instant on-buttons or perhaps a noise clicker. However it is accomplished, the purpose of these procedures is to help clients develop the necessary rapidity of identification that will serve as the foundation upon which clients rest their ability to rapidly change their ongoing speech behavior. With this procedure clients are reinforced for the quickness of the identification to the point where their stopping of the tape recorder or signaling with a light or sounds happens *before* or as close to the beginning of the stuttering as possible. Once again, SLPs should practice this themselves until reasonably confident that they have the ability to quickly and accurately recognize their client's stuttering. At the risk of redundancy, let me restate the clinical axiom: Practice the same tasks yourself that you ask the client to do in therapy (show don't tell). After sufficient practice with a variety of people who stutter, you will find that you will not have to individually prepare this aspect of therapy; however, some homework, on your part, has to be completed prior to your doing this with your client.

On-Line Identification

Once the client is exhibiting 80 percent or greater success at identifying his or her own stutterings on audio and/or audio-video tape recordings, the SLP can begin to help the client identify stutterings during actual or running conversation (a much harder task). Once again, the SLP wants to start with longer, more physically tense and more obvious stutterings. The SLP is also advised to encourage the client for any and all approximations to accurate identification. That is, the client will not immediately be 100 percent successful in the accurate identification of instances of stuttering (as well as other speech disfluencies), and the client's SLP should realize this and reinforce accordingly. Demonstrate to the client that you understand the difficulty of the task and that you appreciate the client's attempts. In the beginning, keep the conversation simple and relating to topics that client is familiar with but less apparent emotionality, for example, talking about fixing squeaky doors or sticky cabinet drawers rather than asking the boss for a raise.

Specify Stutterings to Be Identified. Depending on the frequency and types of stuttering exhibited by the client, the clinician may be able to clearly target this phase of the identification procedure. That is, the SLP may be able to target for the client the specific types of stuttering (longer versus short, sound prolongations versus sound-syllable repetition) he or she wants the client to attend to and identify. As mentioned above, it is a good general rule to start with longer sound-syllable repetitions; but if sound prolongations predominate, then longer rather than shorter instances are best to start this phase of identification with. Remember that (1) many sounds are produced per seconds (possibly as many as ten or more sounds per second) and (2) it takes the unsophisticated listener, like your client in the beginning of therapy, a little bit of time to decide and identify instances of stuttering. Thus, give the client a break, and target longer, more frequently occurring and more obvious stutterings to begin with. This will insure that he or she has that little bit of extra time necessary to make accurate decisions and sufficient enough chances to make it so that you can reinforce for a variety of approximations to accurate identification. With experience the adult who stutters should be able to perceive shorter and shorter instances of speech disfluency until with practice, he or she can perceive very short instances of stuttering that are 250 msec or less in duration (but probably not much shorter than 180 msec, because that is the average reaction time for most adults on these types of tasks).

The Key: Speed of Identification.   As mentioned above, the adult client's ability to *quickly* stop the tape recorder upon perceiving instances of his or her *own* stuttering serves as the bridge or introduction into on-line identification. On-line analysis involves the quick and accurate identification of instances of stuttering *during* the actual production of speech. As previously mentioned, this is no easy task, since adults who stutter must identify their instances of stuttering simultaneously while conducting a conversation with the SLP. The SLP must be very sensitive to the client's feelings about this "multi-tasking"—that it is difficult—and discuss these feelings with the client. The clinician must also realize that the client may find it very *frustrating* to have his or her thoughts or conversation continually interrupted by on-line identification. Naturally, in the beginning, the client may also feel rushed, pressured, or uncomfortable when so much specific attention is being paid to his or her speech production. Again, the SLP must discuss these feelings and let the client know that the SLP respects them. On the other hand, clinicians must not allow such respect to paralyze them or their client from acting in a way that is in the client's best long-range interests no matter how problematic this may be to the client in the short run.

On-Line Identification as Contest Between Client and Clinician.   One way we have successfully employed on-line identification with adults is by a simple contest between the client and ourself. We would begin, after conferring with the client, to specifically target certain speech disfluencies that the client needs to identify in his or her own speech. Then, while we discuss with clients some topics of interest or familiarity, we try to see who is the first one to identify these specific disfluencies. Although we can signal such identity with a simple finger pointing or raising gesture, as mentioned above, a penlight with an instant on-off button is also an effective signaling device. Again, the objective of this contest is the *speed* with which the client can identify the disfluency. Obviously, clinicians can manipulate their latency of signaling to maximize, at least at first, the clients' chances for identifying their own instances *before* clinicians do.

Facilitating On-Line Identification.   To facilitate on-line identification, it is helpful if the clinician selects as a topic of conversation, something that is familiar and of interest to the client. This on-line procedure, at least at first, should be broken up into several short periods, rather than a few long sections within one therapy session. These conversation breaks and discussions of the client's successes and failures with on-line identification enable the SLP to minimize the tension (both physiological and psychological) that may build up when using this therapy method. Better to provide the client with a few successful periods within a therapy session than to spend an entire therapy session working the client so hard that he or she is nearly driven away from therapy. And make no mistake about it, clinicians, no matter how unintentionally, can drive clients away from therapy.

Once again, the clinician's sensitivity regarding the client's ever-changing needs and feelings will dictate the success of this as well as other approaches. With on-line analysis in particular, where the attention to speech-language production is quick, specific, and quite apparent, the client can easily get the feeling that all the clinician is doing is "picking on" the client. It seems in this situation that the essence of the client's reaction is that the clinician only cares about the "mechanics" of speech and not enough about him or her as a person. It is important to recognize this reaction, as it is developing, discuss it, and then possibly mitigate it. The SLP should try, as much as possible, to convey to the client the impression of not only seeing the behavior but the person behind the behavior as well.

Further Reactions to Identification

As the adult client becomes more and more adept at quick and accurate identification, clinician latency can be shortened to make the task more and more challenging for the client. At this point, one of several things may be noticed: (1) clients claim they are stuttering more; (2) clinicians notice the clients' stuttering more (possibly because they are avoiding less and/or repeating more often than producing inaudible sound prolongations or within-word pauses); or (3) the duration of each instance of clients' stutterings seem to be shortening. The third observation, is, as mentioned above, a positive sign that clients are improving in their objective awareness of stuttering that they are already, even without direct modification procedures, beginning to change their speech production. The former two observations, however, are a bit more worrisome to both client and clinician and need some discussion at this point.

Client: I'm Beginning to Stutter More.   As alluded to previously, clients' heightened awareness of their stuttering heightens their awareness! People who stutter can come to believe they stutter more, we believe, because they have become more objectively and accurately aware of their instances of stuttering through identification. The same things, as we'll discuss below, can also happen to their clinicians, that is, through identification, the SLP can actually see and hear more stutterings on the part of the client than he or she originally observed during the diagnostic and first few therapy sessions. The SLP becomes more aware, with exposure to the client, of the depth and breadth of the client's stuttering; that is, in the beginning the SLP may miss some the client's speech disfluencies, because the clinician must attend to a myriad of factors that occur in the development of a reasonable and thorough evaluation and prognosis. The client is not the only person who changes as a result of therapy! Indeed, both the clinician and client change with therapy—both become more adept at perceiving instances of stuttering.

Clinician: Client Does Appear to Be Stuttering More.   However, it may be the case that the client *is* stuttering more now if for no other reason than that he or she talks more as the client–clinician relation develops (that is, the more talking, the greater the chance for stuttering to occur), and that the client has become more willing to enter into (or become less apt to avoid) discussions. What we find of interest in all this is that clinicians often report increases in their client's stuttering and express worry that they—somehow through their therapeutic procedures—have caused these increases! We doubt if they would have the same worry if they noticed after several therapy sessions with a child exhibiting speech misarticulations that the child increased his or her numbers of speech misarticulation. We would also bet that clinicians do not have the same worry when they notice after several sessions with a child with language concerns that there is a decrease in the child's MLU or that there are now apparently more missing grammatical morphemes.

What is being said here is that more stutterings noticed by the clinician after a period of therapy does not necessarily mean that the client has gotten worse, regressed, relapsed, or experienced any other such calamities. This observation may simply mean that: (1) the original estimates of stuttering were inaccurate; (2) the type of stuttering has changed from one that is minimally audible and visible—for example, silent sound prolongations—to one much more audible and visible, such as sound/syllable repetitions; (3) the client is avoiding less, talking more, and in longer units; (4) the situations in which speech is now elicited differ from those used during the original evaluation; and (5) any of these reasons and more in combination. Clinicians must stop flailing themselves when they notice such changes (they must also stop waiting for the other shoe of increased stuttering to drop).

Instead, we should attempt to make the same reactions to increased stutterings that we make to increased articulation errors, missing grammatical morphemes, decreased MLU, or more prevalent hoarseness, and so forth (for further discussion pertinent to this issue see Wingate, 1971). Guilty parents are difficult enough to deal with (e.g., "If we had only given our sixth-grader the Mercedes-Benz convertible he wanted, we know he wouldn't have started to stutter more"); but guilty clinicians, especially when there is little or no reason for such guilty feelings, can be just as problematic. The white-hot spotlight of on-line identification seems to exacerbate these concerns, but it is quite unclear to me how we can assist our adult client change his or her stuttering if the client and ourselves never carefully examine, touch, feel, or hear those behaviors that are interfering with normally fluent speech production and need changing. Perhaps it is much like asking a garage mechanic to fix the engine of our car *without* examining it closely, touching and listening to it during the exam. While it is understandable that people who stutter, unlike some of our political leaders, have met many microphones that they don't love, it is nonetheless important, in a gentle, patient fashion, to focus the limelight of our and our client's attention on their instances of stuttering in attempts to help them change their behavior.

Bridging Between Identification and Modification

The client's ability to temporally beat the SLP at identifying instances of his or her own stuttering *as they occur* during conversation is the bridge between identification and modification. With careful explanation, clients should come to understand and physically *feel* the various things they do inappropriately during speech as they are doing them. I want to stress that the key here is *as the client is producing the stutterings*—not several seconds or five words ago, but during the right here and now. We want the person who stutters to do this right at the exact moment of stuttering. Sooner rather than later. The physical feelings of interfering with speech and the rapidity of these of these behaviors must be carefully examined and accurately recognized. Again, we try to stress to the client (and ourselves) that the problem is NOT within the sound or syllable but involves the strategies used by the adult who stutters to produce those units of speech (as Shakespeare may have expressed it, "the problem is not in our stars but in ourselves").

Spontaneous Modification

For some adults who stutter, simply identifying stutterings as they are being produced is sufficient to enable them to start modifying these very same instances of stuttering. That is, it seems, for some people who stutter, that on-line identification of stuttering—recognizing stutterings as they are occurring—facilitates their attempts to change stuttering. One of the first signs of such facilitation, as previously mentioned, is a decrease in the duration of the instances of stuttering. We have taken this decrease in duration to mean that the person who stutters is beginning to realize that he or she can change his or her stuttering midstream, that he or she can use less physical tension in the production of a particular sound or sound-to-sound transition. Another sign is when the adult who stutters, in the middle of producing a stuttering, stops, perhaps briefly pauses, and then initiates the same sound or syllable in a more appropriate fashion. These signs essentially mean that the client is taking an active, direct approach toward coping with or changing inappropriate speech behavior. By shortening the duration of a stuttering and/or stopping and reinitiating in a more fluent manner, these clients are giving the impression that they are beginning to directly come to grips with their stuttering, that *they* are beginning to *do something* to change their own behavior. These are signs that the adult who stutters is beginning to do battle with his or her stuttering and is taking an active role rather than running and hiding from or avoiding the situation.

To be effective in this battle, we try to provide the adult who stutters with an objective understanding of stuttering as well as an ability to quickly and accurately confront instances of stuttering. Every time I see an adult who stutters begin this self-confrontation process, I am reminded of what I think is a Pogo quote that goes something like "We have met the enemy and he is us." Rather than ducking and weaving, the adult who stutters has started to "face the music" and circumscribe the boundaries of his or her speech problem. The older person who stutters can now begin to operate from a position of understanding rather than ignorance, one of relatively clear vision rather than hazy insight.

If Identification Fails to Develop

Some adults who stutter never seem to develop the ability to identify and subsequently modify instances of stuttering. We are not sure why this is, but several reasons may exist. First, for some, there may be so much emotionality associated with the actual sight, sound, and feel of their stuttering that these individuals find it quite difficult to actually confront occurrences of their own stuttering (Guitar, 1997, discusses such concerns with children who stutter). Many times these clients try to keep therapy on a subjective, fairly abstract discussion basis (cf. Johnson, 1946 for discussion of individuals who employ high levels of verbal abstraction), rather than a get-down-to-specifics approach. Some of these types of clients use an "intellectualization" (cf. Vaillant, 1977, p. 385) method of coping with the problem, and this too gets in the way of their actually coming to terms with their problem. Sometimes, a break from therapy helps, where the clients are given some time to think about whether they are willing and able to specifically confront their instances of stuttering. Second, other adults who stutter do not appear to have the ability to concentrate to the degree and for the length of time necessary to identify and modify instances of stuttering. They may be "tuned-in" to emotional feelings surrounding their stutterings, but the stations they receive broadcast mainly subjective, emotional messages rather than programs that directly and specifically deal with their own behavior. Third, some adults who stutter may be fairly able to see and hear their instances of stuttering but appear relatively unable to physically *feel* these same instances. It is as if this third group of clients are physically as well as emotionally insensitive or out of touch with their own bodily feelings.

Of course, the possibility also exists that the clinician is not very effective in assisting the client to identify instances of stuttering or that the clinician has not sufficiently and clearly explained the rationale for identifying instances of stuttering. We sometimes need to face reality: Some clients cannot or will not easily, readily, or accurately perceive their own instances of stuttering. These clients will either need different approaches or must wait until such time that they are more receptive to our therapeutic approaches.

Individual Therapy for Adults Who Stutter: Modification Phase

Modification of stuttering is actually not that hard, it is just that neither we nor our clients appear to realize this fact! What is hard, on the other hand, is providing the necessary intellectual and/or emotional environment in and around the client which *continually* facilitates, fosters, and encourages the client to modify his or her own speech. Once again, as Williams (1978) suggests, our goal is change of speech *outside* of therapy, not change *within* the therapy room. As we've seen, quick, accurate identification of stuttering is one important aspect of this environment. So is the notion that specific speaking strategies, rather than specific sounds, are the main ingredients of stuttering.

Movement Between Rather Than Movement Within Sounds

The client must be helped to understand that stuttering involves an interference with or disruption of the appropriately timed, smooth, physically easy movements from one articulatory gesture to another. Emphasis is on movement from one articulatory or speech posture to the next (compare to the skiing/pogo stick analogy in Figure 4.2). Attention is placed on movements between sounds rather than the specific nature of the movements needed to produce each sound. We want to facilitate the ability of the adult who stutters to make connections between sounds rather than concentrate on making the specific sounds.

The Problem Relates to the Nature of Speaker's Speech
Behavior Not the Nature of Speech Sounds Spoken

The client needs to realize that speech is something produced by his or her own self as the speaker and, as such, it is something he or she, as the speaker, can modify and change. For example, a simple waltz employed by most couples on a dance floor was not so simple when these various couples were first learning to dance. In the beginning they practiced with and without a partner the basic box, or rectangular, step until they felt reasonably comfortable with it. They practiced the specific movements of body, legs, and feet as well as placement of arms, hands, and feet. They did not practice "waltzing," because this would have been too vague or too macrocosmic an event to learn. Instead, they practiced the specific movements, placements, and postures of their bodies and body parts that constitute the act of waltzing. During practice, the end product—waltzing—was not as important as insuring that each subpart of the act of waltzing (for example, this foot moves here, the arms are placed like so, and leg or the foot follows like that) would be adequate and that with further time and practice, he or she could become a better and better dancer.

Well, this dancing analogy is not exactly identical to changing maladaptive speaking behavior and replacing it with appropriate speaking behavior; however, neither is this analogy that far removed. Like the beginning dancers, the adult who stutters needs to focus on the *specific* postures, movements, contacts, and placements of speech production and be able to initiate them or change them when he or she so desires. If such movements and postures are produced, the end product (speech) will almost take care of itself. The person's speech will be appropriate, perhaps not excellent at first but adequate and, with time and practice, it should get better and better. Helping our adult clients focus on their speech behavior and breaking this behavior down into its constituent parts is one of our primary responsibilities in therapy. Toward these ends, Webster's (1975, 1978) management program, which employs fluency targets, is a move in the right direction. However, only through more empirical research will we be able to more clearly circumscribe those aspects of stuttered speech production most in need of changing as well as those aspects of fluent speech production most in need of adopting.

Where and What to Begin Modifying

As with identification, we first emphasize during the modification phase those aspects of speaking that are the most apparent, longest, and clearly disruptive to the forward flow of fluent speech. While we could start with less apparent, shorter, and less physically tense speech behavior, most of these lesser stutterings will escape the attention of most adults who stutter, at least at the onset of therapy. Thus, we have found it better to start modifying the more easily recognizable stutterings, because once change is effected with these stutterings, it is much more noticeable to the person who stutters and his or her listeners.

Which Stutterings Are Easily Recognizable?   This is not something that is readily explained on paper, but an "easily recognizable" stuttering is most likely to be a longer duration instance of stuttering that is associated with apparent physical tension in and around the face, neck, and upper chest. Along these lines, however, we would like to point

out that it is not usually necessary to *directly* remediate such behaviors as lack of eye contact (e.g., Atkins, 1988; LaSalle & Contour, 1991), turning of the head, or constricting of
the external throat muscles. These inappropriate nonspeech behaviors are most likely a
reaction to, rather than cause of, instances of stuttering (see Conture & Kelly, 1991a, pp.
1051–1053, for a general discussion of possible reasons for inappropriate nonspeech behaviors). Therefore, when modifying stuttering itself (the actual disruptive speech behavior),
the basis for these inappropriate reactions will diminish, which means that the reactions
themselves will drop out.

We must remember that there are just so many hours during the therapy day and that
one must wisely choose his or her battles and battle sites. That is, one must pick and choose
wisely those issues to deal with in order to maximize the effectiveness and efficiency of
such therapy. Thus, starting a therapy program by trying to change the lack of eye contact
of a person who stutters (its obvious nature is apparently one reason it is frequently selected
by beginning SLPs as a behavior to modify) is not an effective use of therapy time when so
many other speech-related events need remedial attention, for example, inappropriate
tongue movement, lip closure, laryngeal abductory gestures, and so forth. However, once
appropriate change of speech behavior is initiated by the client who continues to look down
or away, the clinician can gently but clearly guide the client's eye contact back to the clinician's face for appropriate periods of time (not staring, however) to aid the client in focusing on appropriate changes in ongoing speech behavior.

One Example of an Easily Recognizable Stuttering.   Cessation or fixed- articulatory
posture disfluency types—for example, audible sound prolongation's blocks—are excellent
places to start modification with adult people who stutter. These speech behaviors may
have started when the adult was younger as a reaction to sound-syllable repetition, and thus
it probably has a complex learning history. Careful study will show you that a restricted
number of inappropriate speaking strategies constitute the basic physiologic aspects of
these type of speech disfluencies. You will probably note the relative fixed, stationary, or
stabilized speech production gesture (i.e., there are minimal amounts of the rather wild
oscillations of speech musculature commonly associated with sound-syllable repetitions)
during audible or inaudible sound prolongations and blocks; in particular, with longer
instances of prolongation, you will observe a relatively high degree of physical tension in
the client's speech musculature.

The "Anatomy" of One Easily Recognizable Stuttering.   Listening to these cessation or
fixed-articulatory posture type of speech disfluencies, you may hear: (1) little or no sound
(high probability but not certainty that vocal folds are closed); (2) breathy, whispered, or
noisy vocal quality (high probability of open vocal folds); or (3) a glottal fry-like, popping,
or pulsing sound (closely approximated, but to some degree vibrating vocal folds with
false vocal folds perhaps being medially compressed and/or "loading down" the true vocal
folds). While these various laryngeal behaviors are going on, you'll also probably notice
that the jaw, lips, and/or tongue are "frozen," set, fixed, or stabilized in the posture for the
sound being audibly or inaudibly prolonged; however, these supraglottal structures are not
making the necessary transitional or connecting gesture ("they aren't moving on") to the
next sound. The adult who stutters has "locked" his or her speaking gestures in place on the

sound and is not making the between sound or within syllable transition. During all this, we can make the reasonable assumption that the rib cage and abdomen of the person who stutters are also relatively locked, fixed, stabilized, or, if anything, slowly deflating. All of this detail about these behaviors cannot, of course, be easily explained to the client and in some cases would not be of assistance even if we were to do so. However, you, as the client's SLP, should be clear regarding the nature and frequency of these speaking behaviors because this will help you recognize changes in their quality and quantity as the client progresses through the modification stage of therapy. Furthermore, our rate of speech is quite rapid (two-three words/sec during normal adult speech, [Levelt, Roelofs, & Meyer, 1999]) relative to our ability to identify and modify it. Thus, in the beginning of therapy we are helping the client change inappropriate behavior during, or slightly after, the instance of stuttering. Making these changes during and after the stuttering is not a place of choice, but when starting to modify stuttering it is a place of necessity.

After and Then During the Instance of Stuttering

What to Work on, What Not to Work on.   To begin this discussion, let us assume that an adult who stutters is holding the speech posture for the word-initial /s/ in the word "see" for too long a period of time. This would probably result in an audible sound prolongation on the word-initial /s/. We might see the physical tension in the person's face, particularly the lip area, and neck muscles and possibly the movement of the eyeballs to the left or right together with blinking or closed eyes. However, as mentioned previously, it should be stressed that it is less than helpful to try to modify these "nonspeech" facets of the problem (e.g., eye blinking, facial muscle tension), regardless of their maladaptive nature. Likewise, we hear the air rushing from the lungs, through the larynx and over and through the restricted space formed by the tongue approximating the cutting edge of the central and lateral incisors (teeth). However, it should be stressed that we *not* instruct the adult who stutters to "take a deep breath and start over" because we think he or she has or is about to run out of air.

Instead of these grosser behaviors—facial gestures and air escaping—what we should be observing is the lack of speech posture movement from this posture for the prolonged sound to the next articulatory contact or posture (a lack of transitional or connecting gestures). We should be observing the client's failure to make the necessary movement transition from the word-initial /s/ consonant to the /i/ of the subsequent vowel. The client is probably pressing his or her tongue tip tightly against the alveolar ridge behind the incisors but is not moving it (the tongue) into position for the subsequent sound, in this case a vowel. Again, it needs to be pointed out that we are not witnessing a problem with producing sounds but a problem with connecting or transitioning between sounds—stuttering involves a problem with going from sound to sound, rather than a problem producing particular sounds (similar to Wingate's [1988] "fault line" hypothesis). Perhaps these problems of connection are based on inappropriate strategies. Perhaps they are based on having difficulties with phonological or phonetic encoding. Perhaps with our sound prolongation example one inappropriate strategy has been developed in attempts to override or mask or change another previously developed inappropriate strategy that was used for sound/syllable repetitions. That is, rather than continue the reiterative or repetitive attempts to begin or end a speech posture without making necessary connecting gestures to the next sound (a sound/syllable repetition), the adult who stutters now changes the reiterative gestures to a "frozen," fixed, or stabilized speech gesture (sound prolongation). However, the outcome is the same: The adult who stutters fails to move on to the posture for the next sound. As SLPs we need to work on helping the person who stutters move on to the posture for the next sound, rather than focus on helping him or her move eyeballs or facial muscles in a different fashion.

Modification During and/or After the Stuttering.   Getting back to our example of prolonging the word-initial /s/ by the adult who stutters, we would first try to help him or her change or move on to the next sound while he or she is in the middle of prolonging this sound. This would be our first attempt; however, since many people who stutter do not like to be stopped once they begin talking, it is not unusual for them to continue saying more than a few words rather than to make the necessary change. If this happens, and change during the middle of the stuttered word is not possible, then we would allow the person who stutters to finish the word but immediately repeat the stuttering on this word and encourage change this time. Obviously, this procedure is nothing particularly new (see Starkweather, 1974; Van Riper, 1973); however, what we do believe is slightly but importantly different is that we emphasize in lay person's terms the type of speech production that is being inappropriately used by the adult who stutters. Rather than use such terms as *blocks, pull-outs,* or *bouncing,* which have a place in therapy but can become too vague too quickly, we try to help the client feel, see, and hear the exact thing or things he or she is doing that interfere with speaking (for example, "John, you aren't moving your tongue from the /s/ to the /i/ position and that's why you aren't finishing the word"). We also try to emphasize the common thread that runs through all of these behaviors and focus attention on the client's strategies, rather than the sounds being prolonged or repeated.

Clinician Signals to Client: "Change," "Move on," "Now," or "Easy."   It is not easy to help the client change his or her speech behavior in midstream during running speech, but after a successful period of teaching identification of stuttering, this can be implemented rather successfully. You will want to talk to the client to be sure he or she appears to understand what you want him or her to do ("When you *feel* yourself holding that speech position, let go, move on, slowly and easily, to the next speech posture. With practice, you'll be able to do this quicker and smoother"). Once such understanding is apparent, at the point in time during the stuttering when we have been saying "change" or "move on" to the client, we can, as the client seems to get the point and demonstrates that fact, simply say, "now" at the same point in time. Of course, we have previously spent some time explaining and showing the client what we mean when we say "move on" or "change" (that is, move on to the next sound posture; again, they move onto a sound *posture*, not sound, for the sound that "comes out of the mouth" results from the posture. In essence, it is *postures,* or movement between them, not *sounds* that we change).

In a sense, we become, at this stage, the clients' external monitoring device by helping them tune in and turn on to the type of speech behavior they are producing disfluently and then reminding them when and how to change this behavior by moving on to the next sound(s). Here again, the client and clinician enter into a kind of contest to see who can first recognize the stuttering. Once so recognized, the client is reminded to change and verbally rewarded by the SLP for any and all changes. This procedure requires the SLP to be very supportive and sensitive to the client and his or her feelings. Clients must be verbally rewarded by the SLP for successive approximations to change, and the clinicians at this point must be clear but kind, rapid but not repellent. We do not want to verbally harass clients about their speech the same way everybody else does. Instead, we want to objectively and systematically recognize their instances of stuttering and then help these clients modify (on-line) their inappropriate or stuttered speech production behavior while they are actually producing same. We are not expecting instant success with this and we tell this to the client. We do not expect perfection, but we do tell the client that we expect him or her to give this a try. These "tries" will be greatly facilitated by our support, reinforcement, and understanding for the difficulty that any human being has in changing something about the self. I can easily say that the modification of speech behavior, particularly what has been habituated over a period of several years, is just plain hard work. As the old saying goes, the other half of inspiration is perspiration!

When the Client Fails to Change

If the adult who stutters fails in his or her attempts at changing inappropriate speech behavior when you clearly but in politely as well as supportive tones say, "now," do not perseverate with this procedure. Backtrack and *demonstrate*, once again, for the client the actual or specific change in speech behavior you are referring to; *show* the client how, don't just *tell* the client to change. Far too often we seem reluctant to actually show or demonstrate—through actual positioning as well as moving our own lips, tongue, jaw, and larynx—to the client the inappropriate speech behavior we are talking about and the specific means by which we are asking the client to change this behavior. Perhaps we fear that doing so may be construed by the person who stutters to mean we are criticizing, mocking, or teasing him or her. However, if our feelings are right toward that client, if we have demonstrated good faith to the client in terms of our sincerity to help the client change, then we have little to fear on this score.

Instead, we think that some of our reluctance stems more from our lack of clarity regarding *what* behavior is in need of changing and *what* behavior should be substituted. This is due, in part, to our history of concentrating on "stutterings," "repetitions," "prolongations," or "blocks" without bothering to examine the actual speech production behaviors that create, make up, or underlie our perceptual labels for these behaviors. This concentration on our part reflects the past zeitgeist (spirit of the times) in the field of stuttering, which essentially implied that examination of the speech production of stuttering indicated that the examiner is seeking an organic, physiological, or natural cause of stuttering (see exchange between Cooper & DeNil, 1999, relative to this topic). This zeitgeist, which now with hindsight, we can more objectively evaluate, has led us away from studying a rich source of information regarding stuttering: the actual disruptions in speech-language production that are associated with stuttering as well as the more subtle, perhaps imperceptible disruptions in speech production that may accompany the perceptually fluent speech of people who stutter.

We are only fooling ourselves if we believe that we can more precisely capture the essentials of the stuttered speech production by minimizing our usage of the term *stuttering* in favor of using terms like *sound prolongation, sound-syllable repetition,* or even *block*. This is similar to believing that we have captured the essentials of oranges, lemons, grapefruit, kumquats, and so forth by calling them *citrus fruit*, rather than merely *fruit*. Surely, a term like "sound prolongation" is more of a specific descriptor than "stuttering," but it may still be too broad, still too nonbehavioral, and still too vague to help some of our adult clients help themselves become more fluent, to change their stutterings. We must strive to become more and more *specific* in our understanding of what our stuttering clients *do* when they interfere with their speech production (for an example of a research study that tries to do this, see Caruso et al., 1988). Such specificity should help us to become clearer and clearer when we talk to ourselves about our client's behaviors. It should also help in our talks with our clients (particularly those adult clients who want and need such specificity) regarding what they are and are not doing in terms of the speech-language production behavior they exhibit that listeners label as "stuttering."

When the Client Produces Real Change

We have some clue that our clients are beginning to make significant change when we notice them effecting change in their maladaptive speech production strategies *during* the actual instance of stuttering. This is a rather ethereal event that is quickly over and done with as the client moves on to the next sound, syllable, or word. The SLP must, therefore, quickly recognize such change and clearly and *immediately* reinforce it. Perhaps no other aspect of therapy with adults who stutter places a higher premium on quick and accurate SLP observational abilities than this phase. While the demands on the SLP's observational skills are high, the rewards are great because most clients respond with increased frequency of change.

As mentioned, reinforcement of these client changes by the SLP is quite important. Reinforcement, here as elsewhere, serves to both *confirm* ("Your behavior is correct/good") and *inform* ("That is the type of behavior you and I want to see") the client about his or her exhibited changes. Such reinforcement, particularly during in conversation, can be somewhat disruptive to the forward flow of communication, but it is better to interrupt than to allow to go unnoticed this very positive sign that the client is changing. The actual change during the stuttering may even take longer than if the client had simply "bulled" his or her way through the particular speech posture. However, this is a clear sign that the adult has taken it upon him- or herself to make this change, and the SLP should clearly and emphatically reinforce this self-initiative. Besides, the client's willingness to take slightly more time to make the change, if this is the case, demonstrates an ability to deal with time pressure, to become more independent of real and perceived reasons for "full steam ahead and damn the torpedoes." In essence, these first changes by the adult who stutters are the true beginning of the end of the problem, but this neither implies a cure in the traditional sense of the word (more on the issue of cure toward the end of this chapter) nor a time to relax on the part of the client and clinician (to paraphrase Robert Frost, both still have to travel many miles before either of them sleeps).

Changes in disruptive, inappropriate, or maladaptive speech posture that occurs during the stuttering can then be continually reinforced in restricted utterances ("Tell me everything you know about this ballpoint pen"). During this phase of therapy, try to provide the client with a *restricted* or *closed* set of thoughts, ideas, or topics to deal with so that he or she can concentrate on these changes in stuttering to the exclusion of conjuring up elaborate conversation. Specifically target and demonstrate the change or the types of inappropriate speech behavior you expect or desire the client to modify. The client will be far more successful, at this point, if you don't ask him or her to attempt to change ALL forms of disruptive behavior or every instance of stuttering. Failure, like success, has a way of spreading and influencing its surroundings. We stress to the client (many of whom already believe that they are either all right or all wrong) that consistent change on one specific type of inappropriate speech production, for example, longer sound prolongations, is a very good *first* step and *is* what we would call success at this phase. The adult who stutters may still be holding for too long and with too much physical tension the speech posture needed to produce the word-initial sound, but the client is making real progress if he or she can consistently demonstrate relatively rapid, easier movement into the posture needed for the subsequent sound.

As stated above, it is our believe that much of what we would describe as an instance of stuttering (particularly on the sound prolongation/block variety) results from inappropriate strategies, rather than specific difficulties with particular sounds or syllables. This belief is lent support, we think, by the observation that many clients' abilities to change certain instances of stuttering (for example, reduction in the length of and physical tension of their longer sound prolongations) generalize, and they begin to demonstrate similar changes in other disfluencies. The inappropriate strategy is being replaced by an appropriate one every place the original or inappropriate one was once applied. This can generalize to the point where almost overnight, it seems, the client becomes markedly more fluent. This initial burst of speech fluency maybe what is sometimes called *lucky* or *false fluency* and is not to be confused with increases in speech fluency that result from a more lasting appreciation and ability to apply the "how and the why" of speech modification.

It would, however, seem a bit silly to look a gift horse in the mouth, so to speak, and reject out of hand the initial success the client has demonstrated. At this point in therapy, the client would seem to need words of praise mingled with words of caution as well as discussion of what is going on and why. Try to use the client's initial success to motivate clients toward the further work that must follow, particular the work that is involved in "maintenance" or "carryover" aspects of therapy. What the SLP needs to avoid, however, is premature dismissal from therapy and/or premature expressions of euphoria. Honesty at this juncture is the best short-, medium-, and long-term policy. The client should be supported and encouraged for his or her progress to date but should not have his or her expectations raised to unreasonable heights. When people suddenly fall from heights, no matter how pretty the view, their injuries generally hurt more and last longer than when they stumble over the smaller curbs and potholes of life. The SLP clearly doesn't want to become, as one of our politicians once said, "a nattering nabob of negativism." Instead, he or she will praise the client for present progress as well as facilitate the likelihood of future progress, but at the same time try to help the client understand that Rome wasn't built in a day and occasional setbacks may occur along the road to improved fluency.

Within-Therapy Carryover

Some adults who stutter seem to make change quite easily and effectively when you are monitoring their speaking behavior but seem to do little on their own, even in your presence (this is somewhat similar to discussions of co-dependency [Beattie, 1987] whereby person A gets person B to do their thinking, worrying, and the like for them). Here, we are not talking about a carryover problem in the traditional sense of difficulty transferring or maintaining or carrying over changes in speech behavior from one therapy session to the next; instead, we are discussing carryover problems *within* the therapy session itself.

Client Dependency on Clinician.   An adult who stutters who can quickly and accurately identify and then change during an inappropriate or disruptive speech posture or movement *only* when the SLP is assisting in the monitoring and changing is a client who obviously is *not* ready for dismissal ("I just can't get the feeling of fluency by myself"). The client is dependent on the clinician for changing his or her behavior. This client has a problem, since he or she is not ready to transfer his or her changed speech to the external, everyday environment where the SLP is nonexistent. To understand this situation, we first should examine the client's understanding of the meaningfulness and rationale for your procedure. Ask the client, if he or she knows what is going on and why. If need be, explain again, perhaps using different terms, why you are doing what you are doing and why you think this particular procedure is important. Do not be afraid to retrace your steps and travel over old ground in this case. It is not uncommon that re-explaining "old" issues may give the client new insights, since he or she has now had the time and sufficient experience with which to evaluate these issues afresh.

Second, examine the frequency and manner with which you are reinforcing the client for successful approximations and achievements in his or her own speech and related behavior. Does your reinforcement or reward seem to come too infrequently? Does your reward seem to mean anything to the client? Does he or she seem to understand not only *when* you reward but *what* you are rewarding? Perhaps your rewards are neutral because your relation with the client is rather neutral. Perhaps you are overly businesslike and professional in manner, and the client has trouble relating to this sort of approach. However, this is not to say that you should go completely to the opposite extreme and become the client's buddy. Instead, we are merely suggesting that you study these aspects of your clinical dealings with the client.

Third, do you make it clear what elements of the client's inappropriate strategy must be changed, do you actually *show* the client what aspect of his or her speech behavior must be changed, or do you simply *tell* him or her to change? As we have said before, all too often too many clinicians fail to specifically *show*, or *demonstrate*, or *do* for the client the actual behavior they want the client to exhibit or achieve. Rather, these clinicians do a lot of talking about change, a lot of telling the client to change, or lecturing the client on change. It makes intuitive sense to this writer that a client who is quite hazy about the specifics of changing his or her speech behavior is a client who is very unlikely to make these types of changes and/or put out the necessary effort to make these changes. The client is neither asking for nor should be given a course in the anatomy and physiology of the speech and hearing mechanism; however, the client does want and needs specific instructions on how to change, for example:

> During your sound prolongations, you seem to hold your tongue tip tightly against the roof of your mouth in the front. You then don't move your tongue into the position for the first position for the next sound. During this time, you're also holding open your vocal cords in your voice box. I want you to try to begin to easily close your vocal cords and moving your

tongue tip into position for the next sound when you physically *feel* yourself holding them in that "stuttered" posture. It looks like this (and you slowly and clearly demonstrate several times or until the client seems to have the general idea; for the client to get the specific idea, he or she will have to try it several times him- or herself, with your assistance and/or continual modeling).

Client Failure to Make Change on His Or Her Own. Obviously, even the best-laid clinical plans can go awry: Some clients, for unknown reasons, simply cannot or will not make the shift from clinician-monitored change to client-monitored change. These clients are problematic, but some of them respond better to approaches where they are *given* a procedure to use to change their speech. Such procedures are amply covered elsewhere (e.g., Guitar, 1998; Van Riper, 1973; Wingate, 1976), but they all have a common thread running through them: The client is provided with some internally or externally generated means for minimizing stuttering. The relation these various procedures have to what our present understanding of the speech production characteristics of stuttered/fluent speech is, at best, unclear. Most such procedures are advocated because of their expediency—their ability to improve the client's fluency, if only for a while. The client achieves fluency after a fashion, but this is not to be confused with an approach where the client is viewed as the *perpetrator* (however unintentional) of the stuttering and, as such, has the *ability* or *means* to make the necessary change in speaking behavior (what is done by the adult who stutters, in this case, *can* be undone). In other words, if we take the approach, as we have done throughout this book, that people have the means to effect change within their own speech—without the use of external devices like metronomes, miniaturized or otherwise—then it makes most sense to help them understand and observe what *they* are *doing* that interferes with their speech and see if they can produce more and more of an appropriate strategy for fluent speech ("to do more and more of the things that normally fluent speakers do when they talk"). This does not mean nor are we trying to say that all clients can and will react positively to this approach—it is doubtful that all clients can and will react positively to any approach!—but that this is the conceptual or philosophical base from which we start remediating.

Changing Speech in Conversation

Once the adult client begins to consistently change stuttering (shortening the duration and more physically easily moving on to the next sound) in restricted conversations and situations with the clinician, the clinician can begin to help the client effect change in his or her speech in more natural settings, for example, talking over the phone. Some role playing in the clinical setting of these situations, in advance of their occurrence, may help the client deal with and become appropriately desensitized to the actual speaking situation. Here is where a group therapy situation, which may be conducted in parallel with individual therapy, is quite useful. Both you and the client get a chance to see the extent to which the client can make the change in front of the group. Selected phone calls can also be of help where clients can test their developing ability to change in the presence of time pressure. Having the client order or ask questions in stores (with the cautions mentioned in Chapter 4 regarding this activity) are other good experiences and means of testing the client. Talking to the clinical secretary, school janitor, nurse, librarian, teachers, or fellow clinicians—providing these people have the time, seem willing, and, like the store employees, have been previously briefed by you regarding the nature, purpose, and scope of this procedure—is another good experience and test.

Activities Should Be Brief but Planned.   Remember and try to keep these situations brief, to the point, and allow time for the client and yourself to discuss the results. Do not simply do this to do this. Nothing is less appreciated by clients, particularly adults, than activities that merely take up time in the session, seem to have no real focus or purpose, and appear to be so much "busy work." Instead, plan out in advance these "real-world" conversations and try to reinforce as well as critique, if necessary, the client's performance after each experience. If the client's performance in more than a few phone calls or conversations is less than successful, you may want to return to the therapy room and spend more time on basics. Obviously, this activity, like any other therapy activity, will not work if the client is "sleeping" between therapy sessions.

Trying to Gauge Improvement.   You can get some idea if the client is changing the frequency, duration, type, or severity of his or her stuttering by asking, "What does your wife (husband, father, mother, boss, fellow workers, teacher, and so forth) think about your speech now?" "Has anyone mentioned to you lately anything about your speech?" "Has anyone noticed or said anything to you about your speech since you have been in therapy?" If the client reports that associates, friends, or relatives are starting to notice or mention positive change in his or her speaking behavior, you have some idea, in our experience, that positive change in speaking behavior is starting to occur where it should be occurring, that is, *outside* the confines of the therapy room.

If you can, you might give the client's associates outside of therapy a call and ask their opinions regarding your client's progress. Of course, this presupposes that you have previously established some minimal working relations with them. These calls should not be construed, by the client, as your snooping into his or her personal life but rather as your sincere and honest attempt to determine if other individuals in their environment are beginning to notice positive changes in speaking and related behavior. Often these associates may note positive change when you believe therapy progress to be at a standstill and this, I think, should provide you with some encouragement—clients aren't the only people who need reinforcement!—to keep on keeping on with the client's therapy. Obviously, you would not want to make these phone calls frequently, but they can be made at appropriate times with very positive results on present as well as future therapy plans. Conversely, if such calls indicate little change on the part of the client, but you seem to be noticing considerable change by the client in the therapy room, you have gained valuable information and direction for present and future therapy.

Homework or Further Work Outside Therapy

The Purpose of Homework.   First, the basic reason for doing homework—in the context of therapy for stuttering—is to provide the client practice with and habituation of behavior that is being discussed and dealt with in therapy. Second, such homework assignments foster an acute awareness of speech behavior and the need as well as the means to change speech. Third, homework assignments, especially those that are successfully completed, show clients that they can actually change the way they speak, that they can really do something on their own to help themselves. There is a great deal of truth in two old sayings: "If you want to roll the dice, you gotta pay the price" and "Before you sing the blues, you've gotta pay your dues." Part of the price as well as the dues the adult who stutters must pay to achieve more fluent speech is completion of homework outside the clinic.

Some Realities of Homework Assignments. No one likes to bring homework from the office, and adults who stutter are no exception. Therefore, avoid setting yourself up for frustration, anger, and feelings of resentment: Don't assign your adult client *large* amounts of between-therapy work. Make these assignments short and easily accomplished everyday in a nontherapy setting, for example, the client's bedroom in front of a dressing mirror. Make sure that these assignments are such that the client clearly understands how, why, and when he or she is to do them (helping the client set a *specific* time each day to practice or do homework increases the chance that the practice/homework will get done). Be sure to monitor these assignments—write down at the end of the therapy session what the exact nature of the assignment was—so that the client realizes that you are evaluating his or her completion and relative success with these assignments. If homework assignments involve speaking outside the home, for example, talking to strangers, make sure that during the week the client has an opportunity to encounter strangers! If this is not possible for the client, switch assignments because neglected and impossible assignments will surely influence in-clinic therapy and most clients in a less than positive way.

At the risk of redundancy, homework assignments where the client uses the phone provide excellent opportunities for the client to practice identifying, monitoring, and changing speech behavior. The client's number of calls can be easily be counted; the client can control the length and nature of each call fairly easily, and the exercise can readily be completed at home (and in some cases, at work). Calls don't have to be complex—they can involve the calling of restaurants, pharmacies, department stores, and the like to see when they open or closed. Or calling newspaper ads about items the client knows something about—for example, cars—and asking one or two specific questions—for example, how many miles has the car been driven, does it have front- or rear-wheel drive. Or calling restaurants and asking the price range of their meals. With experience and increasing success, the number, length, and nature of phone conversations can be modified to provide the client with larger quantity and greater diversity of speaking opportunities.

Some Client Reactions to Change

Speech Should Be Automatic; or, Why Do I Have To Think About It All the Time? About the time clients are beginning to change their inappropriate speech strategies more and more on their own, some of them may start to show signs of backsliding. One way or another the client may express the notion that "Your procedure works, but only if I think about it all the time. If I don't think about it, it doesn't work. Am I going to have to think about my speech for the rest of my life?" This is obviously a frustrating state of affairs for both client and clinician.

When Do Conscious Changes in Speech Become Less Conscious or More Automatic. While we do not have good objective information on how long after initial change in speech an adult who stutters needs to continue consciously monitor and change, it does seem that this period of time is longer rather than shorter. That is, there will probably be at least a six- to twelve-month period or longer of behavioral habituation. Some period of time is needed so that the client can generalize his or her increasingly fluent strategy to more and more speaking situations with more and more success. This period of habituation will, therefore, be a period where change in speech strategy is not automatic, where clients will have to be somewhat conscious of their speaking behavior and their relative success or failure at changing and monitoring same. We believe that it is wishful thinking—on both the part of the client and clinician—to expect anything different, to believe and expect establishment of new strategies for speaking in a few months when it has taken several years to establish the other, inappropriate strategies that create the instances of stuttering.

Misleading our clients that change in their speech behavior will be a quick, easy, and painless process is, in my opinion, doing them a great disservice and is more of a sin than providing ineffectual therapy. While we don't subscribe to the modern "no pain no gain" school of thought, we do believe that it is simply going to take some time and effort on the part of the client to change maladaptive, habituated speech strategies that have been used to initiate speech over many years. For example, when beginning speech, the client might habitually fix, lock, or stop the respiratory system during mid-exhalation simultaneously with opening the vocal folds in association with stabilizing the lower jaw and pressing the lips together; this complex of behaviors, this response pattern is going to take sometime to change. One does not learn to drive a car in two weeks but must spend considerable time behind the wheel in various traffic and weather conditions. For example, the process of learning to drive must first involve conscious monitoring of motor behavior until the motor behaviors necessary for steering, accelerating, shifting, and so forth are established, that is, become more automatic. Even when established, these "automatic" behaviors will become continually refined with further experience. Learning never stops, it just becomes less noticeable as refinements and subtleties rather than basic behavioral changes are made.

Creeping Before Walking.   Even though some clients initially exhibit a lack of auto-maticity when changing their speech, these same individuals may want to rush out and use their newly found fluent strategies in ALL situations at ALL times. One can hardly blame them, but the SLP should restrict this tendency somewhat, at least at first, until a client has demonstrated the ability to do this in more controlled situations, in situations where the probability for successful implementation of appropriate strategies is maximized. Once again, back to the car analogy, we explain to the client that after you first learn to drive, you do not want to practice during the time trials for the Indianapolis 500! Instead you practice your driving skills in low-traffic, side-road situations until you get more and more of the feeling for the strategies of driving. We stress patience and try to focus on success in more restricted speaking situations. However, I also tell clients that with time and additional experience, they will be talking in more and more difficult situations. At first, no matter how difficult it may be to restrain oneself, go slow. We must creep before we walk.

Knowing When to Dismiss

In an ideal world, dismissing adults who stutter from therapy should be like the old response parents gave their children when the youngster asked, "Mom, how will I know when I'm in love?" The sage parent supposedly replies, "Don't worry; when it's real love you'll know it." In other words, when an adult who stutters is ready for dismissal from therapy, both the client and clinician should know it. Unfortunately, this is not an ideal world, and we do not always know *when* to dismiss our clients from therapy. Thus, we have to take an educated guesstimation, which is just that: a considered hunch based on our education, training, and clinical experience.

What Sort of Nonspeech, Behavioral "Signs" Does the Client Exhibit? Is the client giving you signs that he or she is ready for a break (either temporary or permanent)? Is he or she calling in more often than in the past with excuses for not coming to therapy? Is he or she more regularly arriving late and leaving early? Do other adults who stutter begin to question why this client continues to come in for therapy because he or she is very fluent now and/or exhibiting little change? Does therapy seem to be playing more and more of a second fiddle to other activities, is therapy becoming less and less of a priority for the client (this may suggest resistance to as well as lack of motivation for further change), even though you continually attempt to remediate the client? Or is the client seemingly interested in helping others with similar speech problems (as mentioned in Conture, 1985, we think that this is always a good sign; for further discussion of "altruism" as a mature coping or adjustive mechanism, see Vaillant, 1977).

What Sort of Speech "Signs" Does the Client Exhibit. Is the client consistently demonstrating in therapy a quick, accurate, and relatively easy ability to identify and change instances of disfluency? Does the frequency of stuttering hover at or below 3 to 5 percent? (Obviously, these sort of percentages would be problematic when we are making decisions with very mild or nearly fluent people who stutter.) Does the clinician have to give minimal or no verbal, auditory, or visual cues before the client begins to change? When the client lapses back into old speech strategies, is he or she able to quickly, easily, and without much emotionality reverse directions and become more fluent again? Do you find yourself, if you have group therapy, using this adult client as a good example or role model for the other adults who stutter?

How Does the Client Manage "Breaks" from Therapy? Does this client, during breaks from therapy, continue to make improvements, albeit small, on his or her own? Do you find that this client, after a longer-than-usual break from therapy (say, three to five weeks or longer), is able to maintain progress to date or has he or she slipped back a couple of rungs? Does the client appear anxious or uncertain about maintaining his or her gains just before a scheduled break from therapy? Sometimes, if you have real doubts about dismissal, a scheduled break from therapy might be a viable alternative, that is, you could terminate therapy for a fixed but relatively brief period of time, say a month, after which the client returns to therapy. Scheduled breaks permit you to observe how the client effects changes on his or her own away from your watchful eye and the "healing" ambience of your clinical situation. As always, of course, make it clear to the client that the door to your clinic will remain open and that you will be willing and able to receive their phone calls and visits.

Dismissal May Result from Lack as well as Demonstration of Success. Dismissal from therapy, for some clients, may not mean that they have been successful in therapy or that their therapy is completed. Some clients may have to be dismissed before they actually achieve normally disfluent speech. These clients may not be able to receive maximal benefit from therapy at this point in their lives for a variety of reasons—for example, too many other professional and personal obligations vying for their attention, concomitant problems that may be ongoing but show signs of future resolution, unavoidable and unresolvable schedule conflicts, and so forth. All of this must be handled carefully by the SLP because he or she does not want to engender hopes of future success (or, conversely, dash all hopes for future improvement) when the SLP is just plain unsure. It is better, in most of these cases, to keep your uncertainties to yourself but make it apparent to the client that the door is always open for further discussion and consultation. In the end, you have to have some faith, which I think you can have, in your client's future ability to many times know when it is right for him or her to reenter speech and language therapy.

Maintenance/Follow-up Therapy

As the various contributors to Boberg's (1993) edited text on the maintenance of fluency indicate, there's much we don't know but would like to find out about maintenance/follow-up therapy. One thing that most clinical investigators do know, however, and that is that some form of maintenance/follow-up therapy is quite important to long-term improvement in stuttering. In essence, once our clients have left therapy, their work has really just begun (again, as Williams [1978] points out, "the goal of therapy is not change within the clinic but change outside the clinic"). The client, in his or her everyday world, now must try to apply the information, insights, and new behavior that have been gained in therapy. For some, this outside-of-clinic effecting of change will go fairly smoothly, but for others it will be problematic. Hopefully, the client has sufficiently developed problem-solving abilities and will be able, although not always 100 percent successfully, to independently change and adjust accordingly to the surroundings.

You Can't Hit a Home Run Every Time up to Bat.   You should let the client know that neither you nor they should expect success each and every time they have to speak. We realize that this instruction may sound a bit heretical because it appears rather pessimistic. It may sound to some that we are saying that the client will stutter forever and ever. Well, perhaps, but this advice is more realistic than pessimistic, in our opinion. It is based on what we believe is the reality of the situation. As previously mentioned, adults who stutter have taken many years to develop their speech problem and their social, emotional, psychological, and intellectual reactions and attitudes to it. The ABCs of stuttering, for some adults, will not be changed overnight, and at this stage we think that the client should be prepared for some future moments, hours, or days of difficulty. We said prepared (forewarned is forearmed), and not excused from attempting to right his or her fluency ship when it is listing and struggling through tough communicative seas.

Follow-up Therapy: Some Logistic Considerations.   The SLP can help the client through the adjustment from daily/weekly therapy to no therapy (i.e., a "normal" schedule) by scheduling follow-up or maintenance therapy sessions. Much of what we know about the number and nature of these sessions has come from experience with clinical practice, but there are very few hard and fast rules in this area. While there is clearly a need for empirical, objective investigations into the quantity and quality of maintenance therapy, there are still a few things that we can pass along at this point—although they are rather imprecise guidelines—that we think may be of help.

First, and perhaps most obvious, maintenance therapy sessions should be spaced far enough apart so that the SLP is not merely duplicating or recapitulating the original therapy schedule, only under a different guise. Second, it is probably better to gradually phase out therapy than to make the client go "cold turkey" and then return. We have used two different plans and prefer the former of the two: (1) once a month, every month for six months following dismissal, then once every two months for six months, followed by once every six months for one year and than periodic phone calls for another twelve to eighteen months or (2) a three- to six-month break from therapy after dismissal, then once every three months for a year, once every six months for one year, and than periodic phone calls for one more year. We prefer the former maintenance schedule because it is more gradual in nature during what we believe is the crucial post-therapy period—the first six months following dismissal. Generally speaking, however, if the client's outside-of-clinic fluency is maintained twelve months post-therapy, then the probability is high that significantly increased fluency will be maintained for the long-term and maintenance sessions can be spaced even farther apart, if the SLP and client so wish. Third, the basic point behind maintenance therapy is that the client not be set adrift, that he or she feels there is a place where contact can be made with a caring, knowledgeable professional who can and will answer questions and help the client work through problems that arise as he or she becomes a more fluent speaker. And, it should be noted, there can be problems.

Problems During Follow-up Therapy.   We've already mentioned the tendency on the part of some clients to feel discouraged during the latter parts of therapy or maintenance therapy, when they are not 100 percent successful in changing their speech and/or speaking more fluently. This problem should be addressed, as stated above, so that the client can learn how to cope with this situation, to be more *tolerant* of mistakes. Another problem that some clients encounter is when the client's newfound fluency begins to influence his or her relations with relatives, friends, and associates. A bit like a child with a new toy, some adults who stutter may begin to use their new, increasingly fluent speech any- and everywhere and at all times, much to the consternation of those around him or her. Whereas before these associates may have felt that the adult client wasn't talking enough, now they may complain—and we've had this occur—that the client is talking too much! Naturally, such problems need to be discussed between client and clinician and, if possible and where necessary, between client and concerned relatives or associates. While these associates must be helped to realize that they can't have it both ways—having the client talk *and* be quiet only when *they* so decree it—the adult client must also realize that normally fluent speakers listen just as well as speak. Their increased fluency is not a license for monologuing, monopolizing the speaking floor, interrupting other speakers, speaking and never listening, and the like. Follow-up sessions provide a natural vehicle for discussing these issues and can be used by clients to tell themselves and others, "I'll ask my speech person what she thinks about that when I see her in a couple of weeks." Of course, when real pressing concerns arise, the telephone can be used with the client being clearly and explicitly told that you will welcome such calls. We have found that it is better to head off little problems at the start, when they occur, before they develop and evolve into bigger ones that require more work on both the part of the client and clinician.

Some Parting Thoughts

"This Is What We Think Needs to Be Considered"

In the two preceding chapters, we discussed our thoughts and those of others regarding the evaluation and remediation of young children and teenagers who stutter. We have tried, in Chapters 3, 4, and 5, as we said at the outset in Chapter 1, not to provide a recipe orientation, but rather a "this is what needs to be considered" approach. Obviously, what we have considered was derived from our clinical and research experience, training, education, and biases regarding stuttering. However, we make no apologies for the selection of our considerations because all that one can do is present what appears most appropriate and important, given his or her considered opinion. Needless to say, other approaches do exist (for example, note Gregory's 1978 description of the "stutter more easily" versus "speak more fluently" forms of therapy or Guitar's, 1998, integration of fluency shaping and stuttering modification approach), and others will continue to be developed and should not be slighted. However, given the present space and orientation of this book, we thought it most appropriate to give the reader a *common thread approach* rather than one fractionated among a variety of approaches.

It's the Therapist, Not Merely the Technique

Regardless of the specific approach, it is the clinician's intensity of purpose, his or her concentration with the task at hand, his or her ability to attend to relevant and screen out nonrelevant detail, his or her ability to listen to the message behind the client's words, and his or her demonstrable caring for the client that will significantly determine the outcome of therapy. While we have come a long, long way from the days when therapy for individuals who stutter (children, teenagers, or adults) was much more of an art form than a science or trained skill, the clinician still remains central to this science and skill. Even though clinicians' personal, experiential, and professional qualities are central to the long-term success of their clients, clinicians must resist the temptation to divorce themselves from the seemingly esoteric world of empirical research. Simply put, the quantity and quality of objective data pertaining to individuals who stutter and stuttering has and will continue to develop to the point where it must, regardless of the clinician's clinical persuasion, be given some consideration by clinicians.

While the art of the clinician—his or her skill in handling people, expressing concern and care for the client, listening to their needs and so forth—can and should never be denied by any thinking individual, neither should clinicians disregard basic, objective empirical evidence regarding stuttering and people who stutter. Granted, not every clinician can and should become an experimentalist testing out this or that hypothesis or collecting this or that normative piece of information. However, as highly trained, educated, and up-to-date practitioners, we should all try to understand the objective information that tells us more and more about the nature of stuttering and people who stutter. Such attempts at understanding are preferable to simply proceeding ahead with clinical game plans derived from databases that have little or no factual support, are reflected by current information, or have had significant doubts cast upon them. Thus, I believe, and am urging, that the future will be a time when the art and the science of stuttering therapy can and should become more closely aligned. As such alignment becomes more and more of a reality, we can begin to hand down, from one generation of clinicians to another, clinical procedures that are based as much on fact as they are on tradition.

Avoid Being Overly Certain About the Uncertain

We have discussed in this and the three preceding chapters some of the complexities, subtleties, and vagaries involved with the clinical management of stuttering. One of the intentions behind these writings, as previously mentioned, was to help people become clear regarding their points of unclarity and confusion. If we have done this, if only in part, then we have contributed to readers' abilities to identify areas of uncertainty, which should, in turn, help us to formulate relevant questions whose answers may truly advance our knowledge. Clarity, however, is not the same as certainty.

If we, on the other hand, are certain about the uncertain—if we think that we have *all* the answers—we will never bother to ask needed questions because we are so certain we understand. We are neither advocating questions nor disagreements for their own sake. Rather, we need to ask ourselves questions. Surrounded by this imperfect world, can we realistically expect that our therapy with people who stutter will be perfect, that they will speak 100 percent fluently, that our therapy approaches will contain within them no points of uncertainty, that ALL of our clients will ALWAYS improve for ALL time? I think not. While we should not and cannot harbor such expectations, we can work toward improving and providing the best possible clinical services. I welcome your joining me in these efforts, for this is the material from which we formulate purposeful and interesting lives as professionals as well as people and help improve the communication of our clients. If we can do this, I am convinced that the best is yet to come for our clients.

Summary

This chapter discusses, relative to adults who stutter, stuttering modification procedures, with particular emphasis on identification and modification (for other excellent overviews and approaches to the treatment of stuttering in adults, see Guitar, 1998; Ham, 1999; Manning, 1996; Shapiro, 1999). As with our discussion of teenagers who stutter, we tried to discuss the broader context of the lives of adults, to better understand "where they are coming from." In this way, we believe, we do not attend solely to the (dis)fluent facet of the adult's life, to the exclusion of all other variables, something that is especially important, in our opinion, when treatment does not work. Regardless of claims to the contrary, there is too much *uncertainty* about the treatment of adults who stutter, especially regarding relapse, maintenance, or long-term recovery, for any clinician to be *certain* that all of the adults who stutter that they treat will always improve for all time.

The chapter also makes the observation that the presence and inter-mingling of the so-called ABCs of stuttering—Affect (A), Behavior (B), and Cognition (C)—are probably most apparent with adults who stutter. Certainly, for adults exhibiting developmental (rather than acquired) stuttering, it seems reasonable to suggest that the B element, the stuttering itself, is more habituated than it is for teens or children who stutter. And, if the adult who stutters is reasonably intact, emotionally and socially, and has been stuttering since, for example, 3 or 4 years of age, it is also reasonable to suggest that there are a number of A as well as C elements included in the melange that constitutes the adult's stuttering problem. In essence, the A and C, at the least, are normal reactions to abnormal B! And while many adults who stutter have previously had less-than-successful experience with treatment for their stuttering, experience that may have left them skeptical about treatment, they still can be very rewarding clients to work with. This is so because their motivation for change can be tremendous; after all, unlike children and most teens, most bring themselves to treatment, they are not brought by someone else. Likewise, their seriousness of purpose, their desire to finally "do something" about and for themselves, and their more refined intellectual and social skills coupled with increased maturity are real pluses in treatment.

Treatment can be individual and/or group (much the same can be said regarding children and teens who stutter),with decisions regarding group, individual, or combined format determined, in large part, by clinician orientation, caseload considerations, and so forth. The chapter makes apparent that one reasonable way to treat adults who stutter involves three interrelated procedures: (1) some form of *discussion* ("talk therapy") dealing with attitudes, beliefs, emotions, and ideas that appear to engender and maintain inappropriate speech production strategies (and/or get in the way of treatment progress, e.g., "I only need to work on my speech during treatment sessions"); (2) objective, nonjudgmental *identification* of those strategies that may interfere with speech production and treatment progress; and (3) systematically *changing* their speaking behaviors to those behaviors that individuals who do not stutter use to produce normally fluent speech. This trilogy of procedures—verbal discussion, identification, and modification—is based on the fact that adults who stutter, like most adults, *behave* in ways that influence the way they think and, conversely, *think* in ways that influence the way they behave. These dynamic interactions between the ABCs of stuttering, while less than tidy, constitute, we believe, the realities of stuttering for adults who stutter.

This chapter makes apparent the author's belief that adults who stutter cannot effectively change, on a long-term basis, speech and related behavior that they do not know how or when they produce. Thus, we believe, especially in the beginning of treatment, adults need to lean to quickly and accurately identify their inappropriate speech production strategies. This knowledge, we attempted to show, must precede and continue together with appropriate forms of modification of these strategies. A key point that we try to make is that the bridge, if you will, between identification and modification, is the adult's ability to *physically feel* what *he* or *she* is *doing* to interfere with *his* or *her* speaking and how those interfering behaviors differ from and can be changed into strategies that can be used to facilitate speaking. Again, we attempt to change the B of the adult who stutters by enlisting elements of their C, and possibly A, to achieve an active- rather than passive-based form of change in stuttering.

The chapter ends by discussing transfer or carryover with adults who stutter. Experience with adults suggests that lasting change from stuttering is generally not rapid. Such change advances, for most adults who stutter, by accretion not quantum. Both client and clinician, therefore, need to have patience for the rather slow manner in which changes occur in adults who stutter. While there is much the clinician can do to help the adult who stutters—and this therapy can be very rewarding for both client and clinician—it is not unreasonable, prior to initiation of therapy, as well as periodically throughout, to help the client become as realistic as possible regarding the length of time the treatment process may entail. Above all, the clinician will want to help the adult who stutters, during the latter phases of treatment, to better appreciate the fact that speech, for all speakers, contains errors, hesitations, and disfluencies. In essence, maintaining a *zero* tolerance for mistakes, disfluencies, or errors of any kind is to be intolerant of the human condition as well as themselves—an attitude, an intolerance that can do nothing but exacerbate and maintain concerns about speech fluency, something we know our clients don't want and are quite capable of learning how to overcome.

CHAPTER

6

Conclusions

Ending is nearly as difficult as beginning. How to organize the unorganizable? So many paths that haven't been traveled enough. However, there are limits to a reader's patience, and end we must. We will do so by presenting (1) our basic assumptions about stuttering, (2) an overview of our approach to the diagnosis and treatment of stuttering, (3) general considerations that we keep in mind when assessing the present status and making future predictions about the field of stuttering, (4) future predictions, and (5) some parting thoughts.

Basic Assumptions About Stuttering

In the preceding chapters, we discussed in detail our approach to the diagnosis and remediation of stuttering in children, teenagers, and adults. This approach rests on and relates to a variety of basic assumptions we make about stuttering and/or the clinical process. What follows, therefore, are some of what we believe are the more important of our *basic assumptions*, assumptions based on a combination of fact, opinion, and philosophy developed from experience, study, and observation.

1. *Stuttering is a disorder of childhood.* The need to understand that developmental stuttering begins, for most people, during childrenhood, generally before 7 years of age (e.g., see Mansson, 2000), and that, over time, the affective, behavioral, and cognitive (ABC) aspects of stuttering in older clients may change and thus differ considerably from those observed in young children.

2. *People who stutter are people first and people who stutter second.* The need to consider that there is much more to a person than the fact that they stutter, and that some of these "other things" may be as important to the person and the person's success in therapy as the stuttering itself.

3. *If stuttering touches parts of the whole person, then the whole of the person may require treatment.* The need to continually strive to understand the ABCs of stuttering, how they interact with one another, how each should be managed, and work toward treatments that integrate traditional with behavioral to maximize long-term change.

4. *People speak to communicate not to be fluent.* The need to consider that the main goal of speaking is communication not fluency.

5. *We typically study groups but we treat individuals.* The need to know what issues are typical for most people who stutter while recognizing important individual differences in etiology and symptomatology among people who stutter, differences that can significantly impact treatment.

6. *The goal of therapy is normal disfluency not total fluency.* The need to understand that normal disfluency not total fluency is the goal (Starkweather, 1987), the only realistic goal, of treatment for stuttering because even people who do not stutter produce disfluencies, some that remarkably resemble instances of stuttering. To have a zero tolerance for speech disfluencies, whether client or clinician, is not only to be unrealistic but to create an atmosphere of intolerance rather than acceptance for the real possibility of occasional human error.

7. *With children, show, not tell, what is desired.* The need to recognize that for children in particular, models and behavioral demonstrations by clinicians and parents speak far louder than all their verbal explanations, instructions, admonitions, and teachings (e.g., see Conture, 1994).

8. *One size therapy may not fit all.* The need to understand that the problem of stuttering is dynamic, multidimensional (e.g., see Smith & Kelly, 1997) and will continue to defy unidimensional explanations and treatment.

9. *Normal reaction to abnormal circumstances.* The need to understand that stuttering is a "layered phenomenon" that evolves over time due to learning and experience so that many behaviors observed result from adaptation to the impairment rather than being part of the basic impairment.

10. *True treatment efficacy involves the ability to use speech in daily communicative situations.* The need to understand that the goal of treatment, effective treatment, is to help the client " . . . speak whenever, about whatever, and to whomever, he or she wants" (Conture & Guitar, 1993, p. 265).

11. *"Average" behavior means that behavior normally varies above and below that average.* The need to understand that while behaviors or events may have a central tendency or average, this can only be possible if there is a "normal" dispersion of values surrounding that central tendency.

12. *Speech/accuracy trade-off during assessment and treatment.* The need to develop the ability to make quick, but accurate behavioral observations of people, their communicative and related activities.

13. *The yin and yang of psyche and soma.* The need to understand how the psyche and soma interact with stuttering and how interactive motor and premotor events (e.g., see Peters & Starkweather, 1990; Starkweather, 1991) may influence stuttering within the context of the psychosocial activities and concerns of the person who stutters.

14. *Stuttering involves premotor as well as motor behaviors.* The need to understand that a person who stutters, just like a person who doesn't, has just as much right to have delays and/or difficulties with syntactic, semantic, and phonological (premotor) (e.g., see Bernstein Ratner, 1997b; Louko, 1995; Paden, Yairi, & Ambrose, 1999; Ratner, 1995; St. Louis, Murray, & Ashworth, 1991) as motor (e.g., see Caruso, Max, & McClowry, 1999; Denny & Smith, 1997; Peters & Hulstijn, 1987; Peters, Hulstijn, &

Starkweather, 1991; Starkweather, 1982—e.g., articulatory execution of speech sounds) processes.

The above assumptions may seem a bit abstract. This abstraction, however, is as much due to the nature of stuttering as it is to the nature of this writer's manner of thought! While abstraction is not necessarily a virtue, neither, in some cases, is specificity. Clearly, it would be preferable to enumerate, quantify, and objectify *all* that we could about stuttering. Such quantitative specificity, however, may presently be neither possible nor feasible, at least for certain aspects of stuttering.

Thus, as aspects of the preceding five chapters indicate, this writer decided not to ignore the reality of such abstract, hard-to-quantify psychosocial factors as anxiety, parental guilt and concern, temperament, coping strategies, motivation, personality variables, and so forth. Ignoring the reality of such nonquantifiable factors would seem to be akin to ignoring the reality of love simply because we have not as yet been able to quantify, measure, or empirically investigate it. Factors like love and motivation may represent some of the untidy, murky details of life but they are, after all, part of life and as such need some, albeit less than objective, consideration.

Evaluation Precedes Remediation

Far too often SLPs begin to remediate individuals who stutter *before* they have a good idea regarding the number and nature of the individual's concerns. While we can never know everything there is to know about our clients, this should not provide us an excuse for beginning our therapy program *before* we carefully evaluate the client, to the best of our ability. We have tried to show that generating an effective therapy plan for stuttering *necessitates* an adequate evaluation of the person who stutters, his or her stuttering speech problem, and related (non)communicative concerns (see Gordon & Luper, 1992a, 1992b; Haynes & Pindzola, 1998; Pindzola, 1986b for overview of appropriate diagnostic assessment/evaluation protocols).

We have also tried to show that besides the speech disfluency problem, SLPs need to recognize that various other speech and nonspeech events should be evaluated—for example, parental standards for child behavior; parental rates of utterance and length and type of turn-switching pauses; the child's articulation, language, voice, hearing, reading and academic abilities; the child's temperament, and so forth. Below we will illustrate how difficult it is to develop such recognition by showing a classic example of the saying, "Do as I say, not as I do." Through this example, I hope to make apparent the that the writer himself has not always recognized that there is more to stuttering than stuttering; that he doesn't always understand that stuttering is not the only or even principal concern of each and every person who stutters that he clinically serves.

Do as I Say Not as I Do: An Example

The following example involves a 7-year-old boy I was remediating for stuttering. He and his parents had been attending our parent–child group regularly on a weekly basis, and while both parties (child and parents) seemed cooperative, interested, and attempting to change, little change was apparent. After consulting with our fellow clinicians who conduct these groups with me (Jennifer H. Ask and Christine L. Adkins), it was decided to enroll the child in individual therapy, a fairly routine recommendation for the approximately 25 to 30 percent for whom the parent–child group seemingly had little or no appreciable benefit. While I had occasionally noticed some extraneous movements and/or lack of attention during the group, we blamed that on the boy's intense curiosity with the world, youthful zeal, and the like. Bent on "correcting" his stuttering, I really did not listen or pay attention to the possibility that the child's activity level and lack of attention might be a problem. Instead, I continued to focus on the child's stuttering. After two or three individual sessions, however, I noticed that he pulled on the collar and sleeves of his shirts to point where a size 10 quickly became a size 14! He sometimes even put the collar or shirt in his mouth, pulling it even further, as we talked. Simultaneous with this, it became clear that he couldn't or wouldn't stay on any one task for much more than five minutes before his attention would drift and shift; extraneous stimuli, no matter how brief or innocuous, even his own shirt/sleeve pulling, would attract his attention off task, away from the treatment activity.

I began to ask the parents about his school performance and behavior at home. It quickly became apparent (e.g., "the teacher feels he is one of the brightest children in the class, but he can't stay on task and his grades are really not very good") that something was going on that was bigger than stuttering. Something that was keeping the child from "absorbing" our therapy, regardless of type (i.e., group versus individual). That something, I suspected, was hyperactivity/attention deficit disorder. In therapy, as certain sports, it is "hard to hit a moving target," especially when that "target" is crawling on and under the table and focusing on everything other than the therapy agenda! Thus, I broke the news to the parents that I suspected he exhibited hyperactivity and/or attention deficit difficulties. Breaking this news to the parents was not easy, because they realized that if the diagnosis was made, this might require drugs. However, they were quite frustrated with the child's progress in school and therapy (as were we) and were willing to try what, after some discussion, seemed like a reasonable course of action.

Referring the child to a child psychologist with whom I've had some very positive interactions eventually resulted in the child being diagnosed as exhibiting "attention deficit disorder," after some interviewing, testing, and the psychologist consulting with the child's pediatrician. The parents, naturally enough, were still reluctant to administer drugs to their child; but after some trials with different drugs and dosage level, a level of medication was reached that brought the child's level of activity and attention well within the range of normalcy. Therapy that had been marginally effective was now showing weekly benefits, and in the space of three months, the boy had made more progress than the entire six to nine months before that! At this writing, his therapy has been shifted to once every month and at this time he is well on his way to becoming a normally disfluent speaker with 1 to 2 percent or fewer stutterings per 100 words. In addition to this, the fluency he exhibits is natural-sounding, he is communicating when, where, and with whom he wants. Furthermore, he has significantly decreased his physical crawling, wiggling, and movement, his cognitive/communicative bouncing from topic to topic, and inattentive behavior. Perhaps most positive, his clinicians, parents, and teachers are now much more capable of interacting with and supporting him in positive, facilitating ways, both in terms of his communicative as well as general behavior. All of this, when I reflected on the situation, reminded of a line in a popular song, "You must be able to see me, before you can learn to read me . . . "

Okay, this is a nice story, with a happy ending, but what is the point? In essence this: If I had not been so focused on the child's stuttering, I would have recognized the child's hyperactivity/inattention concerns much earlier than I did. In fairness to me, these behaviors of the child were not of the gross, constant, or disruptive kind, and within a group setting not as easy to spot as during individual sessions. However, I should have noticed these behaviors sooner, especially when therapy was having little or no influence on his speech fluency. Perhaps, of course, something about the dynamic of individual therapy exacerbated and magnified the child's attention deficit hyperactive disorder, but I really don't think so. Rather, it was my exclusive concern for the child's stuttering that clouded my judgment and kept me from asking some simple but very pertinent questions of the child's father and mother.

My "perceptual sieve" basically obfuscated my observations and thinking, because I had frequently *watched* the child pulling on his shirt, crawling on the table, and not attending to the clinician. However, despite my watching, I didn't actually *see* these behavioral events for what they were—signs of a clinically significant concomitant problem! Fortunately, in this case, an appropriate referral was made and effective treatment was initiated that allowed the child to cooperate and participate with our speech-language therapy in a constructive, positive way. The case, and others like it, make me wonder how many serious and contributory concomitant problems clinicians may overlook in their sincere, but perhaps overly focused, concerns regarding a client's stuttering (or any other speech, voice, or language problem, for that matter). Truly, an objective, thorough evaluation of our clients who stutter is something toward which we continually strive but as yet have not achieved. The need to pigeonhole, categorize, and label all too often blinds us from one of life's basic realities: A person can exhibit more than one problem at the same time! Furthermore, these co-occurring problems can interact to the extent where effective treatment of problem A cannot occur until one initiates effective treatment for simultaneous problem B. Similarly, and just as important, the distracted, inattentive, seemingly uninterested behavior of a child who is pervasively and inappropriately worried and anxious about any and everything can *look like* the inattentive behaviors of ADHD. In brief, when in doubt, the wise SLP refers to a clinical psychologist or pediatrician experienced with the problem and diagnosis of ADHD.

Identification

The Importance of Physically Feeling Behavior That Interferes with Speech-Language Production

We have stressed in the preceding chapters the importance we place on helping people who stutter develop the ability to identify or *physically feel* what they *do* when they interfere with their own speech-language production. If we make the reasonable assumption that the goal of stuttering therapy is to assist people who stutter to transfer their in-clinic fluency to the "real world" outside the clinic, we should try to provide them with a means to insure this transfer. Quick, accurate identification of their own behavior is one means to this transfer ends.

We have previously said it is difficult, at least on a more consistent basis, to change what you do not know that you do when you do it. This specificity—which, as previously mentioned, seems similar to Thorndike's (1913) "specificity doctrine"—that is involved with the identifying or physically feeling of interfering speech behavior can be influenced by such factors as (1) the severity and nature of the stuttering behavior; (2) the client's psycho-social-emotional willingness to come to grips with, subjectively or objectively, what he or she *does* that interferes with forward-flowing, fluent speech-language production; and (3) the client's ability to objectively and analytically assess his or her own behavior, particularly speaking behavior during structured therapy tasks as well as unstructured conversational speech outside of therapy.

The Clinician's Ability to Identify

As previously mentioned, people who stutter can be helped to identify and physically feel their interfering, disrupting, or tensing speech behavior by using audio and audio-video tape recordings, mirrors, magnifying glasses, clickers, buzzers, flashlights, as well as hand gestures or simple statements like "there," "now," or "that's one." These various "devices" have one sole purpose: to help signal to the client the presence and/or occurrence of those interfering speech behaviors we call stuttering. While perhaps obvious, we must stress how important it is for the SLP to have the ability to quickly, accurately, and non-emotionally recognize and point out to the person who stutters his or her inappropriate or interfering speech behavior.

This ability on the part of the SLP really determines, no matter what technology or equipment is used, the success of the identification procedure. And, I hasten to point out, this ability on the part of the SLP can only be developed *if* the clinician spends time listening to audio/videotapes, trying to quickly and accurately identify instances of stuttering as they occur in conversation. For it is during conversation that the clinician must be quickly and accurately aware of instances of stuttering. Why? Well, it is during conversational speech that stuttering must eventually be modified. Being able to identify and/or change stuttering during, for example, an isolated phrase or word is nice, but this is not conversation, and neither client nor clinician should be lulled or fooled into thinking otherwise. People who stutter, like people who don't, typically speak with others through means of running, conversational speech rather than word lists, reading aloud, and board games!

The clinician should also realize that he or she is mainly, if not *only*, using *externally* apparent auditory and visual information to identify stutterings of a person who stutters. However, the person who stutters, besides audition and vision, also has available various *internalized* physically feelings (kinesthesia, deep touch, etc.) associated with his or her stutterings. Therefore, the clinician must make a concerted effort to obtain some degree of appreciation for what instances of stuttering physically feel like as well as sound and look like. The SLP can develop such an appreciation by routinely imitating, as close as possible (in an obviously nonmocking, nonjudgmental, noncritical fashion), the actual instances of stutterings of the person who stutters as well as asking the person if it physically *feels* like thus and so (e.g., "Markus, when I prolong the 's' like you just did—like this [clinician models /s/ prolongation]—I have this tense feeling in the front of my tongue. Is that what it physically feels like to you when you do that?"). An older client, particularly one who is sensitive to the physical aspects of his or her own speech behavior and is reasonably artic- ulate, can help the clinician learn much about what it physically feels like to stutter. As well as having the ability to quickly and accurately identify instances of stutterings, the SLP also needs to be able to provide the person who stutters with some reasonable rationale for iden- tification. And this rationale will generally have to be explained several times until the basic concept is understood. Especially with the silver bullet–seeking client, the SLP will have to repeat this rationale, supplying more detail as the person who stutters progresses through therapy.

Helping the Client Identify Stutterings Should Not Take the Place of Helping the Client Learn to Modify Stutterings

Simply put, identification of stutterings does not and should not take the place of the next phase of treatment, modification of stuttering. They are related processes, but identification is only the beginning of the entire process. Identification is that part of the platform upon which we help the client build a lasting change in speech fluency. Change that passively happens to the client because of what *you make them do* is change that will fade with time. In a client's everyday life, when he or she needs to change his or her speech, the client will need to quickly and nonemotionally recognize how he or she is interfering with the forward flow of speaking behavior. The client must, in my mind, have a reasonably clear rationale for identification. The client must also develop a generalized means of identifying, one that is flexibility enough to be usable in most everyday speaking situations. While it is impor- tant to learn a different, more fluent way of speaking, it is just as important, if not more dif- ficult, to know *when* to appropriately do or demonstrate what is learned. Identification provides some of this knowledge, as well as a means by which the mystery and vagueness of the problem can be removed.

Doing It "to" Clients Versus Having Them Do It "for" Themselves

It is difficult to underestimate the importance of the objective insights gained by the client from a detailed examination of their stutterings and the ability to rapidly identify stuttering after, as well as during, its occurrence. Here, as elsewhere, we want to help the client learn these abilities in an independent, problem-solving fashion. We are *not* interested in the client's becoming dependent upon us for identification and modification of speech. We believe that it is a short-sighted procedure for the SLP to change the clients' speech fluency *for* them, without their objective awareness of what *they do* to interfere with their own behavior and what *they must do* to change. To draw an analogy, let us suppose that you were learning a foreign language. Could we realistically expect that you would be ready and able, by *passively* repeating the words, phrases, and sentences of the foreign language, to effectively use these phrases when the situation calls for you to actually use the foreign language? Conversational speech, above all, is a creative activity. Changes in thought and expression occur on the fly. The number, nature, and complexities of everyday, conversational speaking situations are never predictable, and neither is the learner's emotional-intellectual state at the time when the situation occurs. Thus, learners, to be maximally effective across a wide variety of situations, need to be able to *actively* generate a strategy to effect or change behavior, when they realize the situation demands such action or when they are producing inappropriate behavior.

Modification

Behavior Modification

The 1960s brought to the field of stuttering a panoply of new terms and concepts from the area of learning theory and behavioral therapy (e.g., Brutten & Shoemaker, 1967; Shames & Sherrick, 1963). Although the 1970s witnessed some critical assessment of this approach (e.g., Siegel, 1970), during this time and into the early 1980s, clinical investigators employing behavioral modification methodology with people who stutter seemingly concentrated on refining this methodology (e.g., Martin & Haroldson, 1982; Ryan, 1974, 1978) findings that one may use, it is presumed, to assess the underlying notion that stuttering is learned and/or operates according to the principles and laws of operant conditioning. There has been some thoughtful attempt (e.g., Guitar, 1999) to integrate and/or combine traditional ("stuttering modification") and behavioral modification ("fluency-shaping") approaches when remediating stuttering, as well as rigorous attempts to compare among behavioral and other forms of treatment for school-age children (Ryan & Van Kirk Ryan, 1983). Recent years have witnessed some very creative (e.g., Lincoln & Onslow, 1997) and refined (e.g., Costello & Ingham, 1999; J. Ingham, 1993; R. Ingham, 1999) approaches to behavioral management of stuttering (see Lincoln & Harrison, 1999, for overview of the Lidcombe program, an early intervention for stuttering based on operant tenets).

Although the theory and methodology of *behavior modification* appears to continue to generate interest, particularly with regard to clinical practice, there are, as Prins and Hubbard (1988) indicate, a variety of theoretical issues in this area that still remain unresolved. Whatever the case, behavioral modification, in some form or another, will continue to generate a level of interest and controversy for some time to come (see Guitar, 1998, pp. 89–101; Ingham, 1984, pp. 195–272; Onslow, 1996; Starkweather, 1997, for good overviews of learning/behavioral principles as well as their implications for stuttering). The ability, within the behavioral paradigm, to quantify both what the clinician/researcher and client do, has considerable attraction, especially in this age of accountability.

Behavior modification, broadly defined, is a clinical procedure stemming from conditioning and learning principles used to change a client's behavior. Some have expressed the belief that behavior modification for stuttering is akin to old wine in new bottles (e.g., Sheehan, 1970b), whereas others appear to believe that behavior modification is a sound, more systematic means of remediating stuttering (e.g., Costello Ingham, 1999; Onslow, 1992; Onslow, Andrews & Lincoln, 1994; Onslow, Costa, & Rue, 1990; Ryan, 1978, 1980). There is, as usual, some truth in both opinions; however, we believe that there are other issues that are just as germane, if not more, to the topic of behavior modification of stuttering.

How to Behave Before All the Data Are In

Clearly, the speech of people who stutter needs to be modified, changed, or to coin a term, metamorphosized. Given this need, one could argue that employing behavior modification procedures may make the most sense: These procedures are systematic, relatively quantifiable, and permit reasonably clear communication between clinicians and clients regarding therapy goals and procedure. However, to vociferously promulgate or advocate one specific procedure—whether it be fluency shaping, stuttering modification, or whatever—to the relative *exclusion* of other approaches is inappropriate and unwarranted. This is particularly true given the fact that we are still unclear regarding: (1) the precise behaviors that need modification for long-term recovery and (2) the relative effectiveness of different therapy approaches to bring about long-term recovery from stuttering. We must be careful here, of course. Routine usage of a procedure does not necessarily imply advocation of that procedure and that procedure alone. Rather, it may merely suggest that the clinician knows, believes, and has experience with a certain approach and feels that the relative benefits of the procedure outweigh its costs. *All* treatments, from aspirin to surgery and all points in between, have benefits and costs. Those who believe otherwise—that their treatment is *totally* without *any* cost and/or side effects—exist in a reality this author fails to understand.

Too often, with the treatment of stuttering, we have had to put the cart before the horse and provide therapy without strong justification for its particular use. This, of course, is understandable because we have a practical need to develop workable therapy procedures ("before all the data are in") despite our recognized incomplete understanding of the etiology and nature of stuttering. Indeed, our clients and their families daily stand before us, requesting help, services, and support. It is difficult not to help, not to intervene, even while recognizing the imperfections of such intervention. In this regard, stuttering is similar to cancer, where many possible causes exist but where therapies for the sake of practicality are more often based on what works, what arrests the development of the problem for at least for awhile, than they are on a clear understanding of the cause and true nature of the problem.

Obviously, we must and should continue to provide such clinical services, but we should also, in our writings and lectures, make it apparent to our professional audiences (as well as ourselves) that the present state of the art is less than an exact science. Before all the data are in, we have to help our clients the best way we know how based on our current understanding of available data, accepted practice, and philosophical persuasion. However, we must not confuse what is *expedient* and what most is *appropriate*. Clinical reality requires us to tolerate the former, but it need not make us abandon our continual search for the latter.

Being Able to Modify Stuttering Behavior (in the Present)
Does Not Mean We Know What Stuttering Behaviors
Need Modifying (for Future Success)

Simply put, how can we modify something we don't understand? On the one hand, one can argue that if the behavior goes away or changes, it matters little if we understand the underlying reason for the behavior. The behavior has, simply put, become marginalized or reduced to the point of nonsignificance. But what about when the behavior doesn't change, gets worse, or returns after a more or less long period of relative dormancy? Certainly, adjustments to treatment can be made to try to bring the behavior back under control. However, such approaches still do not make clear why the person is stuttering and/or why stuttering might change, relapse, or worsen, regardless of form of treatment. For answers to these questions, this author believes, researchers must focus their attention in areas other than behavior modification.

Different Behaviors, Different Etiologies: Different Therapies?

Do we really know what an individual does with his or her formulative (semantic, phonologic, and syntactic) and motor execution processes just before and during an instance of stuttering that needs modification (see Stromsta's 1965, 1986 seminal work attempting to describe and characterize the essential elements of speech production associated with stuttering)? Are all behavioral aspects of stuttering equal and resulting from similar underlying processes. (The idea that not all aspects of stuttering are similar is, of course, somewhat consistent with Brutten & Shoemaker's [1967] speculation that some aspects of stuttering, e.g., within-word disfluencies, result from classically conditioned "negative emotion," whereas other aspects—for example, facial gestures—represent adjustive or coping, albeit maladaptive, behaviors that are learned and/or reinforced through instrumental conditioning processes.) We do know, at least behaviorally, that people who stutter do not exhibit similar "constellations" of behaviors (e.g., Schwartz & Conture, 1988; Watson, Freeman, Devous, Chapman, Finitzo, & Pool, 1994)—that is, they significantly differ in terms of their type of speech disfluency, associated nonspeech behaviors, and concomitant problems. Likewise, Van Riper (1971) reported findings, based on clinical reports, that the etiologies of different people who stutter may differ.

Thus, it is more than plausible that one significant reason that our therapies don't always work for all of our clients is that our clients exhibit appreciably different behaviors and etiologies (e.g., Preus, 1981; St. Onge, 1963), differences that may require different therapy (in FUTURE DIRECTIONS, below, we will return to the concept of "subgroups" of stuttering). The problem, however, is that we have a tenuous grasp on what those differences might be as well as what differences make a difference in terms of treatment and how to tailor our treatment accordingly (for an older, but still useful, overview of "types of stutterers," see Van Riper, 1971, Chapter 10). While some may believe that within-group differences between people who stutter have no appreciable influence on treatment outcome, such a belief would appear to fly in the face of what we know about other disorders—for example, attention deficit hyperactivity disorder—where subtle and not so subtle differences in etiologies and manifestations have significant influence on nature and success of intervention. It is one thing, during experimental treatment, to control for level of language development, to restrict untoward influences on the results of treatment. However, in the real world, where clinicians live, such control is not possible. The child who stutters with concomitant language concerns must be treated; to do so without consideration of the co-occurring concerns with language is the clinical equivalent of an ostrich with its head in the sand. Yes, concomitant problems make our diagnosis and treatment more or less ambiguous, but tolerance and dealing with the ambiguous is the hallmark of the educated mind.

Some of the Things We Do Know About STUTTERED Speech Production

It seems to this writer that in our scurry to modify stuttering, we may have lost sight of one important fact: specifically, what aspects of stuttering need to be modified to achieve long-term recovery. Research (e.g., Caruso, Conture & Colton, 1988; Conture, McCall & Brewer, 1977; Conture, Schwartz & Brewer, 1985; Denny & Smith, 1992; Freeman & Ushijima, 1978; Yaruss & Conture, 1993) has provided the *beginnings* of an objective database describing what *actually* happens to speech production *during* stuttering, rather just what we subjectively believe or feel is happening (these *descriptive* of speech production during stuttering are related to but different from more *experimental* studies of the speech production of people who stutter, the latter being designed to discover underlying speech motor processes [and speculate about associated neural centers/mechanisms] that may contribute to stuttering, e.g., see Caruso, Max, & McClowry, 1999, Denny & Smith, 1997, Ingham, 1998, for overviews of such research). For example, research has shown us, among other things, that (1) different types of stuttering may be associated with different types of disrupted speech production; (2) there is a complex relation between the type of stuttering, the phonetic elements being stuttering upon, and the resultant observed speech production behavior; (3) the larynx is clearly a part of stuttering, although there is little evidence to indicate that it "causes" stuttering; (4) the "discoordination" hypothesis (see Van Riper, 1982, pp. 396–453) is not supported by existing empirical findings (e.g., Conture, Colton & Gleason, 1988 and the exchange between DiSimoni, 1990 and Conture, Colton, & Gleason, 1990); and (5) that the underlying dynamics of the speech production processes may differ between people who do and do not stutter (e.g., Peters & Boves, 1988; Smith & Kelly, 1997). Of course, while description of the speech motor/production associated with stuttering has some value for clinicians trying to decide how and what aspects of stuttering to modify, such information has little appreciable explanatory salience (i.e., a behavior can't, at one and the same time, be part as well as cause of a problem). With that in mind, as well as the critiques of Conture (1991) and Ingham (1998) of speech motor control studies of stuttering and cautions of Armson and Kalinowski (1994) that disruptions in the fluent speech of people who stutter may merely be subtle versions of the problem rather than indicators of cause, the pendulum of theoretical interest in stuttering has begun to swing from motor to linguistic (premotor) investigations. Indeed, investigators (e.g., Bernstein Ratner, 1997b; Burger & Wijnen, 1999; Kolk & Postma, 1997; Postma, Kolk, & Povel, 1990b, 1991; Wingate, 1988) are increasingly speculating about and exploring aspects of speech and language production of people who stutter, *above* the level of speech motor execution, for example, lexical access, phonological encoding, and so forth. Where this psycholinguistically oriented research[1] will take us is, of course, unknown at this writing. At least, however, and perhaps like its "speech motor" predecessors, it will at least flesh out the pre-motor (syntactic, semantic, and phonologic) domain that we *must* consider in addition to the motor domain when we theorize about as well as treat stuttering.

---

[1]To assess psycholinguistic literature pertaining to speech errors in people who do not stutter and the theorized cognitive and/or linguistic processes underlying these errors, see, for example, Berg (1986), Blackmer & Mitton (1991), Bredart (1991), Clark & Wasow (1998), Jaeger (1992), and Stemberger (1989).

Starting with "Simple" and Working Toward "Complex" Behavior

Perhaps behavior modification, fluency shaping, or variants thereof might be appropriate for all people who stutter if we knew more precisely what aspects of speech-language production of people who stutter need modification for long-term recovery! (Of course, in the strictest sense, to apply behavior modification methodology and principles to stuttering, we would also have to assume that the stuttering speech behavior results from or behaves in accordance with the laws or principles of conditioning and learning (e.g., see Ingham, 1984, pp. 195–201, for an overview of principles of operant conditioning). A reasonably observant individual can see and hear the person who stutters reiterate, cease, or prolong various speech postures, but what are the *proximal* sources within the brain, brainstem, or vocal tract of these reiterations, cessations, and prolongations? Likewise, where are the *distal* sources that exacerbate, maintain, and perpetuate these behaviors, perhaps temperamental characteristics of the person who stutters (for seminal work in this area, see the work of Kagan, e.g., Kagan, Reznick, & Snidman, 1987; for its possible influence on stuttering, see Guitar, 1998). At present, what too often passes for behavior modification appears to be the result of clinical expediency and/or trial and error experimentation, rather than a clear understanding of what needs modification (it is unfair to level this charge solely at behavior modification, for much could be said about many approaches to stuttering, e.g., stuttering modification). This problem is compounded by some behavioral modification approaches that appear based on very rudimentary, and probably inaccurate, conceptions of the *simple to complex* continuum of speech behavior. Many times this rudimentary understanding appears to be based more on a understanding of written, *orthographic* communication behavior than it does on an understanding of disfluent and fluent speech articulatory, laryngeal, and respiratory behavior (see Faircloth & Faircloth 1973, pp. 77–78, for description of orthographic versus articulatory sounds and syllables).

Spoken Versus Orthographic Behavior

One good example of such rudimentary understanding is typified by clinical approaches that modify speech at the isolated vowel level first and then proceed to the sentence level without apparently once considering if this progression makes sense in terms of *speech and language production*. Given the very elegant models of speech-language production now available (e.g., Levelt, 1989; Levelt, Roelofs, & Meyer, 1999; Levelt & Wheeldon, 1994; Roelefs, 1997), we can and should do better when tailoring the format of our therapies to the actualities of human spoken communication. For example, the primacy/importance of the syllable, as a building block to overt speech production (e.g., Roelefs, 1997), is seldom manifest in many treatment approaches to stuttering. Certainly, one can't quibble with the fact that such a progression (e.g., isolated sound, syllables, words, etc.), at least some of the time, significantly improves the speech fluency of people who stutter. However, one cannot help but wonder if this progression is inappropriate and whether it may somehow contribute to the oft-reported relapse that many people who stutter experience post-therapeutically. It is *speech*, after all, not *orthographic*, behavior that needs modification. It is speech, after all, not orthographic behavior that we use in conversational interactions. Stuttering occurs during speaking not writing. While speech and writing, like walking and running, are related, they are also two distinctly different acts and need to be dealt with accordingly.

Psyche, Soma, and Their Interaction

The idea that stuttering should be treated either *this* way or *that* way is very much related, we think, to our *t'is–t'aint* views of what causes stuttering. Typically, the battle lines have been drawn between the *psyche* (essentially a nurture idea) and the *soma* (essentially a nature idea). One basic premise of the *psyche* philosophy posits that stuttering is caused by nervous overflow into the peripheral speech structures and muscles (perhaps even influencing central processes as well) that results from an individual's subtle to significant psychosocial problems. Thus, for whatever reason, there is some sort of disruption or disturbance in the psyche, attitudes, emotions, and beliefs of the person who stutters, on some level. Therefore, what listeners hear and see as stuttering is nothing more than reflections of these psychosocial problems—that is, the fixations, cessations and repetitive shakings or oscillations of peripheral structures and muscles manifested during other psychosocial problems.

Conversely, the *soma* philosophy views stuttering as the result of some inherent physiological, biochemical, or organic defect (subtle to gross in degree) within the person who stutters that creates, in as yet unknown ways, cessations, fixations, prolongations, and reiterations of speech postures. Such disruptions generally differ in degree and kind from the more profound nervous system damage of problems from cerebral palsy to dysarthria, which also foster certain types of speech dysfunction. Either approach—psyche or soma—seemingly views the problem as having, in essence, a singular cause. Interestingly, however, such categorical thinking is generally not even found in the area of genetics, where environmental factors are almost always taken into consideration along with genetics (see Plomin & DeFries, 1998, for an example of this relative to the genetics of cognition; see Ambrose, Yairi, & Cox, 1993, for an overview of the genetics of stuttering).

A third, perhaps, *equatorial* or *interactionist* approach (an example of which we discussed in Chapter 1) is to view the people who stutter as individuals with a minimal, marginal, subtle, or very difficult to detect difficulties with speech and language processes (semantic, syntactic, phonological, and/or motor execution) during many speaking situations. These difficulties, we believe, are generally of little bother but may become exacerbated—thus disrupting initiation and/or continuation of speech production—when the individual speaks under certain forms of emotional, communicative, or environmental stress. We hasten to add that such stress need not only be *external*—for example, from parents—but *internal* as well—for example, from a child who is intolerant of mistakes of any kind,[2] including speech, who reacts very quickly and strongly to environmental change, and once he or she has so reacted finds it very difficult to quickly modify (i.e., continue) his or her responses to environmental change. What seems to be attractive with this interactionist approach is that it bypasses the t'is-t'aint arguments of the psyche versus soma theory pro-

---

[2]For some of these children such intolerance of mistakes is not limited to speech—for example, the 4-year-old girl who stutters who routinely rips up, crumples up, and throws out a sheet of paper rather than erasing or compensating for one small error made while drawing or writing!

ponents, and even the traditionalist versus behaviorist therapy approach, and assumes that both the person who stutters *and* his or her (internal and external) environment will require attention. While the proportion of attention to psyche versus soma may vary—as we've discussed in Chapters 3, 4, and 5—when dealing with children versus teenagers versus adults who stutter, this middle-ground approach *assumes* interaction between people who stutter and their environments.

Such an approach takes each client as he or she comes, sometimes (1) focusing on one's environment where the environment seems key; other times, (2) concentrating on one's speech-language production strategies when those seem paramount to long-term recovery; and still other times, (3) dealing with *both* the person who stutters and environment when the interaction between the two seems key. While we have previously discussed the elements that we believe are central to changes in actual stuttered speech behavior, we want to make it clear that "focusing on speech" does not mean we disregard the attitudes, beliefs, feelings, and environmental reactions of the person who stutters (and his or her family). Unfortunately, even though these psychosocial and environmental issues are important, we are less clear about commonalties in these issues across people who stutter.

It is quite clear that on the average, people who stutter are *not* markedly different from people who do not stutter, in terms of psychosocial adjustment and development (e.g., Bloodstein, 1995, p. 236). What is beginning to emerge, however, are suggestions and speculations that subtle variations in *temperamental* characteristics (e.g., Amster, 1995; Conture, 1991, pp. 380–381; Glasner, 1949; Guitar, 1997, 1998; Oyler, 1996a, 1996b; Oyler & Ramig, 1995; Zebrowski & Conture, 1998). As mentioned before, it is this writer's opinion, that more than a few children who stutter, particularly those in whom the problem persists, exhibit temperaments that are (1) overly cautious when confronted with novelty or changes in the environment; (2) easily distracted from their ongoing behaviors by environmental stimuli; (3) sensitive to relatively low levels of extraneous stimuli; and (4) unable or slow to quickly modify their reactions to stimuli in more desirable ways. How these characteristics interact, if they do at all, with the child's stuttering is still far from unclear (see Guitar's, 1998, pp. 83–89, speculation in this regard), but we are certain, as we will mention below, that the following years will uncover a great deal in this area, information that should have significant theoretical as well as therapeutic implications. At present, therefore, we should focus on those things we have a better understanding of, in specific, those events that seem the most highly related to changes in stuttering.

Transfer

SLPs Modify Stuttering but Can People Who Stutter Maintain the Modification?

Regardless of the specific approach, therapy that follows the evaluation of stuttering has two general concerns: (1) producing meaningful *in-clinic* change in the nature and number of stuttering and related behavioral events, which then are (2) transferred and maintained *outside the clinic* in a variety of speaking situations. As we've mentioned before, and as Williams (1978) suggested, the goal of our therapy with people who stutter is much more importantly related to transfer of change to the outside environment than change within the therapy setting (for an excellent example of assessment of and attempts to achieve *long-term* outcome, after formal treatment termination, see Lincoln & Onslow, 1997). We believe that effective therapy procedures (i.e., effective = long-term change) involve a systematic monitoring of the client's outside-of-clinic change, for example, surprise or unannounced post-therapy phone calls and actively trying within the clinic to bring about such "real-world" change. Ideally, our therapies should be structured to optimize the bridge between in-clinic change and outside-of-clinic performance. Developing such bridges is, of course, no easy task, but one that should be a main goal of stuttering therapy. Our treatment of stuttering should continually strive to assist people who stutter, should they so choose, to speak as fluently as possible in their *everyday* environment, to effect the necessary behavioral change that will facilitate more fluent speech.

Realistically, even if we are effective in planning for the client's transfer of speech behavior, we should not maintain the hope that each and every one of our clients, particular those with a more habituated stuttering problem, will *immediately* and *dramatically* become fluent outside the clinic. Our experience, which is consistent with Perkins' (1978) comments in this regard, is that real transfer will take longer than any of us would actually like or sometimes even admit to. Speech-language pathologists dealing with people who stutter, particularly those with a more established or habituated problem, would be well advised to develop patience for the length of time it takes a human being to effectively change a central or even peripheral part of themselves, especially when that part is stuttering. Lasting behavioral change is quite possible but seldom easy or quick—especially if the person who stutters, while concerned, fearful, or worried about his or her stuttering, has developed a feeling of near hopelessness that they can be helped and/or the stuttering changed. To compound this, with a teenager, whose friends have all, at least overtly, come to accept the teen who stutters and his or her stuttering, the level of motivation on the part of the teen to put the effort and time into changing his or her speech may be far less than optimal.

Carryover Problems Are Not the Exclusive Domain of Stuttering

In the United States, many of us take French, Spanish, German, and so on in high school and college, for several years. How many of us wind up fluent in these second language as a result of our study? The number, I would wager, is quite small. This is not only an in-class problem but a carryover problem, from class to real world. We must keep in mind, therefore, that stuttering is not all that unique in terms of its relative resistance to change as a result of therapeutic intervention. In fact, human resistance to change appears to be the rule, rather than the exception, no matter if the behavior is cigarette smoking, obsessive compulsive traits, study habits, or sexual dysfunction. For example, Zilbergeld and Evans (1980), in a critical appraisal of Masters and Johnson's (1970) sex-therapy research, state that " . . . the main problem for brief therapy is not inducing change, but maintaining it."[3] Thus, clinicians

[3]B. Zilbergeld & M. Evans (1980). The inadequacy of Masters and Johnson, *Psychology Today, 14*, p. 37. Reprinted by permission of B. Zilbergeld.

dealing with other types of human behavior besides stuttering, in this case sexual dysfunction, are extremely concerned with the amount of relapse or lack of transfer they observe in their clients shortly after termination of therapy. (Studies of sex therapy relapse, not unlike studies of stuttering-therapy relapse, report relapse rates of 37 to 54% relapse after termination of therapy.) SLPs remediating stuttering are not alone in the boat—relapse cuts a wide swath across the human condition.

The point of this comparison of stuttering to other human problems is to caution against our suggesting to ourselves and our clients that we can easily and quickly achieve *long-lasting* change from stuttering. (Quick change? Sure, what is relatively easy can be just as quick to relapse as well!) We've already said that we believe it unethical to encourage our clients, particularly those with a habituated problems, to expect easy, quick cures. Based on current information regarding treatment efficacy (e.g., Conture, 1996; Conture & Wolk, 1990; Cordes, 1998; Fosnot, 1993; Ingham, 1990; Onslow, 1990), this is not, we think, a pessimistic but a realistic approach to stuttering and the individual who stutters. Part of the "slowness" of change, particularly with older clients exhibiting a more habituated problem, is that the ABCs of their problem (discussed elsewhere in this chapter) have become inextricably entwined. And although entwined, the clinician may only focus on one aspect (even one aspect of one aspect!) of the ABC triology, essentially ignoring the other two facets as well as the fact that they are interrelated. At the very least, others (e.g., Burns, 1980) have made clear their view that thoughts (C) and behavior (B) inextricably related.

In this writer's opinion, speech-language pathologists who want to assist people who stutter to produce lasting change must take into consideration the circularity of influence between an individual's thinking (C), feelings (A), and his or her behavior (B). Regardless of which end of the behaviorist-nonbehaviorist continuum a particular therapeutic approach resides, some clients who receive *any* approach will encounter greater to lesser degrees of relapse in stuttering. Indeed, in this writer's opinion, the amount of relapse commonly observed across *all* such approaches—regardless of press releases to the contrary—indicate that a change in approach is needed. We would like to suggest that this change reflects a movement away from the classic t'is-t'aint war waged between behaviorists and traditionalists toward a meld of the "mentalistic" insights and procedures of traditional approaches and the systematic, objective methods and principles of the behavioral approach, as exemplified by the writings of Guitar (1998, 1999), and hopefully this writer as well.[4] Both approaches have something necessary about them, but neither, by itself, appears sufficient.

The Need for Pre- Versus Post-Therapy Research

One difficulty with treatment, in this writer's opinion, is that too many clinicians take their eye off the prize (long-term improvement) in a sincere, but misguided attempt to show "strong first-quarter earnings," that is, rapid results (we will also address the important issue of "transfer," below in the section under FUTURE DIRECTIONS, Treatment Efficacy). A

---

[4]Therapy, of course, is not always necessary for recovery from stuttering, as the thoughtful work of Finn (1996, 1998) on the topic of spontaneous recovery makes clear, even if the process by which this occurs is far from certain.

search for rapid results, by both clinician and client, is quite understandable. The person has a problem and he or she wants to be helped and we want to help them *now*! However, *short-term* is not *long-term*, and what goes away quickly can come back just as quickly.

The above said, it is still unclear, regarding the long-term recovery from stuttering, what aspects of stuttering are the most crucial to modify, relative to long-term recovery. Frequency? Type? Duration? Severity? Associated nonspeech behaviors? Reactions to any or all of these aspects of stuttering? Related to this issue is pre- versus post-therapy research like that exemplified by Metz and others (e.g., Metz et al., 1979, 1983; Robb, Lybolt, & Price, 1985). With this research, Metz and others have attempted to assess what aspects of the acoustic correlates of speech production appear related to therapy-induced changes in stuttering. While it appears that changes in the temporal domain of speech production are most related to improvement in speech fluency, it is still unclear how these acoustic variables relate to *long-term* improvement in stuttering, that is, improvement that lasts five years or longer. Of course, there is always a fly in the ointment! Acoustic measures, in particular, as some have suggested (e.g., Caruso & Burton, 1987) may neither accurately nor precisely reflect underlying supralaryngeal or laryngeal movement. Further, as Atal, Chang, Mathews, and Tukey (1978) reported, it may be difficult to precisely relate changes in acoustic measures to changes in speech production, since the articulatory-acoustic relation is less than simple—for example, *identical* format frequencies and amplitudes in the acoustic signal can be produced by *different* vocal tract shapes. Perhaps we will eventually be able to use instrumental procedures that *directly* measure speech production behavior, like those described by Conture, Colton, and Gleason (1988), Guitar, Guitar, Neilson, O'Dwyer, and Andrews (1988), or Van Lieshout, Peters, Starkweather, and Hulstijn (1993) *in conjunction* with the pre-, during, and post-therapy designs employed by, for example, Metz, Samar, and Sacco (1983) or Robb and colleagues (1985). (For an excellent coverage of designs appropriate for the systematic study of treatment efficacy, see Schiavetti & Metz, 1997.) However, in this writer's opinion, what is needed is a "post-therapy" period that covers the period up to five years after therapy. Onslow and colleagues' reports of evaluation of their Lidcombe program (e.g., Lincoln & Onslow, 1997; see Lincoln & Harrison, 1999, for overview of the Lidcombe program) reflect significant strides in this regard, reporting on their clients *long* after the termination of treatment. This sort of "longitudinal" follow-up work is, of course, difficult as well as expensive; but it is, nevertheless, work that needs to be done.

Again, as with modification, if we knew which aspects of speech-language production are most clearly related to long-term recovery from stuttering as a result of therapy, it would obviate much of the debate regarding what forms of remediation are most appropriate. Indeed, the nature of these behaviors would dictate the nature of our procedures used for modifying stuttering. For example, if research clearly showed us that faster, less hesitant coordinations between laryngeal and supralaryngeal behaviors were the most highly related to long-term improvement in stuttering, then therapies could be designed to maximize changes in these laryngeal-supralayrngeal interactions. Or, for example, if changes in rate of lexical access and use of longer, more complex sentences seemed related to long-term improvement in stuttering, then therapies could be designed to maximize changes in these formulative interactions. Of course, numerous people have already stated what "behaviors" they *believe* are most importantly related to improvement in stuttering. For example, some have suggested that stuttering results from or is related to a conflict in presentation of the role of the self (Sheehan, 1975, 1978); therefore, we should, according to Sheehan, logically employ procedures appropriate to resolving or modifying such a conflict. Unfortunately, while still an interesting idea, we have no evidence that role conflicts or a variety of other behaviors, advocated as "key" for the change of stuttering, are any more or less associated with long-term recovery from the problem, particularly with children.

If we, as SLPs, hope to increase our ability to offer long-term assistance to people who stutter, it seems apparent to this writer that we need to significantly increase our understanding regarding what people who stutter *do*, in terms of the *entirety* (not *merely* motor aspects) of speech and language production when they (1) stutter, (2) appreciably change/modify stuttering, and (3) make long-term recovery from their problem. Telling our clients "You prolong the /s/ when you stutter" is a bit like telling them "You get nervous when you are anxious." An appreciable prolongation of a speech sound in time is almost by definition an example of a stuttering and vice versa; at best, using this approach, we could describe for the client that the acoustic correlate of the sound is *prolonged* while the correlated motor movement has *ceased* or *stopped*. And then try to help the client understand that we evaluate or apply the label *stuttering* to this behavior as well as other behaviors—for example, sound/syllable repetitions. We need to examine what we say to ourselves regarding *how* the person who stutters actually produced the sound prolongation. Do we talk to ourselves like we do to our clients, using this same rather vague almost circular form of reasoning and manner of description? The answer, we are afraid, is all too often *yes*.

Future Directions: General Considerations

The future, it is said, is promised to no one. Certainly, that is true with regard to future theoretical and therapeutic approaches to stuttering. We can only guesstimate, at this point, where the future will take us. Computers, brain-imaging technology, third-party reimbursement, population demographics, research breakthroughs, and the like will all determine where the field of stuttering will go in the next ten years. However, it is both interesting and useful to speculate about future directions—it helps us consider the past and present in light of the future, as well as future areas of seemingly maximal opportunity. To provide context for such speculation, however, some general considerations are in order, to help put our speculations about future directions into context and to provide some framework within which to view present as well as future developments in treatment and theory relative to stuttering.

Change, the One Constant

Complexity is easy. Simplicity, eloquent simplicity, is difficult. Spewing forth a deluge of differing details is far easier than coalescing them into a succinct, summarizing statement that fairly and accurately encapsulates the whole. Developing a phrase, an aphorism, or a principle to capture an era, an age, an issue, or a problem requires the distillation of divergent forces, interests, facts, and opinions. With that in mind, try as I might to capture the current zeitgeist in the field of stuttering, what occurred to me over and over is this: Nothing is as constant as change. Change is inevitable, unless we are standing in front of a vending machine (sorry, I couldn't resist). Indeed, whether in our personal lives, the weather, the economy, the or body politic, change is constant. This seems particularly true in the area of theory and treatment of stuttering. There has been a change since I last wrote these remarks, around 1990. Clearly, the pendulum of professional opinion about the origins and treatment of stuttering has swung in another direction.

Theoretically, the late 1980s through early to mid-1990 witnessed research approaches firmly in the grip of organic, neuromotor, physiological, and speech motor control explanations. In the ensuing ten years, by the late 1990s, the grip of these sorts of explanations had relaxed and the new millennium is witnessing a change toward more psycholinguistic explanations (e.g., see Bernstein Ratner, 1997a, 1997b; Burger & Wijnen, 1999; Melnick & Conture, 2000). Therapeutically, the late 1980s and 1990s still exhibited a heavy emphasis on treating the older person who stutters, while in the late 1990s and into the new millennium, numerous publications (e.g., Onslow & Packman, 1999) suggest that young clients who stutter are increasingly receiving systematic, well-conceived early therapeutic intervention.

Increasingly, both clinicians and researchers alike, when it comes to stuttering, are realizing something that I have previously mentioned: Stuttering is a dynamic, multidimensional disorder (see Smith & Kelly, 1997) that has and will continue to defy unidimensional solutions. Such tolerance for ambiguity, for multiple perspectives, was earlier exemplified, in this writer's opinion, by Van Riper (1971) who suggested, with his now widely known "tracks," that the end called stuttering may be achieved by several different means. At the time, however, although sparking a great deal of discussion, Van Riper's notion that stuttering may result from different paths or tracks was a seemingly lone voice in the wilderness. More recently, models of stuttering such as Smith and Kelly's (1997) and DeNil's (1999) shows the increasing interest in multiple perspectives and considerations. Guitar's (1998) merging of psychosocial with motor/linguistic dynamics is another excellent example of the current zeitgeist in the field, of amalgamation and melding of points of view rather than earlier, more exclusionary frameworks whereby stuttering, in both theory and therapy, is assessed from a unitary or singular perspective.

Drowning in a Sea of Information

As I have mentioned before (Conture, 1990b), perusing textbooks in the area of stuttering (e.g., Bernstein Ratner & Healey, 1999; Bloodstein, 1995; Curlee & Siegel, 1997; Guitar, 1998) strongly suggests that information is pouring into the pool of knowledge about stuttering at an alarmingly fast rate. This is just as true today, at the dawn of the new millennium. Rather than suffer from a lack of information, it sometimes seems that we are in danger of drowning in a sea of facts, figures, and speculation about the problem. Increasingly, the consumer, as well as disseminators of knowledge (i.e., students and their teachers), need to wear a personal flotation device to avoid going under. Hopefully, the guidelines below should help in this regard.

Allowing Information to Cloud Our Judgment

Many of us do not want information to cloud our judgment. This is as true with so-called objective researchers as it is with people on the street when asked their subjective opinions about politics, the economy, or people from other countries. Indeed, many times we have a theory that we systematically look for evidence to support, rejecting all evidence to the contrary. Clearly, the half-life of theories is far longer than that of the strongest facts. For example, there is limited empirical data to support "slowing down" the speaking rate of a child who stutters as well as that of his or her parents. Why, therefore, do clinicians continue to practice this approach? In a word: theory. It seems safe to say that clinicians who engage in this practice have a theory that the child who stutters is speaking and/or selecting sounds, syllables, and words at rates faster than he or she is able to fluently select, encoding and produce them. A decent, good, and reasonable theory, but still a theory nevertheless. And, a theory that requires far more empirical support then it currently enjoys. We hasten to note that we should not single out this theory for blame when so much of our personal and professional practices are theory-rich, but data-poor. So, as students, clinicians, and researchers, we open our professional journals, eager to learn the latest facts and findings. But without some simple guidelines, we may enter a domain that, like a hedgerow maze, quickly turns us every which way but out, burying us in minutia rather than enlightening us with erudition.

Data Are Not Always Reflected in Discussion

First and foremost, as we begin to swim through the sea of information contained in our professional literature, we must recognize, quite clearly, the difference between data and discussions about that data. The former—data—are as factual and as objective as the experimenter could obtain. The latter—the discussion—can be as subjective and as fanciful as the experimenter feels comfortable with and his or her peer reviewers (and journal editors) will tolerate. While discussion can be closely grounded in observable fact, it can also range fairly far afield. Thus, it is important that consumers/readers of research not blur the distinction between data and discussion of same. The common thread that runs through studies should be methods and findings. Once findings have accumulated to a point where a picture starts to emerge, researchers generally find that the speculations contained within their discussions have a more solid base of support.

Science Advances by Small Increments in Knowledge as Much as It Does by Quantal Leaps

Clinicians are people as well as professionals. Thus, it is understandable that clinicians sometimes hope against hope that someday, somehow, someone will find the silver bullet that cures stuttering. Likewise, because researchers are people as well as professionals, it is understandable that they may hope against hope that someday someone will publish the breakthrough study that shows what causes stuttering. While silver bullets and breakthrough studies may indeed emerge, we shouldn't hold our collective breath waiting for that to happen. The trouble with the advancement of knowledge is the trouble with life—both are so daily. Simply put, knowledge advances by accretion.

Our clinical and theoretical knowledge advances gradually as much as it does by quantal steps. Gradually, the story unfolds as independent investigators replicate findings and refine methodology. Sometimes, of course, in the gradual accretion of knowledge, earlier findings get buried in the blitz of intervening journal articles; but that is where careful scholarship, as well as reading, should play a part. For an example of how knowledge advances in small, incremental steps, we will examine one variable, voice onset time (VOT), which was studied for nearly ten years in the area of stuttering.

Early research suggested that there were differences in VOT (i.e., the time between oral release and voicing onset that disguises, e.g., /p/ from /b/) between people who do and do not stutter (e.g., Agnello & Wingate, 1975; Hillman & Gilbert, 1977). However, further study in this area began to report no such difference between the VOTs of people who stutter and their normally fluent peers (for example, Metz, Conture, & Caruso, 1979; Watson & Alphonso, 1982; Zebrowski, Conture, & Cudahy, 1985; Pindzola, 1986a; McNight & Cullinan, 1987). Gradually the story unfolded: To determine whether the VOT of people who stutter significantly differs from those of normals, a great deal of care must be taken when matching subjects as well as when designing speaking material (Adams, 1987; Healey & Ramig, 1986). But the real story, in this writer's opinion, is that looking for differences in VOT is similar to the analogy involving the person who, when asked why he was looking under the corner street lamp for his lost keys, replied, "I'm looking here because the light is better." VOT may be a good street light, but we'll probably have to look elsewhere to find out more about the speech production abilities of people who stutter. There are many examples in the field of stuttering where cults of measurement have development, for example, the repeated use of a measure like VOT is applied to people who stutter and their speech. The measure may, like VOT, be relatively easy to measure, have apparent linguistic significance, and seem related to something people who stutter supposedly have trouble with (temporal interactions between glottal and supraglottal behaviors). And this writer has been as guilty as the next of joining such cults!

In fact, if we had given the study of VOT a moment's thought and considered the fact that if the VOTs of people who stutter were *appreciably* different from those of people who do not stutter, wouldn't this mean that listeners readily perceive, when they listen to a person who stutters, a lot more confusion between their voiced and unvoiced sounds and vice versa? The answer is: Yes, they would note such voiced/voiceless confusions, and no, for people who stutter as a group, listeners do not hear any such confusion. Rather, our gradual build-up of knowledge in this area suggests that other measures and/or aspects of laryngeal-supralaryngeal behavior need to be investigated. This insight took nearly over ten years to develop and has become another brick in the wall of our knowledge about what people do and do not do during speech and language production.

It Is Replication by Independent Researchers Not Size of Sample That Counts in the Long Run

Much is made about the fact that this or that study had one, two, three, or thirty subjects. Should we, as readers of research, disregard findings from studies employing small sample size? While sample size *can* influence the generalizability of findings, the size of the sample is many times related to the question(s) under investigation. Piaget, for example, developed a vast number of observations and a rich theory based on a sample size of one to three subjects (i.e., his own children). Would we denigrate Einstein's theories because they were based on a limited number of observations? Closer to home, in the field of speech science/linguistics, our knowledge of "normal" VOT values was, for many years, based on a total sample size of well under ten subjects, but this did not stop many investigators from positing elaborate speculations and theories based on these findings. This is neither a call for small sample sizes nor a dismissal of the importance or relevance of sample size to the generalizability of findings. Rather, it is an attempt to help us to see that sample size is not as much the issue as whether independent researchers obtain similar findings.

Indeed, replication by independent researchers was one of the decision rules applied by Andrews and his colleagues (1983) in their review of stuttering research. To my mind, it is more impressive that identical findings were reported in three *independently* conducted studies, each containing only three subjects apiece, than findings from one study of ten subjects that is never replicated. If our understanding of stuttering advances by an accretion of knowledge, it also advances when more than one investigator observes the same phenomenon. If this sort of agreement requires 3 or 33 or 103 subjects, so be it. Big is not necessarily better.

We started out with this section on by talking about change, and that is a fitting way to close it as well. For the past ten years or so have witnessed considerable change in the area of stuttering, both theoretically and therapeutically. And some of these changes, this writer predicts, will continue well into the first ten years of the new millennium. It is these areas of potential growth, where change has already occurred, that have become prominent and are likely to remain prominent for some time that we would like to note at this point. Thus, it is only fitting that we begin with the beginning, children, for this is where the problem typically starts, at least for developmental stuttering.

Future Directions: Opportunities

Children

If we know nothing else about stuttering, we know, for the vast majority of people who stutter, that it begins in childhood (so-called developmental stuttering, to distinguish it from acquired stuttering, the latter typically observed in adults, and usually after some physical and/or psychosocial trauma). By 7 years of age, most of those people who are going to stutter have begun to do so. As we mentioned previously, some children will continue to begin after 7 and before 12, but these are in the minority (recently we evaluated a 10-year-old boy who, as far as we could tell, began when he was 8 years old and in the second grade). And some adults will begin in their teenage or adult years, after physical and/or psychosocial difficulties or trauma, but this adult onset stuttering is generally of the so-called "acquired" variety. The bulk of the problem that begins in childhood is described as "developmental," and it is these developmental problems that we are talking about in this space.

First, until the last few years, even though stuttering sees its origins in childhood, it was, with some notable exceptions, predominantly studied in adulthood (for critical assessment of this approach, see Yairi, 1993, p. 198). While the ground-breaking work of the 1950s in the study of childhood stuttering by Johnson and colleagues (e.g., Johnson, 1955; Johnson & Associates, 1959) opened wide the door in this area, it quickly seemed to be shut in the sense that few followed Johnson's lead and walked into the land of childhood to study stuttering. Until the past ten years or so.

Beginning around 1980, first at Syracuse University and now at Vanderbilt University, from a speech science/motor perspective, with my colleagues and students, I began to systematically study children who stutter, a perspective that has slowly but surely changed to include a predominantly premotor or psycholinguistic perspective. Our work is cited throughout this text and there is no need, at this point, to delve into it further (the reader might obtain some overviews of our research-oriented thinking in this area by examining, e.g., Conture, 1991; Logan & Conture, 1997; Yaruss & Conture, 1996; and our treatment-oriented thinking in this area by reading Conture, 1997; Conture & Melnick, 1999).

At about the same time, at the University of Illinois, Champagne-Urbana, Ehud Yairi, his associates, and students began a similar program of study into childhood stuttering, initially building from the base provided by Johnson's efforts. And now have have considerably expanded, extended, and refined it well beyond Johnson's beginning efforts. Yairi has widely published his findings (e.g., Ambrose & Yairi, 1999; Yairi & Ambrose, 1999; Yairi, Ambrose, Paden, & Throneberg, 1996), but perhaps two of the better, in this writer's opinion, overviews of this work and thinking may be found in Yairi (1997a, 1997b).

Second, the surface of an understanding of children who stutter has just been scratched. In our opinion, much of the reticence of researchers to study children who stutter have been the children themselves! Young children simply aren't as attentive, cooperative, mature, and rational as adults—there is just no other way to say it than that! Experimentally, as in real life, children are a handful! However, childhood is the soil from which stuttering grows and, like it or not, we are going to have to get our hands real dirty, if we are ever to understand the root causes of stuttering. Children are vulnerable and reactive to the influences of their environment in ways that adults aren't. Their speech and language production is a work in progress, unlike the relative stability of that of teenagers and adults. Children are physically, psychologically, motorically, and neurologically growing in ways that adults aren't. Their level of education, understanding, and knowledge is vastly different from that of adults. Many of them, for example, do not read, making certain means of studying them difficult, to say the least! Their involvement in therapy is a decision made by others, while adults who enter treatment do so on their own accord. Children stand on the dependence side of the dependence/independence divide, a chasm that most adults have leapt over long ago. And the stuttering behavior of children, by and large, has been in existence far less time so that frequency, severity, type, duration, and so on are many times different from that exhibited by adults with developmental stuttering (obviously, an adult who, shortly after head injuries suffered in a car crash, began to stutter would also have a brief history; however, such *acquired* stuttering is not the focus of our discussion in this section).

Thus, our best chance to understand the variables that underlie stuttering is to study it in childhood, before the problem has had a chance to add layers of behaviors, attitudes, and feelings due to experience, learning, and reaction. Not easy, that is correct. Not simple, that is also correct. But germane, important, and necessary to our growth as a field, that is also correct. Indeed, I look for the work begun by Yairi, ourselves, and others to continue in the work of our students, their students and others. Why?

Third, there are many reasons why. For example, advances in psycho-linguistic models, computational and otherwise; advances in understanding of speech and language in general; and advances in genetics, particularly behavioral applications and advances in neuro-imaging, will make it easier and more attractive to ask the difficult questions and do the difficult study of children who stutter. And as our knowledge of childhood stuttering grows, this knowledge will attract more knowledge and individuals interested in furthering this needed body of information. Adults have and will continue to be studied, for many good and important reasons, but just as no one would take information collected on 5-year-olds and apply that to a 35-year-old, the reverse is true. To do otherwise is to defy all that we know about development from related fields like psychology.

Fourth, and I will return to this later, the issues of comorbidity (i.e., two or more problems co-occuring in one person) in children who stutter will, I predict, continue to be assessed and better understood. Likewise, the nature and time course of speech disfluencies in all children, not just children who stutter, will become clearer and clearer. In particular, the relation of speech fluency to syntax, semantics, and phonology will become clearer, together with the role various parts of the brain play in such speaking events. The notion of "tracks" (e.g., Van Riper, 1971) and "subgroups" (e.g., Schwartz & Conture, 1988), whether etiological or behavioral in nature, will continue to be explored. Above all, significant inroads will be made into early and more effective treatments for young children who stutter (e.g., Conture & Melnick, 1999; Ramig, 1993; Ramig & Bennett, 1997; Runyan & Runyan, 1999; Rustin, 1996; Rustin, Botterill, & Kelman, 1996), such children are at an age where we reasonably believe that our assistance can make a positive difference and alleviate the needless "holding pattern" that many children go through when given the well-intended, but misinformed guidance to "wait, he'll outgrow it."

Subgroups

We wrote in this space, almost ten years ago, that "more and more workers will try to uncover—on perceptual, acoustic, physiological, and other levels—differences *among* people who stutter that make a difference" (Conture, 1990b, pp. 287–288). So much for our powers of prediction! Actually, relatively little research has been conducted on this topic during the past ten years, although theorization by Smith and Kelly (1997), for example, implies that there are different ends to the same means of becoming someone who stutters. Such differences, as speculated about by Smith and Kelly, lead to what can best be termed "etiological" (i.e., different cause, same behaviors) subgroups. Likewise, our speculation and research into concomitant developmental concerns (e.g., Rustin & Purser, 1991) and speech and language problems (e.g., Yaruss and Conture, 1996) imply the possibility of "etiological" subgroups. What has received more attention, I believe, is the possibility of "behavioral" subgroups (i.e., roughly similar cause, different behavior), as advocated by Daly (1981), Preus (1981), Schwartz and Conture (1988) and Van Riper (1971). This work leads me to suggest that " . . . childhood stuttering may not only begin from different origins but once begun the problem may develop along parallel but different routes" (Conture, 1990a, p. 10).

Second, I would urge that while this area—subgroups of people who stutter—has not received a great deal of direct research attention in the past ten years, it should not be dismissed. At the very least, knowing something about the number and nature of these various "subgroups" of people who stutter should be very useful to researchers in terms of subject selection and matching and to clinicians' trying to differentially diagnose stuttering and plan therapy accordingly. Indeed, these potentially appreciable *within-group* (i.e., within the group of people who stutter) differences should help us explain why some of our *between-group* differences (i.e., between people who do and do not stutter) are minimized. In other words, the differences *within* the group of people who stutter may be greater, for some measures, than the difference *between* people who do and do not stutter, nullifying our ability to assess differences between people who stutter and people who do not.

Third, one excellent reason for the study of subgroups relates to the issue of persistent stuttering versus unassisted/spontaneous recovery from stuttering (see Finn, 1996, 1998; Yairi et al., 1996, for detailed discussion of this issue). It is not too farfetched to suggest that certain etiologies and behaviors are more apt to be associated with children whose stuttering *persists* than for children whose stuttering *remits*. These within-group differences directly pertain to subgroups among people who stutter. Our tendency to approach stuttering as a monolithic rather than diverse entity may cause us to overlook and blur some *very* important distinctions among these individuals, distinctions that unless we attend to them may cause us to misdiagnose, mistreat, and misunderstand.

Attention Deficit Hyperactivity Disorder (ADHD)

It is fitting that we mention ADHD soon after discussing children because much of the diagnosis of ADHD involves children. Why? Well, one of the criteria for ADHD is that some of its symptoms (e.g., often does not seem to listen when spoken to directly) must appear before the age of 7. Sound familiar? That is, below 7 years of age is exactly the age range during which stuttering typically begins. Does this mean that stuttering is but a manifestation of ADHD? Hardly, but in this writer's opinion, due to our historical tendency to research stuttering in adults, we have missed an important issue of childhood, ADHD, which has *real* potential for, at the least, disrupting any treatment for childhood stuttering we try to employ.

To begin, we recommend to those readers trying to get an overview of ADHD, particularly as it relates to the pragmatics (social use) of language, that they review Camarata and Gibson (1999). These authors provide a nice overview of the two areas (ADHD and pragmatics of language) and offer seemingly reasonable suggestions, based on a transactional (bidirectional) model of language development, of how ADHD could interfere and/or interact with pragmatic language behavior and development. At the least, for the child and/or parent with ADHD (yes, parents could have been ADHD as children and still exhibit, more or less, ADHD behaviors and/or disruptions in pragmatics of speech perhaps related to these behaviors), we need to consider how ADHD may manifest itself behaviorally during diagnosis and how it may influence the nature and course of treatment for stuttering.

First and foremost, we need epidemiological (e.g., incidence/prevalence) research describing the prevalence of ADHD among children who stutter. At present, we do know that there is a high comorbidity (45%) between language disorders and attention deficit disorder (ADD), based on a large sample (3,208) of children 6 to 11 years of age (Tirosh & Cohen, 1998). Is the prevalence this high between stuttering and ADD or ADHD? I do not know, but given the high co-occurrence of ADD and language disorders, I would expect that as many as 10 to 20 percent of children who stutter exhibit ADD/ADHD, to some degree.

Second, we need information about how children who stutter, who also exhibit varying degrees of ADD/ADHD, respond to treatment. Poorly, I would think, and experience tells me, if we consider how, for example, the inattentive aspect of ADD/ADHD interferes with school or academic progress. This is not a call for developing different treatments for children who stutter with ADHD, but for treatments to adjust to the circumstances that ADHD imposes—for example, breaking procedures into short blocks of time, with brief breaks between blocks to activities.

Third, we need information about whether some of the behaviors we may attribute to stuttering, for example, having difficulty waiting turns, might not, at least for some children who stutter, be better laid at the doorstep of ADD/ADHD. Similarly, we need to know more about the mothers and fathers of children who stutter, in terms of their own history of ADD/ADHD, whether diagnosed or not. It is entirely possible that what we have thought were interfering parental communicative behaviors (i.e., behaviors that make it difficult for the child to initiate and/or maintain fluent speech) originate from the parents' *own* (un)diagnosed ADD/ADHD concerns. In particular, the presence of *impulsivity* (an aspect of ADHD, predominantly hyperactivity-impulsive type)—for example, an individual who often interrupts or intrudes on others—would seem to warrant exploration in our opinion. These are the parents who, despite careful, clear, and repeated instructs to the contrary by the SLP, continue to ask and then answer questions for their child, blurt out answers to the child's question *before* the child is finished, have difficulty waiting their speaking turn, and so forth. Such continued behavior on the part of the parent may not be due to their inability to learn, uncooperativeness, and the like but by a condition that the person has little apparent knowledge and/or control over. The same, of course, can be said of the child who stutters. Whether child, parent, or both, much more needs to be known about how ADHD interacts with and/or exacerbates stuttering.

Temperament

In 1991, we made our first mention in print (Conture, 1991, pp. 380–381) of the possible role of temperament in stuttering, but well before that (e.g., Glasner, 1949) one can find empirical evidence that the most common temperamental characteristic of children who stutter is a distinct "hypersensitivity." Perhaps encouraged by the significant contributions of Kagan (1994) to understand and explain childhood temperamental characteristics, others in the field of stuttering have recently researched (e.g., Amster, 1995; Oyler, 1996a, 1996b; Oyler & Ramig, 1995; Rustin & Purser, 1991) and speculated (e.g., Conture & Melnick, 1999; Guitar, 1997, 1998; Zebrowski & Conture, 1998) about the role of temperament in stuttering. Guitar (1997, 1998), perhaps, has done the most to go beyond the mere description of temperament in relationship to stuttering, offering a preliminary model of how these selected aspects of temperament may interact with speech fluency.

First, what is needed, using modern, standardized test instruments (e.g., McDevitt and Carey's [1995] *Behavioral Style Questionnaire*, for 3- to 7-year-old children) is the collection of epidemiological information regarding the temperamental characteristics of children who stutter in relationship to their age- and sex-matched nonstuttering peers. In our opinion, this is large-scale research, requiring at least 30 children in both groups (stuttering and nonstuttering). Why? In our experience, attempting to use such scales as the *Behavioral Style Questionnaire*, any one child who stutters or doesn't stutter may show extremely behaviorally inhibited behavior. But we must, as the old caution in law goes, "beware the study based on a series of one." Generalizations about temperament in the population of people who stutter are interesting to make, but they will require a good deal of data, collected by several independent researchers, based on many subjects (across ages, severity levels, etc.). Further, there is the real possibility, given that temperament is not immutable to the influences of the environment, that what we observe temperamentally with children, may not be what we observe with the temperament of adults. Likewise, researchers who engage in this type of research should be *very* sensitive to the possibility that there is *no* one size fits all temperament for people who stutter and that there may be subgroups where temperament plays more of a role in stuttering than for other subgroups. For an example of how "subgroups of temperament" may play different roles in stuttering, let us consider Adams's (1992) observation that childhood stuttering may be influenced by "positive emotions," for example, the excitement related to anticipating a future trip to Disneyworld. Adams's observation is consistent with our own, but we think it may not be as applicable for some children who stutter as it for others. For example, for the behaviorally expressive child who stutters, such anticipation or change in routine may have minimal influence on his or her stuttering; however, a child of sensitive or behaviorally inhibited temperament may unduly react with overall physical tension and agitation, reactions that may make it difficult to speak in a fluent fashion. Again, temperament *must* be viewed in context—in this case, the context of a complex interaction between normal environmental stressors or change (see Hill, 1999) *and* the inherent characteristics or tendencies of the person who stutters, interactions that are undoubtedly variable in terms of their influence on stuttering across the population of people who stutter.

Second, Guitar's (1997, 1998) attempt to model the relationship of temperament and stuttering is a good start. His notion of temperamental variables interacting with linguistic/motoric variables is an attractive idea, although this author is more inclined to emphasize linguistic (premotor) than motor variables. But that is not the point. Temperament *must* interact with some other variable(s) to contribute to stuttering, otherwise all the behaviorally inhibited people of the word would stutter, something that is hardly the case! Clearly, more such modeling of the role of temperament in stuttering needs to take place. In particular, a model that would predict *what* aspects of speech and language temperamental characteristic might influence, how, and in what direction. I mean why only speech fluency? Why not speed of lexical access? Phonological accuracy? Speed of morphosyntactic construction? For example, perhaps children who show an inability to quickly modify their reactions to stimuli (a temperamental characteristic) might exhibit longer duration stutterings, that is, they find it difficult, once they have "made a mistake," to rapidly change their initial reaction, and "let go" and "move on," as it were. Whatever the case, a correlation, no matter how strong, between certain temperamental characteristics and stuttering does not an explanation make. We need models of the relationship between specific temperamental characteristics and specific aspects of speech-language production, models that lead to testable, nontrivial experimentation exploration.

Third, and as alluded to above, it *must* be recognized that behavioral inhibition readily exists in the population of children who do not stutter. Behavioral inhibition is *not* the exclusive domain of people who stutter, not by a long shot. Kagan, for example, seldom, to this writer's knowledge, studies children who stutter and yet clearly finds indications of behavioral inhibition! So what? Well, if children who do not stutter also exhibit the temperamental characteristics we believe are related to stuttering (and they do—some of the most behaviorally inhibited children this author has tested to date, as part of his research, have been children who do not stutter), then these characteristics, by themselves, cannot "cause" stuttering! However, no thoughtful worker in this area, I believe, would suggest that certain temperamental characteristics "cause" stuttering. Indeed, temperamental characteristics, by themselves, would not seem to be able to cause, but perhaps they significantly perpetuate or maintain stuttering. So, whatever temperamental characteristics we posit contribute to stuttering, we must, on the basis of the evidence before us, also posit some other, nontemperamental characteristics that actually cause the instances of stuttering in the first place. What might those "other" characteristics be? For an answer to that question, we turn to the area of psycholinguistics.

Linguistic Activities and Behavior (e.g., Syntactic, Semantic, and Phonological Encoding)

The field of psycholinguistics has been around since before this author was in graduate school, in the late 1960s to early 1970s. Thus, psycholinguistics, as a discipline, is not particularly new. What is new, perhaps, is its emergence as the source of some of the preeminent, modern models of speech and language across all disciplines (e.g., Dell, 1986; Levelt, 1989; Roelofs, 1997). Fueled by its close ties to the growing field of cognitive psychology, the work of such individuals as the Dutch psycholinguist Levelt (1989), with colleagues (e.g., Levelt, 1991; Roelofs, 1997) and students, has done much to clarify the complex process of converting thought to spoken word. And it has been to this field and work of such psycholinguistic scholars as Levelt (e.g., Levelt et al., 1999), Dell (1986), Kolk and Postma (1997), and others (e.g., Bernstein Ratner, 1997b) that this writer has turned for the answer to the question above: What other, nontemperamental characteristics might "cause" stuttering?

Of course, we have no answer at this point, but we truly believe, based on our own work, that of others, and psycholinguistic theory and research, that the "proximal source" for instances of stuttering will be found in those processes that occurred *between* thought and motor execution of that thought. The evidence is just too overwhelming for it to be otherwise—for example, the clear indication that the length and complexity of the utterance is significantly related to instances of singleton and/or clustered stutterings (e.g., Bernstein Ratner & Sih, 1987; Gaines, Runyan, & Meyers, 1991; Logan & Conture, 1995; Logan & LaSalle, 1999; Weiss & Zebrowski, 1992; Yaruss, 1999b). This is not to suggest that motor execution has nothing to do with stuttering, or that difficulties with motor execution do not have the potential to exacerbate the duration, tension, and severity of the stuttering, once it starts. Subtle motor slowness, clumsiness, or incoordination may also make it more difficult for some people to quickly and efficiently perform the types of behaviors SLPs are teaching in therapy. However, to this writer's way of thinking, it would seem that only elements of the processes *above* the level of motor execution—syntactic, semantic and phonological—are fast enough, rule-governed enough, and creative enough to account for what we know about stuttering (e.g., it is most apt to occur on function words in children, more apt to occur on longer, more grammatical complex utterances, most apt to occur during unstructured, conversational, propositional speech etc.). Perhaps Wingate (1988) puts it best when he says:

. . . stuttering is a defect in the language production system, a defect that extends beyond the level of motor execution. . . . There is ample evidence to indicate that the defect (stuttering) is not simply one of motor control or coordination, but that it involves more central functions of the language production system (p. 239).

First, there is a need for systematic descriptive and experimental study of the syntactic, semantic, and phonological processes of people who stutter (see Bock & Levelt, 1994; Levbelt, Schriefers, Vorberg, Meyer, Pechman, & Havinga, 1991; Levelt & Wheeldon, 1994, for overview of some current thinking regarding syntactic, semantic, and phonological processing, respectively, in people who do not stutter). While standardized tests can lead the way, so to speak, to give us some general idea of the formulative abilities of people who stutter, they are not sufficiently dynamic and too divorced from the realities of conversational speech to explain, for example, how a subtle delay in word retrieval might produce an instance of speech disfluency. Rather, to best understand how these syntactic, semantic, and phonological processes may influence stuttering, we need to manipulate them and assess how people who do and do not stutter respond to these manipulations, in particular how these manipulations might influence their ongoing speech fluency.

Second, there is a need for models (e.g., Karniol, 1995; Perkins, Kent, & Curlee, 1991; Postma & Kolk, 1993) that attempt to explain how disruptions in formulative processes (i.e., syntactic, semantic, and phonologic encoding) contribute to instances of speech disfluency (for earlier empirical attempts to assess relationship between speech fluency and "formulative"/linguistic aspects of speech, see Colburn & Mysak, 1982; Bernstein Ratner & Sih, 1987). There is particular need, in this writer's opinion, for these models to be consonant with contemporary, major psycholinguistic models (e.g., Bock, 1982; Dell, 1986; Levelt, 1989; Roelefs, 1997). The latter models have led to a tremendous amount of empirical testing (e.g., Levelt et al., 1999; Meyer & Schriefers, 1991) and deserve serious consideration by those interested in the relationship between formulative, linguistic processes and stuttering. Just as important, at this point, it would seem that further description of the prevalence of these disruptions (e.g., more phonological problems in children who stutter) will not tell us a great deal more. Further research showing, for example, that X study reports 25 percent and Y study reports 31 percent of children who stutter also exhibit disordered phonology will not really add to our store of information in this area. The point is not that one sample differs somewhat from another sample in terms of percentage prevalence of phonological problems, but that children who stutter are *significantly* more apt to exhibit mild to severe phonological concerns than those who do not. Of even greater importance, we must get beyond the notion that these phonological concerns *must* be clinically significant to be of consequence to conversational speech. Instead, it is entirely possible that rather than exhibit clinically significant formulative problems (e.g., expressive language disorder), what may be the case is that children who stutter are in the lower end of normal limits in terms of syntactic, phonological, and semantic processes (an innate ability that could be out of step with internal as well as external requirements to speak quickly, adult-like, and flawlessly). Indeed, if children who stuttered had to have clinically significant formulative problems in order to stutter, this would have been apparent a long time ago and treatment would have been adjusted accordingly! Having formulative processes within the lower ends of normal limits together with a tendency on the part of the child to use and/or strive for flawless, rapid, complex, adult-like grammar, words, pronunciation, and so on could result in a higher frequency than normal speech disfluency rate. This would be even more the case if the child's tendency was aided and abetted by a mother/father who encouraged, modeled, or required nearly error-free, adult-like communication.

Third, and finally, we need to consider that the *speed*, not just subtle/gross *errors* in formulative processes, might be a factor in stuttering. In other words, if stuttering is a problem with the *temporal* aspects of speech production perhaps this is because it reflects problems with temporal activation of formulative processes and not errors in these processes (or as Kent, 1984, suggests, the very definition of stuttering as a disruption in the rhythm or fluency of speech indicates that stuttering results from a disturbance in temporal processes). Indeed, for example, some types of "word-finding" may not be a search for the word, per se, but a "waiting" for the word to be activated, to be inserted or "slotted" into the appropriate syntactic frame. Likewise, perhaps, for people who stutter, it is simply that these formulative processes "go too slowly," something in running speech that would naturally cause hesitations, pauses, or stoppages in the forward flow of production. If we assume that only 100 msec (one-tenth of second) are required to select the word with which to name an object (Levelt et al., 1991)—the entire process, from selection to actual overt naming taking about 500 to 600 msec (.5 to .6 second) for adult speakers—if a person who stutters takes 200 to 300 msec to make the same word selection, this could have a definite influence on the rapidity with which the person eventually overtly produces the word. Again, this problem could be compounded if this subtle but significant delay in semantic activation (an *automatic* process, not within the person's ability to directly control) is coupled with the person's tendency to select words even faster than the norm (a *controlled* process, something the person can actually regulate).

Concomitant Speech and Language Problems of People Who Stutter

As the review by Louko, Conture, and Edwards (1999, Table 7-1) suggests, there is considerable evidence to suggest that children who stutter are apt to exhibit phonological disorders. Similarly, Paden, Yairi, and Ambrose (1999) have recently found that those children for whom stuttering persists, when compared to those who recover from stuttering, exhibit lower/poorer scores on several measures of phonology (e.g., mean percentage of error, relative level of severity impairment, etc). Indeed, in the nearly ten years since I wrote about this topic in this space, a great deal of information has been collected, and debated, about the concomitant problems of people who stutter, in particular phonological problems (e.g., see review of Louko et al., 1999). Indeed, while subject selection as well as methodological problems clearly exist in this area (e.g., Nippold, 1990), the overwhelming evidence suggests that one of the more common problems that people who stutter exhibit is phonological difficulties, particularly in children. Such concomitant problems have tremendous salience to our understanding of stuttering because they suggest areas that may be problematic in terms of overall speech and language production, areas that many contribute to stuttering. Already we can see one theory (Postma & Kolk, 1993) that attempts to explain how one aspect of formulation, phonological encoding, may contribute to stuttering (see

Butterworth, 1992, for further discussion of how disruptions in phonological encoding can disturb speech-language production). Perhaps, as it becomes clearer that a given percentage of children who stutter also exhibit lower ends of normal limits to below normal limits phonological abilities, we will gain further insights into the etiological/behavioral subgroups discussed above.

Likewise, we have some suggestion from the longitudinal study of young children who stutter that those who persist—that is, do not spontaneously recover—may be more apt to score more poorly on indices of phonological development (e.g., Paden, Yairi, & Ambrose, 1999). We have already shown elsewhere (Conture, Louko, & Edwards, 1993) that children who stutter and exhibit phonological problems may require different types of treatment. We anticipate that "special" therapies to manage people who stutter with concomitant problems will be developed and rest some of their rationale on information gathered from tests like the *OMAS* test developed by Riley and Riley (1986). Above all, we believe that consideration of the entirety of speech–language production, not merely speech fluency, brings the problem of stuttering further within body of the larger knowledge and treatment arena of speech and language in general rather than continually considering stuttering as some isolate divorced from mainstream understanding and treatment of human communication problems.

Cortical Activity and Structure of People Who Stutter

In the nearly ten years since I wrote about this area of opportunity, technology has considerably advanced, leading to many opportunities to assess the cortical *activity* of people who stutter (e.g., DeNil, Kroll, Kapur, & Houle, in press; Ingham, Fox, Ingham, Zamarripa, Martin, Jerabek, & Cotton, 1996; Watson & Freeman, 1997). Likewise, similar technological advances have led to renewed interest in cortical structure of people who stutter (Foundas, 1998). Perhaps, however, to put modern approaches to cortical activity/structure of people who stutter, a brief historical review is in order.

Although Orton (1927) and Travis (1931) are generally cited as being among the first to explore and suggest possible differences between people who stutter and their normally fluent peers in terms of central nervous system (CNS) function, it is only within the past fifteen to twenty years that advances in technology for the study of CNS function have permitted the type of investigations necessary to seriously assess Orton and Travis's earlier speculations. (For an overview of such technology see Fincher, 1984; Krasuski, Horowitz, & Rumsey, 1996; Sochurek, 1987.) Moore (1984, 1993) and Moore and Boberg (1987) have nicely summarized the earlier electroencephalographic (EEG) and related work in this area; indeed, Moore himself has contributed much of the recent empirical work in this area (e.g., Moore, 1986).

This area, in this writer's opinion, truly deserves continued "replication by independent researchers." I believe that replicating observations of cortical activities/processes of people who stutter (e.g., Fox et al., 1996; Ingham et al., 1996; Moore, 1993; Pool et al., 1991; Pool, Freeman, & Finitzo, 1987; Wu, Maguire, Riley, Fallow, LaCasse, et al., 1995) is particularly critical for at least two reasons. First, one can make the reasonable assumption that cortical activities/processes vary as much as linguistic and motor activities/ processes, both between and within speakers. If this is so, and we have no reason to believe it is not, many independent investigations of many people who stutter (who vary by age, length of problem, severity, etc.) will be required before we develop a clearer, more certain understanding of the central tendency and variation of cortical activity/processes associated with stuttered and fluent speech-language production of people who stutter. Second, the findings from this area have such broad, important, overarching implications for our fundamental understanding of stuttering that we must be patient, to get this "right" before drawing conclusions based on too few, restricted, etc. observations and/or subjects. If we can achieve further independent replication and be cautious and patient in our interpretation of evolving findings in this area, the future of this line of investigation is bright, albeit not without methodological and conceptual concerns, some of which I discuss immediately below.

First, in the past ten years, with advances in technology, work in this area has moved from electroencephalographic (EEG) recording of the "brain waves" of people who stutter (e.g., Wells & Moore, 1990) to the use of various neuroimaging procedures (e.g., positron emission tomography [PET] used by Ingham et al., 1996). Some endeavors will continue, I believe, to explore differences in *structural* as well as *functional behavioral* asymmetries in the brains of people who stutter relative to those who do not. In particular, this writer is hopeful that researchers will focus their attention on differences—between people who do and do not stutter—in cortical activity/behavioral asymmetries during *active* processing or handling of meaningful speech or linguistic stimuli. With this line of research, like many others, we need to keep our eye on the prize: People who stutter mainly do so during unstructured, propositional conversational speech, particularly with a listener. While differences may be found in nonspeech activities, it is very difficult, in this writer's opinion, to ascertain how such differences contribute to actual instances of stuttering. Thus, various nonspeech behavioral (e.g., finger tapping) tasks using electrophysiological procedures (e.g., study of hemispheric alpha wave asymmetries via means of EEG) means will continue to be used to study the neurological activity of people who stutter. However, in this writer's opinion, it is most likely that future breakthroughs in this area will come through the application of neuroimaging technologies (e.g., PET or functional magnetic resonance imaging [fMRI]) during *actual* speech-language production, production that approximates, as much as possible, the syntactic, semantic, phonological, and motoric processes that occur during conversational speech.

Second, this area of research is *not* without concerns. Three of the more apparent to this author are as follows: (1) speed of temporal resolution of neuroimaging relative to time course of speech events of interest; (2) adequate models for what cortical activities one might expect people who stutter to exhibit; and (3) the difficulties with applying neuroimaging to 3- to 6-year-old children, the time period during which stuttering is most apt to begin.

About the first concern, *temporal resolution of neuroimaging*: As mentioned before, adults can easily see a picture and correctly name the same within 550 to 650 msec (about one-half second), while certain of the neuroimaging procedures could take up to two full minutes to resolve or display a picture (although some of the newer procedures, like functional magnetic resonance imaging, fMRI, take less than 1 second). Likewise, adults can readily produce 10 sounds per second. What this means, therefore, is that the resulting neuroimage can be a composite or "smear" across many different speech events. While the temporal resolution of these neuroimaging procedures is rapidly advancing (e.g., fMRI), at present this is still a concern Why? Well, let's speculate that one of the difficulties people who stutter have is quickly accessing the mental lexicon (dictionary). Let's assume, for argument's sake, that the average normally fluent speaker takes 100 msec to select a word after seeing a picture to name while a person who stutters takes 300 msec. Also assume that such activity has a cortical correlate that we might be able to detect on a neuroimage. Now, if it takes say several seconds to produce a neuroimage, many other events could have taken place during that timeframe, over and beyond the selection of a word—for example, thinking about what's for lunch, thinking about whether the person just pronounced the word right, asking the experimenter a question, and so forth. It is a certainty that the time course of many speech and language events are well under a second, in particular, these events are *extremely rapid* during connected speech. Why? Well, how else could we produce 10 or so sounds per second, that is, call up and then overtly articulate a word in one-half second? Thus, it is speech events occurring within this brief timeframe that we must account for, like it or not, if we are to account for "why" people stutter and where within the brain such process or processes may go awry. We are not at a point, I think, where we can do this, but we will be, and shortly.

The second concern, *models for brain activity during stuttering*: This, perhaps, is the Achilles heel of this area of research (as well as other areas of research in stuttering). While the level of description is elegant in many of these studies, it is often nontheory driven. This is, of course, understandable, but regrettable at the same time. Without some a priori notion, speculation or theory of where within (1) the process of syntactic, semantic, and phonological processes events are likely to go awry to initiate an instance of stuttering, and (2) the brain such activities might take place, results become an elegant cataloguing of interesting observations, with no clear indication of how they account for instances of stuttering. One can find laudable, creative procedures for more closely relating specific speech disorders (e.g., apraxia) with specific cortical activities/structures (e.g., Dronkers, 1996); likewise, we can find similarly laudable post hoc attempts to account for neuroimaging findings relative to specific aspects of speech and language production (e.g., Liotti, Gay, & Fox, 1994). However, what we don't often find in this area—and hopefully we will see more of this—is where the researchers a priori suggest, for example, that phonological encoding is problematic in people who stutter and then go through, ideally in an experimental way, manipulating salient aspects of phonological encoding, all the while assessing the activity of particular areas of the brain thought to be involved with phonological encoding. Such an approach has the potential for ruling in or out various facets of speech and language formulation relative to stuttering.

The third concern, using *neuroimaging with young children*: Anyone who has tested, studied, or treated young children (3 to 6 years of age) can readily attest to their "ability" to quickly fatigue, lose interest in a task, lose attention, and become uncooperative and fearful about events that pose no real threat to them. Thus, bringing such children into an atmosphere—for example, fMRI—that produces a lot of noise and where they must sit/lie still and cooperate for a period of time, can be quite problematic. At the John F. Kennedy Center for Research on Human Development (at my university, Vanderbilt), researchers have taken on this difficult task with neuroimaging simulators, to "get the children used to" these procedures. However, no one expects this to be an easy task, and much of the success of these procedures with young children will be dependent on a complex interaction between parental cooperation, child cooperation, and experimenter expertise as well as sensitivity to the concerns and needs of young children and their families. This type of work must go forward, however, for it is only at the level of childhood that we can study stuttering and/or processes that may contribute to it in their "purest" forms, before the contaminating influences of development, experience, treatment, and learning have been layered onto and interact with basic stuttering behavior and/or causes. Furthermore, given the commonly agreed on assumption that, as a rule, adults who stutter, when compared to children who stutter, are more apt to have developed attitudinal, emotional, etc. reactions to stuttering, one could predict that the cortical activities/areas/processes associated with (dis)fluent speech may differ between adults and children. During this relatively early stage of this research, there appears to be little concern and/or control for these cognitive-emotional reactions (reactions that surely have neurophysiological correlates) in brain-imagining studies of adults who stutter. However, such control seems eventually necessary to minimize the potential that cortical activity correlates of emotions/reactions have for obfuscating cortical activity associated with (dis)fluent speech-language production.

Motor Activity and Behavior (e.g., Temporal Coordination of Tongue and Jaw Movements During Speech)

Without a doubt, in the past ten to fifteen years, some of the more eloquent, well-controlled studies in the area of stuttering have been in the area of speech motor control and motor execution (e.g., Van Lieshout, 1995; Van Lieshout, Starkweather, Hulstijn, & Peters, 1995). And, with continued technological advances in this area, we see no reason why such research will abate in the next few years. Information about various aspects of speech production that heretofore was extremely time-consuming and laborious to collect, analyze, and process now, with computer-assisted or even computer-automated methodology, becomes more "doable" within a reasonable period of time. While the number of subjects assessed in any one study of speech production is generally, for the foreseeable future, never as large as that studied via perceptual means, the sizable number of data points typically gathered per subject, the relative stability of speech production, and nature of questions asked in this area generally permit smaller sample sizes. However, in this writer's opinion, this area of research, despite considerable, diligent efforts by individuals in this area, has not lived up to its bright promise of the early to mid 1980s. Why?

First of all, this area is still plagued with what I've described before as the *looking-for-keys-under-the-lamplight syndrome*. In brief, it's night, and an individual who has had a bit too much to drink is seen looking around on the ground under a lamplight near his front porch. A friend, seeing this, asks the person what he is doing. The person replies, "Looking for my keys." "Where did you lose them?" asks the friend. "Oh," the inebriated one replies, "over there on my porch, but the light's better here!" In essence, even though it is quite clear that stuttering is a disorder of childhood, most of the high sophisticated research in this area, exploring motor correlates of stuttering, has concentrated on adults. Why? Simply put, its easier, for the same reasons I mentioned above: Children can be quick to fatigue, rapidly lose interest in a task before it is completed, lose attention if they feel stressed, mentally challenged, become uncooperative and fearful about events that pose no real threat to them, and so on. Why put up with this hassle, where you might lose as many as 50 percent of your young subjects to lack of cooperation and the like, when there are relatively cooperative adults? Adults, while not uniformly cooperative and attentive, can at least be reasoned with and talked to. Try doing that with a 4-year-old who has decided that those tiny surface electromyographic (EMG) electrodes need to be taken off him, despite the fact they don't in any way hurt or pose a threat to him! Furthermore, in all fairness, some of the technologies in this area have either simply not been adapted or are not suitable for young children, something that is a project unto itself. This field, in my opinion, will only really move forward towards narrowing down the motor correlates of stuttering when it routinely assesses these correlates in 3- to 7-year-old children who stutter.

Second, putting aside the tendency to study adults rather than children, *what has this area of endeavor shown us to date?* That is very unclear (see critical review of Ingham, 1998). Again, in all fairness to this area, whatever differences are found or uncovered, relative to the motor execution abilities of people who stutter, are most likely subtle, imperceptible to human eyes and ears (see Armson & Kalinowski, 1994, for discussion of whether these "differences" relate to cause or merely subtle aspects of stuttering itself). Thus, we should not expect to see gross, dramatic, readily apparent differences and disabilities in motor execution in people who stutter—their overall speech and even their stutterings are just not that aberrant. Indeed, brief, subtle motoric disruptions, if they could be shown to be routinely associated with, leading to, or causing fluency failure in conversational speech, would probably be sufficient to support the claims of some that motoric disruptions contribute to stuttering. However, to date, no such subtle, brief disruptions have been found in the majority of people who stutter when they stutter during conversational speech that appears to be, albeit peripheral or distal, the "cause" of instances of stuttering. On the whole, we are not talking about individuals who are dysarthric or aphasic. We are talking about individuals who exhibit more of certain kinds of speech disfluencies than others. Succinctly put, if there were *gross* differences in motor behavior in the speech of people who stutter, we would have discovered that long ago.

All that said, what subtle, imperceptible differences has this area uncovered? I think the record will show that the main findings in this area relate to: slower reaction times, seemingly related to *motor* (e.g., movement of tongue from a rest position to a position for articulating a speech sound) rather than linguistic (e.g., syntax, semantics, etc.) events , increased variability/instability of motor processes, and subtle temporal disruptions/relationships in the acoustic speech signal. Okay, fine, but how, unless we see similar behaviors across the developmental lifespan, can these behaviors/disruptions be interpreted? I mean, is it not possible that these subtle disruptions in adults who stutter are the results, the residuals of nearly a lifetime of adjusting, avoiding, escaping, tensing, and so on in reaction to speech disfluencies? Might not the person who stutters—like an individual with a cleft palate who learns lingual-velar (e.g., /g/) contact for lingual-alveolar (e.g., /d/) sounds to compensate for nasal emission/hypernasality—also "compensate" for stuttering by "botching up" their motor processes to the point where the entirety of their motor execution for speech is different from normal? Again, in fairness to this area of endeavor, there are signs that investigators are seriously starting to assess children who stutter and that at least in the acoustic signal there may be signs that across the lifespan, children, teens, and adults who stutter may exhibit subtle difficulties in temporal control for speech production (e.g., Chang, Ohde, & Conture, 1999; Robb & Blomgren, 1997).

A third area, the area of motor execution, just like cortical activity and structure of speech, needs a model that explicitly spells out, in a testable manner, *how motor processes can and do cause the speech disfluencies called stuttering*. While laudable attempts have been made to weave the fabric of motor processes into a theory of stuttering, they fall short, in this author's mind. I say this because these theoretical explanations do not explicitly tell us how X motor disruption or process results in the Y speech disfluency, for example, sound/syllable repetitions, which we call stuttering. Suggesting that motor disruptions or instability contributes to or "causes" hesitations, disruptions, and breakdowns in speech fluency are not sufficient, in my opinion. Any truly viable model of stuttering must explain, I believe, if at all possible, what causes the essential behavior we call stuttering that is most often manifest in sound/syllable repetitions, sound prolongations, monosyllabic whole-word repetitions, blocks, and some "tense pauses" between words. Not the myriad of psychosocial (e.g., frustration), nonspeech (e.g., blinking of eyelids), and so forth reactions, but the essential behaviors we perceive and label as stuttering.

Fourth, motor models of stuttering *must* begin to acknowledge the nearly overwhelming evidence that *linguistic* (premotor) *events* (e.g., longer, more grammatically complex sentences) *are highly correlated to stuttering*; similarly, models from a premotor (syntactic, semantic, and/or phonological) perspective must readily acknowledge the possibility that motor processes could very well interact with and/or exacerbate any theorized difficulties in premotor processes exhibited by people who stutter. Indeed, given the rapid advances in knowledge that have and will continue in the field of psycholinguistics, especially in the area of cognitive/formulative processes, I predict that present and future motor models of stuttering will become increasingly marginalized if they eschew linguistic events, trying to remain totally physiological in their explanations of stuttering, and thus disregard evidence suggesting premotor involvement in stuttering.

Fifth, in 1990, I wrote in this space about the *"temporal discoordination hypothesis"* (see Van Riper, 1971; Perkins et al., 1976), a concept that has been revisited, albeit in a revised form, by Perkins and colleagues (1991). No matter how seemingly attractive or high in face validity the notion of "temporal discoordination," the theory has received very minimal support from empirical studies of the speech production of people who stutter (e.g., Caruso, Conture, & Colton, 1988; Conture, Colton, & Gleason, 1988; Prosek, Montgomery, & Walden, 1988). However, some research (e.g., Conture, Rothenburg, & Molitor, 1986) is suggestive of the notion that at transitions between sounds, children who stutter may do so, at least at the laryngeal level, in a manner subtly but significantly different and perhaps less efficient from their peers who don't stutter (an issue we will return to below).

Clearly, the terminology, concepts, and methods used to describe and study the "discoordination" hypothesis needs refinement, in light of present data. For example, it is possible that "discoordinations" can occur *within* one speech structure—for example—the lips, as well as *between* different structures—for example, the laryngeal and supralaryngeal systems. Likewise, it is apparent that "coordination" and "discoordination" represent terms that are widely used but just as often misused, and definitions of these terms must encompass thinking and work from related areas of speech motor control and the like. Research increasingly makes it clear that speech structures move not only through time but space as well and both aspects—time and space—will have to be considered when investigating and theorizing regarding speech production abilities of people who stutter. Speaking of time, we have already mentioned the fact that time encompasses much more than the mere durations and transitions of speech production gestures and that the perceptions of people who stutter (see Zimmerman's [1980a, 1980b] early attempts to do this) in terms of passing time during speech and nonspeech behavior plays a role in this problem.

Sixth, *failure to learn from critical appraisal* is a problem for all of us. While we have learned, on descriptive as well as experimental levels, a good deal more about the speech production of people who stutter (e.g., Conture, Colton, & Gleason, 1988; Denny & Smith, 1997; Prosek, Montgomery, & Walden, 1988; Smith & Kelly, 1997; Van Lieshout, 1995), including their stuttered speech production (e.g., Caruso, Conture, & Colton, 1988; Denny & Smith, 1992; Yaruss & Conture, 1993; Zimmerman, 1980a), Armson and Kalinowski's (1994) and Ingham's (1998) critiques raise a number of appropriate cautions and concerns with speech motor control and related research in the area of stuttering. A wise person, I believe it was Wendell Johnson, once said that to be completely positive about the unconfirmable shows not stubbornness, but a fear of the uncertain. Those who persist seeking *purely* motoric explanations of stuttering, without reference to the myriad of co-occurring processes, suggest that they may have such fear. For as we have mentioned previously (Conture, 1991), no one single behavior(s) has emerged from this work as being most often associated with stuttering or changes in stuttering during treatment, particularly with children.

One reason, we submit, is that studies of speech motor control and stuttering have been hampered is due to a bias to study the periphery (however, workers in this area clearly and appropriately speculate about central or neural issues, e.g., Denny & Smith, 1997). This is logical, of course, because, after all, an instance of stuttering, at a most fundamental level of description, is a disruption in the motor execution of speech. However, so is right-sided paralysis, but would any thoughtful modern-day neurologist look to the muscles of the paralyzed arm or leg for clues as to their source? We think not. What is needed is a wider field of vision. Vision must be expanded beyond the motor to include the domain of the premotor system to assess interactions between motor and premotor processes (e.g., Peters & Starkweather, 1990). After all, the resulting motor disruptions could just as easily start with difficulties with word selection, morphosyntactic construction, and phonological encoding as they do with peripheral difficulties with motor execution. It is time to stop eschewing central processes while solely focusing on peripheral processes when trying to understand stuttering. In essence, we must realize that unless central processes occur, there is nothing for the peripheral processes to execute!

Finally, we hope that the information collected in the research labs about motor execution and its role in stuttering can be used to write computer programs, programs that will find their way increasingly into the clinic first in the form of acoustic feedback of articulatory, then laryngeal behavior (via means of EGG methodology), and finally through feedback of muscle tensions/activity through surface electromyography (at this writing, some beginning, commercially available products in this area are emerging). The potential of crossover, cooperative endeavors between those who study speech motor execution and those who treat people who stutter, particular adults, is an area that having some potential to advance clinical practice. At the least, application of the findings and technology of speech motor research to actual clinical practice, particularly with teenagers and adults who stutter, is something I believe clinicians who treat stuttering will want to continue to monitor through journal articles and conference presentations in the years ahead.

Again, I believe, at least for clinical purposes, that one important contribution that the area of speech motor control research can make is a thorough documentation of exactly what people who stutter do articulatorily, laryngeally and respiratorily before, during, and after stuttering. Granted, such research is mainly descriptive not theory-driven in nature, and granted there will be a good deal of individual variation in the manifestations of instances of stuttering (see, e.g., Hutchinson, 1974, for an early attempt to do such work, and the degree of individual variation he observed); however, clinicians really need a much clearer, objective idea than they have about what actually occurs at the periphery (e.g., mouth, larynx, etc.) during instances of stuttering. Why? Well, these are the exact speaking behaviors that clinicians try to identify and change, regardless of whether these behaviors have central, peripheral, or combined origins. So much treatment goes on with people who stutter, and yet there is so little objective information about the exact nature of the behavior we are trying to assess, identify, and treat. Having such information, based on a large sampling of stutterings exhibited by a representative sample of people who stutter, is vital to an accurate, effective program of treatment based on identification and modification of instances of stuttering. In brief, it seems clear to this writer that clinicians could find value in such information in terms of both assessment and intervention.

Transitions

Within the literal cornucopia of facts regarding speech production of stuttering lies one seemingly hidden verity: People who stutter appear to exhibit difficulties making smooth, rapid transitions between speech sounds. On the surface, such difficulties would appear to be a motor execution, perhaps phonetic, even phonological problem. However, as we will mention at the end of this section, it is quite possible that concerns "upstream" of these events—for example, semantic and/or syntactic encoding—contribute to difficulties people who stutter seem to have with transitions between sounds.

That researchers and clinicians alike have long speculated about the possibility that transitions between sounds are problematic for people who stutter can be observed in the remarks, in 1861, of James Hunt who wrote:

> What is it then that distresses the stutterer, surely not the initial explosive (read: word-initial stop plosive consonant)? Why, it is the enunciation of the following sound, be it a vowel or a consonant, which is his difficulty; he cannot join them, and it is this which makes him repeat the explosive, until the conjunction is effected. It is, therefore, during the *transition* (italics added) from one mechanism to another that the impediment chiefly takes place. (p. 22)

More recently, in 1976, Wingate suggested much the same thing:

> We can achieve a major simplification in understanding stuttering by considering the ele-mental features as the distinction "markers" of a stutter.
>
> It is a mistake to consider them to *be* the stuttering. They are more properly under-stood as marking an event which is the essence of stuttering. This event is a failure in pho-netic *transition* (italics added), i.e., a failure to move to the next phoneme in the required sequence. "Failure" is only a superficial description of what actually happens. The fact that the speaker does not move forward in spite of clear intention to do so makes it appropriate to view the failure as *inability* to continue in the phonetic sequence. (p. 253)

Wingate's suggestion (that he had previously discussed [1969]) although seemingly grounded in a more phonetic/motor execution point of view, is consistent with Blood-stein's (1975) comment that "When stutterers prolong a sound or attack it with effort, they also tend to break its natural transition into the next sound," that when a person who stut-ters expects difficulty on an upcoming sound that ". . . he (the person who stutters) tends to prepare himself to say the sound as a fixed articulatory position rather than as a normal movement leading into the rest of the world" (p. 6).

Thus, whether due to inherent delays or difficulties with speech production, learned and/or psychosocial reactions to speaking, more than a few scholars have suggested that transitions between sounds are problematic for people who stutter. However, is there evi-dence to support such speculation? In our opinion, the answer is yes. In essence, after reviewing this area, there are sufficient empirical observations of transition difficulties to warrant further investigation of this topic.

One of the more well-known observations in this area is that of Stromsta (1965, 1986) who reported, on the basis of a longitudinal study of children who stutter, that the speech disfluencies of these children were characterized by "abnormal formant transitions and abnormal terminations of phonation" (Stromsta, 1986, p. 4). These are obviously poten-tially important findings, if they can be independently verified with other children who stut-ter (particularly for CWS without demonstrable delays and/or disorders in speech sound articulation or phonology). Unfortunately, most of the work in this area has been con-ducted with adults, individuals (as we've mentioned before) who have had considerable opportunity to develop a variety of psychosocial and/or physiological reactions to stutter-ings. In our opinion, such reactions, regardless of how they have developed, make it diffi-cult to study any facet of the speech production of adults who stutter without also studying the "overlay" of reactions to difficulties with speaking. In essence, acoustic assessment of adult speech-language production, when compared to that of children, may more often wind up studying *reaction to* rather than *contribution to* or *cause of* instances of stuttering. Be that as it may, there are numerous reports of missing or atypical formant transitions in the fluent and disfluent speech of adults who stutter (e.g., Harrington, 1987; Howell & Vause, 1986; Howell, Williams, & Vause, 1987; Montgomery & Cooke, 1976; Robb & Blomgren, 1997). For example, Howell and Vause (1986) reported that "85% of the spec-trograms of the fluent speech [of adults who stutter] were judged as lacking transitions between initial consonant and the medial vowel and 84.8% of the disfluent productions" (p. 1572). Likewise, studies of the influence of treatment on stuttering (e.g., Metz, Samar, & Sacco, 1983) have reported an association between stuttering frequency and silence in the voiced stop consonant intervocalic interval, with Metz and colleagues speculating that this association relates to disruptions in the regulation of timing for voiced stop consonant production. More recently, Robb and Blomgren (1997), studying the fluent speech of adults who do and do not stutter, found that adults who stutter, when compared to adults who do not stutter, exhibited significantly larger slopes or trajectories of F2 transition after consonantal release. Robb and Blomgren took this finding to suggest that that adults who stutter exhibit" . . . greater or quicker movement of the tongue body within the oral cavity in transitioning from closing-to-opening-to-closing vocal tract gestures" than their normally fluent peers.

With regard to children who stutter, what little research that has been conducted suggests CWS also exhibit difficulties with transitions between sounds. For example, Zebrowski, Conture, and Cudahy (1985) found that while CWNS, during perceptibly fluent transitions between consonant and vowel, exhibit an inverse relationship between stop gap and aspiration duration (e.g., as stop gap duration lengthens, aspiration duration shortens), CWS do not. This finding suggests that CWS produce the temporal aspects of speech in less than an optimally efficient fashion. Similarly, Conture, Rothenberg, and Molitor (1986) reported that CWS, when compared to CWNS, produced significantly less typical glottal activity during perceptibly fluent consonant-vowel and vowel-consonant transitions. Likewise, Yaruss and Conture (1993) found that the F2 transition durations during instances of stuttering of "high-risk" (for continuing to stutter) CWS were different than those of CWNS. And most recently, Chang, Ohde, and Conture (1999) reported that during perceptibly fluent utterances CWS, when compared to CWNS, produced significantly smaller differences in F2 transition rates between bilabial and alveolar places of articulation.

What does all the above mean? First, this is an area, particularly with children, that warrants further study with larger number of subjects, with rigorous controls on subject selection, matching between children who do and do not stutter across a variety of speaking tasks, from single-word lists to conversational speech. This if, of course, a large undertaking, but this area will not be clarified, if it is possible to do so, by continually studying only small samples of subjects—for example, five people who stutter and five people who do not stutter. Second, explanations of why the transitions of people who stutter may be problematic should not be limited to motoric or phonetic accounts because the phonetic plan that the motor system must execute may itself be problematic. In other words, rather than motoric difficulties, the problem may lie with the phonetic plan of people who stutter, a plan resulting from the complex interplay of syntactic, semantic, and phonologic processes. In other words, if the plan is awry, particularly the phonological portion, this may create subtle difficulties in the motor system's ability to efficiently, quickly, and smoothly execute speech-language production. Third, it is reasonable to suggest that Kent's (1984) notion that stuttering is associated with disruptions of temporal processes is consistent with the above observations that people who stutter exhibit difficulties with transitions during speech-language production. However, it is just as reasonable to suggest that time is not merely a property of the peripheral level of speech-language production, time is also very salient to the initiation and development of the phonetic plan, a plan that must be generated "centrally" for the peripheral motor system to subsequently execute. In this writer's opinion, only by realizing, like the old song said, that the ankle bone is connected to the knee bone, the knee bone connected to the leg bone, that *motor execution* is connected to the *planning of speech-language production* will we ever achieve the depth and breadth of perspective needed to comprehensively understand stuttering.

Treatment Efficacy

Several have recently reviewed treatment efficacy in the field of stuttering (e.g., Conture, 1996; Cordes, 1998; Ingham & Cordes, 1999; Ingham & Riley, 1998; Yaruss, 1998b), and, perusing such reviews, one can fairly say that a great deal more needs to be done in this area, from all perspectives. While some seemingly wave their flags from the battlements, urging those who would rally around and follow them to exercise rigor, whatever that is, they sometimes unfortunately do so in a manner more suggestive of mortis than rigor. In this writer's opinion, rather than these my-way-or-the-highway, one-size-fits-all means of conducting treatment efficacy research, the wisdom of time and the realities of developmental differences and nontreatment variables (e.g., ADHD) in children, teenagers, and adults will make it crystal clear that researchers in this area will need to maneuver according to circumstances. Is this ambiguous? Yes, but as I say elsewhere in these pages, a tolerance for ambiguity rather than insistence on certainty is the hallmark of the educated mind. Be that as it may, like many health-related fields, we are a long way from adequately documenting how our treatments ameliorate the disability and handicap of stuttering, although tremendous strides have been made in this direction (e.g., see Ingham & Riley, 1998, for suggested guidelines for documenting treatment efficacy for children who stutter).

First, let us look at *consensus agreement regarding designs to study treatment efficacy* (see Schiavetti & Metz, 1997, pp. 120–148, for an excellent overview of designs germane to treatment efficacy research and Couture's, 1999a, suggestions regarding application of these designs to stuttering). If at all possible, we need to agree on several viable designs for the assessment of treatment of stuttering in children, teens, and adults. Some of these designs will be group in nature, others single-subject, still others perhaps combinations of group with follow-up single-subject studies of group exemplars. While double-blind studies with placebo and control groups may be feasible with adults when using drugs (see Brady, 1991, for overview of drug intervention for stuttering), such designs may be all but impossible for preschool children who stutter, whose anxious parents having read literature, talked to friends and other professionals, want therapy sooner than later and have little or no interest in participating in experimental invention when they sincerely and strongly believe that their child's (future) development is at stake. In essence, treatment study designs that work for adults may not necessarily work when applied to children; other, hopefully as rigorous, approaches will have to be developed that are suitable for children.

It is not sufficient to argue that statistical textbooks contain adequate designs for work in this area; if we, as a field, cannot generally agree on the most appropriate designs, use and adapt them to the treatment of stuttering, we will continue to argue about such events as presence/absence of control groups, length of time post-treatment needed to establish maintenance, number of measures per treatment session required, and the like. And as long as such nonproductive argument continues, we may continue to remain the professional equivalent of the cultural remnants of the former Yugoslavia—fractionated, building ourselves up by tearing others down, swearing allegiance to our tribe, and disregarding the efforts of all other tribes.

The second area of concern is the *blurring of the emotional edges between clinical investigator and his or her intervention technique*. Clinicians work long and hard to develop a method, a procedure and format that works for each of them. Naturally, therefore, when they test their approaches, they are not exactly dispassionate, they are emotionally invested. For they must be passionate and invested, otherwise the time-consuming, labor-intensive work of developing a treatment approach simply doesn't get done if the clinician lacks emotional motivation. This is reality, for even the most objective among us. And, in my opinion, individuals who do not recognize this reality of human nature need to, in the vernacular, "get a grip." The problem is not that lack of objectivity exists, the problem is how do we recognize that fact and do our level best to minimize undue subjectivity when evaluating the fruits of our clinical labors? I have no easy answers for this, merely note this concern in passing.

What I will say, though, is that I find it increasingly difficult to put a great deal of credence in reports of treatment efficacy with people who stutter that contain little or no report of failure. This failure to report failures does not help move us beyond the my-therapy-is-better-than-your-therapy stage that we have been mired in for far too long. For many people, stuttering is a difficult problem to turn around and for some it takes many attempts before they become reasonably normally disfluent. To read about treatments, no matter how eloquent, seemingly factual, carefully developed, and objectively reported, which contain *no* indication that some of the subjects failed, at least to some degree, is, in my experience, pushing the credibility envelope to the point of breaking. Indeed, we learn as much if not more about our abilities to intervene/treat by our failures than we do our successes. And we must learn to describe our failures with as much detail and clarity as we do our successes.

Third, we need to look at the *notion that all therapies are alike regardless of their theories*. If this is true, we need more explicit, documented evidence describing the commonalties among our clinical approaches and the rationale for same. If there are important commonalties among therapies, it would decrease our tendency to eagerly claim novelty for any one clinical procedure, since they all may be manipulating the same variables only through different means. Conversely, we should not be too eager to totally cast aside procedures like rhythmic stimulation—which may shed needed light on the variables of import—simply because these procedures have been kicking around the back drawers of our clinical desks for years (and/or have been misused by charlatans and mountebanks). These procedures deserve, at the least, continued, careful empirical study as well as systematic clinical investigation. We also need to subject "tried-and-true" procedures to objective empirical assessment—for example, the influence of parental speaking rate on a child's speech fluency (Stephenson-Opsal & Bernstein Ratner, 1988).

If all therapies for people who stutter are so much alike, we need studies and critical reviews that make explicit to each clinician, researcher, and student alike how our treatments are similar, instead of giving the appearance of vast differences in approach when, in fact, the names may be different but the game essentially the same. One early, meaningful attempt at exploring commonalties among various stuttering theorists and/or therapies can be found in an edited book by Gregory (1978). Gregory and his contributing authors discuss their various approaches to stuttering, and by so doing the reader gains the knowledge that these workers do share certain common ideas despite their more well-known differences of opinion (much might be said of a more recent book by Onslow & Packman,

1999, where different treatment approaches are provided for the reader, to compare and contrast similarities and differences). Guitar (1999), through their attempt to meld behavioral and traditional approaches, as well as Guitar (1998), also show the desire to explore the commonalties of stuttering therapy to integrate approaches. However, in recent years, attention has turned from searching for commonalties among treatments to more general issues pertaining to the need for as well as problems with treatment efficacy research for people who stutter (e.g., Conture, 1996; Cordes & Ingham, 1998).

While there are many forces, practical as well as theoretical, that have and will continue to foster this focus on treatment efficacy, one word of caution is in order. If we create a cottage industry centered on *treatment efficacy that has no apparent, obvious, or visible ties to theories* that seem best able to explain the cause(s) of stuttering, we may come, in the long run, to a situation where we are *long on empirical evidence* and *short on explanatory support*. For without explanation for *why* something works, not merely the fact that it does work, then there is no way to explain why it *doesn't* work! And with stuttering, we can be sure that even the best of our treatments won't work some of the time for some people. Failing to explain why our treatments do not work, both in the eyes of the public as well as funding agencies, has the real potential for casting serious doubts on the diligent efforts of those who study treatment efficacy, regardless of their scientific rigor and efforts to do well. Make no mistake about it, theoretically motivating our various treatment approaches, regardless of how objective, data-oriented, and systematic they may be, is no small undertaking. It is a chasm, the divide between modern-day theorization about stuttering and modern-day treatment of stuttering that must be bridged for the field as a whole to move forth.

A fourth important area is the need to develop *clinical databases*. With the proliferation of the computer in every facet of our daily personal and professional lives, clinicians will start to develop their own databases on the clients they evaluate and remediate (e.g., Yaruss, LaSalle, & Conture, 1998). While some will raise various concerns with the specific manner and nature of collecting, reporting, and interpreting such information (see exchange between Cordes, 2000; Yaruss, Conture, & LaSalle, 2000), the reporting of "clinical records" is a long-standing, common practice in many fields. Individuals in our field (e.g., Doehring, 1996; Lubker & Tomblin, 1998) apparently believe that so-called records-review studies can provide us with a variety of insights into the clinical process. Obviously, clinicians have always had access to these databases in the form of clinical records and folders; however, the computer, with its ability to rapidly count, sort, and organize, has greatly expanded the accessibility of these records. Subtle and not-so-subtle trends can emerge as clinicians scroll through these databases looking for past clients similar to those they are currently confronted with. For example, when examining the records of children whose stuttering persists, phonological processes may emerge as variables highly associated with either protracted therapy or relapse. Some of this clinically based data may challenge widespread clinical hunches about stuttering. I, for one, will be interested to see whether clinicians and researchers alike will allow factual information to ruin "good" theory, for as Kurlansky (1998, p. 187) suggests, ". . . theory cannot be killed by mere experience."

Fifth, we need to develop a generalized understanding of *transfer* that could apply to all therapies, or at least for those treatments for preschoolers, school-age children, teenagers and adults who stutter. While some rightfully include this as one of the basic three elements of treatment (e.g., baseline, acquisition, and extinction of behavior), its centrality to the long-term success of treatment cannot be overlooked (also, what cannot be overlooked are reliable indexes of instances of stuttering, e.g., see Ingham, Cordes, & Finn, 1993, for attempts to develop same and Ambrose & Yairi, 1999, for attempts to develop metrics distinguishing child who do and do not stutter). Indeed, good transfer is good therapy; conversely, poor transfer means, regardless of the depth and breadth of treatment, poor therapy. Transfer *is* where the client lives, not in treatment; thus, much, much more needs to be known about the elements of this familiar but poorly understood process. At least to begin, this needs to be a content-free or therapy-blind investigation, that is, not driven by proving that this or that treatment is better than another in terms of transfer. Instead, what is needed is a systematic investigation of what things different treatments/clients share that are associated of true transfer, true relapse, and short-term "slips" in behavior. It is tempting to draw parallels between stuttering therapy and other therapies used to remediate human disorders, for example, sexual dysfunction, where it has become increasingly apparent that changing of behavior is much less difficult than maintaining it. Description and criteria need to be developed to help clinicians understand, identify, and distinguish between true relapses and relatively short-term "slips" in behavior, so that they can help themselves and their clients understand that such relatively temporary "slips" or reverting to old, inappropriate behavior does not a relapse make. Again, what is needed here is a therapy-blind study of common problems with relapse and transfer, to move this most important aspect out of this "this therapy is better than that therapy" realm into "these are the elements a treatment needs if it is to maximize long-term treatment." Of course, it is quite possible that elements of treatment associated with transfer may differ depending on the developmental level of stuttering, that is, with children, teenagers, or adults. Changes in stuttering, in terms of frequency, nature, associated nonspeech behaviors, and affective and cognitive reactions may mean, simply put, that what are effective transfer procedures with school-age children who stutter may not be with college-age adults who stutter. Further, it may turn out that with children, significantly involving their parents (e.g., Conture & Melnick, 1999; Lincoln & Onslow, 1997; Ramig, 1993; Starkweather, Gottwald, & Halfond, 1990) in intervention may lead to the best long-term maintenance (a possibility, of course, that must await empirical verification).

Sixth, as mentioned above, there is a continued need to meld traditional therapies (e.g., Cooper & Cooper, 1985) and behavioral as well as direct and indirect (e.g., Ramig & Bennett, 1997) therapies. Why? Humans neither live by behavior nor thought/feeling alone. The ABCs of stuttering (that we have touched on earlier, e.g., see Siegel, 1999 for an interesting discussion of the ABCs of stuttering) can oftentimes best be addressed when bringing together traditional (sometimes called "stuttering modification") with behavioral (sometimes called "fluency shaping") approaches. It is clear that the purists in both camps, will dismiss such a suggestion, but the less pure, such as this author, feel that such rigid ideologies serve neither the public nor the profession well. Stuttering and the people who exhibit it are just too much of a diverse bundle of behavior, emotions, and thought to ever be effectively understood and treated solely from one rigid perspective.

Although not a meld of behavioral and traditional therapies, we can find "combined" interventions such as Ramig and Bennett (1997) that involve a mixing of indirect and direct treatment approaches for school-age children who stutter. Such an approach is appropriately eclectic, seemingly taking the best from both approaches to address the realities of treating school-age children. Such combining or melding would seem to recognize that thought, feeling, and attitudes can influence behavior *and* that behavior can influence thought, feeling, and attitudes (see Guitar, 1997, for excellent example of such a clinical approach). A blend or mix of behavior and traditional therapies might involve mixing the insightful, perhaps sometimes a bit abstract, approach of the traditionalists with the more empirical, sometimes unnecessarily specific approach of the behaviorists. This melding or meshing of approaches is quite consistent with the growing trend in some physical sciences—for example, biology and physics—toward more humanistic approaches to science. While the pendulum of thought in the field of stuttering will probably never completely stop in the middle, it is believed that the extent of its swing from one side to another will never again be as great as has been observed in the past. Inhabiting this middle ground, as it were, means that students, in both their academic and clinical training, will need to be exposed to and learn about divergent bodies of information—for example, behavioral versus humanistic studies, principles, and practices. It will also mean that students and clinicians alike will need to become and remain knowledgeable regarding both premotor and motor aspects of speech and language production (e.g., see Bosshardt & Fransen, 1996, pp. 785–787, for discussion of coordination between premotor and motor levels of speech–language production). Such knowledge will be essential in order to read present/future literature, meaningfully attend workshops and conferences, as well as apply such information to the evaluation and remediation of stuttering.

Finally, as I have suggested elsewhere (Conture, 1999a), we need to explore how our treatment influences the handicap of stuttering, for example vocational disadvantages of stuttering (see, e.g., Prins, 1991; Yaruss, 1998a, 1998b, for an overview of how the concepts of impairment, disability, and handicap may apply to stuttering). If our treatments lead to improvement in fluency, but no improvement in academic, social, and vocational interactions, we need to know this, and not just for stuttering but all speech and language disorders. Conversely, if our treatments do not appreciably influence fluency but permit, for whatever reason, the person who stutters to interact whenever, wherever, and with whomever he or she wants across most to all academic, social, and vocational situations, we want to know that as well. It is particularly hoped that by assessing stuttering, the behavior in relation to stuttering, and the social disadvantages, we can come to a more realistic appraisal of the role stuttering plays in people's lives and that a zero tolerance for stuttering is good for neither client nor clinician.

Naturalness, Suitability, and Utility of Speech

What good is having a broken leg bone completely mended if the leg is not usable? The form may be correct, but function still missing. It should come as no surprise, therefore, that the *benefit* of increased fluency resulting from many therapy procedures may also *cost* in terms of changes in other aspects of speech and language production. For example, significant increments in the fluency of people who stutter (for example, Shames & Florance, 1980; Webster, 1975, 1978) may result from reducing the rate of movement between and within sounds and encourage the use of more gradual onsets and offsets of speech with less physical tension. Although, at least initially other aspects of speech behavior are changed—for example, fundamental frequency—these changes often drop out. However, if they do not, they may contribute to the perceived "unnaturalness" of speech some of these therapies seem to create (see Manning, 1996, pp. 222–228, for a good overview of "naturalness" as it relates to stuttering).

Within the past ten to fifteen years, considerable attention has been paid to the "naturalness" of speech exhibited by people who stutter, in general, and in specific with regard to how treatment for stuttering may influence the entirety, not merely fluency, of speech of people who stutter (e.g., Franken, 1987; Ingham, Ingham, Onslow, & Finn, 1989; Ingham & Onslow, 1985; Kalinowski, Noble, Armson, & Stuart, 1994; Metz, Schiavetti, & Sacco, 1990; Runyan, Bell, & Proseck, 1990). Franken and colleagues (1997) have investigated a related topic, the "suitability" of communication, across various speaking situations by people who stutter. Perhaps Manning (1996, p. 227) best summarizes one important implications of these studies when he suggests that ". . . the goal of treatment may be considerably more complex than just producing perceptually fluent speech."

Another way to summarize these studies is to suggest that researchers recognize that the cure, fluency, for some therapies, for some people who stutter, may be worse than the stuttering bite. It is clear that more than "fluency" is being changed during therapy; researchers have, in the past ten to twenty years, begun to seriously assess how treatment influences the "naturalness" of the speech of people who stutter. And a good deal more needs to be done in this general area. In particular, whether, after therapy, the person who is speaking significantly more fluently is also speaking more, with more people, and in more situations than pretherapy. Does this relate to "naturalness" or "suitability" or "utility" or all three? We don't know, but it is information we desperately need to prove that our treatments positively impact the *daily life activities* of people we treat. Again, *fluency is not the goal of speaking—communication is the goal of speaking* and our treatments must recognize this fact and evaluate whether they improve communication as well as fluency.

Put in other terms, we might ask, have some treatments won the fluency battle but lost the functionally useful speech war? Clearly, some therapies achieve increased fluency but decreased *naturalness*, especially in the prosodic aspects of speech—for example, variations in pitch, loudness, and duration; and less spontaneity in communication when every utterance must be monitored, scanned and "scoured clean" of speech errors/disfluencies. Indeed, clinicians may concentrate on improving the fluency of someone who stutters even though that person may be much more interested in the naturalness rather than amount of fluency he or she achieves.

While it is true that increased fluency may make a person who has been stuttering for many years feel like his or her speech "doesn't sound or feel right," we are not talking about that here. We are talking about a manner of speaking employed to increase speech fluency that does so by creating a form of speaking that looks and sounds to both listener and speaker alike as a drone, without normal prosodic variation or liveliness, a form of speech that appears overly controlled and/or hesitant. It is small wonder, therefore, that people who stutter who learn such a procedure quickly revert back to stuttering, for at least that contains greater degrees of normalcy in terms of prosody than the nearly, at its worse, robotic-like "drone" created by some treatments. For clients and clinicians alike, therefore, ". . . we must not only consider the *product* of therapy but the *utility* or *usability* of that product to the person receiving the therapy" (Conture & Guitar, 1993, p. 276). For, if after treatment, the person is reasonably fluent but to achieve that fluency he or she must speak in such a way that he or she essentially dislikes, that person still suffers from a "disability," that is, he or she refuses to use the telephone, something that leads to a "handicap," that is, the person doesn't participate in society to the fullest extent (Yaruss, 1998a).

Self-Help Organizations

Manning (1996, p. 250) suggested that self-help/support organizations, ". . . play an important, often critical role, in providing individuals with an opportunity for support and encouragement that is essential for long-term success following treatment." I strongly agree, although at first, I was not sure. My initial formal contact with self-help organizations for people who stutter was in the mid to late 1980s, and in the intervening years professionals like myself have watched this movement grow in breadth and depth in the field of stuttering. Besides stuttering, it was my impression during my initial contacts with self-help organizations, that many individuals who attended these groups had experienced greater or lesser degrees of failure in treatments. Some of these failures, I thought, were due to a combination of factors: the treatment itself, the person administering the treatment, the person receiving treatment, and/or for most, some complex interaction between treatment and the person. At that time, I felt that more than a few of the individuals I met at such support group conferences were less than convinced of Johnson's (1961, p. 185) notion that "To be helped you must be helpable, and to be helpable you must work with those who are trying to work with you. Other persons can hardly do more than make it possible for you to help yourself."

First, *positive, constructive change in self-help organizations* is quite apparent. In recent years, these organizations and the members who participate in them have become more numerous, better organized, and increasingly sophisticated in terms of the complexity of stuttering and treatment of same. Furthermore, the membership has seemingly diversified to include people who have experienced tremendous success in therapy, individuals who beautifully and cogently write about the problem (e.g., Carlisle, 1985; Jezer, 1997), the parents of children who stutter, and even children who stutter. Truly, to work in the field of stuttering, for the present and foreseeable future, one *must* know something about, and if appropriate, contribute to the good and welfare of these self-help organizations. Such exposure and knowledge should begin during the preservice training of speech–language pathologist and should be assumed to be, in my opinion, one of the professional, if not personal, obligations clinicians assume when they become a speech–language pathologist—for example, where possible, attendance at self-help meetings, subscribing to self-help newsletters, and the like. Just as our treatments are not without concerns, self-help organizations are not without concerns, but it is quite clear that self-help organizations have arrived, are thriving, and have great potential for helping not only those who participate but the field in general.

In particular, I recently presented (Conture, 1999b) at a self-help group and was especially gratified to see a dramatic lessening in the "them" versus "us," (i.e., clinicians versus clients) attitudes I initially perceived in the 1980s. There has been, I believe, increasing, genuine, and constructive dialogue between the professionals and the lay people, attempts to understand where each was coming from, and so forth. What I had witnessed formerly, seeming internecine warfare, was counterproductive and diluted our overall effort, which must be united to attract the federal and private dollars, not to mention rightfully deserved insurance reimbursement, to help study, prevent, and inform about this problem. Is all sweetness and light between clinician and client? No, of course not. Nirvana will probably never be reached in terms of client/clinician relations. Indeed, some degree of natural tension between the two is probably necessary for both parties to remain objective about one another. However, strides have and will continue to be made to bridge the gap between people who stutter and those who professionally serve them, and I expect the self-help organization has and continues to play a leadership role in this regard. This is a truly bidirectional effort, however, with clinicians encouraging and expecting, at least from time to time, members from self-help organizations to attend and present at their conferences, and people who stutter expecting and encouraging speech-language pathologists to attend and present at their conferences, and not only on the topic of treatment. The need for consumers—consumers who stutter—to know about what the products of basic and applied research should be, in my opinion, is something self-help organizations discuss during at least one portion of each of their conferences. Conversely, I think our professional conferences should—and we have made strides in this direction—have a forum during each conference where self-help organizations can interact and present as well as interact with the professionals who attempt to serve them.

Second, self-help organizations can be *antidotes to charlatans*. As the public—particularly that sector of the public that attends and participates in self-help organizations—grows in number and sophistication, those individuals who continue to claim clinical and theoretical monopolies on the truth will find it increasingly difficult to operate. Why? Because the public will slowly come to recognize and discriminate between the reputable professional and the mountebank. While everyone would like to have the silver bullet, as the true complexities, nuances and subtleties of stuttering are made increasingly apparent to the public, professionals alike, and self-help groups, it will become increasingly difficult for any one individual to try to claim a clinical or theoretical monopoly on the truth regarding the cause and remediation of stuttering. Such phrases as "overnight success," "100% success rate," "complete cure" and the like will more likely become repellants as the membership of such self-help organizations becomes more and more adept at seeing through the smokescreen and mirrors of the latter-day "great and powerful Oz."

It is believed that the facts relating to stuttering theory and therapy will simply be so much better understood by the lay public, due in part of the influence of self-help groups. This understanding will weigh so heavily against the "great and powerful Oz," as more and more individuals will recognize the untenable nature of such a therapeutic or theoretical monopoly. Ultimately, thorough this process, fewer and fewer will dare to claim such omnipotence, and those who do will receive scant attention. This widespread recognition of stuttering's complexities and nuances by the lay public, fueled in part by self-help organizations and other not-for-profit organizations like the *Stuttering Foundation of America*, should help counter the inappropriate, self-inflated approaches of a few. As such charlatans are debunked, it should mark the true advancement of stuttering from an interesting object to be kicked around among different disciplines into a recognized sub-disciplines within speech-language pathology, with its own standards, approaches, and body of knowledge, based on objects clinical and laboratory endeavor. Our clients deserve no less.

Finally, we need to seriously examine the matter of *insurance reimbursement*. People who stutter are people who pay insurance premiums. Thus, collectively they should have some voice, some clout, when contacting insurance companies to be more reasonable in terms of rates and length of time clinical services are covered. This is not an issue that can or will be solved by an individual person who stutters, but by a collection of people who stutter. And it is the consumer, not the service provider, whom the insurance companies will listen and respond to. Speech-language pathologists can provide facts and figures about the need, efficacy, type, and length of treatment and explain the difficulties typically faced in receiving appropriate reimbursement from insurance companies; but in this writer's opinion, the consumers are in the driver's seat. They pay insurance premiums, just like everyone else, and their collective voice should be heard and attended to by the people who collect those premiums, the insurance companies. Because schools have nurses and psychologists, does this mean that parents of children who stutter, for example, should not be reimbursed for appropriate, needed outside-of-school services for medical or psychosocial adjustment? We think not. Again, adding this issue, at least for continued discussion, to the many worthwhile projects self-help organizations have and will continue to tackle would be a benefit to consumers and professionals alike.

Some Parting Thoughts

The Future Is a Carte Blanche We Write on with Hope

The team that loses the championship game is many times quoted as saying, ". . . wait until next year." The future is a carte blanche that we often write on with hope. Things are always going to work or turn out for the better in the future. We, too, as speech–language pathologists who work with people who stutter continually anticipate and hope that new approaches and information "just around the bend and over the horizon" will improve our clinical acumen, methodology, and treatment outcome. While, as the saying goes, tomorrow is promised to no one, our field has been paying its dues and the future appears to hold bright promise for those who stutter and those who professionally manage them.

Two Trains Running in Parallel

Like many facets of speech–language pathology, we must realize one basic fact about individuals who work in the area of stuttering: The employment setting dictates much of what these professionals do and think about with regard to stuttering. While professional conferences, journal articles, books, and the like continually bring these professionals together throughout the year, there can be no denying the fact that individuals who clinically serve people who stutter and individuals who empirically research people who stutter have related, but different perspectives, interests, and needs (for further discussion of the preparation and practices of school-based SLPs relative to stuttering, see Kelly, Martin, Baker, Rivera, Bishop, Krizizke, Stettler, & Stealy, 1997). It's as if there were two trains running on parallel tracks whose passengers occasionally look out the window and wave at one another or who even disembark and mingle together at common stops but who get back on the train and ride toward their separate destinations. Clinicians have an interest and need to know about the most effective way to manage stuttering, and researchers have an interest and need to know the most they can about stuttering, whether or not such information has immediate application to treatment.

Granted, there are scientific clinicians as well as clinical scientists who routinely bridge the gap between treatment and theory (see, Goldberg, 1997, pp. 311–321) between applied and basic science, but most workers *daily* find themselves on one side or the other. We mention this distinction since future directions will probably come not only from the laboratory but will also result from clinical practice. Thus, scientists will need to monitor the results of clinical practitioners just as clinicians will want to monitor the findings of experimentalists. The complexities of stuttering are such that neither group of workers can afford to ignore the efforts of one another.

Nature INTERACTING with Nurture

For those of you who have read this book from the beginning, realize that I am fully supportive of any and all attempts to better understand the very difficult-to-understand *interactions* between the person who stutters and his or her environment, particularly in children. Such studies must not only address *initial, originating,* or *precipitating* causes but *maintaining, perpetuating, exacerbating,* and *aggravating* factors as well. Increasingly, I believe, studies of mother–child, father–child, mother–father–child interactions with children between 3 and 7 years of age (see Kelly, 1993, 1994, 1995 for a series of studies germane to this topic) will show that mothers and fathers of children who stutter are grossly similar to mothers and fathers of children who don't stutter. However, this same research, we believe, will uncover relatively subtle differences in verbal and nonverbal behavior for *some* families of children who stutter—for example, mothers and/or fathers who more frequently than normal answer their child's questions for him or her. These differences, we predict, will be more apt to be associated with those children for whom stuttering persists than for whom it improves due to treatment and/or unassisted development! Documenting the number and nature of these predictors of chronicity/continuation of stuttering in both the children and their families is an area desperately in need of study. Although there are many difficulties in conducting this work in a careful, meaningful way, the potential rewards in terms of new information and insights are truly great.

Explicating a Common Thread Gives the Lay Public Something to Hold onto

While differences may be healthy, lead to constant exploration, and are the stuff that fosters theoretical as well as therapeutic progress, unnecessary differences can also give the lay public the impression that no one really knows what is going on with stuttering. If everybody is right but different, then everybody must be wrong! However, despite this public impression, nothing could be farther from the truth.

As mentioned throughout this book, much has been and continues to be discovered in the area of stuttering. This fact needs to be made apparent to the lay public, our students, and, not the least, ourselves! Again, as mentioned directly above, we also need to clarify and explicate the degree of similarities among our various approaches. The mountebanks and charlatans of the world thrive on unnecessary ambiguity. These people have far less chance of treating people who stutter, for the most part, if those of us who diligently study and conscientiously deliver clinical services to people who stutter would put more of a concerted effort into explaining how much consistency there really is among approaches to stutterings used by SLPs who specialize in this disorder.

The common thread among our therapies must be there because too many seemingly different therapeutic approaches appear to have a similar ameliorative influence on the speech of people who stutter. If nothing else, keeping this common thread notion in mind when we evaluate and remediate people who stutter should help us, as individual SLPs, clarify what variables most of our colleagues are trying to manipulate or modify. Of course, clarification of these parameters is not a solution for same, but at least it is a start.

What Can Be Changed, What Can't, and the Ability to Recognize the Difference

We have stated elsewhere (e.g., Conture, 1996) that the harbingers for the future of remediation of stuttering are quite bright while fully recognizing the many concerns and issues we still have to contend with when conducting and reporting research on treatment efficacy. We have gained considerable more basic understanding of stuttering in recent years (e.g., Logan & Conture,. 1997; Van Lieshout, 1995; Yairi, 1997a, 1997b) and become increasing sophisticated in our abilities to systematically and objectively evaluate claims of therapeutic success (e.g., Cordes, 1998; Ingham & Cordes, 1999; Ingham & Riley, 1998; Metz, Onufrank, & Ogburn, 1979; Metz, Samar, & Sacco, 1983; Metz, Schiavetti, & Sacco, 1990; Robb, Lybolt, & Price, 1985; Sacco & Metz, 1987; Samar, Metz, & Sacco, 1986; Yaruss, 1998b). These increases in our basic knowledge and understanding of clinical process in the area of stuttering can only lead to more appropriate and effective approaches to the diagnosis and remediation of stuttering and to the development of research projects that should bring us ever closer to understanding the truth about stuttering.

It will be recalled from the front of this book, that readers of these pages were offered *NO* guarantees, recipes, quick fixes, or total solutions for curing stuttering; and, to this writer's knowledge, none were given. Guarantees, cures, and total solutions for complex human problems like stuttering are ideals to which one might like to aspire; however, one must also recognize that such ideals are not compatible with the present state of the human condition. While an overly realistic view might actually have a depressive influence on a person, an altered state of consciousness resulting from an overly optimistic feeling does not provide sufficient motivation to improve our lot. Instead, recognizing the imperfections of the human condition, while certainly no panacea, at least provides us with a reasonable backdrop against which we can develop (and hopefully work towards improving) our understanding as well as diagnosis and remediation. We are quite confident that in the future, speech–language pathologists will develop a better and better understanding of the human condition that everybody shares, including people who stutter. In this way, we believe that in their daily dealings with people who stutter, they will come to realize, as Niebuhr (1934; in Bingham, 1961, p. iii) suggested, ". . . what cannot be changed . . . what should be changed, and wisdom to distinguish the one from the other."[5]

Hammers Versus Swiss Army Pocketknives

Above all, what would seem to be imperative, regardless of our personal or professional interest in stuttering, is to remind ourselves that people who stutter occupy the same large temperate zone that most of us inhabit, a land where psyche and soma freely mingle and commingle. And because we are fellow inhabitants of this region, it is not always easy for us to clearly discern the totality and diversity of the forces that come together to cause, exacerbate, and perpetuate behaviors like stuttering. Some of us, therefore, in a misguided attempt to reduce the variability of what they must account for, observe, measure, and explain when studying and/or treating stuttering, often reach for one tool, the hammer, to pound their world into a semblance of order.

Disagreeing with all who attempt to employ instruments more suited for a diversity of circumstances, hammer wielders fail to realize that they ". . . make their observations through the perceptual filters provided by their theories—and the less aware they are of this reason for disagreeing the more they disagree" (Johnson, 1958, p. xx). It's almost as if they approach the study and treatment of stuttering as a game of whack-a-mole. It's not. Rather, to study and treat stuttering is to experience continual opportunity to maneuver according to circumstances, to employ the personal and professional equivalent of a Swiss Army pocket knife, a tool designed from the ground up to cope with a diverse set of challenges. Some may, of course, continue to construe the many facets of stuttering, as so many nails, thus justifying, in their minds, the use of a hammer. Contrary to such nonproductive practices, nothing would give this author more satisfaction than having those who peruse and read his current meanderings decide to employ the mental and professional equivalent of Swiss Army pocket knives rather than hammers when studying, assessing, and treating stuttering.

[5]J. Bingham, *Courage to change: An Introduction to the life and thought of Reinhold Niebuhr* (Boston: Little, Brown, 1961), p. iii.

APPENDIX A

Interview Questions for the Parent(s) of a Disfluent Child

Remember: These questions are a *guide* for you. It is *your* job to organize the questions in a logical sequential manner for each individual client. Furthermore, they may be adapted and modified for use with older children and adults.

Introduction

What can we do to help you? or Tell us (me) about why you are here today? or Tell us (me) about the (your child's) problem? or What seems to be the matter or the problem?

How did you find out about our clinic?

General Development

Tell us a little about his/her general development from birth to present. (Don't strive for detail at this point.)

How does this compare with his/her sister's and brother's development?

Other children his age that you may know?

Are you satisfied with his/her development?

Family History

Are there any speech, hearing, or language problems in other family members (mother's *and* father's side?)

(If so) did they receive speech therapy or other professional assistance (help)?

Speech Language Development and History

When did he/she begin to babble? (You may need to define the term babbling.)

Begin to imitate (non)speech sounds?

Begin to say first words?

Begin to say first phrases, for example, "milk all gone."

Does he/she have any articulation or language problems? (May need to explain these terms.)

Academic Information

How is he/she progressing in school? (Be sure to know if child is in school before asking this question.)

Which subjects does he/she like the best?

How does he/she do in the subjects?

Which subjects does he/she like the least?

How does he/she do in these subjects?

Social Behavioral

What are his/her interests or hobbies?

Who are his/her playmates? Ages? Younger or older?

(At this time you may present selected items of the Vineland Social Maturity Scale or else intersperse them during the interview.)

Is there anything (other than speaking) that particularly concerns you about your child?

How would you best describe your child (e.g., shy, sensitive, extroverted, easy-going, etc.)?

History/Description of Problem: Part 1

Describe what you see to be your child's speaking problems(s) at this time.

When did this start?

Who noticed the problem first? Under what circumstances?

Were you worried or concerned about it at the beginning?

What was your reaction at that time?

Did you being this "problem" to his/her attention?

What did you call it?

When did *you* begin to use the word "stuttering"? If not you, *who* did, if anyone?

Did you or do you ever notice the same behavior in your other children at any time?

Children or relatives, neighbors, or others?

Speech/Language Abilities

Did your child have any trouble saying words? Sounds? Syllables? Letters? (Or, does he/she have any speech articulation problems?)

Can you *describe* (and/or show me by demonstration) your child's speech (stuttering) behavior when you first noticed the problem?

Is it the same now?

Has it changed? That is, is the duration, type, frequency cyclically changing or stabilized? (It may be necessary to provide examples, for example, sound repetitions, sound prolongations, word, part-word or phrase repetition. Clinician should know how (and be prepared) to produce these various disfluency types.

History/Description of Problem: Part 2

Any body movements? Before? Now? Other concomitant behaviors?

Eye contact? Has this changed since beginning of problem?

Facial grimaces?

What aspect of the problem concerns you the most?

What was/is different that he had/has never done before?

Since the "onset" of this speech problem has your child done this every time he/she has spoken? Is he/she ever fluent?

Anxiety Situational Hierarchy

a) In certain situations?

b) On any particular words? Sounds? Letters?

c) With certain listeners? For example, authority figures

d) Strangers, friends, mother, father, and so forth.

Does he avoid any situation to avoid speaking?

Why do you think the problem developed?

Do you think it will change?

How?

If it were to change, do you think there would be any other changes in various aspects of his/her behavior? Would the child be different, for example, in his interactions if he/she didn't stutter?

What have you been told previously about your child's "stuttering"? Other problems? (Advice from relatives, teachers, friends, doctor, speech pathologist, etc.)

Has your child had any speech therapy? Other counseling? Has anyone else in your family had any kind of counseling, for example, psychological? Academic?

History/Description of Problem: Part 3

What have you done to help your child stop stuttering?

Does/did it help?

Who recommended this procedure to help your child?

Why do you do this?

Do you think that your child reacts to his speech behavior? Does he/she get embarrassed or show concern?

Is he/she aware? How do you know?

How does he/she react to your recommendations, promptings, "help"?

Does he/she try to improve his/her speech?

Results?

How do you react to your child's stuttering? (For instance, looking away, speaking for him, interrupting, punishing?)

How do children, relatives, friends, strangers, and others react to/comment about his or her speech?

Is someone more critical or his or her speech?

How do you react when your child is speaking in front of others?

Do other children ever comment on or tease your child about his or her speaking? How does he or she react to this teasing? How do you react? Does this teasing hurt you?

Family Interaction

What kinds of things do you do as a family? What things does your child enjoy the most? The least?

Do you talk with your child very much? (read, play, etc.?) Your spouse? (This is a important question—dwell on it if there is any hint of inadequate communication.)

How does the child get along with sister(s) and brother(s)? Any hostilities or jealousies or rivalries?

How do you (or spouse) handle these?

Social/Behavioral

Does your child play well by him- or herself?

Does he/she have many friends? Do they visit him/her at home? Does he/she visit them?

Does the child require much attention? More than normal? Needs more from mother or father?

Does your child seem more active than children his or her age? Give an example.

How does he or she adjust to a new environment, situation? Sensitive to changes in environment? Routine? Discipline?

How does the child react to discipline? How do you, in general, discipline? (Stress need for information and that you are not going to discipline them for their discipline procedures.)

Does he or she do what you ask? Complete chores, and so forth?

Does he or she do anything that particularly annoys you or anyone else?

Why does it annoy you? How have you attempted to resolve this problem?

Wrap Up

If you could wish for three things for your child (the sky is the limit), what would you wish for?

Note to a Beginning Speech–Language Pathologist

Clinicians as People

Before we became speech and language clinicians, we were people, and we will be people after we stop being clinicians. We need to know as much about ourselves as people as we do about communicative disorders if we really want to become effective clinicians. This is not a plea for encounter sessions, T-groups, psychoanalysis, or the like (even though some of us, from time to time, may need and seek such experiences). Rather, it is a plea for the need to consider ourselves as people, people with frailties, people with strengths, people who are constantly learning how to facilitate learning in other people and hopefully, ourselves.

Many of the problems that parents bring to us are problems we still wrestle with within ourselves. Many of our young clients' concerns are ones we had as children ourselves or ones we have with our own youngsters. We should not feel helpless knowing these things. Instead, we may feel some relief that our clients share in the same human condition that we are experiencing.

Starting from a base where we recognize our humanness and all that it entails, we have a lot less farther to fall when we come up against the difficulties of changing certain aspects of the human condition. Let us then consider some aspects about ourselves that will be factors in our dealings with clients with communicative disorders.

A Clinician's Need to Be Self-Analytical

Somewhere between total oblivion to our mistakes and complete paralysis if a mistake is made is the area that clinicians should strive for. Happy-go-lucky clinicians who bumble through diagnosis and management are constantly amazed that their performances are not always the best. Conversely, clinicians who are paralyzed with fear that they will make a mistake are constantly amazed that they ever do anything right.

The ability to be appropriately self-analytical is a skill that is not easily acquired, but it is a skill well worth the acquisition. Clinicians who are continually growing, in the professional sense, are the clinicians who are capable of turning the errors they produce back into the system. Many clinicians resist the development of self-appraisal skills for a variety of reasons, not the least of which is the real threat to self that such personal scrutiny represents. Such clinicians are often confused between their *self* (personality) and their *behavior*. These clinicians can advise Mrs. Jones to tell Tommy, "I do not like having orange peels thrown on the rug," instead of the usual, "Tommy, why are you such a bad boy?" However, these same clinicians do not seem able to apply this logic to their own self-analysis.

Knowing when you are going in the right or wrong direction is fundamental to your continued improvement as a clinician. Surely, other professionals and personnel will tell you how you are doing and if they like or dislike your work, but if you are *totally* dependent upon them for your feedback and monitoring of performance, it is going to be a long, long time before you start to see substantial improvement in your performance. You really have to work at developing an objective appraisal system for your own performance. It will not come overnight. You will have to develop sensitivity for other people's unspoken feelings, ideas, and so forth, and change your performance accordingly. You will have to be a better reader of clinical situations and adapt yourself appropriately.

Obviously, self-analysis will, from time to time, indicate to you that you are in error. Knowing you are in error will require you to modify your performance. Your ability to modify and entertain the notion that you are in error will take maturity and compromise on your part. The temptation to negate your errors and assign the blame to your client, the parents, your supervisor, your professors, the system, and so forth, will be great. However, such passing of the buck will not allow you to fully develop to the greatest extent possible. You will have to shoulder the responsibility for your errors and performance and attempt to modify them appropriately.

The monitoring of your clinical performance requires diligence but not necessarily paranoid caution. You can be relatively flexible in clinical situations as long as you realize that you are capable of changing your inappropriate clinical procedures. Your ability to monitor and change is as much an assumption for you as for your client: If you cannot monitor and modify your own behavior, how do you expect your client to do so?

A Personality "Suitable" for Becoming a Clinician

Interpersonal relations are obviously of importance to the speech–language pathologist. The personality of the clinician does enter into the clinical equation that equals effective diagnosis and management. But what personalities are best? What are the necessary interpersonal relations that go into effective clinical operations? To begin, we must distinguish between the personality we *are* and the personality we *become* in the clinical setting. It has been said somewhere that we wear many masks for the different people we interact with. That is, we modify, to some degree, our interpersonal relations depending upon the person(s) we deal with. Consequently, different people may get different ideas or perceptions about our personalities.

We must realize that our *basic personality* may not be the reason we have clinical difficulties; however, our ability to play a role (personality) appropriate for the therapy setting may be less than adequate. We may not be putting on a wardrobe suitable to wear into the therapy room. And I am not talking about jeans versus a skirt or a T-shirt versus a shirt and tie. I am talking about the type of person you come across to your client as being while you are interacting with him or her in the clinical environment.

Now, it is also obvious that the larger the discrepancy between your *everyday* or *basic personality* and your *clinical personality*, the more uncomfortable your clinical duties will become. However, who ever said that you should feel comfortable all the time? Aren't you entitled to your moments of unease and uncertainty? We said that certain clinical roles will facilitate therapeutic endeavors, but we did not say it would always be easy or comfortable for you to enact those roles.

Your clinical personality should be as nonjudgmental as possible. You must become as sensitive a listener as possible, as objectively critical and at the same time appropriately reinforcing as you can be. You must convey belief that the person can and will change. You must convey an interest in the person as a person, and not just as a person who stutters or as a set of interesting behaviors. Rogers' clinical tenet of *unconditional positive regard* is a good facet to add to your clinical personality. You must be able to open yourself up to a client's questions, about who and what you are, but at the same time realize when you need to take charge and shift the focus of the therapy interaction. Above all, your personality must convey to the client a sincere interest in his or her welfare, without becoming emotionally involved to the point where your objectivity vanishes and your ability to assist the person diminishes.

Do you have to be outgoing to be a good clinician, or can you be the shy, retiring type and still be effective? This question is inappropriate. Let us see what you do in the clinical setting. If you are continually cracking jokes to maintain attention, running off at the mouth, and being in general a hail-fellow-well-met, but giving clients no indication that you care about them or their problems, your clinical personality is inappropriate. Clients are apt to say of such clinicians, "Well, he's a nice person, but I don't think he understands me and my problem." On the other hand, if you religiously run through your clinical exercises, give minimal exposure to your personal frailties, and are basically standoffish, then you have problems. Of these clinicians clients usually say," They seem to know about my problems, but they really don't care about me, the person." In essence, your clinical personality, whatever its form (and this form may have to be changed depending upon the client or clinical setting), must convey and reflect some of the following:

1. Interest in the client as a person
2. Knowledge about the problem(s) at hand
3. Ability to assist the client in making change and belief that such change is possible
4. Objective assessment of behaviors, situations, and personal variables and minimal judgmental statements
5. Sensitivity towards the client's and your involvement in the human condition first and his or her problem(s) second

The Development of a Clinician: From Classroom to Clinic

We take courses (short and long), sit through endless lectures, participate in seminars, and involve ourselves in independent studies. Our education is long and demanding. And then, one day, we step into the clinic for our first diagnostic or therapy session.

Suddenly, it seems, we are in another realm. We face a different world of real people with real problems who want our help and guidance and comfort. Gone are the books discussing hypothesis A versus hypothesis B. No more do we engage in the fascinating seminar discussions on whether a particular problem is learned or innate. We are on the line with a client, and time must be spent in a professional way. The way we spend this time, however, is the crux of our professional abilities.

Not all information we achieve in our education is readily applicable to the clinical process. This does not mean the information is useless, but sometimes clinicians express this opinion. What they appear to fail to realize is that education develops particular thought processes as well as provides specific course content. Instead of accepting black or white approaches to the world, education tells us that many events are situated along a continuum. Such a relativistic notion does not excuse clinicians from making decisions; however, it should influence the type of decisions they make. Similarly, education instructs that problem solving—which asks answerable questions, tests them, and rejects and/or accepts hypotheses on the basis of findings—is more appropriate than waiting for the answer from the expert(s).

Education expands horizons and our abilities to deal with change; it does not simply fill empty vessels. Surely, you cannot think in a vacuum. No one expects you to deal with communicative disorders without certain basic facts, figures, information, and concepts, but somewhere along the way, it is up to *you* to bridge the gap between classroom and clinic.

We often hear the claim, by clinicians in trouble. "If I'd only had so and so in such and such course then I'd be all right." The truth is, however, that these clinicians are not *applying* even the limited amount of information they do have. They appear to see no relation between what they learned and what they must do in the clinic. They seem to expect the clinical process to take care of itself ("All I need is experience"). Experience, in and of itself, will lead them nowhere if the experience does not involve their active participation. Practice does not make perfect. Perfect practice makes perfect.

Student–clinicians having trouble in the clinic do not seem able to transfer from academic to clinical setting. This lack of transference may result from a number of things: They did not really learn the content of their courses, (classroom excellence is often reflected in clinical excellence) or they did not really change their thought processes as a result of their education (they are still waiting around to be shown how to do whatever they have to do).

Many times such clinicians seem unable to compartmentalize their personal from their professional lives. Problems at home creep into and interfere with their clinical performance ("I couldn't concentrate on therapy because I'm worried about getting my car fixed").

Problem student–clinicians avoid evaluations by their supervisors and professors with the claim, "I tried to reach you but you weren't in." Interestingly, student–clinicians *without* clinical concerns always seem to find their supervisors and professors in their offices. The less than adequate student–clinician claims, "No one told me I was doing poorly." Perhaps this is so, but often they were told and they did not hear or listen. Short of being told, "We are flunking you out," problem student–clinicians do not seem to understand their supervisors when they say there are concerns or problems with the student's performance. Such students appear to lack the ability to self-analyze and to receive and act upon objective criticism they receive from their supervisors and professors.

A really unfortunate situation arises when student–clinicians who have received negative objective evaluations of their clinical performance begin to rely too much on supervisor–professor input for their clinical endeavors. They seem to be looking to some big person for help, because they have received negative evaluation; they become tremendously unsure of how to proceed. This fosters a vicious cycle where supervisors begin to see clinicians as overly dependent on feedback for clinical performance. Student–clinicians, in turn, come to rely too much on this feedback and do not develop the ability to problem solve and perform independently. Such cycles are difficult to break once started; we need to be aware of their potential for development so that we can head off their very existence.

Looking to others for assistance and suggestions is reasonable and appropriate, but when it becomes routine and habitual, it has the real potential for thwarting personal growth and independence. Self-responsibility for our lives, while never easy, is an absolute must for the development of an independent clinician. We all lapse back into stages of dependence, but hopefully we pick ourselves up off the floor and try to regain self-responsibility for our acts. It is our responsibility to apply course content to clinical endeavor. We must be the person to employ the necessary problem-solving orientation to the clinical situation. An active role is needed on the part of the clinician; passivity will result in little change and growth. Although it may be a comfort to blame external factors for our inabilities, in the long run it is we ourselves who must come to grips with the demands of the clinical interaction and try to rise to the challenge.

Self-analysis, problem solving, dedication to the task at hand, independence of thought and action, creative reactions to new situations, and the ability to transfer information from class to clinic are some of the more important hallmarks of a good student–clinician. Although very few people achieve all these hallmarks to the ideal degree, many people are working to achieve such goals. They are at least aware of the presence of these goals and believe them to be of importance. We can become all the clinician we can become as long as we realize that we are the ones who have to do the becoming.

How Much Training You Have Had

There is great temptation to become defensive when a patient or client asks you how much training you have had. There are times when we do not like people poking around into our professional credentials. How we handle such questions, however, reflects as much on our training as it does on our maturity, experience, and so forth.

First, if at all possible, find out why you are being questioned. Maybe you say to the person, "I understand your interest, but why do you ask?" In any case, try to find out why you are being questioned about your credentials. Sometimes clients are shopping around for the best (in their opinion) clinician, and other times they are simply testing you. It is important to distinguish between the two motivations.

Second, look to yourself. What signals are you giving that elicit such a question? Is it your apparent uncertainty, or is it your lack of ease with a client, or what? Remember to keep in mind the difference between your uncertainty as a clinician–person and your uncertainty regarding the handling of a particularly unique, difficult, or unclear case. If you are young (especially your physical appearance and manner of expression), you can just expect more queries about your credentials or experiences. There is no need to become defensive. Remember, experience comes from going through the experiences you are going through.

Finally, have your past successes (or lack thereof) with a particular age client, parent, or communicative disorder finally caught up with you? Perhaps, if time or money permit, a course in the area of concern (no matter if you have had a course with the same title or not) may be a wise investment. We are never, thank goodness, too old to learn or relearn. If nothing else, start picking up books and journals and read.

"My Child's Been with You for Three Months and I Don't See Any Change"

Lack of progress, or no apparent new behavior, is often the beginning of the end of a therapy program. Parents who do not see any progress become less likely to chauffeur little Johnny in for his twice-a-week therapy. Johnny, likewise, is apt to become frustrated, less willing to work, and less motivated if he detects lack of progress, and the clinician, poor person, becomes depressed at the living testimony to his or her ineptness.

Surely, one does not want to whitewash incompetent methods that have resulted in minimal clinical progress. Just as surely, however, one does not want to excuse the reluctant client and his or her parents who will not or cannot cooperate in the therapy process to bring about a change. We must, however, realize when lack of progress is really telling us something about the problems(s) we are dealing with.

First, have we evaluated and diagnosed the situation correctly and completely? Are we ignoring some important variable—for example, a limited attention span—because we believe the client can rise above such trivia and exert enough will power to improve? Therapy, it has been said, is a continual diagnostic experience; however, many times we forget this in the rush to fill the therapy hour with methods to effect the cure.

Second, does lack of progress really indicate that perhaps we are expecting change prior to change being possible? Are we becoming unnecessarily anxious with the slowness of the behavioral change process? Parents, particularly, are susceptible to wanting to speed up the pace of their child's development. Parents give us important clues to this when they tell us that Billy's stuttering "is holding him back and if he can lick this thing he'll be able to do much . . . he has so much potential . . . he's got to change it now before it's too late." They become impatient with our procedures, especially when those procedures do not work on his speech. As mentioned in the text, it is our role to tell parents, from the beginning, approximately how long therapy will take and what steps it will involve. Children must crawl before they walk, and parents must be made to understand this. Not matter how much they love their child and desire for their child's well being, the learning process cannot be sped up. There are no free lunches.

Third, clients may become depressed at the rate of progress because they envisioned you as the guru who was going to lift the stuttering burden off their shoulders without any sweat, pain, work, and travail on their part. It comes as a surprise to them when they learn that behavioral changes require them to work and practice every day at changing their speech. What is wrong, they think; it is not supposed to be this hard. I thought this speech doctor was supposed to cure me. Some doctor!

The client, like the impatient parent, must realize that change takes time, work, and patience. The longest journey begins with a single step. We, as clinicians, must clearly articulate to the clients our goals and subgoals and the time frame within which such goals will be realized. We must set our clients up for the inevitable wall of inertia they will meet when they begin to try to change their old, well-learned, but inappropriate behavior. If we expect more stuttering before less stuttering, we should tell the client and the parents. We might explain that for change to occur, the client must diminish his or her circumlocutions and avoidances and actually stutter. Likewise, we should tell the client and parents what they might look for in terms of signs of early improvement, for example, decreased duration of stuttering.

Even the most seemingly depressing situation like that of a no-progress client is an opportunity for developing our clinical skills and assisting our client. Asking questions about the whys of the no-progress evaluation will provide the opportunity. Looking for answers from the experts and books will provide us some assistance, but we may maximize the potential of the opportunity. Our progress as clinicians, like that of our clients, has a certain price, but fortunately all of us have the potential to pay this price.

APPENDIX C

An Example of a Diagnostic Report for a Child Who Stutters

Vanderbilt Bill Wilkerson Center

Division of Speech/Language Services

Summary of Fluency Evaluation

Client:	Johnny Shoemaker
Birthdate:	5/5/91
Parents:	Mr. and Mrs. Shoemaker
Address:	1030 Heel Lane
	Nashville, TN 44098

Date of Evaluation: 7/6/99
Age at Evaluation: 8;2 (years;months)

SUMMARY STATEMENT

On July 6, 1999, Johnny Shoemaker, accompanied by his mother, was seen at the Vanderbilt Bill Wilkerson Center (VBWC) for a speech and language evaluation due to concerns regarding disfluent speech. Johnny began receiving speech therapy services for stuttering at school when he was in preschool (at approximately 3 years of age). On 1/14/98, Johnny was assessed by Joan Smith, M.S., CCC-SLP, at VBWC. At that time (1/14/98), Johnny produced an average of 12 speech disfluencies per 100 words of conversational speech and received an overall score of 27 on the *Stuttering Severity Instrument-3*, a severity rating of moderate to severe. Johnny received individual speech therapy services (one hour/week) at VBWC for approximately eight months and was discharged on 8/27/98 with recommendations to continue speech therapy with Bonnie Wilson, Speech-Language Pathologist (SLP), at Valley Elementary School, Nashville, TN.

During the present (7/6/99) evaluation, Johnny produced an average of 15.51 speech disfluencies per 100 words of conversational speech (range: 14-17 disfluencies per 100 words), which included the following speech disfluency types (from most to least frequent): audible sound prolongations, whole-word repetitions, sound/syllable repetitions, phrase repetitions, and revisions. Approximately 90% of these 15.51 speech disfluencies were stuttered-like (e.g., sound/syllable repetitions). The average duration of Johnny's speech disfluencies was 0.70 seconds (range: 0.47-0.88 seconds). Johnny's expressive/receptive language skills were average for his chronological age (8;2).

Based on results of this evaluation, it was recommended that Mr. and Mrs. Shoemaker use fluency-enhancing strategies with Johnny (see "Recommendations") and enroll him in an individual speech therapy program with Dr. Edward Conture at VBWC (one-hour/week) beginning in July 1999.

BIRTH HISTORY
Reportedly unremarkable.

MEDICAL HISTORY
Reportedly remarkable for:
1. abnormally large tonsils
2. difficulty feeding as an infant and chewing meat as a young child
3. two instances of strep throat in 1997

DEVELOPMENTAL HISTORY
Johnny reached all developmental milestones (e.g., motor, speech, and language) within expected age limits, according to parental report.

FAMILY HISTORY
Reportedly remarkable for:
1. a maternal cousin who exhibited speech disfluencies as a child

OTHER SIGNIFICANT INFORMATION:
According to Mrs. Shoemaker, Johnny is a charming, easygoing, and interesting child who has been described by his teachers as articulate and hard working. Mrs. Shoemaker reported that, following the discontinuation of speech therapy at VBWC in August 1998, Johnny made good progress in school speech–language therapy with his speech fluency until approximately February 1999, after which his speech became more disfluent (in February 1999, his school SLP, Bonnie Wilson, reportedly left school employment due to a maternity leave). Mrs. Shoemaker reported that she continues to work on using appropriate fluency-enhancing pragmatic skills, such as not trying to interrupt or answer questions for Johnny. Mrs. Shoemaker stated that both she and her husband feel that improving Johnny's speech fluency is a primary concern now, since Johnny will be entering the 3rd grade with children less familiar to him and who may be less tolerant of his disfluent speech.

FINDINGS

Behavior: Johnny was alert, pleasant, and cooperative during this evaluation. However, it was quite apparent that Johnny tended to be highly concerned about making mistakes and/or how many answers he got right during testing.

Hearing: A hearing screening test, which was performed at school (5/21/97), revealed that Johnny's hearing is within normal limits.

Speech Mechanism: Informal observation indicated structure and function adequate for speech production.

Voice and Resonance: Informal observation revealed normal vocal quality and resonance properties.

Language: Administration of three standardized language tests, the *Clinical Evaluation of Language Fundamentals Screening Test- 3rd edition* (CELF-3), *Peabody Picture Vocabulary Test- 3rd edition* (PPVT-III), and the *Expressive Vocabulary Test* (EVT), indicated that Johnny's expressive/receptive language abilities are within normal limits. On the CELF-3, which is a screening test of expressive and receptive language ability, Johnny received a total score of 19, placing him 3 points above criterion. On the EVT (a test of expressive vocabulary), Johnny received a standard score of 102, placing him at the 55th percentile. Results from the PPVT-III, which is a test of receptive vocabulary, revealed that Johnny scored at the 61st percentile, with an age equivalent of 8;9.

Articulation: Speech sound articulation was subjectively perceived to be within normal limits. Speech intelligibility (i.e., the ability to be understood in conversational speech) was judged to be good, even when the context was unknown.

Fluency: A 200-word spontaneous speech sample was obtained during a conversational interaction between Johnny and his mother. Johnny produced an average of 15.51 disfluencies per 100 spoken words (range from 14 to 17 disfluencies). Of these 15.51 disfluencies, 89% were stutter-like disfluencies (e.g., whole-word repetitions and sound prolongations) and 11% were non-stuttered or normal disfluencies (e.g. phrase repetitions, interjections, and revisions). The vast majority (86%) of his stuttered-like disfluencies were sound prolongations and/or blocks. Analysis of disfluency types is as follows:

Stuttering Disfluencies:	Total	% of sample
Sound/syllable repetitions (e.g., "tea,tea,teacher")	2	1.00%
Whole-word repetitions (e.g., "the, the boy")	2	1.00%
Audible sound prolongations (e.g., "dddddog")	24	12.00%
Total: __28__		__14.00%__

Normal Disfluencies:

Phrase repetitions	2	1.00%
(e.g., "the dog went, the dog went home")		
Revisions	1	0.51%
(e.g., "the dog , the cat is big")		
Total:	<u>3</u>	<u>1.51%</u>
Total Disfluencies:	**<u>31</u>**	**<u>15.51%</u>**
(stuttering+normal disfluencies)		

Speech fluency was also evaluated using the *Stoker Probe Technique*, which associates the level of communicative responsibility with the frequency of speech disfluencies. Results revealed a total of 8 disfluent response to 25 questions (32%) asked in reference to common objects. Johnny's speech disfluencies were most common at levels III (e.g., "Where can you buy it?"), IV (e.g., "Tell me all about it"), and V (e.g., "Tell me your own story about it"). This suggests that the frequency of Johnny's disfluencies is somewhat influenced by the type of questions asked of him (e.g., one word response to a question [low communicative responsibility] vs. an open-ended question [high communicative responsibility]).

The *Stuttering Severity Instrument-3* (SSI-3) was administered to determine the severity of Johnny's stuttering behavior. Johnny received an overall score of 15, which is equivalent to a severity score in the "mild" range. The *Sound Prolongation Index* revealed that Johnny produces sound prolongations for 9 out of 10 stuttered words.

A measure of Mrs. Shoemaker's *articulatory rate of speech* revealed a mean rate of 220 words per minute (range: 197 to 262 wpm). Johnny's *articulatory rate of speech* revealed a mean rate of 215 words per minute (range: 174 to 250 wpm). Both Johnny and Mrs. Shoemaker exhibit a very rapid speech rate compared to the "ideal" speech rate of 160–180 wpm.

The rate of Johnny's word/lexical access was assessed using 30 white-on-black line drawing pictures of simple objects (e.g., a boat). The time between picture exposure and Johnny's fluent verbal response was recorded for each picture and averaged across all 30 pictures. On average, Johnny's speech reaction time for picture naming was 965.14 ms (approximately nine-tenths of a second), approximately 300 ms slower than the average normally fluent adult speaker, a factor that may make it difficult for him to quickly access or "call up words," especially when such words are uncommon to him and/or he is trying to speak too rapidly. All of Johnny's single-word responses on this test were perceived to be fluent and correctly articulated.

The *Carey Temperament Scale* (Middle Childhood) (CTS) was completed by Mrs. Shoemaker prior to this evaluation to achieve some general idea regarding Johnny's temperament. Overall, Johnny appears to be a behaviorally expressive child, however, his CTS profile suggests that his temperament is characterized by a slow/gradual ability to modify his reactions to stimuli or changes in the environment.

DIAGNOSIS/IMPRESSIONS

Johnny Shoemaker, an eight-year, two-month-old male, was found to exhibit stuttered-like speech disfluencies in the mild to moderate range of severity. These disfluencies were categorized primarily by audible sound prolongations, but also by combinations of sound/syllable repetitions, whole-word repetitions, phrase repetitions, and revisions. Johnny's speech disfluencies may be related to a combination of various factors: a relatively slower rate of (lexical) word access, an overly rapid speaking rate, a slow/gradual ability to change reaction to environmental stimuli, and/or heightened sensitivity to making mistakes and/or need to be "correct" in all he does.

RECOMMENDATIONS

Based on results of this evaluation and interview, it was recommended that:

1. Johnny be enrolled in an individual speech therapy program with Dr. Edward Conture and Danielle Jones at VBWC (one-hour/week) beginning in July 1999.
2. Mr. and Mrs. Shoemaker continue to use the following fluency enhancing techniques when interacting with Johnny:
    a. a slower rate of speech
    b. model shorter and simpler sentences during time when Johnny is stuttering
    c. minimize answering questions for and/or interrupting when Johnny is talking
    d. pause (1 second) after Johnny's utterances (i.e., avoid "talking over" Johnny's utterances).
    e. avoid asking Johnny a lot of questions, especially during periods of marked speech disfluency.
3. Mr. and Mrs. Shoemaker view the videotape, *Stuttering and Your Child: A Videotape for Parents* [Stuttering Foundation of America (SFA)]. SFA materials may be ordered by calling 1-800-992-9392. The price is $10.00.

DISPOSITION

The above recommendations were explained to Mrs. Shoemaker and she appeared to agree with these recommendations. Please contact us at (615) 936-5100 if there is any other information we can provide.

Danielle Jones, M.A., CCC-SLP
Speech-Language Pathologist

Edward G. Conture, Ph.D., CCC-SLP
Speech Language Pathologist
TN License #2010 Faculty Supervisor

Twelve Minus One Report-Writing Concerns

(1) *The unquoted comment.* A parent says, "Johnny's throat tightens up and he squeezes the sound out when he stutters."

Incorrectly reported: Mrs. Jones remarked that when Johnny stutters he tightens up his throat and squeezes the sound out **OR** when Johnny stutters he tightens up his throat and squeezes the sound out.

Correctly reported: The mother (or Mrs. Brown) reported that when Johnny stutters ". . . he tightens up his throat and squeezes the sound out."

(2) *The conversational or colloquial phrase.* The child is observed to produce facial grimaces during instances of stuttering.

Incorrectly reported: Eye twitching was viewed a lot during stuttering. **OR** Johnny twisted up or screwed up or scrunched up his face quite a bit.

Correctly reported: The examining clinician observed that during Johnny's instances of stuttering he blinked his eyes, contracted the facial muscles on the right side of his face, and looked away from his listener.

Although the warden of Cool Hand Luke might have said, in describing colloquial language usage during report writing, "What we got here is a failure to communicate," you shouldn't use the same level of description. As I've often said to beginning clinicians, "You are not writing an email or letter to a friend, you are trying to clearly document and express to your fellow colleagues your professional observations, opinions, findings, and recommendations." The report you write will be a reflection of your level of clinical knowledge, expertise in expressing that knowledge, and your basic ability to think and organize complex issues.

(3) *Ambiguous reference(s).* A father lists several concerns he has about his son, for example, "Tommy is lazy, selfish, and perfectionistic."

Incorrectly reported: You write, in reference to the father's expressed concerns, "This problem is very troublesome to the parent." **OR** "These are frequent problems or concerns." **OR** "That, and nothing else, was a big concern."

Correctly reported: "The third concern, Tommy's perfectionistic manner, was often mentioned by the father." **OR** "The father's expressed concern regarding Tommy's "selfishness" was supported by a similar comment by Tom's mother. Generally speaking, sentences that begin with *that, those, these, this, them, there*, and the like are going to result, for the purposes of the clinical report, in an ambiguous referent. Remember that vaguely stated remarks generally beget vague responses.

(4)   *Cause and effect relations versus associations, correlations and relations.* A father mentions that middle-ear problems and stuttering co-exist within his child.
Incorrectly reported: Middle-ear problems seem to cause stuttering. **OR** Middle-ear problems probably don't cause stuttering. **OR** (to use another frequently abused situation) Stuttering is caused by inappropriate language or articulation or voice or communication abilities or radioactive carrots. Where is it written that any of the above "cause–effect" relations exist?
Correctly reported: Johnny's middle-ear problems, according to the father, appear to be (not to be) *related* to OR correlated with OR associated with Johnny's stuttering. **OR** The father reported an apparent relation OR association OR correlation between Johnny's expressive language errors and his frequency of stuttering.

(5)   *Chronology mythology.* The parents report a normal pregnancy and delivery followed by the child's normal attainment of developmental milestones. Sometime following these events, the parents reported the onset of "stuttering."
Incorrectly reported: The child began to stutter around three and a half years of age. Pregnancy was normal and developmental milestones were all normal. The parents stated that delivery was normal.
The above inappropriate listed chronology is one of the most very frequently occurring problems seen in student-written reports.
Correctly reported: "The parents reported that Sally's mother's pregnancy and delivery were normal OR without incident OR unremarkable. Sally, in the first two years of her life, exhibited normal development of motor, neurologic, cognitive, and communicative behavior. Subsequently, when Sally was about 3;5 years of age, the parents reported that they noticed that she began to stutter."

My stylistics in the above "correct" example are not as important as the chronology of events. *Start* at the *beginning* and *end* at the *end.* Give the reader a break and assist him or her to follow the chain of events from beginning to end. Provide the reader with a temporal skeleton to hang the myriad of events upon. It is not that there is too little information, but that there is too much information and that the reader needs assistance in knowing what to attend to and when. *The chronology of events is one of the more frequently botched up sections of beginning clinician reports.*

(6)   *Obfuscation through jargonation.* The child reads, three times in succession, a series of seven sentences with each sentence ranging from three to six words in length. (This happens with other areas *not only* adaptation).
Incorrectly reported: The adaptation sentences were read by Johnny OR Adapting to the adaptation sentences was marginally adequate considering the consistency of the loci OR Simple, declarative sentences were adapted OR The adaptation sentences were orally read by Johnny in attempts to examine the adaptation effect.

Correctly reported: Johnny read, three times in succession, a series of seven sentences (each sentence consisting of three to six words in length). "The adaptation sentences," "The Stocker," "The CAI," "The oral periph," and the like are phrases that often appear in beginning clinician reports. These phrases assume that ALL readers know what the "Stocker" refers to and this assumption, I can assure you, is not very valid. Instead of showing the report writer's erudition and sophistication, these phrases confuse the reader and generally reflect negatively on the report writer. Try, whenever possible, to give referents for specialized tests and procedures. I realize it is bulky, but it does communicate.

(7) *The passive phrase.* The client's sister Jane constantly teases the client.
Incorrectly reported: Constantly teased in the situation is Jimmy Brown by his sister Jane. **OR** By pulling on his hair and sticking her tongue out, Jim Brown is constantly teased by Jane Brown.
Correctly reported: The mother reported that her daughter Jane "constantly teases" her son Jim. **OR** Jane Brown, according to the mother, "constantly teases" her brother Jim.

REMEMBER:

Subject, verb; subject, verb; subject, verb. "The boy throws the rock" rather than "The rock is thrown by the boy." "The mother expressed concern about her son's speech" rather than "Concern was expressed regarding the son's speech by the mother." Noun, verb; noun, verb; etc. Simple, declarative sentences. The sentence, for the most part, should not begin or end in a preposition. Student-written reports should consist of active mode sentences.

(8) *The reader is supposed to understand what is in the writer's head. One of writers' most common problems.* For example, a child exhibits severe articulatory distortion of /s/ and /r/, receptive language difficulties and 9 within-word disfluencies per 100 words spoken.
Incorrectly reported: "The child had a great deal of difficulty communicating" OR "The child has a big speech problem." **OR** "The child has noticeable speech problems." How can anyone know what you are referring to in these statements? This problem is the ambiguous reference problem in the extreme.
Correctly reported: "The child's communicative difficulties are witnessed by her articulatory distortion of /s/ and /r/, her receptive language deficits, and her frequent (9 per 100 words spoken) within-word disfluencies."

Don't expect the reader to know what is in your head unless you put it down on paper. Don't assume, write it out. I believe that you can't learn how much is enough until you've done more than enough—at least in terms of report writing. Remember that as you write, you are silently talking to yourself, as it were, and that you sometimes think what you silently said to yourself was what you wrote out on paper. Check the paper and see whether you did indeed write out your silent thoughts.

(9)   *Lack of attention to detail.* Missing pagination, tables, and figures that are referenced in the prose but are not attached to the manuscript, incorrectly spelling words like "course," "these," and so forth. Along with this problem is the report that is so messily written or typed that it takes a magnifying glass and two tons of patience to read. Why should a reader pay attention to a report that is sloppily written, consisting of frequent spelling errors, missing tables and figures, lines that are left out or missing words and the like? Why should a reader pay any attention to detail in your report when it is obvious, from the form of your report, that you don't pay any attention to its detail? A bit of compulsiveness and pride in workmanship as well as sweat is what is needed. Try incorrectly reporting some father's or mother's age and see what sort of reaction you'll get!

(10)   *Poor proofreading.* What can I say to get people to improve this skill? Clearly, (9) above is directly related to this problem. My critique is an attempt to get you to be more analytical and careful in your writing out. In effect, I'm trying to get you to critique your report before you hand it out for dissemination. You will learn, hopefully, to achieve a balance between lackadaisical report writing and the report-writing paralysis whereby you are afraid to commit anything to prose for fear that someone may critique it. Proofreading is particularly difficult when you've spent hours and hours on a piece of work; however, if you don't do it, who will? Surely, not your employer or colleagues; all they will do is comment on your shoddy work. Learn to proofread now, while there are some people around who can help you develop this skill.

(11)   *Yes, Virginia, report writing is hard work.* Into every life some rain must fall, and the arduousness of report writing will be part of your personal cloudburst. I believe that report writing can be successfully developed and honed; however, I never said it would be easy. It will get easier if you keep with it, but a crunch will come somewhere along the way whereby you feel you just can't do it, aren't smart enough, don't really want to become a clinician after all, and the like. All I can say is that many others have come before you and have prevailed and many others will come after you and likewise prevail. Why should be you different? Each skill we achieve requires that we pay a certain price, and for some the cost may be too dear. Don't assume that just because you can talk you should be able to write. The two relate, but are nowhere near a 1-to-1 relationship. One thing I'm sure of, however, is that this diagnostic experience will provide you with the beginnings of a foundation upon which to build the skill of writing your clinical observations of communicative disorders/processes and related matters.

APPENDIX E

Ten Common Mistakes Observed During a Diagnostic

(1) *Little or no reinforcement/feedback.* A child has been literally sweating his way through 5 to 10 diadochokinetic tasks. He looks tired and frustrated; however, he keeps on performing.

Incorrectly Handled: The clinician dutifully records the elapsed time and number of syllables produced. The clinician is very intent on correct test administration; other than test instructions, she provides little encouragement, praise, smiles, words of kindness, and so forth. Her "robotic" performance, however, is not taken as positive reinforcement.

Correctly Handled: Interspersed with appropriate test administration, instructions and recording keeping, the clinician recognizes that a **PERSON** is taking the test and so she praises, smiles, encourages and the like. She is heard to say such things as "You are doing fine (or a good job or good work)" **OR** "Not much longer now, you're doing fine." She doesn't sacrifice accurate test administration for human support for the oftentimes scared and frightened client. She provides *words of encouragement* ("OK, fine; you're doing all right"), *indexes of progress* ("Fine, we are about halfway") and of *how much further to go* ("We're almost done"). She is ready to give understandable explanation for client's question about test or test material ("Oh, this thing? This is a fancy stopwatch that I use to time or record these events or exercises or tasks").

Beginning clinicians frequently forget that they are testing people. Their lack of confidence in their ability to administer a test OR all tests OR their clinical skills OR themselves OR some combination of these factors makes them concentrate on the test to the exclusion of the person taking the test.

(2) *Inability to quickly/accurately score test(s).* A child with a suspected reading problem has just taken a complete *Woodcock Reading Mastery Test.* The mother and father have expressed concern that maybe the child should be referred to a reading clinic.

Incorrectly Handled: The test is still unscored 0.5 hours after complete administration. The clinician gives, as an excuse, the statement, "I'm sorry I can't score the test because this is the first time I've given it. Maybe next time, OK?" The child leaves the clinic without the information necessary to make the best possible recommendation regarding referral to a reading clinic.

Correctly Handled: The clinician has given and scored the Woodcock to at least two other people **BEFORE** the day of the diagnostic. (S)he is familiar with the scoring charts and tables and has a general idea how to fill out the test results forms **BEFORE** the evaluation. The parents receive the information **BEFORE** they leave the clinic. Once again, there is no substitute for previous experience with test scoring. You may think you can fake it, but you can't. Your lack of familiarity with the test will be apparent. Nothing can take the place of prior experience with the test(s). Walking in cold and giving a client a test without ever having practiced the test before is a major reason for beginning clinician failure in diagnostics.

(3) *Time wastage, or we've got all the time in the world.* A clinician is interviewing parents regarding their child's development of a recent three- to four-month period.
Incorrectly Handled: The father says, "We took a vacation to Yellowstone and you should have seen the bears." The clinician replies, "Well, how did your son like the bears?" The father says "fine" and the clinician says "Did he see the geysers?" The father says, "Yes." And the clinician says "Did he like them?" The father says "Oh yes and then we went fishing." And the clinician says . . .
Correctly Handled: The father says, "We took a vacation to Yellowstone and you should have seen the bears." The clinician says, "Yes, I imagine those bears and Yellowstone are really something to see. Sounds like real fun; tell me, after you got back from your vacation, how was your son's speech?"
When time is limited, conversation should be as germane as possible to the purpose of the diagnostic. While you don't want to ignore human concerns and interests, not everything that happens to family is of relevance to or needs to be covered in the diagnostic. Excessively long and frequent tangents waste time and, even more important, they can tire as well as confuse both client and clinician. They also give the client the impression he or she is providing information when in fact the information that transpires is many time of little consequence. Recognize these invitations for small talk and avoidance of salient issues for what they are and don't get yourself continually off track. You *don't* have all the time in the world. In the end you'll have to draw conclusions, and these conclusions will have to be based on substance, not one or two anecdotes or a series of non-germane topics of conversation.

(4) *Your son just hijacked a 707? That's nice, now tell me about when he first began to walk.* A mother has just been telling you, with a great deal of emotion in her voice and manner, that she's afraid that her leaving her son in a daycare center somehow caused him to stutter.
Incorrectly Handled: The clinician says, "There is no evidence that daycare centers cause stuttering." **OR** "That's interesting; now what about toilet training?" **OR** "We're going to have to move along now Ms. Smith."
Correctly Handled: The clinician senses the mother's concern and says, "That must make you feel pretty sad (or unhappy or upset or bad); however, I know that you love your child and want to do the best for him/her. Although I understand your concern about the daycare center—I can see how bothered you are by it—I don't think you need to be too overly concerned or worried. It is likely that the daycare experience had no significant relation to your child's stuttering; in fact, playing with his peers/friends on a daily basis is a good foundation/experience for kindergarten."

(5) *Destandardize, standardize what's the difference? Why be so compulsive about test-ing? Who has time for such picky detail?* A clinician is employing the *MacDonald Deep Test* for the screening of a client's speech articulation.
Incorrectly Handled: The clinician lets the client say the two words or syllables as separate entities. Or the clinician says each test item just *before* the client says the test item. Whatever the case, this problem reflects the clinician's lack of preparation, familiarity with the test, and general ineptness.
Correctly Handled: The clinician administers and scores and reports the *Deep Test* according to the test manual instructions/common clinical practice.

(6) *Fluency? Well, no, I can't tell you much about his fluency, but I can tell you his score on the Quick, Tempin-Darley, or Vineland Test or the color of his eyes!* The begin-ning clinician has tested and been observing the child; the clinician's colleague or supervisor then asks the student clinician for an evaluation of fluency.
Incorrectly Handled: Well, he sure does (or does not) stutter. He really gets stuck a lot doesn't he? Did you see his score on the *Vineland* (or *Quick* or *Templin-Darley* or *Woodcock* or *Peabody* or whatever)? Really depressed, isn't he!
Correctly Handled: He stutters about 3 to 4 words per every 10 words. Most of these stutterings tend to be part-word repetitions; yes, I think part-word repetitions pre-dominate. I've stopwatched about 20 stutterings and they average about 1 second in duration with a range of 0.50 to 4.5 seconds. I think a lot of the stutterings are asso-ciated with breathy voice quality; he seems to be consistently stuttering on word-ini-tial stops. And so forth and so on.

(7) *Yes, Mr. Jones, the adaptation scores of his supraglottal stuttering in conjunction with MLU deficits strongly indicate incipient fluency problems beyond a primary state of evolution. Quite impressed, aren't you? You should hear me order from a restaurant's wine list.* The father asks what the problem is concerning his son's speech and language behavior.
Incorrectly Handled: His locatives are deleted from most of his embedded phrases and when they appear they are disfluently produced with excessive glottal tension.
Correctly Handled: Your son sometimes stutters (repeats and prolongs sounds and syllables). He doesn't stutter too often and the length of each of his stutterings is not too long, but we will want to keep in touch. No need for panic, but here are a few things that might help. . . .

(8) *See how nervous or neurotic or how little self-confidence he has or how shy he is or how confused he is or how any other relatively negative layperson description he is? It's obvious that my glittering generality explains the cause of the stuttering.* During the course of the evaluation, the client's hands are splotched, visibly shaking, he clears his throat a lot, and frequently licks his lips.
Incorrectly Handled: Mr. Jones, why are you so nervous? (You're making me ner-vous and I can't test you when I'm nervous.) **OR** It's so obvious: Nervous people stutter. **OR** If he could only learn to relax he'd stop stuttering.

Correctly Handled: Mr. Jones may have a lot to test anxiety—concern over being evaluated. I wonder what we can say and do to alleviate some of this anxiety. Perhaps there is a relation here between the stuttering and obvious anxiety/emotional concerns, but other aspects also need exploration.

(9) *He began to stutter, the parents say, when he witnessed his Ken doll divorcing his Barbie doll. It's obvious that such trauma generally causes stuttering.* The mother reports that Johnny was in a car accident and that shortly thereafter he began to stutter.
Incorrectly Handled: Have you seen a psychiatrist about this? **OR** Well, accidents do happen and they are known to cause stuttering; I suggest you keep him out of cars and away from streets for a while. **OR** We see a *lot* of these type of cases/problems.
Correctly Handled: Ms. Smith, we sometimes hear from people who stutter or their parents that such and such an event was associated with the beginnings of the stuttering. Our experiences, and that of others, just don't indicate that these events generally cause stuttering. Heck, so many people experience these same events that if they caused stuttering then a great deal more people would be stuttering. No, I think what happens is that people look for situations and events to explain things they don't understand and if that thing is a problem then it is natural for a person to look for explanations in other associated problems (for example, car accidents, personal injuries and so forth). It's just natural to pin the blame for one problem on another problem outside of our control. I said natural, but not necessarily correct, since in the vast majority of cases, the onset of stuttering is associated with no known trauma.

(10) *While I'm busy administering these tests or asking these questions, don't you dare have any human concerns or needs!* The clinician is administering the *Stocker Probe* to an 18-year-old who is obviously becoming concerned and anxious over the test in terms of its apparent appropriateness and purpose.
Incorrectly Handled: Just a few more items now and we'll be all done and then we can have some fruit juicy. Now, won't that be nice? **OR** Don't worry about it, just keep on going. **OR** Come on now, big boys don't cry!
Correctly Handled: I know you must feel a little silly and perhaps embarrassed answering some of these questions, but I'd like to have your responses to them because they will help me help you. **OR** Some of these objects might appear a little young or silly for someone your age, but I'm just interested in your speech/language (communication) when you talk about them. I'm not interested in your intelligence or some deep, dark psychological problem; I'd just like to hear/listen/study/examine your communication (speech/language) during these structured speaking tasks. I know some of it may appear silly—it is sorta—but I'd just like you to try your best and give me a verbal response to each of the questions. Thanks a lot for your help.

NOTE: The "correctly handled" responses for numbers 9 and 10 are rather expansive because I wanted to give you a variety of ways of dealing with these common clinical situations.

A P P E N D I X   F

Children Who Stutter: Suggestions for the Classroom Teacher

From time to time, classroom teachers will have children who stutter in their class. What follows is information as well as suggestions that should better help teachers understand and deal with these children.

(1) *Children who stutter should be treated similarly to their peers.* Teachers should try to deal with children who stutter as they would any other "normally" developing child. While all children have special needs, "special" classroom activities do not need to be created to deal *routinely* with children who stutter. Neither should these children be *routinely excluded* from specific classroom activities. Treat the child who stutters, *as much as possible*, like the other children in the classroom.

(2) *Some kinda help is the kinda help these kids can do without.* Teachers should make every attempt to cease and desist in any and all direct corrections of the young stutterer's pronunciation of speech sounds, expressive language usage, or speech disfluencies (that is, stutterings) *while* the child is routinely conversing with the teacher or other children. These corrections seem to make intuitive sense—they are frequently used by parents and other listeners—but if they really helped, there would be little reason for therapy with stutterers. Of course, a teacher should feel free to help young stutterers who misspell a word while writing, mispronounce a word while reading aloud during reading class or who, during a grammar lesson, use incorrect syntax. These corrections are the type that the teacher uses with *all* children in class. However, teachers should try to avoid any and all corrections that, although well intended, call undue or inappropriate attention to the child's speech and language problem. Sometimes these corrections can wind up becoming part of the problem rather than part of the solution.

(3) *Accentuate the positive, eliminate the negative.* As much as possible, on days when the child who stutters seems particularly fluent (that is, doesn't stutter), the teacher should try to draw the child out and encourage him or her to talk and read. Conversely, on days when he or she is particularly disfluent (that is, stuttering a lot), the teacher should call less frequently on the child to talk, recite, or read aloud in class. Encouraging the child to talk is best done on good (fairly fluent) days, while encouraging quiet or nontalking activities is best done on bad (frequently stuttering) days.

(4) *Once children begin to speak, they should be allowed to finish.* Teachers should try—just as they do when normally fluent children speak—to let the child who stutters complete or finish his or her words, phrases, or sentences. Interrupting and filling in words for the child, correcting the child's vocabulary or grammar usage, telling him or her to "repeat it like this," and so forth *while* the child is talking may seem as if it helps, but it does not. These interruptions convey a *less than positive* message to the child about both his or her speaking abilities as well as the teacher's evaluation of them. Teachers and other adult listeners can't expect the peers of the child who stutters to listen and not interrupt if they, as adults, model and continue to do the opposite.

(5) *Use as much group speaking, singing, or reading as possible.* Where and whenever possible, teachers should try to incorporate choral or group reading aloud, speaking, or singing in the classroom. These should not be special activities, but appropriate for and consistent with classroom activities and objectives. These acts maximize the chances of the child who stutters for producing speech just like that produced by his or her normally fluent peers and should contribute to positive feelings about self and speaking abilities.

(6) *If you can't master the subject, master the other kids.* Some children tease or mock other children for a variety of reasons; for example, (a) they themselves are having trouble mastering subject material, so they try to "master" other children by ridiculing and/or putting them down; (b) they may feel that any attention is better than no attention at all and, to them, other people's negative reactions to their teasing are worth it if they get increased attention; and (c) they are uncomfortable with differences and really don't understand that their mocking, teasing, or ridiculing hurts the other child. Whatever the case, if the situation arises where another member of the class *frequently* or *routinely* teases the child who stutters about his or her speech or related matters, the teacher should intervene.

First, when the child who stutters is out of the room, the teacher should give a short lecture to the class discussing how different people develop in different ways when learning different skills—for example, riding a bike, throwing a ball, learning to talk, read, write, and the like. This talk may need to be given a few times, each time while the young child is out of the room, and the teacher should observe the lectures' influence on the child(ren) doing the teasing. Second, if, after such lectures, the teasing continues, the teacher should take aside the child doing the teasing and have an "information-sharing" conversation with the child. This conversation should describe the various ways in which children differ in their development and how teasing and ridicule do not help children who are different; it just makes them feel bad. The teacher should try to deliver this message in a firm but polite manner and minimize the teasing child's sense that he or she is being punished. This conversation may have to take place more than once. Any improvement in the ways in which the child who teases interacts with the child who stutters should be subtly but clearly reinforced by the teacher.

REFERENCES

Abwender, D., Trinidad, K., Jones, K., Como, P., Hymes, E., & Kurlan, R. (1998). Features resembling Tourette's syndrome in developmental stutterers. *Brain and Language, 62,* 455–464.

Ackermann, H., Hertrich, I., Ziegler, W., Bitzer, M., & Bien, S. (1996). Acquired dysfluencies following infarction of the left mesiofrontal cortex. *Aphasiology, 10,* 409–417.

Adams, L. H. (1955). A comparison of certain sound wave characteristics of stutterers and nonstutterers. In W. Johnson & R. Leutennegger (Eds.), *Stuttering: In children and adults* (pp. 398–401). Minneapolis, MN: University of Minnesota Press.

Adams, M. R. (1977). A clinical strategy for differentiating the normally nonfluent child and the incipient stutterer. *Journal of Fluency Disorders, 2,* 141–148.

Adams, M. (1980). The young stutterer: Diagnosis, treatment and assessment of progress, *Seminars in Speech Language and Hearing, 1,* 289–299.

Adams, M. (1987). Voice onsets and segment durations of normal speakers and beginning stutterers, *Journal of Fluency Disorders, 12,* 1333–1400.

Adams, M. (1990). The demands and capacities model I: Theoretical elaboration. *Journal of Fluency Disorders, 15,* 135–141.

Adams, M. (1991). The assessment and treatment of the school-age stutterer. *Seminars in Speech and Language, 12,* 279–290.

Adams, M. (1992). Childhood stuttering under "positive" conditions. *American Journal of Speech-Language Pathology, 1,* 5–6.

Adams, M. (1993). The home environment of children who stutter. *Seminars in Speech and Language, 14,* 185–191.

Adams, M., Freeman, F., & Conture, E. (1984). Laryngeal dynamics of stutterers. in R. Curlee & W. Perkins (Eds.), *Nature and treatment of stuttering: New directions* (pp. 89–129). San Diego, CA: College-Hill Press.

Adams, M., Guitar, B., & Conture, E. (1979). A review of biofeedback procedures for school-age stutterers. *Journal of Childhood Communication Disorders, 3,* 8–12.

Agnello, J., & Wingate, M. (1975). Voice onset and voice termination features of stuttering. In L. M. Webster & L. C. Furst (Eds.), *Vocal tract dynamics and stuttering.* New York: Speech and Hearing Institute.

Ainsworth, S., & Fraser, J. (Ed.). (1988). *If your child stutters: A guide for parents* (3rd ed.). Memphis, TN: Speech Foundation of America.

Ambrose, N., & Yairi, E. (1995). The role of repetition units in the differential diagnosis of early childhood incipient stuttering. *American Journal of Speech and Language Pathology, 4,* 82–88.

Ambrose, N. G., & Yairi, E. (1999). Normative disfluency data for early childhood stuttering. *Journal of Speech, Language, and Hearing Research, 42,* 895–909.

Ambrose, N., Yairi, E., & Cox, N. (1993). Genetic aspects of early childhood stuttering. *Journal of Speech and Hearing Research, 36.*

Ambrose, N., Yairi, E., & Cox, N. (1997). The genetic basis of persistence and recovery in stuttering. *Journal of Fluency Disorders, 40,* 567–580.

Amster, B. (1995). Perfectionism and stuttering. In C. Starkweather & H. Peters (Eds.), *Stuttering: Proceedings of 1st World Congress on Fluency Disorders* (pp. 540–543, Vol. II). Nijmegen, The Netherlands: University Press Nijmegen.

Anderson, J., & Conture, E. (2000). *Language abilities of children who stutter.* Manuscript submitted for publication.

Andrews, G., & Craig, A. (1988). Prediction of outcome after treatment for stuttering, *British Journal of Psychiatry.*

Andrews, G., Craig, A., Feyer, A., Hoddinott, A., Howie, P., & Neilson, M. (1983). Stuttering: A review of research findings and theories circa 1982, *Journal of Speech and Hearing Disorders, 48,* 226–246.

Andrews, G., & Cutler, J. (1974). Stuttering therapy: The relationship between changes in symptom level and attitudes. *Journal of Speech and Hearing Disorders, 39,* (3), 312–319.

Andrews, G., & Ingham, R. (1971). Stuttering: Considerations in the evaluation of treatment. *British Journal of Disorders of Communication, 6,* 427–429.

Andrews, G., Neilson, M. (November, 1981). *Stuttering: A state of the art seminar.* Paper presented to Annual Conference of Speech-Language-Hearing Association, Los Angeles, California.

Armson, J., & Kalinowski, J. (1994). Interpreting results of the fluent speech paradigm in stuttering research: Difficulties in separating cause from effect. *Journal of Speech and Hearing Research, 37,* 69–82.

Atal, B., Chang, J., Matthews, M., & Tukey, J. (1978). Inversions of articulatory-to-acoustic transformation in the vocal tract by computer-sorting technique. *Journal of Acoustical Society of America, 63,* 1535–1555.

Atkins, C. (1988). Perceptions of speakers with minimal eye contact: Implications for stutterers. *Journal of Fluency Disorders, 13,* 429–436.

Au-Yeung, J., & Howell, P. (1998). Lexical and syntactic context and stuttering. *Clinical Linguistics & Phonetics, 12,* 67–78.

Au-Yeung, J., Howell, P., & Pilgrim, L. (1999). Phonological words and stuttering on function words. *Journal of Speech, Language & Hearing, 41,* 1019–1030.

Axline, V. M. (1947). *Play therapy.* Boston: Houghton Mifflin.

Bahill, T., & Curlee, R. (1993). *User's guide to childhood stuttering: A second opinion.* Tucson, AZ: Bahill Intelligent Computer System.

Bailey, A., & Bailey, W. (1982) Managing the environment of the stutterer. *Journal of Childhood Communication Disorders, 6,* 26–39.

Bakker, K. (1999). Technical solutions for quantitative and qualitative assessments of speech fluency. *Seminars in Speech and Language, 20*(2), 185–196.

Barr, H. (1940). A quantitative study of the specific phenomena observed in stuttering, *Journal of Speech Disorders, 5,* 277–280.

Bates, E. (1976). Pragmatics and sociolinguistics in child language. In D. Morehead & A. Morehead (Eds.), *Normal and deficient child language.* Baltimore: University Park Press.

Baumgaertel, A., & Wolraich, M. (1998). Practice guideline for the diagnosis and management of attention deficit hyperactivity disorder. *Ambulatory Child Health, 4,* 45–58.

Baumgartner, J. (1999). Acquired psychogenic stuttering. In R. Curlee (Ed.), *Stuttering and related disorders of fluency* (pp. 269–288). New York: Thieme.

Beattie, G. (1983). *Talk.* Milton Keynes, England: Open University Press.

Beattie, M. (1987). *Codependent no more.* New York: Harper/Hazelton.

Beech, H., & Fransella, F. (1968). *Research and experiment in stuttering.* Oxford England: Pergamon Press.

Beecher, H. K. (1955). The powerful placebo. *Journal American Medical Association, 159,* 1602–1606.

Beitchman, J., Nair, R., Clegg, M., & Patel, P. (1986). Prevalence of speech and language disorders in 5-year-old kindergarten children in the Ottawa-Carleton region. *Journal of Speech and Hearing Disorders, 51,* 98–110.

Benson, H. (1976). *The relaxation response,* New York: Avon Books.

Benson, H., & Epstein, M. D. (1975). The placebo effect: A neglected asset in the care of patients. *Journal American Medical Association, 232,* 1225–1227.

Benson, H., & McCallie, D. (1979). Angina pectoris and the placebo effect. *New England Journal of Medicine, 300,* 1424–1429.

Berg, C., Rapoport, J., & Flament, M. (1986). The Leyton Obsessional Inventory-Child Version. *Journal of the Americas Academcy of Child and Adolescent Psychiatry, 25,* 84–91.

Berg, T. (1986). The aftermath of error occurrence: Psycholinguistic evidence from cut-offs. *Language and Communication, 6,* 195–213.

Bernstein Ratner, N. (1993). Atypical language development. In J. Berko Gleason (Ed.), *The development of language* (3rd ed.; pp. 325–368). Columbus: Merrill.

Bernstein Ratner, N. (1997a). Linguistic behaviors at the onset of stuttering. In W. Hulstjn, H. F. M. Peters, & P. H. H. M. Van Lieshout (Eds.), *Speech production: Motor control, brain research and fluency disorders* (pp. 585–593). Amsterdam: Elsevier Science B.V.

Bernstein Ratner, N. (1997b). Stuttering: A psycholinguistic perspective. In R. Curlee & G. Siegel (Eds.), *Nature and treatment of stuttering: New directions* (2nd ed., pp. 99–127). Boston: Allyn & Bacon.

Bernstein Ratner, N., & Healey, E. (Eds.). (1999). *Stuttering research and practice: Bridging the gap.* Mahwah, NJ: Lawrence Erlbaum Associates.

Bernstein Ratner, N., & Sih, C. (1987). Effects of gradual increases in sentence length and complexity on children's dysfluency. *Journal of Speech and Hearing Disorders, 52,* 278–287.

Bettleheim, B. (November, 1985). Punishment versus discipline: A child can be expected to behave well only if his parents live by the values they teach. *Atlantic, 256,* 51–56.

Bingham, J. (1961). *Courage to change: An introduction to the life and though of Reinhold Niebuhr.* Boston: Little, Brown.

Blackmer, E., & Mitton, J. (1991). Theories of monitoring and the timing of repairs in spontaneous speech. *Cognition, 39,* 173–194.

Blood, G., & Conture, E. (1998). Fluency disorders. In C. Frattali (Ed.), *Outcome measurement in speech-language pathology* (pp. 387–405). New York: Thieme Medical Publishers.

Bloodstein, O. (1960a). The development of stuttering: I. Changes in nine basic features, *Journal of Speech Hearing Disorders, 25,* 219–237.

Bloodstein, O. (1960b). The development of stuttering: II. Developmental phases, *Journal of Speech and Hearing Disorders, 25*, 366–376.

Bloodstein, O. (1961). The development of stuttering: III. Changes in nine basic features. *Journal of Speech and Hearing Disorders, 26*, 67–82.

Bloodstein, O. (1975). Stuttering as tension and fragmentation. In J. Eisenson (Ed.), *Stuttering: A Second Symposium*. New York: Harper & Row.

Bloodstein, O. (1987). *A handbook on stuttering* (4th ed.). Chicago: National Easter Seal Society for Crippled Children and Adults.

Bloodstein, O. (1988). Science in communication disorders: Letter to the editor. *Journal of Speech and Hearing Research, 53*, 347–348.

Bloodstein, O. (1993). *Stuttering: The search for a cause and a cure*. Boston: Allyn & Bacon.

Bloodstein, O. (1995). *A handbook on stuttering* (5th ed.). San Diego, CA: Singular Publishing Group.

Boberg, E. (Ed.). (1993). *Neuropsychology of stuttering* (pp. 39–72). Edmonton, Alberta: The University of Alberta Press.

Bock, J. (1982). Towards a cognitive psychology of syntax: Information processing contributions to sentence formulation. *Psychological Review, 89*, 1–47.

Bock, K., & Levelt, W. J. M. (1994). Language production: Grammatical encoding. In M. A. Gernsbacher (Ed.), *Handbook of psycholinguistics*. Orlando, FL: Academic Press.

Boehmler, R. (1958). Listener responses to non-fluencies. *Journal of Speech and Hearing Research, 1*, 132–141.

Borden, G., Baer, T., & Kenney, M. (1995). Onset of voicing in stuttered fluent utterance. *Journal of Speech and Hearing Research, 28*, 363–372.

Bosshardt, H-G. (1993). Differences between stutterers and nonstutterers' short-term recall and recognition performance. *Journal of Speech and Hearing Research, 36*, 286–293.

Bosshardt, H-G., & Fransen, H. (1996). Online sentence processing in adults who stutter and adults who do not stutter. *Journal of Speech and Hearing Research, 39*, 785–797.

Bosshardt, H-G., & Nandyal, I. (1988). Reading rates of stutterers and nonstutterers during silent and oral reading. *Journal of Speech and Hearing Disorders, 13*, 407–420.

Botterill, W., Kelman, E., & Rustin, L. (1991). Parents and their pre-school stuttering child. In L. Rustin (Ed.), *Parents, families and the stuttering child* (pp. 59–71). San Diego, CA: Singular Publishing Group.

Bouwen, J. (June, 1999). Personal communication. Schoonhoven, The Netherlands.

Brady, J. (1991). The pharmacology of stuttering: A critical review. *American Journal of Psychiatry, 148*, 1309–1316.

Brazelton, T. (1974). *Toddlers & parents*. New York: Dell.

Brazelton, T. (1983). *Infants & parents*. New York: Bantam/Delcorte.

Bredart, S. (1991). Word interruption in self-repairing. *Journal of Psycholinguistic Research, 20*, 123–138.

Brown, R. (1973). *A first language/The early stages*. Cambridge, MA: Harvard University Press.

Brutten, G., & Dunham, S. (1989). The communication attitude test: A normative study of grade-school children. *Journal of Fluency Disorders, 14*, 371–377.

Brutten, G., Bakker, K., Janssen, P., & van der Meulen, S. (1984). Eye movements of stuttering and non-stuttering children during silent reading. *Journal of Speech Hearing Research, 27* (4), 562–566.

Brutten, E., & Shoemaker, D. (1967). *The modification of stuttering*. Englewood Cliffs, NJ: Prentice-Hall.

Burger, R., & Wijnen, F. (1999). Phonological encoding and word stress in stuttering and nonstuttering subjects. *Journal of Fluency Disorders, 24*, 91–106.

Burns, D. (1980). *Feeling good: The new mood therapy*. New York: NAL Penguin.

Butterworth, B. (1992). Disorders of phonological encoding. *Cognition, 42*, 261–286.

Camarata, S., & Gibson, T. (1999). Pragmatic language deficits in attention-deficit hyperactivity disorders (ADHD). *Mental Retardation and Developmental Disabilities Research Reviews, 5*, 207–214.

Canning, B., & Rose, M. (1974). Clinical measurement of the speech, tongue, and lip movements in British children with normal speech. *British Journal of Disorders of Communication, 9*, 45–50.

Canter, G. (1965). Speech characteristics of patients with Parkinson's disease: III. Articulation diadochokinesis, and overall speech adequacy. *Journal of Speech and Hearing Disorders, 30*, 217–224.

Cantwell, D., & Baker, L. (1985). Psychiatric and learning disorders in children with speech language disorders: A descriptive analysis. *Advances in Learning and Behavioral Disabilities, 4*, 29–47.

Carlisle, J. (1985). *Tangled tongue: Living with a stutter*. Toronto: University of Toronto Press.

Caruso, A., Abbs, J., & Gracco, V. (1988). Kinematics analysis of multiple movement during speech in stutterers. *Brain, III*, 439–455.

Caruso, A., & Burton, E. (1987). Temporal acoustic measures of dysarthria with amgotrophic lateral sclerosis. *Journal of Speech and Hearing Research, 30*, 80–87.

Caruso, A., Conture, E., & Colton, R. (1988). Selected temporal parameters of coordination associated with stuttering in children, *Journal of Fluency Disorders, 12,* 57–82.

Caruso, A., Max, L., & McClowry, M. (1999). Perspectives on stuttering as a motor speech disorder. In A. Caruso & E. Strand (Eds.), *Clinical management of motor speech disorders in children* (pp. 319–344). New York: Thieme.

Chang, S., Ohde, R., & Conture, E. (1999). *Coarticulation in preschool children who stutter: A locus equation approach.* Paper presented at Annual Conference of American Speech-Language and Hearing Association, San Francisco, CA.

Childers, D., & Krishnamurthy, A. (1984). A critical review of electroglottography. *CRC Critical Reviews in Biomedical Engineering, 12,* 131–161.

Childers, D., Naik, J., Larar, J., Krishanmurthy, A., & Moore, G. (1983). Electroglottography, speech and ultra-high speed cinematography. In I. Titze & R. Scherer (Eds.), *Vocal fold physiology; Biomechanics, Acoustics and phonatory control* (pp. 202–220). Denver, CO: Denver Center for the Performing Arts.

Churchill, W. (1939). In P. Knowles (Ed.), *The Oxford dictionary of quotations* (5th ed.; p. 216). Oxford, UK: Oxford University Press.

Clark, H., & Wasow, T. (1998). Repeating words in spontaneous speech. *Cognitive Psychology, 27,* 201-242.

Colburn, N., & Mysak, E. (1982). The co-occurrence of disfluency with specified semantic-syntactic structures. *Journal of Speech and Hearing Research, 15,* 421–427.

Colton, R., & Conture, E. (1990). Problems and pitfalls in the use of electroglottography. *Journal of Voice, 4,* 10–24.

Conture, E. (1974). Some effects of noise on the speaking behavior of stutterers. *Journal of Speech and Hearing Research, 17,* 714–723.

Conture, E. (1982). *Stuttering* (1st ed.). Englewood Cliffs, NJ: Prentice-Hall.

Conture, E. (1983). The general problem of change. In J. Fraser-Gruss & H. Gregory (Eds.), *Stuttering therapy: Transfer and maintenance* (pp. 13–28). Memphis, TN: Speech Foundation of America.

Conture, E. (1987b). Studying young stutterers' speech production: A procedural challenge. In H. Peters & W. Hulstijn (Eds.), *Speech motor dynamics in stuttering* (pp. 117–139). Wien/New York: Springer-Verlag.

Conture, E. (1987c). Fluency & beyond: Self-help mutual aid, *Speak Easy Newsletter,* 6–7.

Conture, E. (1990a). Childhood stuttering: What is it and who does it? In J. Cooper (Ed.), *Research needs in stuttering: Roadblocks and future directions* (ASHA Reports 18, pp. 2–14). Rockville, MD: American Speech-Language-Hearing Association.

Conture, E. (1990b). *Stuttering* (2nd ed.). Englewood Cliffs, NJ: Prentice-Hall.

Conture, E. (1991). Young stutterers' speech production: A critical review. In H. Peters, W. Hulstjn, & C. Starkweather (Eds.), *Speech motor control and stuttering* (pp. 365–384). Amsterdam: Elsevier Science Publishers.

Conture, E. (1994). (Producer). *Stuttering and your child: A videotape for parents* (30-min video). Memphis, TN: Stuttering Foundation of America.

Conture, E. (1996). Treatment efficacy: Stuttering. *Journal of Speech and Hearing Research, 39,* S18–S26.

Conture, E. (1997). Evaluating childhood stuttering. In R. Curlee & G. Siegel (Eds.), *Nature and treatment of stuttering: New directions* (2nd ed.; pp. 239–256). Boston: Allyn & Bacon.

Conture, E. (1999a). Bridging the gap between stuttering research and practice: An overview. In N. Bernstein Ratner & E. Healey (Eds.), *Stuttering research and practice: Bridging the gap* (pp. 1–12). Mahwah, NJ: Lawrence Erlbaum Associates.

Conture, E. (1999b). Change, the one constant. *Speak Easy Newsletter, 19,* 1, 8, & 12.

Conture, E., & Caruso, A. (1978). Book review: The Stocker Probe technique for diagnosis and treatment of stuttering in young children (a test developed by Beatrice Stocker). *Journal of Fluency Disorders, 3,* 297–298.

Conture, E., & Caruso, A. (1987). Assessment and diagnosis of childhood disfluency. In L. Rustin & H. Purser (Eds.), *Progress in the treatment of fluency disorders* (pp. 57–82). London: Taylor and Francis.

Conture, E., Colton, R., & Gleason, J. (1988). Selected temporal aspects of coordination during fluent speech of young stutterers. *Journal of Speech and Hearing Research, 31,* 640–653.

Conture, E., Colton, R., & Gleason, J. (1990). Author's reply to DiSimoni's "comment." *Journal of Speech and Hearing Research, 33,* 404–405.

Conture, E., & Fraser, J. (Eds.) (1989). *Stuttering and your child: Questions and answers.* Memphis, TN: Speech Foundation of America.

Conture, E., Fraser, J., Guitar, B., & Williams, D. (Co-producers). (1995). *Stuttering and your child: A videotape for parents* [30-min videotape]. Memphis, TN: Stuttering Foundation of America.

Conture, E., & Guitar, B. (1993). Evaluating efficacy of treatment of stuttering: School-age children. *Journal of Fluency Disorders, 18,* 253–287.

Conture, E., Guitar, B., & Fraser, J. (Co-producers) (1997). *Therapy in action: The school-age child who stutters* [38-min videotape]. Memphis, TN: Stuttering Foundation of America.

Conture, E., & Kelly, E. (1991a). Young stutterer's non-speech behaviors during stuttering. *Journal of Speech and Hearing Research, 34,* (5) 1041–1056.

Conture, E., & Kelly, E. (1991b). Young stutterers' speech production: Some clinical implications. In L. Rustin (Ed.), *Parents, families and the stuttering child.* (pp. 25–39). San Diego, CA: Singular Publishing.

Conture, E., Louko, L., & Edwards, M. L. (1993). Simultaneously treating childhood stuttering and disordered phonology: Experimental therapy, preliminary findings. *American Journal of Speech-Language Pathology, 2,* 72–81.

Conture, E., McCall, G., & Brewer, D. (1977). Laryngeal behavior during stuttering, *Journal of Speech and Hearing Research, 20,* 661–668.

Conture, E., & Melnick, K. (1999). Parent-child group approach to stuttering in preschool and school-age children. In M. Onslow & A. Packman (Eds.), *Early stuttering: A handbook of intervention strategies* (pp. 17–51). San Diego, CA: Singular Press.

Conture, E., Rothenberg, M., & Molitor, R. (1986). Electroglottographic observations of young stutterers' fluency. *Journal of Speech and Hearing Research, 29,* (3) 384–393.

Conture, E., Schwartz, H., & Brewer, D. (1985). A further study of laryngeal behavior during stuttering. *Journal of Speech and Hearing Research, 28,* 233–240.

Conture, E., & van Naerssen, E. (1977). Reading abilities of school-age stutterers, *Journal of Fluency Disorders, 2,* 195–300.

Conture, E., & Wolk, L. (1990). Efficacy of intervention by speech-language pathologists: Stuttering. *Seminars in Speech and Language, 11,* 200–211.

Conture, E., & Yaruss, S. (1993). *Handbook for childhood stuttering: A training manual.* Tucson, AZ: Bahill Intelligent Computer Systems.

Conture, E., & Zebrowski, P. (1992). Can childhood speech disfluencies be mutable to the influencies of speech-language pathologists, but immutable to the influences of parents? *Journal of Fluency Disorders, 17,* 121–130.

Cooper, E. (1979) *Understanding stuttering: Information for parents.* Chicago: National Easter Seal Society for Crippled Children and Adults.

Cooper, E. (February, 1980). Etiology and treatment of stuttering. *Ear, Nose and Throat Journal.*

Cooper, E., & Cooper, C. (1985). *Personalized fluency control therapy.* Allen, TX: DLM.

Cooper, E., & DeNil, L. (1999). Is stuttering a speech disorder? *ASHA, 41,* 10–11.

Cooper, E. B. (1978). Intervention procedures for the young stutterer. In H. Gregory, *Controversies about stuttering therapy.* Baltimore: University Park Press.

Cordes, A. (1998). Current status of the stuttering treatment literature. In A. Cordes & R. Ingham (Eds.), *Treatment efficacy for stuttering: A search for empirical bases* (pp. 117–144). San Diego, CA: Singular Publishing Group.

Cordes, A. (2000). Comments on Yaruss, LaSalle, and Conture (2000). *American Journal of Speech-Language Pathology, 9,* 162–165.

Cordes, A., & Ingham, R. (1995). Stuttering includes both within-word and between-word disfluencies. *Journal of Speech and Hearing Research, 38,* 382–386.

Cordes, A., & Ingham, R. (Ed). (1998). Treatment efficacy for stuttering: A search for empirical bases. San Diego, CA: Singular Publishing Group.

Cordes, A., Ingham, R., Frank, P., & Ingham, J. (1992). Time-interval analysis of interjudge and intrajudge agreement for stuttering event judgments. *Journal of Speech and Hearing Research, 38,* 382–386.

Costello, J., & Ingham, R. (1984). Assessment strategies for stuttering. In R. Curlee and W. Perkins (Eds.), *Nature and treatment of stuttering: New directions* (pp. 303–303). Boston: College-Hill Press.

Costello, J., & Ingham, R. (1999). Behavioral treatment of young children who stutter: An extended length of utterance method. In R. Curlee (Ed.), *Stuttering and related disorders of fluency* (2nd ed.; pp. 80–109). New York: Thieme.

Costello Ingham, J., & Riley, G. (1998) Guidelines for documentation of treatment efficacy for young children who stutter. *Journal of Speech, Language and Hearing Research, 41,* 753–770.

Cox, N. (1988). Molecular genetics: The key to the puzzle of stuttering. *ASHA, 30,* 36–40.

Craig, A., & Andrews, G. (1985). The prediction and prevention of relapse in stuttering. *Behavior Modification, 9,* 427–442.

Craig, A., Franklin, J., & Andrews, G. (1984). A scale to measure loss of controlled behavior. *British Journal of Medical Psychology, 57,* 173–180.

Culatta, R., & Goldberg, S. (1995). *Stuttering therapy: An integrated approach to theory and practice.* Boston: Allyn & Bacon.

Cullinan, W. (1988). Consistency measures revisited. *Journal of Fluency Disorders, 13,* 1–10.

Curlee, R. (1980). A case selection strategy for young disfluent children. *Seminars in Speech, Language and Hearing, 1*(4), 277–287.

Curlee, R. (1981). Observer agreement on stuttering and disfluency. *Journal of Speech and Hearing Research, 24,* 595–600.

Curlee, R. (1993). Evaluating treatment efficacy for adults: Assessment of stuttering disability. *Journal of Fluency Disorders, 18,* 319–331.

Curlee, R., & Siegel, G. (1997). *Nature and treatment of stuttering: New directions* (2nd ed.). Boston: Allyn & Bacon.

Curlee, R., & Yairi, E. (1997). Early intervention with early childhood stuttering: A critical examination of the data. *American Journal of Speech-Language Pathology, 6,* 8–18.

Curtis, J. (1967). Disorders of articulation. In W. Johnson, S. Brown, J. Curtis, C. Edney, & J. Keaster (Eds.), *Speech handicapped school children* (3rd ed.; pp. 111–174). New York: Harper & Row.

Czikzentmihaly: M. (1975). *Beyond boredom and anxiety.* San Francisco: Jossey-Bass.

Daly, D. (1981). Differentiation of stuttering subgroups with Van Riper's developmental tracks: A preliminary study. *Journal of the National Student Speech and Hearing Association, 9,* 89–101.

Daly, D. (1988). A practitioner's view of stuttering. *ASHA, 30,* 34–35.

Daly, D., & Burnett, M. (1996). Cluttering: Assessment, treatment planning and case study illustration. *Journal of Fluency Disorders, 21,* (3–4) 239–248.

Daly, D., & Burnett, M. (1999). Cluttering: Traditional views and new perspectives. In R. Curlee (Ed.), *Stuttering and related disorders of fluency* (2nd ed.; pp. 222–254). New York: Thieme Medical Publishers.

Davis, D. M. (1939). The relation of repetitions in the speech of young children to measures of language maturity and situational factors: Part I. *Journal of Speech and Hearing Disorders, 4,* 303–318.

Davis, D. M. (1940). The relation of repetitions in the speech of young children to measures of language maturity and situational factors: Parts II & III, *Journal of Speech and Hearing Disorders, 5,* 235–246.

Dell, C. W. (1980). *Treating the school age stutterer: A guide for clinicians.* Memphis, TN: Speech Foundation of America.

Dell, G. (1986). A spreading-activation theory of retrieval in sentence production. *Psychological Review, 93,* 283–321.

Dell, G., & Julliano, C. (1991). Connectionist approaches to the production of words. In H. F. M. Peters, W. Hulstijn, & C. W. Starkweather (Eds.), *Speech motor control and stuttering.* Amsterdam: Exerpta Medica.

Dembrowski, J., & Watson, B. (1991). An instrumental method for assessment and remediation of stuttering: A single-subject case study. *Journal of Fluency Disorders, 16,* 241–273.

DeNil, L. (1999). Stuttering: A neurophysiological perspective. In N. Bernstein Ratner & E. C. Healey (Eds.), *Stuttering research and practice: Bridging the gap* (pp. 85–102). Mahwah, NJ: Lawrence Erlbaum Associates.

DeNil, L., & Brutten, G. (1991). Speech-associated attitudes of stuttering and non-stuttering children. *Journal of Speech and Hearing Research, 34,* 60–66.

DeNil, L., Kroll, R., Kapur, S., & Houle, S. (in press). A position emission tomography study of silent and oral single word reading in stuttering and nonstuttering adults. *Journal of Speech, Language and Hearing Research.*

Denny, M., & Smith, A. (1992). Graduations in a pattern of neuromuscular activity associated with stuttering. *Journal of Speech, Language and Hearing Research, 35,* 1216–1229.

Denny, M., & Smith, A. (1997). Respiratory and laryngeal control of stuttering. In R. Curlee & G. Siegel (Eds.), *Nature and treatment of stuttering: New directions* (2nd ed.; pp. 99–127). Boston: Allyn & Bacon.

DiSimoni, F., (1990). Comment on Conture et al. (1988) and Prosek et al. (1988). *Journal of Speech and Hearing Disorders, 33,* 402–403.

Dodson, F. (1970). *How to parent.* New York: Signet.

Doehring, D. G. (1996). *Research strategies in human communication disorders* (2nd ed.). Austin: TX: Pro-Ed.

Douglas, E., & Quarrington, R. (1952). The differentiation of interiorized and exteriorized secondary stuttering. *Journal of Speech and Hearing Disorders, 17,* 377–385.

Dronkers, N. (1996). A new brain region for coordinating speech articulation. *Nature, 384,* 159–161.

Dunn, L., & Dunn, L. (1997). *Peabody Picture Vocabulary Test* (PPVT-III). (3rd ed.). Circle Pines, MN: American Guidance Service, Inc.

Eckel, F., & Boone, D. (1981). The s/z ratio as an indication of laryngeal pathology. *Journal of Speech and Hearing Disorders, 46,* 147–149.

Edwards, M., & Shriberg, L. (1983). *Phonology: Application in communication disorders.* San Diego: College-Hill Press.

Egolf, D., & Chester, S. (1973). Nonverbal communication and disorders of speech and language. *ASHA, 15,* 511–518.

Ekman, P. (1982). Methods for measuring facial action, in K. Scherer and P, Ekman, (Eds.), *Handbook of methods in nonverbal behaviors.* Cambridge, England: Cambridge University Press.

Erickson, R. L. (1969). Assessing communication attitudes among stutterers. *Journal of Speech and Hearing Research, 12,* 711–724.

Faircloth, S., & Faircloth, M. (1973). *Phonetic science: A program of instruction.* Englewood Cliffs, NJ: Prentice-Hall.

Farmer, A., & Brayton, E. (1979). Speech characteristics of fluent and dysfluent Down's syndrome adults. *Folia Phoniatrica, 31,* 284–290.

Felsenfeld, S. (1997). Epidemiology and genetics of stuttering. In R. Curlee & G. Siegel (Eds.), *Nature and treatment of stuttering: New directions* (2nd ed.; pp. 3–23) Boston: Allyn & Bacon.

Fincher, J. (1984). New machines may soon replace the doctor's black bag. *Smithsonian*, 64–71.

Finn, P. (1996). Establishing the validity of recovery from stuttering without formal treatment. *Journal of Speech and Hearing Research, 39*, 1171–1181.

Finn, P. (1998). Recovery without treatment: A review of conceptual and methodological consideration across disciplines. In A. Cordes & R. Ingham (Eds.), *Treatment efficacy for stuttering: A search for empirical bases* (pp. 3–25). San Diego, CA: Singular Publishing Group.

Fletcher, S. (1972). Time-by-count measurement of diadochokinetic syllable rate. *Journal of Speech and Hearing Research, 15*, 763–770.

Fluharty, N. (1974). The design and standardization of a speech language screening test for use with preschool children. *Journal of Speech and Hearing Disorders, 39*, 75–88.

Fluharty, N. (1978). *Preschool Speech & Language Screening Test.* Hingham, MA: Teaching Resources Corporation.

Flynn, P. T. (1978). Effective clinical interviewing. *Language Speech and Hearing Services in Schools*, IX, 256–271.

Fosnot, S. (1993). Research design for examining treatment efficacy in fluency disorders. *Journal of Fluency Disorders, 18*, 221–251.

Foundas, A. (November, 1998). Biological bases of stuttering. *ASHA Leader, 3* (16), 124.

Fox, P., Ingham, J., Hirsch, T., Downs, H., Martin, C., Jerabek, P., Glass, T., & Lancaster, J. (1996). A PET study of the neural systems of stuttering. *Nature, 382*, 158–162.

Frances, A., First, M., & Pincus, H. (1995). *Diagnostic and statistical manual-IV guidebook* (4th ed.). Washington, DC: American Psychiatric Press.

Franken, M. (1987). Perceptual and acoustic evaluation of stuttering therapy. In H. Peters & W. Hulstijn (Eds.), *Speech motor dynamics in stuttering* (pp. 285–294). Wien/New York: Springer-Verlag.

Franken, M. C., van Bezooijen, R., & Boves, L. (1997). Stuttering and communicative suitability of speech. *Journal of Speech Language and Hearing Research, 40*, 83–94.

Fraser, J., & Perkins, W. H. (Eds.). (1987). *Do you stutter: A guide for teens.* Memphis: Speech Foundation of America.

Freeman, F., & Ushijima, T. (1978). Laryngeal muscle activity during stuttering. *Journal of Speech Hearing Research, 21*, 538–562.

Fudala, J. (1970). *The Arizona Articulation Proficiency Scale.* Beverly Hills, CA: Western Psychological Services.

Gaines, N., Runyan, C., & Meyers, S. (1991). A comparison of young stutterers' fluent versus stuttered utterances on measures of length and complexity. *Journal of Speech and Hearing Research, 34*, 37–42.

German, D. (1989). *Test of Word Finding (TWF).* Allen, TX: DLM Teaching Resources.

German, D. (1991). *Test of Word Finding in Discourse.* Allen, TX: DLM Teaching Resources.

Ginott, H. (1969). *Between parent and teenager.* New York: Avon.

Gladwell, M. (1998, August 17). Do parents matter? *The New Yorker*, LXXIV, (24), 54–65.

Glasner, P. (1949). Personality characteristics and emotional problems in stutterers under the age of five. *Journal of Speech and Hearing Disorders, 14*, 135–138.

Goldberg, S. (1997). *Clinical skills for speech-language pathologists.* San Diego, CA: Singular Publishing Group.

Goldman, R., & Fristoe, M. (1986). *Goldman-Fristoe Test of Articulation (GFTA).* Circle Pines, MN: American Guidance Services.

Goldsmith, H., Buss, A., Plomin, R., Rothbart, M., Thomas, A., Chess, S., Hinde, R., & McCall, R. (1987). Roundtable: What is temperament? Four approaches. *Child Development, 58*, 505–529.

Gordon, P., & Luper, H. (1992a). The early identification of beginning stuttering I: Protocols. *American Journal of Speech-Language Pathology, 1*, 43–53.

Gordon, P., & Luper, H. (1992b). The early identification of beginning stuttering II: Problems. *American Journal of Speech-Language Pathology, 1*, 54–55.

Goyer, R., Reading, S., & Rickey, J. (1968). *Interviewing principles and techniques.* Dubuque, IA: William C. Brown.

Gray, M. (1940). The X family: A clinical and laboratory study of a "stuttering" family. *Journal of Speech Disorders, 5*, 343–48.

Gregory, H. (Ed.) (1978). *Controversies about stuttering therapy.* Baltimore: University Park Press.

Gregory, H., & Gregory, C. (1999). Counseling children who stutter and their parents. In R. Curlee (Ed.), *Stuttering and related disorders of fluency* (2nd ed; pp. 43–64). New York: Thieme.

Gregory, H., & Hill, D. (1980). Stuttering therapy for children. In W. Perkins (Ed.), *Stuttering disorders.* New York: Thieme-Stratton.

Guitar, B. (1975). Reduction of stuttering frequency using analog electro/myographic feedback, *Journal of Speech and Hearing Research, 18*, (4) 672–685.

Guitar, B. (1984). Indirect treatment of childhood stuttering. In J. Costello (Ed.), *Speech disorders in chil-*

dren: Recent advances (pp. 291–311). San Diego, CA: College-Hill Press.

Guitar, B. (1988). Is it stuttering or just normal language? *Contemporary Pediatrics*, 1–10.

Guitar, B. (1997). Therapy for children's stuttering and emotions. In R. Curlee & G. Siegel (Eds.), *Nature and treatment of stuttering: New direction* (2nd ed.; pp. 28–29). Boston: Allyn & Bacon.

Guitar, B. (1998). *Stuttering: An integrated approach to its nature and treatment* (2nd ed.). Baltimore, MD: Williams & Wilkins.

Guitar, B. (1999). *Stuttering: An integration of contemporary therapies.* (2nd ed.). Memphis, TN: Stuttering Foundation.

Guitar, B., Adams, M., & Conture, E. (1979). Clinical feedback. *Journal of Childhood Communication Disorders*, *3*, 3–12.

Guitar, B., & Conture, E. (1988). *If you think your child is stuttering . . .* (a pamphlet). Memphis, TN: Speech Foundation of America.

Guitar, B., & Conture, E. (1991). *The child who stutters: To the pediatrician.* Memphis, TN: Speech Foundation of America.

Guitar, B., & Conture, E. (Co- Producers). (1996). *Do you stutter: Straight talk for teens* (35-min video). Memphis, TN: Stuttering Foundation of America.

Guitar, B., Guitar, C., Neilson, P., O'Dwyer, T., & Andrews, G. (1988). Onset sequencing of selected lip muscles in stutterers and non-stutterers. *Journal of Speech and Hearing Research*, *31*, 28–35.

Guitar, B., & Peters, T. (1980). *Stuttering: An integration of contemporary therapies.* Memphis, TN: Speech Foundation of America.

Guitar, B., & Peters, T. (1999). *Stuttering: An integration of contemporary therapies* (2nd ed.). Memphis, TN: Stuttering Foundation of America, Publication No. 16.

Guyton, A. (1971). *Textbook of medical physiology* (4th ed.). Philadelphia: Saunders.

Hall, E. (1966). *Help wanted? A guidebook for parents and therapists dealing with young non-fluent children.* Evanston, IL: Junior League of Evanston.

Hall, E. (1977). The occurrence of disfluencies in language-disordered school-age children. *Journal of Speech and Hearing Disorders*, *42*, 364–369.

Hall, N. (1996). Language and fluency in child language disorders: Changes over time. *Journal of Fluency Disorders*, *21*, 1–32.

Hall, N., Yamashita, T., & Aram, D. (1993). Relationship between language and fluency in children with developmental language disorders. *Journal of Speech and Hearing Research*, *36*, 568–579.

Ham, R. (1986). *Techniques of stuttering therapy*, Englewood Cliffs, NJ: Prentice-Hall.

Ham, R. (1999). *Clinical management of stuttering in older children and adults.* Gaithersburg, MD: Aspen Publishers.

Hancock, K., Craig, A., McCready, C., McCaul, A., Costello, D., Campbell, K., & Gilmore, G. (1998). Two- to six-year controlled-trial stuttering outcomes for children and adolescents. *Journal of Speech, Language, and Hearing Research*, *40*, 1242–1252.

Hanson, B., Gronhond, K., & Rice, P. (1981). A shortened version of the Southern Illinois University Speech Situation Checklist for the identification of speech related anxiety. *Journal of Fluency Disorders*, *6*, 351–360.

Hardy, J. (1970). Development of neuromuscular systems underlying speech production. In *Speech and the denofacial complex: The state of the art. ASHA Reports*, *5*, 49–68.

Hardy, J. (1978). Basic concepts neural processes of speech and language. in J. Curtis (ed.), *Processes and disorders of human communication.* New York: Harper & Row.

Harrington, J. (1987). Coarticulation and stuttering: An acoustic and electropalatographic study. In H. Peters & W. Hulstijn (Eds.), *Speech motor dynamics in stuttering* (pp. 381–392). Wien/New York: Springer Press.

Harris, T. (1967). *I'm OK—you're OK.* New York: Harper & Row.

Hayhow, R. (1983). The assessment of stuttering and the evaluation of treatment, in P. Dalton (Ed.), *Approaches to the treatment of stuttering.* London: Croom Helm.

Haynes, W., & Pindzola, R. (1998). *Diagnosis and evaluation in speech pathology* (5th ed.). Boston: Allyn & Bacon.

Healey, C. (1982). Speaking fundamental frequency characteristics of stutterers and non-stutterers. *Journal of Communication Disorders*, *15*, 21–29.

Healey, C. (1984). Fundamental frequency contours of stutterers' vowels following fluent stop consonant productions. *Folia Phoniatrica*, *36*, 145–151.

Healey, E. C., Grossman, F., & Ellis, G. (1988). Behavioral characteristics of adult stutterers: Implications for determining treatment strategies. Poster presentation to Annual Conference of American Speech Hearing Language Association.

Healey, E., & Ramig, P. (1986) Acoustic measures of stutterers' and nonstutterers' fluency in two speech contexts. *Journal of Speech and Hearing Research*, *29*, 325–331.

Helm-Estabrooks, N. (1999) Stuttering associated with acquired neurological disorders. In R. Curlee (Ed.), *Stuttering and related disorders of fluency* (2nd ed.; pp. 269–288). New York: Thieme.

Hilgard, E., & Bower, G. (1966). *Theories of learning* (3rd ed.). New York: Appleton-Century-Crofts.

Hill, D. (1999). Evaluation of child factors related to early stuttering: A descriptive study. In N. Bernstein Ratner & E. Healey (Eds.), *Stuttering research and practice: Bridging the gap* (pp. 145–174). Mahwah, NJ: Lawrence Erlbaum Associates.

Hill, W. F. (1997). *Learning: A survey of psychological interpretation* (6th ed.). New York: Harper & Row.

Hillman, R., & Gilbert, H. (1977). Voice onset time for voiceless stop consonants in the fluent reading of stutterers and non-stutterers, *Journal of Acoustical Society of America* , *61*, 610–611.

Hixon & Hardy, J. (1964). Restricted motility of the speech articulators in cerebral palsy. *Journal of Speech and Hearing Disorders*, *29*, 293–306.

Howell, P., Au-Yeung, J., & Pilgrim, L. (1999). Utterance rate and linguistic properties as determinants of lexical dysfluencies in children who stutter. *Journal of Acoustical Society of America*, *105* (1), 1–10.

Howell, P., Au-Yeung, J., & Sackin, S. (1999). Exchange of stuttering from function to content words with age. *Journal of Speech, Language, and Hearing Research*, *42*, 345–354.

Howell, P., Au-Yeung, J., & Sackin, S. (2000). Internal structure of content words leading to lifespan differences in phonological difficulty in stuttering. *Journal of Fluency Disorders*, *25*, 1–20.

Howell, P., Hamilton, A., & Kryiacoupoulos, A. (1984). Automatic detection of repetitions and prolongation in stuttered speech. *Journal of Acoustical Society of America*, *79*, 1571–1579.

Howell, P., Sackin, S., & Glenn, K. (1997a). Development of a two-stage procedure for the automatic recognition of dysfluencies in the speech of children who stutter: I. Psychometric procedures appropriate for selection of training material for lexical dysfluency classifiers. *Journal of Speech, Language, and Hearing Research*, *40*, 1073–1084.

Howell, P., Sackin, S., & Glenn, K. (1997b). Development of a two-stage procedure for the automatic recognition of dysfluencies in the speech of children who stutter: II. ANN recognition of repetitions and prolongations with supplied word segment markers. *Journal of Speech Language and Hearing Research*, *40*, 1085–1096.

Howell, P., & Vause, L. (1986). Acoustic analysis and perception of vowels in stuttered speech. *Journal of Acoustical Society of America*, *79*, 1571–1579.

Howell, P., Williams, M., & Vause, L. (1987). Acoustic analysis of repetitions in stutterers' speech. In H. Peters & W. Hulstijn (Eds.), *Speech motor dynamics in stuttering*. Wien/New York: Springer Press.

Howie, P. (1981). Concordance for stuttering in monozygotic and dizygotic twin pairs. *Journal Speech and Hearing Research*, *24*, 317–321.

Hresko, W., Reid, D., & Hammill, D. (1991). *Test of Early Language Development-2*. Austin, TX: Pro-Ed.

Hubbard, C., & Prins, D. (1994). Word familiarity, syllabic stress pattern and stuttering. *Journal of Speech and Hearing Research*, *37*, 564–571.

Hubbard, C., & Yairi, E. (1988). Clustering of disfluencies in the speech of stuttering and non-stuttering preschool children. *Journal of Speech and Hearing Research*, *31*, 228–233.

Hull, F., Mielke, P., Timmons, R., & Willeford, J. (1971). The national speech and hearing survey: Preliminary results, *ASHA* , *13*, 228–233.

Hunt, J. (1967). *Stammering and stuttering, their nature and treatment*. New York: Hatner Publishing Company. (Original work published in 1861).

Hutchinson, J. (1974). Aerodynamic patterns of stuttered speech. In M. Webster & L. Furst (Eds.), *Vocal tract dynamics and dysfluency* (pp. 71–123). New York: Speech and Hearing Institute of New York.

Ilg, F., & Ames, L. (1960). *Child behavior*. New York: Dell.

Ingham, J. C. (1993). Current status of stuttering and behavior modification I: Recent trends in the application of behavior modification in children and adults. *Journal of Fluency Disorders*, *18*, 27–55.

Ingham, J., & Riley, J. (1998). Guidelines for documentation of treatment efficacy for young children who stutter. *Journal of Speech, Language, and Hearing Research*, *40*, 753–770.

Ingham, R. (1984). *Stuttering and behavior therapy: Current status and experimental foundations*. San Diego, CA: College-Hill Press.

Ingham, R. (1985). Assessment of stuttering in children. In J. Gruss (Ed.), *Stuttering therapy: prevention and early intervention*. Memphis, TN: Speech Foundation of America.

Ingham, R. (1990). Research on stuttering treatment for adults and adolescents: A perspective on how to overcome a malaise. In J. Cooper (Ed.), *Research needs in stuttering: Roadblocks and future directions* (ASHA Reports 18, pp. 91–97). Rockville, MD: American Speech-Language-Hearing Association.

Ingham, R. (1998). On learning from speech-motor control research on stuttering. In A. Cordes & R. Ingham (Eds.), *Treatment efficacy and stuttering: A search for empirical bases* (pp. 67–102). Singular Publishing Group.

Ingham, R. (1999). Performance-contingent management of stuttering in adolescents and adults. In R. Curlee

(Ed.), *Stuttering and related disorders* (2nd ed.; pp. 200–221). New York: Thieme.

Ingham, R., & Cordes, A. (1997). Self-measurement and evaluating stuttering treatment efficacy. In R. Curlee & G. Siegel (Eds.), *Nature and treatment of stuttering: New directions* (2nd ed.; pp. 413–437) Boston: Allyn & Bacon.

Ingham, R., & Cordes, A. (1999). On watching a discipline shoot itself in the foot: Some observation on current trends in stuttering treatment research. In N. Bernstein Ratner & E. Healey (Eds.), *Stuttering research and practice: Bridging the gap* (pp. 211–230) Mahwah, NJ: Lawrence Erlbaum Associates.

Ingham, R., Cordes, A., & Finn, P. (1993). Time-interval measurement of stuttering: Systematic replication of Ingham, Cordes & Gow (1993). *Journal of Speech and Hearing Research, 36,* 1168–1176.

Ingham, R., Fox, P., Ingham, J., Zamarripa, F., Martin, C., Jerabek, P., & Cotton, J. (1996). Functional-lesion investigation of developmental stuttering with positron emission tomography. *Journal of Speech and Hearing Research, 39,* 1208–1227.

Ingham, R., Ingham, J., Onslow, M., & Finn, P. (1989). Stutterers' self-ratings of speech naturalness: Assessing effects and reliability. *Journal of Speech and Hearing Research, 32,* 419–431.

Ingham, R., & Onslow, M. (1985). Measurement and modification of speech naturalness during stuttering therapy. *Journal of Speech and Hearing Disorders, 50,* 261–268.

Jaeger, J. (1992). 'Not by the chair of my hinny hin hin': Some general properties of slips of the tongue in young children. *Journal of Child Language, 19,* 335–366.

Jaffe, J., & Feldstein, S. (1970). *Rhymes of dialogue.* New York: Academic Press.

Janssen, P., Kraaimaat, F., & van der Meulen, S. (1983). Reading ability and disfluency in stuttering and non-stuttering elementary school children, *Journal of Fluency Disorders, 8,* 39–53.

Jezer, M. (1997). *Stuttering: A life bound up in words.* New York: Basic Books/Harper & Row.

Johnson, W. (1946). *People in quandries.* New York: Harper & Row.

Johnson, W. (1955). A study of the onset and development of stuttering. In W. Johnson (Ed.), *Stuttering in children and adults.* Minneapolis: University of Minnesota Press.

Johnson, W. (1958). The six mean and the stuttering. In J. Eisenson (Ed.), *Stuttering: A symposium,* (pp. xi–xiv). New York: Harper & Row.

Johnson, W. (1961). *Stuttering and what you can do about it.* Minneapolis: University of Minnesota Press.

Johnson, W., & Associates (1959). *The onset of stuttering.* Minneapolis: University of Minnesota Press.

Johnson, W., Brown, S., Curtis, J., Edney, C., & Keaster, J. (1967). *Speech handicapped school children* (3rd ed.). New York: Harper & Row.

Johnson, W., Darley, F., & Spriestersbach, D. (1963). *Diagnostic methods in speech pathology.* New York: Harper & Row.

Kadi-Hanifi, K., & Howell, P. (1992). Syntactic analysis of the spontaneous speech of normally fluent and stuttering children. *Journal of Fluency Disorders, 17,* 151–170.

Kagan, J. (1994). *Galen's progeny: Temperament in human nature.* New York: Basic Books.

Kagan, J., Reznick, J., & Snidman, N. (1987). The physiology and psychology of behavioral inhibition in children. *Child Development, 58,* 1459–1473.

Kagan, J., & Snidman, N. (1991). Temperamental factors in human development. *American Psychologist, 46,* 856–862.

Kail, R., & Leonard, L. (1986). Word-finding abilities in language impaired children. *ASHA Monograph, 25.*

Kalinowski, S., Noble, S., Armson, J., & Stuart, A. (1994). Pretreatment and posttreatment speech naturalness ratings of adults with mild and severe stuttering. *American Journal of Speech-Language Pathology, 3,* 61–66.

Karniol, R. (1995). Stuttering, language, and cognition: A review and a model of stuttering as a suprasegmental sentence plane alignment (SFA). *Psychological Bulletin, 117.*

Kelly, E. (1993). Speech rates and turn-taking behaviors of children who stutter and their parents. *Seminars in Speech and Language, 14*(3), 203–214.

Kelly, E. (1994). Speech rates and turn-taking behaviors of children who stutter and their fathers. *Journal of Speech and Hearing Research, 37*(6), 1284–1294.

Kelly, E. (1995). Parents as partners: Including mothers and fathers in the treatment of children who stutter. *Journal of Communication Disorders, 28*(2), 93–105.

Kelly, E., & Conture, E. (1988). Acoustic and perceptual correlates of adult stutterers' typical and imitated stutterings. *Journal of Fluency Disorders, 13,* 233–252.

Kelly, E., & Conture, E. (1991). Intervention with school-age stutterers: A parent-child fluency group approach. *Seminars in Speech and Language, 12,* 309–322.

Kelly, E., & Conture, E. (1992). Speaking rates, response time latencies, and interrupting behaviors of young stutterers, nonstutterers, and their mothers. *Journal of Speech and Hearing Research, 35,* (6) 1256–1267.

Kelly, E., Martin, J., Baker, K., Rivera, N., Bishop, J., Krizizke, J., Stettler, D., & Stealy, J. (1997). Academic and clinical preparation and practices of school speech-language pathologists with people who stutter. *Language, Speech and Hearing Services in Schools, 28*, 195–212.

Kent, R. (1984). Stuttering as a temporal programming disorder. In R. Curlee & N. Perkins (Eds.), *Nature and treatment of stuttering: New directions* (pp. 283–302). San Diego: College-Hill Press.

Kidd, K. (1983). Recent progress of the genetics of stuttering. In C. Ludlow & J. Cooper (Eds.), *Genetic aspects of speech and language*. New York: Academic Press.

Kidd, K. (1984). Stuttering as a genetic disorder. In R. Curlee & W. Perkins (Eds.), *Nature and treatment of stuttering: New directions* (pp. 149–169). San Diego, CA: College-Hill.

Kolk, H. (1991). Is stuttering a symptom of adaptation or impairment? In H. Peters, W. Hulstijn, & C. W. Starkweather (Eds.), *Speech motor control and stuttering* (pp. 131–140). Amsterdam: Elsevier Science.

Kolk, H., Conture, E., Postma, A., Louko, L. (1991). *The covert-repair hypothesis and childhood stuttering.* Paper presented at Annual Conference of American Speech-Language-Hearing Association, Atlanta, GA.

Kolk, H., & Postma, A. (1997). Stuttering as a covert repair phenomenon. In R. Curlee & G. Siegel (Eds.), *Nature and treatment of stuttering: New directions* (2nd ed; pp. 182–203). Boston: Allyn & Bacon.

Kosinski, J. (1966). *The painted bird.* New York: Pocket Cardinal Books.

Krasuski, J., Horowitz, B., & Rumsey, J. (1996). A survey of functional and anatomical neuroimaging techniques. In G. Lyons & J. Rumsey (Eds.), *Neuroimaging: A window to the neurological foundations of learning and behavior in children.* Baltimore: Paul H. Brookes.

Krause, R. (1982). A social psychological approach to the study of stuttering. In C. Fraser & K. Scherer (Eds.), *Advances in the social psychology of language.* Cambridge, England: Maison des Sciences de l'Homme and Cambridge University Press.

Krupski, A. (1986). Attention problems in youngsters with learning handicaps. In J. K. Torgesen & B. Y. L. Wond (Eds.), *Psychological and educational perspectives on learning disabilities.* (161–192). New York: Academic Press.

Kully, D., & Langevin, M. (1999). Intensive treatment for adolescents. In R. Curlee (Ed.), *Stuttering and related disorders of fluency* (2nd ed.; pp. 139–159). New York: Thieme.

Kurlansky, M. (1998). *Cod.* New York: Penguin Books.

Lange, A., & Jakubowski, P. (1976). *Responsible assertive behavior.* Champaign, IL: Research Press.

LaSalle, L., & Conture, E. (1991). Eye contact between young stutterers and their mothers. *Journal of Fluency Disorders, 16*, 179–199.

LaSalle, L., & Conture, E. (1995). Disfluency clusters of children who stutter: Relation of stutterers to self-repairs. *Journal of Speech and Hearing Research, 38*, 965–977.

LeFrancois, G. (1972). *Psychological theories and human learning: Kingor's report.* Monterey, CA: Brooks/Cole.

Le Shan, E. (1963). *How to survive parenthood.* New York: Warner Paperback Library.

Levelt, W. J. M. (1989). *Speaking: From intention to articulation.* Cambridge, MA: MIT Press.

Levelt, W. J. M. (Ed.). (1991). *Lexical access in speech production.* Cambridge, MA: Blackwell.

Levelt, W., Roelofs, A., & Meyer, A. (1999). A theory of lexical access in speech production. *Behavioral and Brain Sciences, 22*, 1–75.

Levelt, W., Schriefers, H., Vorberg, D., Meyer, A., Pechman, T., & Havinga, J. (1991). The time course of lexical access in speech production: A study of picture naming. *Psychological Review, 98*, 122–142.

Levelt, W., & Wheeldon, L. (1994). Do speakers have access to mental syllabury? *Cognition, 50*, 239–269.

Lewis, S. (1920). *Main street.* New York: Harcourt Brace.

Lincoln, M., & Harrison, E. (1999). The Lidcombe program. In M. Onslow & A. Packman (Eds.), *The handbook of early stuttering intervention* (pp. 103–118). San Diego, CA: Singular Publishing Group.

Lincoln, M., & Onslow, M. (1997). Long-term outcome of early intervention for stuttering. *American Journal of Speech-Language Pathology, 6*, 51–58.

Liotti, M., Gay, C., & Fox, P. (1994). Functional imaging and language: Evidence from positron emission tomography. *Journal of Clinical Neurophysiology, 11*, 175–190.

Logan, K., & Conture, E. (1995). Length, grammatical complexity, and rate differences in stuttered and fluent conversational utterances of children who stutter. *Journal of Fluency Disorders, 20*, 35–61.

Logan, K., & Conture, E. (1997). Selected temporal grammatical and phonological characteristics of conversational utterances produced by children who stutter. *Journal of Speech and Hearing Research, 40*, 107–120.

Logan, K., & LaSalle, L. (1999). Grammatical characteristics of children's conversational utterances that contain disfluency clusters. *Journal of Speech, Language, and Hearing Research, 42*, 80–91.

Logan, K., & Yaruss, J. (1999). Helping parents address attitudinal and emotional factors with young children who stutter. *Contemporary Issues in Communication Science and Disorders, 26*, 69–81.

Louko, L. (1995). Phonological characteristics of young children who stutter. *Topics in Language Disorders, 13*(3), 48–59.

Louko, L., Conture, E., & Edwards, M. L. (1999). Treating children who exhibit co-occurring stuttering and disordered phonology. In R. Curlee (Ed.), *Stuttering and related disorders of fluency* (2nd ed.; pp. 124–138). New York: Thieme Medical Publishers.

Louko, L., Edwards, M. L., & Conture, E. (1990). Phonological characteristics of young stutterers and their normally fluent peers. *Journal of Fluency Disorders, 15*, 191–210.

Lubker, B. B., & Tomblin, E. (1999). Epidemiology: Informing clinical practice and research on language disorders of children. *Topics in Language Disorders, 19*, (1) 1–26.

Luper, H. (1982). Intervention with the young stutterer. *Journal of Childhood Communication Disorders, 6*, 3–4.

Luper, H., & Mulder, R. (1964). *Stuttering therapy for children*. Englewood Cliffs, NJ: Prentice-Hall.

MacKay, D., & McDonald, M. (1984). Stuttering as a sequencing and timing disorder. In W. Perkins & R. Curlee (Eds.), *Nature and treatment of stuttering: New directions*. San Diego, CA: College-Hill Press.

MacDonald, J., & Martin, R. (1973). Stuttering and disfluency as two reliable and unambiguous response classes. *Journal of Speech and Hearing Research, 16*, 691–699.

Mahr, G., & Leith, W. (1992). Psychogenic stuttering of adult onset. *Journal of Speech and Hearing Research, 35*, 283–286.

Manning, W. (1996). *Clinical decision making in the diagnosis and treatment of fluency Disorders*. Albany, NY: Delmar Publishers.

Mansson, H. (2000). Childhood stuttering: Incidence and development. *Journal of Fluency Disorders*.

Martin, R., & Haroldson, S. (1982). Contingent self-stimulation for stuttering. *Journal of Speech and Hearing Disorders, 47*, 407–413.

Martin, R., Haroldson, S., & Triden, K. (1984). Stuttering and speech naturalness. *Journal of Speech and Hearing Disorders, 49*, 53–58.

Martin, R., Parlour, S., & Haroldson, S. (1990). Stuttering and level of linguistic demand: The Stocker Probe. *Journal of Fluency Disorders, 15*, 93–106.

Masters, W., & Johnson, V. (1970). *Human sexual inadequacy*. New York: Little, Brown.

Mastrud, B. (1988). T*he Oxfordshire fluency programme for adolescent stutterers*. Paper presented to Second Oxford Dysfluency Conference, Oxford, England.

McDevitt, S., & Carey, W. (1995). *Behavioral style questionnaire*. West Chester, PA: TemperaMetrics.

McDonald, E. (1964). *Articulation testing and treatment: A sensory-motor approach*. Pittsburgh: Stanwix House.

McDowell, E. (1928). *The educational and emotional adjustments of stuttering children*. New York: Columbia University Teachers College.

McGregor, K. (1997). The nature of word-finding errors of preschoolers with and without word-finding deficits. *Journal of Speech, Language and Hearing Research, 40*, 1232–1244.

McGregor, K., & Leonard, L. (1989). Facilitating word-finding skills in language-impaired children. *Journal of Speech and Hearing Disorders, 54*, 141–147.

McNight, R., & Cullinan, W. (1987). Subgroups of stuttering children: Speech and reaction times, segments duration and naming latencies. *Journal of Fluency disorders, 12*, 217–233.

Melnick, K., & Conture, E. (2000). Relationship of length and grammatical complexity to the systematic and nonsystematic speech errors and stuttering of children who stutter. *Journal of Fluency Disorders, 25*, 21–45.

Merits-Patterson, R., & Reed, C. (1981). Disfluencies in the speech of language-delayed children. *Journal of Speech and Hearing Research, 24*, (1) 55–58.

Metz, D., Conture, E., & Caruso, A. (1979). Voice onset time, frication and aspiration during stutterers' fluent speech, *Journal of Speech Hearing Research, 22*, 649–656.

Metz, D., Onufrak, J., & Ogburn, R. S. (1979). An acoustical analysis of stutterers' speech prior to and the termination of therapy. *Journal of Fluency Disorders, 4*, 249–254.

Metz, D., Samar, V., & Sacco, P. (1983). Acoustic analysis of stutterers' fluent speech before and after therapy. *Journal of Speech and Hearing Research, 26*, 531–536.

Metz, D., Schiavetti, N., & Sacco, P. (1990). Acoustic and psychophysical dimensions of the perceived speech naturalness of nonstutterers and posttreatment stutterers. *Journal of Speech and Hearing Disorders, 55*, 516–525.

Meyer, A., & Schriefers, H. (1991). Phonological facilitation in picture-word interference experiments: Effect of stimulus onset asynchrony and types of interfering stimuli. *Journal of Experimental Psychology: Learning, Memory, and Cognition, 17*, 1146–1160.

Meyers, S., & Freeman, F. (1985a). Are mothers of stutterers different? An investigation of social-communicative interaction. *Journal of Fluency Disorders, 10,* 193–210.

Meyers, S., & Freeman, F. (1985b). Interruptions as a variable in stuttering and disfluency. *Journal of Speech and Hearing Research, 28,* 428–435.

Meyers, S., & Freeman, F. (1985c). Mother and child speech rates as a variable in stuttering and disfluency. *Journal of Speech and Hearing Research, 28,* 436–444.

Miller, N. (1944). Experimental studies of conflict. In J. Hunt (Ed.), *Personality and the behavior disorders.* New York: Ronald Press.

Montgomery, A., & Cooke, P. (1976). Perceptual and acoustic analysis of repetitions in stuttered speech. *Journal of Communication Disorders, 9,* 317–330.

Moore, W. H., Jr. (1984). Central nervous system characteristics of stutterers, in R. Curlee & W. Perkins (Eds.), *Nature and treatment of stuttering: New directions.* San Diego, CA: College-Hill Press.

Moore, W. H., Jr. (1986). Hemispheric alpha asymmetries of stutterers and non-stutterers for the recall and recognition of words and connected reading passages: Some relations to severity of stuttering. *Journal of Fluency Disorders, 11,* 71–89.

Moore, W. H. Jr. (1993). Hemisphere processing research. In E. Boberg (Ed.), *Neuro-psychology of stuttering* (pp. 39–72). Edmonton, Alberta: The University of Alberta Press.

Moore, W., & Boberg, E. (1987). Hemispheric processing and stuttering. In L. Rusting, H. Purser and D. Rowley (Eds.), *Progress in the treatment of fluency disorders.* London: Taylor & Francis.

Morley, M., (1957). *The development and disorders of speech of childhood.* New York: Ronald Press.

Murphy, A., & FitzSimons, R. (1960). *Stuttering and personality dynamics.* New York: Ronald Press.

Murray, H., & Reed, C. (1977). Language abilities of preschool stuttering children. *Journal of Fluency Disorders, 2,* 171–176.

Mutti, M., Sterling, H., & Spaulding, N. (1978). *Quick Neurological Screening Test. Revised Edition.* Novato, CA: Academic Therapy Publications.

Neelley, J., & Timmons, R. (1967). Adaptation and consistency in the disfluent speech behavior of young stutterers and stutterers. *Journal of Speech and Hearing Research, 10,* 250–256.

Neill, A. (1960). *Summerhill: A radical approach to child rearing.* New York: Hart Associates.

Neilson, M. (1980). *Stuttering and the control of speech: A system analysis approach.* Ph.D. dissertation, University of New South Wales, Australia.

Neilson, M. (1999). Cognitive-behavioral treatment of adults who stutter: The process and the art. In R. Curlee (Ed.), *Stuttering and related disorders of fluency* (2nd ed.; pp. 181–199). New York: Thieme.

Neilson, M., & Neilson, P. (1987). Speech motor control and stuttering: A computational model of adaptive sensory-motor processing. *Speech Communications, 6,* 325–333.

Netsell, R. (1973). Speech physiology. In R. Minifie, T. Hixon, & F. Williams (Eds.), *Normal aspects of speech, hearing and language.* Englewood Cliffs, NJ: Prentice-Hall.

Newcomer, P., & Hammill, D. (1997). *Test of Language Development Primary – Third Edition (TOLD-P:3).* Austin, TX: Pro-Ed.

Newman, P., Harris, R., & Hilton, L. (1989). Vocal jitter and shimmer in stuttering. *Journal of Fluency Disorders, 14,* 87–95.

Niebuhr, R. (1968). Prayer (1934). In E. M. Beck (Ed.), *Bartlett's familiar quotations* (14th ed.). Boston: Little, Brown.

Nippold, M. (1990). Concomitant speech and language disorders in stuttering children: A critique of the literature. *Journal of Speech and Hearing Disorders, 55,* 51–60.

Olswang, L., & Bain, B. (1994). Data collection: Monitoring children's treatment progress. *American Journal of Speech-Language Pathology, 3,* 55–66.

Onslow, M. (1990). Treatment efficacy: The breadth of research. In L. Olswang, C. Thompson, S. Warren, & N. Minghetti (Eds.), *Treatment efficacy research in communication disorders* (pp. 99–104). Rockville, MD: American Speech-Language-Hearing Foundation.

Onslow, M. (1992). Choosing a treatment procedure for early stuttering: Issues and future directions. *Journal of Speech and Hearing Research, 35,* 983–993.

Onslow, M. (1996). *Behavior management of stuttering.* San Diego, CA: Singular Publishing Group.

Onslow, M., Andrews, C., & Lincoln, M. (1994). A control/experimental trial of an operant treatment for early stuttering. *Journal of Speech and Hearing Research, 37,* 1244–1259.

Onslow, M., Costa, L., & Rue, S. (1990). Direct early intervention with stuttering: Some preliminary data. *Journal of Speech and Hearing Disorders, 55,* 405–416.

Onslow, M., & Packman, A. (Eds.). (1999). *The handbook of early stuttering intervention.* San Diego, CA: Singular Publishing Group.

Orton, S. (1927). Studies in stuttering. *Archives of Neurology and Psychiatry, 18,* 671–672.

Oyler, M. E. (1996a). *Vulnerability in stuttering children* (No. 9602431). Ann Arbor, MI: UMI Dissertation Services.

Oyler, M. E. (1996b, December). *Temperament: Stuttering and the behaviorally inhibited child.* Seminar presented at the American Speech-Language-Hearing Association Annual Convention, Seattle, WA.

Oyler, M., & Ramig, P. (1995, December). *Vulnerability in stuttering children.* Seminar presented at the American Speech-Language-Hearing Association Annual Convention, Orlando, FL.

Paden, E. (1998, Fall). When should we recommend phonological remediation for children prone to otitis media? *Hearsay,* 70–73.

Paden, E., Matthies, M., & Novak, M. (1989). Recovery from OME-related phonologic delay following tube placement. *Journal of Speech and Hearing Disorders,* 54, 94–100.

Paden, E., Novak, M., & Beiter, A. (1987). Predictors of phonologic inadequacy in young children prone to otitis media. *Journal of Speech and Hearing Disorders,* 52, 232–242.

Paden, E., & Yairi, E. (1996). Phonological characteristics of children whose stuttering persisted or recovered. *Journal of Speech and Hearing Research,* 39,987–990.

Paden, E., Yairi, E., & Ambrose, N. (1999). Early childhood stuttering II: Initial status of expressive language abilities. *Journal of Speech Language Hearing Research,* 42, 1113–1124.

Pellowski, M., & Conture, E. (1999, November). *Changes in speech disfluencies in relationship to chronological age.* Paper presented to Annual Conference of American Speech Language and Hearing Association, San Francisco, CA; manuscript in preparation (2000).

Pellowski, M., Conture, E., & Anderson, J. (2000). *Articulatory and phonological assessment of children who stutter.* Paper to be published in the Proceedings of the Third World Congress on Fluency Disorders, Nyborg, Denmark.

Pellowski, M., Conture, E., Roos, J., Adkins, C., & Ask, J. (2000). A parent-child group approach to treating stuttering in young children: treatment outcome data. Presented to Annual Treatment Efficacy Conference, Vanderbilt University, Nashville, TN.

Perkins, W. H. (1970). Physiological studies. In J. G. Sheehan (Ed.), *Stuttering: Research therapy.* New York: Harper & Row.

Perkins, W. H. (1978). From psychoanalysis to discoordination. In H. H. Gregory (Ed.), *Controversies about stuttering therapy.* Baltimore: University Park Press.

Perkins, W., Kent, R., & Curlee, R. (1991). A theory of neuropsycholinguistic function in stuttering. *Journal of Speech and Hearing Research,* 34, 734–752.

Perkins, W., Rudas, J., Johnson, L., & Bell, J. (1976). Stuttering: Discoordination of phonation with articulation and respiration. *Journal of Speech Hearing Research,* 19, 509–522.

Peters, H., & Boves, L. (1988). Coordination of aerodynamic and phonatory processes in fluent speech utterances of stutterers. *Journal of Speech Disorders,* 31, 352–361.

Peters, H. F. M., & Hulstijn, W. (Eds.). (1987). *Speech motor dynamics in stuttering.* Wien/New York: Springer-Verlag.

Peters, H., Hulstijn, W., & Starkweather, C. W. (Eds.). (1991). *Speech motor control and stuttering.* Amsterdam: Exerpta Medica.

Peters, H., & Starkweather, C. (1990). The interaction between speech motor coordination and language processes in the development of stuttering: Hypotheses and suggestions for research. *Journal of Fluency Disorders,* 15, 115–125.

Peters, J., Romine, J., & Dykman, R. (1975). A special neurological examination of children with learning disabilities. *Developmental Medicine and Child Neurology,* 17, (1) 63–78.

Pindzola, R. (1986a). Acoustic evidence of aberrant velocities in stutterers' fluent speech. *Perceptual and Motor Skills,* 62, 399–405.

Pindzola, R. (1986b). A description of some selected stuttering instruments. *Journal of Childhood Communication Disorders,* 9, 183–200.

Pindzola, R., Jenkins, M., & Lokken, M. (1989). Speaking rates of young children. *Language, Speech and Hearing Services in the Schools,* 20, 133–138.

Pindzola, R., & White, D. (1986). A protocol for differentiation the incipient stutterer. *Language, Speech and Hearing Services in the Schools,* 17, 2–15.

Plomin, R., & DeFries, J. (May, 1998). The genetics of cognitive abilities and disabilities. *Scientific American,* 278 (3), 62–69.

Podrouzek, W., & Furrow, D. (1988). Preschoolers' use of eye contact while speaking: The influence of sex, age, and conversational partner. *Journal of Psycholinguistic Research,* 17, 89–98.

Pool, K., Finitzo, T., Devous, M., Watson, B., & Freeman, F. (1991). Regional cerebral blood flow in developmental stutterers. *Archives of Neurology,* 48, 509–512.

Pool, K., Freeman K., & Finitzo, T. (1987). Brain electrical activity mapping: applications to vocal motor control disorders. In H. Peters & W. Hulstijn (Eds.),

Speech motor dynamics in stuttering (pp. 151–160). Wien/New York: Springer-Verlag.

Postma, A. (1991). Stuttering and self-correction: On the role of linguistic repair processes in disfluencies of normal speakers and stutterers. Nijmegen, The Netherlands: Nijmeegs Instituut voor Cognitie-Onderzoek en Informatietechnologie (NICI), NICI Technical Report 91–104.

Postma, A., & Kolk, H. (1993). The covert repair hypothesis: Prearticulatory repair processes in normal and stuttered disfluencies. *Journal of Speech and Hearing Research, 36,* 472–487.

Postma A., Kolk, H., & Povel, D-J. (1990a). On the relation among speech errors, disfluencies, and self-repairs. *Language and Speech, 33,* 19–29.

Postma, A., Kolk, H., & Povel, D-J. (1990b). Speech planning and execution in stutterers. *Journal of Fluency Disorders, 15,* 49–59.

Postma, A., Kolk, H., & Povel, D-J. (1991). Disfluencies as resulting from covert self-repairs applied to internal speech errors. In H. Peters, W. Hulstijn, & C. Starkweather (Eds.), *Speech motor control and stuttering* (pp. 141–148). Amsterdam: Elsevier Science Publishers.

Preus, A. (1981). *Attempts at identifying subgroups of stutterers.* Olso, Norway: University of Norway Press.

Prins, D. (1974). Motivation/part one. In C. Starkweather (Ed.), *Therapy for stutterers.* Memphis, TN: Speech Foundation of America.

Prins, D. (1991). Theories of stuttering as event and disorder: Implications for speech production processes. In H. Peters, W. Hulstijn, & C. W. Starkweather (Eds.), *Speech motor control and stuttering* (pp. 571–580). Amsterdam: Elsevier Science Publishers.

Prins, D., (1999). Describing the consequences of disorders: Comments on Yaruss (1998). *Journal of Speech, Language and Hearing Research, 42,* 1395–1397.

Prins, D., & Hubbard, C. (1988). Response contingent stimuli and stuttering: Issues and implications. *Journal of Speech and Hearing Research, 31,* 696–709.

Prins, D., & Lohr, F. (1972). Behavioral dimensions of stuttered speech. *Journal of Speech and Hearing Research, 15,* 61–71.

Prins, D., Main, V., & Wampler, S. (1997). Lexicalization in adults who stutter. *Journal of Speech, Language and Hearing Research, 40,* 373–384.

Prosek, R., Montgomery, A., & Walden, B.(1988). Constancy of relative timing stutterers and nonstutterers. *Journal of Speech and Hearing Research, 25,* 29–33.

Purser, H. (1987). The psychology of treatment evaluation. In L. Rustin, H. Purser, & H. Rowley (Eds.),

Progress in the treatment of fluency disorders (pp. 258–272). London: Taylor & Francis.

Ragsdale J., & Sisterhen, D. (1984). Hesitation phenomena in the spontaneous speech of normal and articulatory-defective children. *Language and Speech, 27,* 235–244.

Ramig, P. (1993). Parent-clinician-child partnership in the therapeutic process of the preschool and elementary-aged child who stutters. *Seminars in Speech and Language, 14,* (3), 226–237.

Ramig, P., & Bennett, E. (1995). Working with 7- to 12-year-old children who stutter: Ideas for intervention in the public schools. *Language, Speech and Hearing Services in Schools, 26,* 138–150.

Ramig, P., & Bennett, E. (1997). Clinical management of children: Direct management strategies. In R. Curlee & G. Siegel (Eds.), *Nature and treatment of stuttering: New directions* (pp. 292–312). Boston: Allyn & Bacon.

Ramig, P., Krieger, S., & Adams, M. (1982). Vocal changes in stutterers and nonstutterers when speaking to children. *Journal of Fluency Disorders, 7,* 369–384.

Ratner, N. (1995). Treating the child with concomitant grammatical or phonological impairment. *Language, Speech and Hearing Services in Schools, 2,* 180–186.

Read, C., Buder, E., & Kent, R. (1990). Speech analysis systems: A survey. *Journal of Speech and Hearing Research, 33,* 363–374.

Read, C., Buder, E., & Kent, R. (1992). Speech analysis systems: An evaluation. *Journal of Speech and Hearing Research, 34,* 314–332.

Rees, N. (1980). Learning to talk and understand. In T. Hixon, L. Shriberg, & J. Saxman (Eds.), *Introduction to communication disorders.* Englewood Cliffs, NJ: Prentice-Hall.

Rickenberg, H. (1956). Diadochokinesis in stutterers and non-stutterers. *Journal of the Medical Society of New Jersey, 53,* 324–326.

Rieber, R. W. (1977). *The problem of stuttering: Theory and therapy.* New York: Elsevier.

Rieber, R. & Wollock, J. (1977). The historical roots of the theory and therapy of stuttering. *Journal of Communication Disorders, 10,* 3–24.

Riley, G. (1980). *Stuttering Severity Instrument for Children. and Adults* (rev. ed.). Austin, TX: Pro-Ed.

Riley, G. (1981). *Stuttering Prediction Instrument for Young Children* (3rd ed.). Austin, TX: Pro-Ed.

Riley, G. (1994a). *Stuttering Severity Instrument for Young Children* (SSI-3) (3rd ed.). Austin, TX: Pro-Ed.

Riley, G. (1994b). *Stuttering Severity Instrument for Young Children* (3rd ed.). Austin, TX: Pro-Ed.

Riley, G., & Riley, J. (1979). A component model for diagnosing and treating children who stutter. *Journal of Fluency Disorders, 4*, 279–293.

Riley, G., & Riley, J. (1986). *Oral motor assessment and treatment*. Tigard, OR: CC Publications.

Riley, G., & Riley, J. (1988). Looking at a vulnerable system. *ASHA, 30* 32–34.

Robb, M., & Blomgren, M. (1997). Analysis of F2 transitions in the speech of stutterers and nonstutterers. *Journal of Fluency Disorders, 21*, 1–16.

Robb, M., Blomgren, M., & Chen, Y. (1998). Formant frequency fluctuation in stuttering and nonstuttering adults. *Journal of Fluency Disorders, 23*, 73–84.

Robb, M., Lybolt, J., & Price, H. (1985). Acoustic measures of stutterers' speech following an intensive therapy program, *Journal of Fluency Disorders, 10* 269–279.

Robbins, J., & Klee, T. (1987). Clinical assessment of oropharyngeal motor development in young children. *Journal of Speech and Hearing Disorders, 52*, 271–277.

Robinson, F. (1964). *Introduction to stuttering*. Englewood Cliffs, NJ: Prentice-Hall.

Roelofs, A. (1997). The WEAVER model of word-form encoding in speech production. *Cognition, 64*, 249–284.

Rosenbek, J., Messert, B., Collins, M., & Wertz, R. (1978). Stuttering following brain damage. *Brain and Language, 6*, 82–96.

Rothenberg, M. (1981). Some relations between glottal airflow and vocal fold contact area. In C. L. Ludlow & M. O. Hart (Eds.), *Proceedings of the Conference on the Assessment of Vocal Pathology*. Rockville, MD: ASHA Reports, 31, 88–95.

Rothenberg, M., & Mahshie, J. (1988). Monitoring vocal fold abduction through vocal fold contact area. *Journal of Speech and Hearing Research, 31*, 338–351.

Runyan, C., Bell, J. & Prosek, R. (1990). Speech naturalness ratings of treated stutterers. *Journal of Speech and Hearing Disorders, 25*, 29–33.

Runyan, C., & Runyan, S. (1999). Therapy for school-age stutterers: An update on the fluency rules program. In R. Curlee (Ed.), *Stuttering and related disorders of fluency* (pp. 101–114). New York: Thieme Medical Publishers.

Rustin, L. (1987). The treatment of childhood dysfluency through active parental involvement. In L. Rustin, & H. Rowley (Eds.), *Progress in the treatment of fluency disorders*. London, England: Taylor & Francis.

Rustin, L. (1995). *The management of stuttering in adolescence: A communication skills approach*. San Diego, CA: Singular Publishing Group.

Rustin, L. (1996). *Assessment and therapy for young dysfluent children: Family Interaction*. San Diego, CA: Singular Publishing Group.

Rustin, L., Botterill, W., & Kelman, E. (1996). *Assessment and therapy for young dysfluent children*. London: Whurr Publishers.

Rustin, L., Cook, F., & Spence, R. (1995). *The management of stuttering in adolescence: A communication skills approach*. London: Whurr Publishers.

Rustin, L., & Purser, H. (1991). Child development, families, and the problem of stuttering. In L. Rustin (Ed.), *Parents, families and the stuttering child* (pp. 1–24). San Diego, CA: Singular Publishing Group.

Ryan, B. (1974). *Programmed therapy for stuttering in children and adults*. Springfield, IL: C.C. Thomas.

Ryan, B. (1978). Stuttering therapy in a framework of operant conditioning and programmed learning. In H. Gregory (Ed.), *Controversies about stuttering therapy*. Baltimore: University Park Press.

Ryan, B. (1980). *Programmed therapy for stuttering children and adults*. (3rd ed.). Springfield, IL: Charles C. Thomas.

Ryan, B. (1992). Articulation, language, rate and fluency characteristics of stuttering and nonstuttering preschool children. *Journal of Speech and Hearing Research, 35*, 333–342.

Ryan, B., & Van Kirk Ryan, B. (1983). Programmed stuttering therapy for children: Comparisons of four establishment programs. *Journal of Fluency Disorders, 8*, 291–321.

Sacco, P., & Metz, D. (1987). Changes in stutterers' fundamental frequency contours following therapy. *Journal of Fluency Disorders, 12*, 1–8.

Sacco, P., & Metz, D. (1989). Comparison of period by period fundamental frequency of stutterers and nonstutterers over repeated utterances. *Journal of Speech and Hearing Research, 32*, 439–444.

Samar, V., Metz, D., & Sacco, P. (1986). Changes in aerodynamic characteristics of stutterers' fluent speech associated with therapy, *Journal of Speech and Hearing Research, 29*, 106–113.

Schiavetti, N. (1975). Judgments of stuttering severity as function of type and focus of type of disfluency. *Folia Phoniatrica, 27*, 26–37.

Schiavetti, N., & Metz, D. (1997). *Evaluating research in communicative disorders* (3rd ed.). Boston: Allyn & Bacon.

Schindler, M. (1955). A study of educational adjustment of stuttering and nonstuttering child. In W. Johnson & R. Leutenegger (Eds.), *Stuttering in children and adults* (pp. 348–360). Minneapolis, MN: University of Minnesota Press.

Schum, R. (1986). *Counseling in speech and hearing practice.* Rockville, MD: National Student Speech Language Hearing Association, Clin. Series No. 9.

Schwartz, H. D. (1999). *A primer for stuttering therapy.* Boston: Allyn & Bacon.

Schwartz, H. D., & Conture, E. (1988). Sub-grouping young stutterers: Preliminary behavioral perspectives. *Journal of Speech and Hearing Research, 31,* 62–71.

Schwartz, H. D., Zebrowski, P., & Conture, E. (1990). Behaviors at the onset of stuttering. *Journal of Fluency Disorders, 15,* 77–88.

Semel, E., Wiig, E., & Secord, W. (1996). *Clinical Evaluation of Language Fundamentals Screening Test-Third Edition (CELF-3).* San Antonio, TX: The Psychological Corporation, Harcourt Brace & Company.

Shames, G., & Egolf, D. (1976). *Operant conditioning and the management of stuttering.* Englewood Cliffs, NJ: Prentice-Hall.

Shames, G., & Florance, C. (1980). *Stutter-free speech: A goal for therapy.* Columbus, OH: Chas. E. Merrill.

Shames, G., & Sherrick, C. (1963). A discussion of nonfluency and stuttering as operant behavior. *Journal of Speech and Hearing Disorders, 28,* 3–18.

Shapiro, A. (1964). Factors contributing to the placebo effect: Their implications for psychotherapy. *American Journal of Psychotherapy, 18,* Suppl. 1, 73–88.

Shapiro, A. (1980). An electromyographic analysis of the fluent and dysfluent utterances of several types of stutterers. *Journal of Fluency Disorders, 5,* 203–231.

Shapiro, D. (1999). *Stuttering intervention: A collaborative journey to fluency freedom.* Austin, TX: Pro-Ed.

Shaywitz, B., Shaywitz, S., & Byrne, T. (1983). Quantitative analysis of computed tomographic brain scans in children with attention deficit disorder, *Neurology, 33,* 1500–1503.

Shaywitz, S., & Shaywitz, B. (1985). Attention deficit disorders. In J. O. Cavenar, et al. (Eds.), *Psychiatry,* Vol. 2. 1–15.

Shaywitz, S., & Shaywitz, B. (1988). Attention deficit disorder: Current perspectives. In J. Kavanagh, T. Truss, Jr. (Eds.), *Learning disabilities: Proceedings of the national conference* (pp. 367–523). Parkton, MD: York Press.

Sheehan, J. (1958). Conflict theory of stuttering. In J. Eisenson (Ed.), *Stuttering: A symposium.* New York: Harper & Row.

Sheehan, J. (1970a). Reflections on the behavioral modification of stuttering. In C. Starkweather (Ed.), *Conditioning in stuttering therapy.* Memphis, TN: Speech Foundation of America.

Sheehan, J. (1970b). Personality approaches. In J. G. Sheehan (Ed.), *Stuttering: Research and therapy.* New York: Harper & Row.

Sheehan, J. (1975). Conflict Theory and avoidance-reduction therapy. J. Eisenson (Ed.), *Stuttering: A second symposium.* New York: Harper & Row.

Sheehan, J. (1978). Current issues on stuttering and recovery. In H. Gregory (Ed.), *Controversies about stuttering therapy.* Baltimore: University Park Press.

Sheehan, J., & Martyn, M. (1970). Stuttering and its disappearance. *Journal of Speech Hearing Research, 13,* 279–289.

Shriberg, L., & Kwiatkowski, J. (1982). Phonological disorders I: A diagnostic classification system. *Journal of Speech and Hearing Disorders, 47,* 226–241.

Shriberg, L., & Smith, A. (1983). Phonological correlates of middle-ear involvement in speech-delayed children: A methodological note. *Journal of Speech and Hearing Research, 26,* 293–297.

Shriberg, L., & others. (1975). The Wisconsin Procedure for Appraisal of Clinical Competence (W-PACC): Model and data. *ASHA, 17,* 158–165.

Siegel, G. (1970). Punishment, stuttering and disfluency, *Journal of Speech Hearing Disorders, 13,* 677–714.

Siegel, G. (1999). Integrating affective, behavioral and cognitive factors in stuttering. In N. Bernstein Ratner & E. C. Healey (Eds.), *Stuttering research and practice: Bridging the gap.* (pp. 113–122). Mahwah, NJ: Lawrence Erlbaum Associates.

Silverman, F. (1996). *Stuttering and other fluency disorders* (2nd ed.). Boston: Allyn & Bacon.

Silverman, S., & Bernstein Ratner, N. (1997). Syntactic complexity, fluency and accuracy of sentence imitation in adolescents. *Journal of Speech, Language and Hearing Research, 40,* 95–106.

Skinner, B. F. (1953). *Science and human behavior.* New York: Macmillan.

Smith, A. (1999). Stuttering: A unified approach to a multifactorial, dynamic disorder. In N. Bernstein Ratner & E. C. Healey (Eds.), *Stuttering research and practice: Bridging the gap* (pp. 27–44). Mahwah, NJ: Lawrence Erlbaum Associates.

Smith, A., & Kelly, E. (1997). Stuttering: A dynamic, multifactorial model. In R. Curlee & G. Siegel (Eds.), *Nature and treatment of stuttering: New directions* (2nd ed.; pp. 204–217). Boston: Allyn & Bacon.

Smith, A., & Weber, C. (1988). The need for an integrated perspective on stuttering, *ASHA, 30,* 30–31.

Sochurek, H. (1987). Medicine's new vision. *National Geographic, 171,* 2–41.

Sommers, R., et al. (1959). Training parents of children with functional articulation. *Journal of Speech and Hearing Research, 2,* 258–265.

Spock, B. (1946). *Pocketbook of baby and child care.* New York: Pocket Books.

Spock, B. & Rothenberg, M. (1985). *Dr. Spock's baby and child care* (Fortieth Anniversary Edition). New York: Dutton.

St. Louis, K. (Ed.). (1996). Research and opinion on cluttering. *Journal of Fluency Disorders, 21*, Nos. 3 & 4, 171–371.

St. Louis, K., & Hinzman, A. (1988). A descriptive study of speech, language and hearing characteristics of school-aged stutterers. *Journal of Fluency Disorders, 13*, 357–373.

St. Louis, K., Murray, C., & Ashworth, M. (1991). Coexisting communication disorders in a random sample of school-aged stutterers. *Journal of Fluency Disorders*, 16, 13–23.

St. Onge, K. (1963). The stuttering syndrome. *Journal of Speech and Hearing Research*, VI, 195–197.

Starbuck, H. (1974). Motivation/part two. In C. Starkweather (Ed.), *Therapy for stutterers.* Memphis, TN: Speech Foundation of America.

Starkweather, C. (1974). *Therapy for stutterers.* Memphis, TN: Speech Foundation of America.

Starkweather, C. W. (1982). *Stuttering and laryngeal behavior.* Rockville, MD: *ASHA Monographs, 21.*

Starkweather, C. W. (1987). *Fluency and stuttering.* Englewood Cliffs, NJ: Prentice-Hall.

Starkweather, C. (1991). Stuttering: The motor-language interface. In H. Peters, W. Hulstijn, & C. Starkweather (Eds.), *Speech motor control and fluency.* Amsterdam: Excerpta Medica.

Starkweather, C. (1997). Learning and its role in stuttering development. In R. Curlee & G. Siegel (Eds.), *Nature and treatment of stuttering: New directions,* (2nd ed.; pp. 79–95). Boston: Allyn & Bacon.

Starkweather, C. W. & Gottwald, S. (1990). The demands and capacities model II: Clinical applications. *Journal of Fluency Disorders, 15*, 143–157.

Starkweather, C., Gottwald, S., & Halfond, M. (1990). *Stuttering prevention: A clinical method.* Englewood Cliffs, NJ: Prentice-Hall.

Stemberger, J. (1989). Speech errors in early child language production. *Journal of Memory and Language, 28*, 164–188.

Stephenson-Opsal, D., & Bernstein Ratner, N. (1988). Maternal speech rate modification and childhood stuttering. *Journal of Fluency Disorders, 13*, 49–56.

Stocker, B. (1976). *Stocker Probe Technique for diagnosis and treatment of stuttering in young children.* Tulsa, OK: Modern Education Corporation.

Stromsta, C. (1965). A spectrographic study of disfluencies labeled as stuttering by parents. *De therapy voices et loquelae.* Proceedings of the 13th Congress of the International Association of Logopedics and Phoniatrics, Vienna, Austria, Vol. 1: 317–320.

Stromsta, C. (1986). *Elements of stuttering.* Oshtemo, MI: Atsmorts Publishing.

Tanner, D., & Cannon, N. (1978). *Stuttering: Parental Diagnostic Questionnaire.* Tulsa, OK: Modern Education Corporation.

Tate, M., & Cullinan, W. (1962). Measurement of consistency of stuttering. *Journal of Speech and Hearing Research, 5*, 272–283.

Tetnowski, J. A. (1998). Linguistic effects on disfluency. In R. Paul (Ed.), *Exploring the speech-language connection* (Vol 8., pp. 227–247). Paul H. Brookes Publishing Co.

Thielke, H., & Shriberg, L. (1990). Effects of recurrent otitis media on language, speech and educational achievement in Menominee Indian Children. *Journal of American Indian Education*, 25–25.

Thomas, M., & others. (1972). *Free to Be . . . You and Me.* New York: Bell Records.

Thompson, J. (1983). *Assessment of fluency in school-age children.* Resource Guide. Danville, IL: Interstate Printers and Publishers.

Thorndike, E. (1913). *The psychology of learning* (Educational psychology, II). New York: Columbia University's Teacher College.

Thorner, R., & Remein, Q. (1982). Principles and procedures in the evaluation of screening for disease. In J. Chaiklin, I. Ventry, & R. Dixon (Eds.), *Hearing measurement: A book of readings* (4th ed.). Reading, MA: Addison-Wesley Publishing.

Throneburg, R., Yairi, E., & Paden, E. (1994). Relation between phonologic difficulty and the occurrence of disfluencies in the early stages of stuttering. *Journal of Speech and Hearing Research, 37*(3), 504–509.

Thurnes, K., & Caruso, C. (1994). Parents' perceptions of the effects of ear infections on their children's speech-language behavior. *National Student Speech Language Hearing Association Journal, 21*, 65–73.

Tirosh, E., & Cohen, A. (1998). Language deficit with attention-deficit disorder: A prevalent comorbidity. *Journal of Child Neurology, 13*, 493–497.

Travis, L. (1931). *Speech pathology.* New York: Appleton-Century-Crofts.

Turner, P. (1969). *Clinical aspects of autonomic pharmacology.* Philadelphia: Lippincott.

Vaillant, G. (1977). *Adaptation to life.* Boston: Little, Brown.

Van Borsel, J., Van Lierde, K., Van Cauwenberge, P., Guldemont, I., & Van Orshoven, M. (1998). Severe acquired stuttering following injury of the left supplementary motor region: A case report. *Journal of Fluency Disorders, 23*, 49–58.

Van Lieshout, P. (1995). *Motor planning and articulation in fluent speech of stutterers and nonstutterers.* Ph.D. dissertation, University of Nijmegen, Nijmegen, The Netherlands

Van Lieshout, P. H. H. M., Peters, H. F. M., Starkweather, C. W., & Hulstijn, W. (1993). Physiological differences between stutterers and nonstutterers in perceptually fluent speech: EMG amplitude and duration. *Journal of Speech and Hearing Research, 36,* 55–63.

Van Lieshout, P. H. H. M., Starkweather, C. W., Hulstijn, W., & Peters, H. F. M. (1995). The effects of linguistic correlates of stuttering on EMG activity of nonstuttering speakers. *Journal of Speech and Hearing Research, 38,* 36–372.

Van Riper, C. (1954) *Speech correction: Principles and methods* (3rd ed.) Englewood Cliffs, NJ: Prentice-Hall.

Van Riper, C. (1963). *Speech correction: Principles and methods* (4th ed.). Englewood Cliffs, NJ: Prentice-Hall.

Van Riper, C. (1970). Historical approaches, In J. Sheehan (Ed.), *Stuttering: Research and therapy.* New York: Harper & Row.

Van Riper, C. (1971). *The nature of stuttering.* Englewood Cliffs, NJ: Prentice-Hall.

Van Riper, C. (1973). *The treatment of stuttering.* Englewood Cliffs, NJ: Prentice-Hall.

Van Riper, C. (1974). Modification of behavior. In C. Starkweather (Ed.), *Therapy for stutterers.* Memphis, TN: Speech Foundation of America.

Van Riper, C. (1975). The stutterer's clinician. In J. Eisenson (Ed.), *Stuttering: A second symposium.* New York: Harper & Row.

Van Riper, C. (1982). *The nature of stuttering* (2nd ed.). Englewood Cliffs, NJ: Prentice-Hall.

Vanryckeghem, M., & Brutten, G. (1992). The communication attitude test: A reliability investigation. *Journal of Fluency Disorders, 3,* 177–190.

Vanryckeghem, M., & Brutten, G. (1997). The speech-associated attitude of children who do and do not stutter and the differential effect of age. *American Journal of Speech-Language Pathology, 6,* 67–73.

Wall, M., & Myers, F. (1995). Clinical management of childhood stuttering (2nd ed.). Austin, TX: Pro-Ed.

Watkins, R., Yairi, E., & Ambrose, N. (1999). Early childhood stuttering III: Initial status of expressive language abilities. *Journal of Speech Language Hearing Research, 42,* 1125–1135.

Watson, B., & Alphonso, P. (1982). A comparison of LRT and VOT values between stutters and nonstutterers. *Journal of Fluency Disorders, 7,* 219–242.

Watson, B., & Freeman, F. (1997). Brain imaging contributions. In R. Curlee, & G. Siegel (Eds.), *Nature and treatment of stuttering: New directions* (pp. 143–166). Boston: Allyn and Bacon.

Watson, B., Freeman, F., Chapman, S., Miller, S., Finitzo, T., Pool, K., & Devous, M. (1991). Linguistic performance deficits in stutterers: Relation to laryngeal reaction time profiles. *Journal of Fluency Disorders, 16,* 85–100.

Watson, B., Freeman, F., Devous, M., Chapman, S., Finitzo, T., & Pool, K. (1994). Linguistic performance and regional cerebral blood flow in persons who stutter. *Journal of Speech and Hearing Research, 37,* 1221–1228.

Webster, R. (1975). *The Precision Fluency Shaping Program: Clinician's program guide.* Blacksburg, VA: University Publications.

Webster, R. (1978). Empirical considerations regarding stuttering therapy. In H. Gregory (Ed.), *Controversies about stuttering therapy.* Baltimore: University Park Press.

Weiss, A., & Zebrowski, P. (1991). Patterns of assertiveness and responsiveness in parental interactions with stuttering and fluent children. *Journal of Fluency Disorders, 16,* 125–41.

Weiss, A., & Zebrowski, P. (1992). Disfluencies in the conversations of young children who stutter: Some answers to questions. *Journal of Speech and Hearing Research, 35,* 1230–1238.

Weiss, A., & Zebrowski, P. (1994). The narrative productions of children who stutter: A preliminary view. *Journal of Fluency Disorders, 19,* 39–63.

Wells, B., & Moore, W. (1990). EEG alpha asymmetries in stutterers and nonstutterers: Effects of linguistic variables on hemispheric processing and fluency. *Neuropsychologica, 28,* 1295–1305.

Westby, C. (1979). Language performance of stuttering and nonstuttering children. *Journal of Communication Disorders, 12,* 133–145.

Williams, D. E. (1957). A point of view about stuttering. *Journal of Speech Hearing Disorders, 22,* 390–397.

Williams, D. E. (1971). Stuttering therapy for children. In L. E. Travis (Ed.), *Handbook of speech pathology and audiology.* Englewood Cliffs, NJ: Prentice-Hall.

Williams, D. E. (1978). A perspective on approaches to stuttering therapy. In H. Gregory (Ed.), *Controversies about stuttering therapy.* Baltimore: University Park Press.

Williams, D. E. (1985). Talking with children who stutter. In J. Fraser (Ed.), *Counseling stutterers.* Memphis, TN: Stuttering Foundation of America.

Williams, D. E., Melrose, B., & Woods, C. (1969). The relationship between stuttering and academic achievement. *Journal of Communication Disorders, 2,* 87–98.

Williams, D. E., & Kent, L. (1958). Listener evaluations of speech interruptions, *Journal of Speech Hearing Research, 1,* 124–131.

Williams, D. E., & Silverman, F. (1968). Note concerning articulations of school-age stutterers. *Perceptual and Motor Skills, 27,* 713–714.

Williams, D. E., Silverman, F. H., & Kools, J. A. (1968). Disfluency behavior of elementary school stutterers and nonstutterers: The adaptation effect. *Journal of Speech and Hearing Research, 11,* 622–630.

Williams, D. E., Silverman, F., & Kools, J. (1969). Disfluency behavior of elementary-school age stutterers and nonstutterers: The consistency effects, *Journal of Speech and Hearing Research, 12,* 301–307.

Williams, K. (1997). *Expressive Vocabulary Test (EVT).* Circle Pines, MN: American Guidance Services, Inc.

Wingate, M. E. (1964). A standard definition of stuttering. *Journal of Speech Hearing Disorders, 29,* 484–489.

Wingate, M. (1969). Stuttering as a phonetic transition defect. *Journal of Speech and Hearing Disorders, 34,* 107–108.

Wingate, M. E. (1971).The fear of stuttering. *ASHA, 13,* 3–5.

Wingate, M. E. (1976). *Stuttering theory and treatment.* New York: Irvington Publishers.

Wingate, M. E. (1988). *The structure of stuttering: A psycholinguistic analysis.* New York: Springer-Verlag.

Winitz, H. (1961). Repetitions in the vocalizations of children in the first two years of life. *Journal of Speech and Hearing Disorders,* Monogra Supplies, 7, 55–62.

Winn, M. (1977). *The plug-in drug.* New York: Viking.

Wolk, L. (1990). *An investigation of stuttering and phonological difficulties in young children.* Unpublished doctoral dissertation, Syracuse University, Syracuse, NY.

Wolk, L., Edwards, M., & Conture, E. (1993). Coexistence of stuttering and disordered phonology in young children. *Journal of Speech and Hearing Research, 36,* 906–917.

Woods, C. L., & Williams, D. E. (1971). Speech clinicians' conceptions of boys and men who stutter. *Journal of Speech and Hearing Disorders, 36,* 225–234.

Woods, C. L., & Williams, D. E. (1976). Traits attributed to stuttering and normally fluent males. *Journal of Speech and Hearing Research, 19,* 267–278.

Wu, J., Maguire, G., Riley, G., Fallow, J., LaCasse, L., Chin, S., Klein, E., Tang, C., Cadwell, S., & Lottenberg, S. (1995). A positron emission tomography [18F] deoxyglucose study of developmental stuttering. *Neuroreport, 6,* 501–505.

Yairi, E. (1981). Disfluencies of normally speaking two-year old children, *Journal of Speech and Hearing Research, 24,* 490–495.

Yairi, E. (1982). Longitudinal studies of disfluencies in two-year old children, *Journal of Speech and Hearing Research, 25,* 155–160.

Yairi, E. (1993). Epidemiologic and other considerations in treatment efficacy research with preschool-age children who stutter. *Journal of Fluency Disorders, 18,* 197–220.

Yairi, E. (1997a). Disfluency characteristics of childhood stuttering. In R. Curlee & G. Siegel (Eds.), *Nature and treatment of stuttering: New directions* (2nd ed.; pp. 49–78). Boston: Allyn & Bacon.

Yairi, E. (1997b). Home environments and parent-child interaction childhood stuttering. In R. Curlee & G. Siegel (Eds.), *Nature and treatment of stuttering: New directions* (2nd ed.; pp. 3–23). Boston: Allyn & Bacon.

Yairi, E., & Ambrose, N. (1992). A longitudinal study of stuttering in children: A preliminary report. *Journal of Speech and Hearing Research, 35,* 755–760.

Yairi, E., & Ambrose, N. (1999). Early childhood stuttering I: Persistence and recovery rates. *Journal of Speech Language Hearing Research, 42,* 1097–1112.

Yairi, E., Ambrose, N., & Cox, N. (1996). Genetics of stuttering : A critical review. *Journal of Speech Language and Hearing, 39,* 771–784.

Yairi, E., Ambrose, N., & Niermann, B. (1993). The early months of stuttering: A developmental study *Journal of Speech and Hearing Research, 36,* 521–528.

Yairi, E., Ambrose, N., Paden, E., & Throneburg, R. (1996). Predictive factors of persistence and recovery: Pathways of childhood stuttering. *Journal of Communication, 29,* 51–77.

Yairi, E., & Carrico, D. (1992). Early childhood stuttering: Pediatricians' attitudes and practices. *American Journal of Speech-Language Pathology, 1,* 54–62.

Yairi, E., & Clifton, N. F., Jr. (1972). Disfluent speech behavior of preschool children, high school seniors, and geriatric persons. *Journal of Speech Hearing Research, 15* 714–719.

Yairi, E., & Hall, K. (1993). Temporal relations within repetitions of preschool children near the onset of stuttering: A preliminary report. *Journal of Communication Disorders, 26,* 231–244.

Yairi, E., & Jennings, S. (1974). Relationship between the disfluent speech behavior of normal speaking preschool boys and their parents. *Journal of Speech and Hearing Research, 17,* 94–98.

Yairi, E., & Lewis, B. (1984). Disfluencies at the onset of stuttering. *Journal of Speech and Hearing Research, 27,* 154–159.

Yaruss, J. S. (1997a). Clinical implications of situational variability in preschool children who stutter. *Journal of Fluency Disorders, 22,* (3) 187–203.

Yaruss, J. (1997b). Clinical measurement of stuttering behaviors. *Contemporary issues in communication science and disorders, 24,* 33–43.

Yaruss, J. (1998a). Describing the consequences of disorders: Stuttering and the international classification of impairments, disabilities and handicaps. *Journal of Speech, Language and Hearing Research, 41,* 249–257.

Yaruss, J. (1998b). Treatment outcomes in stuttering: Finding value in clinical data. In A. Cordes & R. Ingham (Eds.), *Treatment efficacy for stuttering: A search for empirical bases,* (pp. 213–242). San Diego, CA: Singular Publishing Group.

Yaruss, J. (1999a). Disfluency frequency counter [Computer Software]. Pittsburgh, PA: Author.

Yaruss, J. (1999b). Utterance length, syntactic complexity and childhood stuttering. *Journal of Speech, Language, and Hearing Research, 42,* 329–344.

Yaruss, J. S. (in press). Converting between word and syllable counts in children's conversational speech samples. *Journal of Fluency Disorders.*

Yaruss, J., & Conture, E. (1993). F2 transitions during sound/syllable repetitions of children who stutter and predictions of stuttering chronicity. *Journal of Speech and Hearing Research, 36,* 883–896.

Yaruss, J., & Conture, E. (1995). Mother and child speaking rates and utterance lengths in adjacent fluent utterances: Preliminary observations. *Journal of Fluency Disorders, 20,* 257–278.

Yaruss, J., & Conture, E. (1996). Stuttering and phonological disorders in children: Examination of the covert repair hypothesis. *Journal of Speech and Hearing Science, 39,* 349–364.

Yaruss, J., LaSalle, L., & Conture, E. (1998). Evaluating young children who stutter: Diagnostic data. *American Journal of Speech-Language Pathology, 7,* 62–76.

Yaruss, J., Logan, K., & Conture, E. (1995). Speaking rate and diadochokinetic abilities of children who stutter. In C. W. Starkweather & H. F. M. Peters (Eds.), *Stuttering: Proceedings of the First World Congress on Fluency Disorders* (pp. 283–286) Nijmegen, Netherlands: University Press.

Yaruss, J., Max, M., Newman, R., & Campbell, J. (1998). Comparing real-time and transcript-based techniques for measuring stuttering. *Journal of Fluency Disorders, 23,* (2) 137–151.

Yaruss, S. (1999). Impairment and disability is stuttering: A response to Prins. *Journal of Speech, Language and Hearing Research, 42,* 1397–1399,

Yaruss, S., LaSalle, L., & Conture, E. (2000). Understanding stuttering in children: A response to Cordes. *American Journal of Speech-Language Pathology, 9,* 165–171.

Young, E., & Perachio, J. (1993). *Patterned Elicitation Syntax Test.* Tucson, AZ: Communications Skill Builders.

Young, M. (1984). Identification of stuttering and stutterers. In R. Curlee and W. Perkins (Eds.), *Nature and treatment of stuttering: New directions.* San Diego: CA: College-Hill Press.

Zebrowski, P. (1991). Duration of the speech disfluencies of beginning stutterers. *Journal of Speech and Hearing Research, 34,* 483–491.

Zebrowski, P. (1994). Duration of sound prolongations and sound/syllable repetition in children who stutter: Preliminary observations. *Journal of Speech and Hearing Research, 2,* 254–263.

Zebrowski, P., & Conture, E. (1989). Judgments of disfluency by mothers of stuttering and normally fluent children. *Journal of Speech and Hearing Research, 32,* 625–634.

Zebrowski, P., & Conture, E. (1998). Influence of non-treatment variables on treatment effectiveness for school-age children who stutter. In A. Cordes & R. Ingham (Eds.), *Treatment efficacy for stuttering: A search for empirical bases.* San Diego, CA: Singular Publishing Group.

Zebrowski, P., Conture, E., & Cudahy, E. (1985). Acoustic analysis of young stutterers' fluency, *Journal of Fluency Disorders, 10,* 173–192.

Zilbergeld, B., & Evans, M. (1980). The inadequacy of Masters and Johnson. *Psychology Today, 14,* 28–43.

Zimmerman, G. (1980a). Articulatory dynamics of fluent utterances of stutterers and nonstutterers. *Journal of Speech Hearing Research, 23,* 108–121.

Zimmerman, G. (1980b). Articulatory behaviors associated with stuttering: Cinefluorographic analysis. *Journal of Speech and Hearing Research, 23,* 95–107.

Zimmerman, J., Steiner, V., & Pond, R. (1979). *Preschool Language Scale Revised Edition.* Columbus, OH: Charles E. Merrill Co.

Zwitman, D. (1978). *The disfluent child.* Baltimore: University Park Press.

AUTHOR INDEX

Abbs, J., 53, 312

Abwender, D., 107

Ackermann, H., 19, 286

Adams, L.H., 100, 101, 162

Adams, M.R., 10, 26, 31, 32, 59, 79, 99, 162, 181,
241, 266, 269, 347, 353

Adkins, C., 174, 175, 176, 177

Agnello, J., 347

Ainsworth, S., 134, 235

Alphonso, P., 347

Ambrose, N.G., 5, 13, 14, 15, 21, 25, 28, 38, 54, 70,
81, 87, 89, 90, 91, 129, 136, 154, 155, 158, 159,
258, 328, 339, 349, 351, 356, 357, 370

Ames, L., 153

Amster, B., 148, 340, 352

Anderson, J., 25, 98, 259

Andrews, C., 334

Andrews, G., 24, 25, 78, 81, 86, 113, 181, 343, 348

Aram, D., 98

Armson, J., 372

Arnson, J., 337, 361, 363

Ashworth, M., 328

Ask, J., 174, 175, 176, 177

Atal, B., 343

Atkins, C., 308

Au-Yeung, J., 18, 31, 38, 111, 223

Axline, V.M., 151

Baer, T., 99

Bahill, T., 92, 153

Bailey, A., 167

Bailey, W., 167

Bain, B., 131

Baker, K., 375

Baker, L., 158, 159

Bakker, K., 83, 104

Bates, E., 181

Baumgaertel, A., 105, 106

Baumgartner, J., 286

Beattie, M., 90, 313

Beech, H., 285

Beecher, H.K., 253

Beitchman, J., 71, 93, 158

Beiter, A., 103

Bell, J., 53, 362, 372

Bennett, E., 143, 287, 350, 370

Benson, H., 212, 253, 273

Berg, C., 107

Berg, T., 337n

Bernstein Ratner, N., 20, 25, 32, 37, 96, 97, 157, 181,
328, 337, 345, 354, 355, 368

Bettleheim, B., 148, 178

Bien, S., 19, 286

Bingham, J., 378

Bishop, J., 375

Bitzer, M., 19, 286

Blackmer, E., 337n

Blomgren, M., 100, 362, 366

Blood, G., 2

Bloodstein, O., 3, 15, 23, 24, 25, 26, 27, 30, 89, 93,
100, 129, 136, 150, 161, 166, 173, 222, 235, 267,
274, 285, 340, 345, 365

Boberg, E., 320, 357

Bock, J., 355

Bock, K., 355

Boehmler, R., 8, 11

Boone, D., 81, 102

Borden, G., 99

Bosshardt, H-G., 25, 104, 372

Botterill, W., 134, 167, 350

Bouwen, J., 287

Boves, L., 13, 246, 273, 337, 372

Bower, G., 298

Brady, J., 367

Brayton, E., 166

Brazelton, T., 153

Bredart, S., 337n

Brewer, D., 99, 100, 194, 240, 264, 337

Brown, R., 157

Brown, S., 147, 160, 167

Brutten, G., 15, 72, 79, 81, 92, 104, 197, 237, 334,
336

Buder, E., 62

Burger, R., 337, 345

Burnett, M., 56

Burns, D., 288, 342

Burton, E., 343
Buss, A., 115, 137
Butterworth, B., 357

Cadwell, S., 357
Camarata, S., 351
Campbell, J., 12, 81
Campbell, K., 186
Canning, B., 109
Cannon, N., 69
Canter, G. 109
Cantwell, D., 158, 159
Carey, W., 117, 352
Carlisle, J., 373
Carrico, D., 135
Caruso, A., 53, 59, 92, 96, 102, 111, 134, 180, 240,
    312, 328, 337, 343, 347, 362, 363
Caruso, C., 103
Chang, J., 343
Chang, S., 362, 366
Chapman, S., 157, 336
Chen, Y., 100
Chess, S., 115, 137
Chester, S., 16
Childers, D., 102, 269
Chin, S., 357
Clark, H., 337n
Clegg, M., 71, 93, 158
Clifton, N.F., Jr., 14
Cohen, A., 351
Colburn, N., 355
Collins, M., 286
Colton, R., 53, 102, 240, 269, 337, 343, 362, 363
Como, P., 107
Conture, E., 2, 5, 6, 8, 9, 10, 11, 15, 16, 20, 23, 25, 38,
    42, 44, 45, 46, 49, 50, 52, 53, 54, 56, 59, 60, 72,
    79, 86, 87, 88, 89, 90, 92, 93, 94, 95, 96, 97, 98,
    99, 100, 102, 104, 109, 111, 115, 121, 122, 133,
    134, 135, 137, 139, 143, 144, 145, 148, 155, 156,
    157, 158, 159, 160, 162, 166, 167, 168, 174, 175,
    176, 177, 180, 181, 186, 187, 188, 194, 210, 215,
    216, 222, 223, 224, 240, 241, 259, 264, 266, 269,
    308, 319, 328, 336, 337, 340, 342, 343, 345, 347,
    349, 350, 352, 356, 357, 362, 363, 366, 367, 369,
    370, 371, 373, 377
Cook, F., 218, 224, 254, 259, 260
Cooke, P., 365
Cooper, C., 370
Cooper, E.B., 134, 148, 241, 311, 370

Cordes, A., 6, 7, 8, 121, 274, 342, 367, 370, 377
Costa, L., 334
Costello Ingham, J., 174
Costello, D., 186
Costello, J., 59, 334
Cotton, J., 357, 358
Cox, N., 21, 28, 38, 70, 136, 137, 339
Craig, A., 24, 25, 113, 181, 186, 348
Cudahy, E., 347, 366
Culatta, R., 59
Cullinan, W., 89, 347
Curlee, R., 2, 5, 6, 8, 31, 33, 34, 59, 92, 153, 345, 355,
    362
Curtis, J., 147, 160, 167
Cutler, J., 72, 81, 113
Czikszentmihalyi, M., 248

Daly, D., 56, 124, 158, 159, 350
Darley, F., 15, 59, 79, 86, 89, 92, 258, 274
Davis, D.M., 14
DeFries, J., 339
Dell, C.W., 161
Dell, G., 35, 354, 355
Dembrowski, J., 241
DeNil, L., 72, 79, 81, 92, 241, 311, 345, 357
Denny, M., 240, 328, 337, 363
Devous, M., 157, 336, 357
DiSimoni, F., 337
Dodson, F., 153, 184
Doehring, D.G., 369
Douglas, E., 124, 257
Downs, H., 357
Dronkers, N., 359
Dykman, R., 109, 110

Eckel, F., 81, 102
Edney, C., 147, 160, 167
Edwards, M.L., 25, 71, 92, 93, 94, 95, 97, 121, 135,
    156, 158, 160, 259, 356, 357
Egolf, D., 16, 240, 254
Ekman, P., 90
Ellis, G., 113
Epstein, M.D., 253
Erickson, R.L., 72
Evans, M., 341

Faircloth, M., 338
Faircloth, S., 338
Fallow, J., 357

Farmer, A., 166
Feldstein, S., 122
Felsenfeld, S., 21, 28, 115, 136
Feyer, A., 24, 25, 181, 348
Fincher, J., 357
Finitzo, T., 157, 336, 357
Finn, P., 342n, 351, 370, 372
First, M., 107, 114
FitzSimons, R., 151
Flament, M., 107
Fletcher, S., 109
Florance, C., 371
Fluharty, N., 96
Flynn, P.T., 67, 68, 70, 75
Fosnot, S., 342
Foundas, A., 357
Fox, P., 357, 358, 359
Frances, A., 107, 114
Frank, P., 7, 8
Franken, M.C., 13, 246, 273, 372
Franklin, J., 113
Fransella, F., 285
Fransen, H., 371
Fraser, J., 134, 148, 216, 224, 235
Freeman, F., 46, 99, 157, 240, 269, 336, 337, 357
Fristoe, M., 94, 160
Fudala, J., 94

Gaines, N., 157, 354
Gay, C., 359
German, D., 111
Gibson, T., 351
Gilbert, H., 347
Gilmore, G., 186
Ginott, H., 224, 254, 257, 270
Gladwell, M., 254
Glasner, P., 340, 352
Glass, T., 357
Gleason, J., 337
Glenn, K., 7, 8, 240
Goldberg, S., 59, 376
Goldman, R., 94, 160
Goldsmith, H., 115, 137
Gordon, P., 59, 329
Gottwald, S., 31, 32, 181, 370
Goyer, R., 67
Gracco, V., 53, 312
Gray, M., 150

Gregory, C., 135
Gregory, H., 135, 228, 294, 322, 368
Gronhond, K., 72
Grossman, F., 113
Guitar, B., 24, 37, 59, 72, 115, 121, 134, 136, 148, 188, 215, 216, 218, 224, 238, 240, 241, 245, 252, 254, 266, 288, 305, 315, 322, 323, 328, 334, 338, 340, 342, 343, 345, 352, 353, 369, 371, 372
Guitar, C., 343
Guldemont, I., 19
Guyton, A., 197

Halfond, M., 370
Hall, E., 160, 228, 229, 232
Hall, K., 88
Hall, N., 98
Ham, R., 59, 86, 224, 323
Hamilton, A., 240
Hammill, D., 96
Hancock, K., 186
Hanson, B., 72
Hardy, J., 108, 109
Haroldson, S., 13, 181, 274, 334
Harrington, J., 365
Harris, R., 100
Harris, T., 130
Harrison, E., 334, 343
Havinga, J., 355
Hayhow, R., 59
Haynes, W., 61, 66, 75, 329
Healey, C., 100, 101, 162
Healey, E.C., 113, 347
Helm-Estabrooks, N., 286
Henley, E., 345
Hertrich, I., 19, 286
Hilgard, E., 298
Hill, D., 177, 228, 353
Hill, W.F., 16
Hillman, R., 347
Hilton, L., 100
Hinde, R., 115, 137
Hinzman, A., 71, 93, 99, 159
Hirsch, T., 357
Hixon, T., 109
Hoddinott, A., 24, 25, 181, 348
Horowitz, N., 357
Houle, S., 357
Howell, P., 7, 8, 18, 31, 38, 111, 157, 223, 240, 365
Howie, P., 24, 25, 70, 181, 348

Hresko, W., 96
Hubbard, C., 334
Hull, F., 71, 93, 158
Hulstijn, W., 328, 329, 343, 360
Hunt, J., 364
Hutchinson, J., 240, 364
Hymes, E., 107

Ilg, F., 153
Ingham, J.C., 2, 7, 8, 147, 174, 334, 357, 358, 367, 372
Ingham, R., 6, 7, 8, 59, 72, 86, 129, 274, 294, 334, 337, 342, 357, 358, 363, 367, 369, 370, 372, 377

Jaeger, J., 337n
Jaffe, J., 122
Jakubowski, P., 220
Janssen, P., 104
Jenkins, M., 43
Jennings, S., 14
Jerabek, P., 357, 358
Jezer, M., 131, 373
Johnson, L., 53, 362
Johnson, V., 341
Johnson, W., 9, 10, 14, 15, 28, 59, 79, 86, 89, 92, 134, 135, 147, 150, 151, 160, 167, 206, 248, 258, 274, 348, 373, 378
Jones, K., 107
Juliano, C., 35

Kadi-Hanifi, K., 157
Kagan, J., 115, 136, 338, 352
Kail, R., 111
Kalinowski, J., 337, 361, 363
Kalinowski, S., 372
Kapur, S., 357
Karniol, R., 31, 355
Keaster, J., 147, 160, 167
Kelly, E., 15, 16, 29, 31, 32, 49, 52, 54, 56, 72, 79, 89, 122, 134, 135, 139, 166, 167, 168, 240, 308, 328, 337, 345, 350, 363, 375, 376
Kelman, E., 134, 167, 350
Kenney, M., 99
Kent, L., 8, 11
Kent, R., 31, 33, 34, 62, 355, 362, 366
Kidd, K., 21, 28, 136
Klee, T., 109
Klein, E., 357

Kolk, H., 31, 33, 35, 36, 37, 38, 40, 41, 42, 44, 45, 337, 354, 355, 356
Kools, J.A., 14, 81
Kosinski, J., 225
Kraaimaat, F., 104
Krasuski, J., 357
Krause, R., 15, 89
Krieger, S., 162
Krishnamurthy, A., 102, 269
Krizizke, J., 375
Kroll, R., 357
Krupski, A., 105
Kryiacoupoulos, A., 240
Kully, D., 224, 287
Kurlan, R., 107
Kurlansky, M., 59, 369
Kwiatkowski, J., 103

LaCasse, L., 357
Lancaster, J., 357
Lange, A., 220
Langevin, M., 224, 287
Larar, J., 102
LaSalle, L., 9, 15, 54, 86, 89, 92, 99, 109, 121, 122, 139, 143, 144, 155, 186, 308, 354, 369
Le Shan, E., 123, 135, 151
LeFrancois, G., 16
Leith, W., 19
Leonard, L., 111
Levelt, W.J.M., 29, 309, 338, 354, 355, 356
Lewis, B., 14, 79, 87
Lewis, S., 7
Lincoln, M., 334, 341, 343, 370
Liotti, M., 359
Logan, K., 20, 25, 109, 112, 157, 181, 354, 377
Lohr, F., 15, 56, 89
Lokken, M., 43
Lottenberg, S., 357
Louko, L., 25, 44, 71, 92, 93, 94, 95, 97, 121, 135, 155, 156, 159, 160, 259, 328, 356, 357
Lubker, B.B., 369
Luper, H., 59, 134, 329
Lybolt, J., 343, 377

MacDonald, J., 7
MacKay, D., 31, 33, 34
Maguire, G., 357
Mahr, G., 19

Mahshie, J., 269
Main, V., 111
Manning, W., 323, 372, 373
Mansson, H., 327
Martin, C., 357, 358
Martin, J., 375
Martin, R., 7, 13, 181, 274, 334
Martyn, M., 129
Masters, W., 341
Mastrud, B., 218
Matthews, M., 343
Matthies, M., 103
Max, L., 328, 337
Max, M., 12, 81
McCall, G., 99, 100, 194, 240, 264, 337
McCall, R., 115, 137
McCallie, D., 212, 253
McCaul, A., 186
McClowry, M., 328, 337
McCready, C., 186
McDevitt, S., 117, 352
McDonald, E., 207
McDonald, M., 31, 33, 34
McDowell, E., 159
McGregor, K., 111
McNight, R., 347
Melnick, K., 52, 115, 134, 135, 143, 144, 157, 166,
        167, 168, 181, 210, 216, 345, 349, 350, 352, 370
Melrose, B., 25, 89
Merits-Patterson, R., 97, 157
Messert, B., 286
Metz, D., 14, 162, 243, 343, 347, 365, 367, 372, 377
Meyer, A., 29, 309, 338, 354, 355, 356
Meyers, S., 46, 157, 354
Mielke, P., 71, 93, 158
Miller, N., 254
Miller, S., 157
Mitton, J., 337n
Molitor, R., 99, 102, 162, 269, 362, 366
Montgomery, A., 362, 363, 365
Moore, G., 102
Moore, W.H., Jr., 357, 358
Morley, M., 159
Mulder, R., 134
Murphy, A., 151
Murray, C., 328
Murray, H., 25, 157
Mutti, M., 81, 110

Myers, F., 31, 59, 134
Mysak, E., 355

Naik, J., 102
Nair, R., 71, 93, 158
Nandyal, I., 104
Neelley, J., 89
Neill, A., 152
Neilson, M., 24, 25, 102, 181, 287, 288, 348
Neilson, P., 102, 181, 343
Netsell, R., 197
Newcomer, P., 96
Newman, P., 100
Newman, R., 12, 81
Niebuhr, R., 378
Niermann, B., 5, 14, 15, 54, 89, 90, 91, 129, 154
Nippold, M., 25, 93, 156, 356
Noble, S., 372
Novak, M., 103

O'Dwyer, T., 343
Ogburn, R.S., 243, 343, 377
Ohde, R., 362, 366
Olswang, L., 131
Onslow, M., 134, 216, 334, 341, 342, 343, 345, 369,
        370, 372
Onufrak, J., 243, 343, 377
Orton, S., 357
Oyler, M.E., 24, 81, 115, 136, 340, 352

Packman, A., 134, 216, 345, 369
Paden, E., 25, 87, 88, 93, 103, 156, 158, 159, 258,
        328, 349, 351, 356, 357
Parlour, S., 181, 274
Patel, P., 71, 94, 158
Pechman, T., 355
Pellowski, M., 174, 175, 176, 177, 187, 223, 259
Perachio, J., 128
Perkins, W.H., 31, 33, 34, 53, 224, 274, 341, 355,
        362
Peters, H.F.M., 328, 329, 337, 343, 360, 363
Peters, J., 109, 110
Peters, T., 72
Pilgrim, L., 111, 223
Pincus, H., 107, 114
Pindzola, R., 43, 59, 61, 66, 75, 329, 347
Plomin, R., 115, 137, 339
Pond, R., 96

Pool, K., 157, 336, 357
Postma, A., 31, 33, 34, 35, 36, 37, 38, 40, 41, 42, 44, 45, 337, 354, 355, 356
Povel, D-J., 38, 337
Preus, A., 56, 166, 336, 350
Price, H., 343, 377
Prins, D., 5, 15, 56, 69, 89, 111, 124, 212, 236, 371
Prosek, R., 362, 363, 372
Purser, H., 28, 115, 350, 352

Quarrington, R., 124, 257

Ragsdale, J., 93
Ramig, P., 24, 81, 115, 136, 143, 162, 287, 340, 347, 350, 352, 370
Rapoport, J., 107
Ratner, N., 328
Read, C., 62
Reading, S., 67
Reed, C., 25, 97, 157
Rees, N., 181
Reid, D., 96
Remein, Q., 10, 11
Reznick, J., 338
Rice, P., 72
Rickenberg, H., 109
Rickey, J., 67
Rieber, R.W., 27, 260
Riley, G., 13, 15, 43, 71, 79, 86, 92, 105, 109, 121, 158, 159, 174, 222, 357
Riley, J., 2, 43, 71, 105, 109, 121, 147, 158, 159, 174, 357, 366, 367
Rivera, N., 375
Robb, M., 101, 343, 362, 366, 377
Robbins, J., 109
Robinson, F., 276
Roelofs, A., 29, 276, 309, 338, 354, 355, 356
Romine, J., 109, 110
Roos, J., 174, 175, 176, 177
Rose, M., 109
Rosenbek, J., 286
Rothbart, M., 115, 137
Rothenberg, M., 99, 102, 153, 162, 269, 362, 366
Rudas, J., 53, 362
Rue, S., 334
Rumsey, J., 357
Runyan, C., 157, 350, 354, 372
Runyan, S., 350

Rustin, L., 115, 134, 167, 218, 224, 254, 259, 260, 350, 352
Ryan, B., 43, 93, 156, 157, 159, 232, 334

Sacco, P., 162, 243, 343, 365, 372, 377
Sackin, S., 7, 8, 18, 31, 111, 240
Samar, V., 243, 343, 365, 377
Schiavetti, N., 8, 11, 14, 343, 367, 372, 377
Schindler, M., 159
Schriefers, H., 355
Schum, R., 61
Schwartz, H.D., 15, 56, 72, 86, 89, 90, 99, 100, 113, 194, 218, 219, 224, 232, 240, 246, 252, 264, 336, 337, 350
Secord, W., 96
Semel, E., 96
Shames, G., 232, 240, 254, 334, 371
Shapiro, A., 240, 253
Shapiro, D., 59, 224, 323
Shaywitz, B., 105, 108
Shaywitz, S., 105, 108
Sheehan, J., 16, 111, 129, 243, 254, 274
Sherrick, C., 232, 334
Shoemaker, D., 15, 72, 197, 237, 334, 336
Shriberg, L., 61, 94, 103
Siegel, G., 297, 334, 345, 370
Sih, C., 20, 157, 354, 355
Silverman, F., 14, 20, 24, 71, 81, 158, 159, 181
Sisterhen, D., 93
Skinner, B.F., 16
Smith, A., 27, 29, 31, 32, 54, 56, 103, 235, 240, 328, 337, 345, 350, 363
Snidman, N., 115, 338
Sochurek, H., 357
Sommers, R., 167
Spaulding, N., 81, 110
Spence, R., 218, 224, 254, 259, 260
Spock, B., 153
Spriesterbach, D., 15, 59, 79, 86, 89, 92, 258, 274
St. Louis, K., 71, 93, 99, 159, 328
St. Onge, K., 336
Starbuck, H., 69, 212, 236
Starkweather, C.W., 31, 32, 55, 58, 181, 310, 328, 329, 334, 343, 360, 363, 370
Stealy, J., 375
Steiner, V., 96
Stemberger, J., 337n
Stephens-Opsal, D., 368
Sterling, H., 81, 110

Stettler, D., 375
Stocker, B., 79, 92, 180, 274
Stromsta, C., 336, 365
Stuart, A., 372

Tang, C., 357
Tanner, D., 69
Tate, M., 89
Tetnowski, J.A., 25, 97
Thielke, H., 103
Thomas, A., 115, 137
Thomas, M., 73, 153, 180
Thompson, J., 69, 71, 158, 159, 274
Thorndike, E., 332
Thorner, R., 10, 11
Throneburg, R., 25, 87, 88, 156, 159, 349, 351
Thurnes, K., 103
Timmons, R., 71, 89, 93, 158
Tirosh, E., 351
Tomblin, E., 369
Travis, L., 357
Triden, K., 13
Trinidad, K., 107
Tukey, J., 343
Turner, P., 197

Ushijima, T., 240, 337

Vaillant, G., 113, 306, 319
van Bezooijen, R., 13, 246, 273, 372
Van Borsel, J., 19
Van Cauwenberge, P., 19
van der Meulen, S., 104
Van Kirk Ryan, B., 334
Van Lierde, K., 19
Van Lieshout, P.H.H.M., 343, 360, 363, 377
van Naerssen, E., 104
Van Orshoven, M., 19
Van Riper, C., 22, 33, 54, 61, 113, 130, 133, 134, 143,
    151, 156, 160, 180, 183, 208, 212, 228, 232, 236,
    243, 260, 266, 274, 280, 298, 310, 315, 336, 337,
    345, 350, 362
Vanryckeghem, M., 72
Vause, L., 365
Vorberg, D., 355

Walden, B., 362, 363
Wall, M., 31, 59, 134
Wampler, S., 111

Wasow, T., 337n
Watson, B., 157, 241, 336, 347, 357
Weber, C., 27
Webster, R., 243, 307, 371
Weiss, A., 157, 182, 354
Wells, B., 358
Wertz, R., 286
Wheeldon, L., 338, 355
White, D., 59
Wiig, E., 96
Wijnen, F., 337, 345
Willeford, J., 71, 93, 158
Williams, D.E., 8, 11, 14, 25, 50, 59, 71, 81, 89, 134,
    141, 142, 148, 158, 159, 179, 205, 208, 225, 227,
    240, 243, 245, 284, 306, 320, 340
Williams, K., 97, 128
Williams, M., 365
Wingate, M.E., 3, 31, 33, 34, 37, 97, 103, 110, 225,
    304, 315, 337, 347, 354, 364, 365
Winitz, H., 14
Winn, M., 185, 233
Wolk, L., 42, 43, 81, 110, 156, 342
Wollock, J., 27
Wolraich, M., 105, 106
Woods, C.L., 25, 50, 89, 284
Wu, J., 357

Yairi, E., 2, 9, 11, 13, 14, 21, 25, 26, 28, 38, 57, 70,
    79, 81, 83, 84, 85, 87, 88, 91, 93, 122, 135, 136,
    139, 143, 154, 155, 156, 158, 159, 186, 258, 328,
    339, 348, 349, 351, 356, 357, 369, 377
Yamashita, T., 98
Yaruss, J.S., 5, 9, 12, 20, 25, 38, 42, 44, 45, 49, 54, 79,
    81, 86, 87, 88, 92, 99, 109, 112, 121, 122, 139,
    143, 144, 146, 156, 186, 222, 229, 240, 274, 287,
    288, 337, 350, 354, 363, 367, 370, 373, 377
Yaruss, S., 59
Young, E., 128
Young, M., 85, 225

Zamarripa, F., 357, 358
Zebrowski, P., 6, 8, 15, 59, 79, 87, 89, 115, 137, 157,
    182, 340, 347, 352, 354, 366
Ziegler, W., 19, 286
Zilbergeld, B., 341
Zimmerman, G., 240, 362, 363
Zimmerman, J., 96
Zwitman, D., 69, 134, 233

SUBJECT INDEX

ABCs of stuttering, 287–289, 370

Activity, 115

Age grouping for therapy, young children, 144–145

Air pressure *vs.* muscle tension, 197

Air stoppers, 195–197

Analogies
assembly-line, 40–41
barrel bridge, 200, 202
blown-up balloon, 199–200
closed-fist-to-relaxed-hand, 201–205
cursive writing, 208–210
garden hose, 193–198
jumping into swimming pool, 191–192
lily pad, 200, 201
log jam, 196–198
out of sight, out of mind, 189–190
skier *vs.* pogo stick, 267–268
thumb and opposing fingers, 200–201, 203
touching hot stove burner, 192–193
what has to be changed, 268–269

Arizona Articulation Proficiency Scale, 94

Articulation disordered, 93

Articulation/phonological behavior of children who
stutter, 93–96

Articulation problem, presence of, 158–160

Assembly-line analogy, 40–41

Assessment and evaluation, 59–128
basic beliefs, 60
components of evaluation, 64–78
assessment, 78–118
intake form, 65–66
interview procedure, 66–78
written report, 65
equipment, 62–64
audio recordings, 62–63
video recordings, 63–64
examiner, examining the, 60–61
facilities, 61–62
informed consent; client's right-to-know, 64
perspective of client's unique circumstances, 60
referral to therapy, 118–125

Attention Deficit Disorder (ADD), 351

Attention Deficit Hyperactivity Disorder (ADHD),
105–107, 277–278, 351–352

Audio recordings, 62–63
child's reaction to, 206–207
microphone placement, 62

"Barbs" or fluency inhibitors, 230–231

Barrel bridge analogy, 200, 202

Basal fluency level, 229

Behavioral Style Questionnaire (BSQ), 117, 352

Behavior modification, 334

Beta phase, 87

Bidirectional
communication, 17–18
conversational speech, 46

Blown-up balloon analogy, 199–200

Brown's stage IV, 157

Carryover, 271–273, 313–315
problems, 341–342

Cessation disfluencies, 222

Change, 14–15, 344–345

Charlatans, 262

Children's Attitudes Towards Talking-Revised, 91

Closed-fist-to-relaxed-hand analogy, 201–205

Clinical Evaluation of Language Fundamentals-3,
Screening Test, 96

Comcomitant speech and language problems of people
who stutter, 356–357

Common thread approach, 322, 376

Communicative and related behaviors, assessing,
78–118
academic ability and status, 104–105
Attention Deficit Hyperactivity Disorder (ADHD),
105–107
expressive/receptive language
syntax, 96–97
vocabulary, 97–99
comparable vocabulary and language scores,
98
vocabulary higher than language scores, 98
vocabulary lower than language scores, 98
fluency, 78–92
consistency of disfluency, 89–90
disfluency types, 86–88
duration of disfluency, 87–89

Communicative and related behaviors, fluency, (continued)
  frequency of stuttering, 79–84
  noticeable nonspeech behaviors, 91–92
  number and variety of associated nonspeech behaviors, 90–91
  sample size, 85
  stuttered words *vs.* syllables, 85–86
  hearing, 102–103
  (in)formal testing of stuttering, 92–96
  neuromotor speech and nonspeech behavior, 108–110
    diadochokinesis (alternating motion rate), 108–109
    screening tests for neuromotor functioning, 110
    stuttering on DDK, naming, or single-word responses, 110
  psychosocial adjustment, 111–115
    concerns that may hinder speech therapy, 112–113
    issues that warrant concerns to mental health professionals, 113–114
    motivation, 112
    oppositional-defiant behavior, 114–115
  reading, 103–104
  temperament, 115–118
  Tourette's syndrome, 107–108
  voice, 99–102
    hyperfunctional voice usage, 101–102
    jitter, shimmer, and formant frequency fluctuations, 100
    variations in fundamental frequency, 100
  word finding, 110–111
Conversation, changing speech in, 315–316
Cortical activity and structure of people who stutter, 357–360
Covert repair hypothesis, 35–37
Cursive writing analogy, 208–210

Demands and capacities model, 32
Desensitization, 228–235
Diadochokinesis, 108–110
Diagnostic report for child who stutters, example, 391–404
Differences in people and behavior
  recognizing, 51–53
  tolerating, 53–55
Disfluencies, examples of, table, 6
Dismissing from therapy, 318–320

Down syndrome, 166
Dyssynchronous syllable frames and segment content model, 34–35

"Effortless-avoidance" continuum, 12–13
Electroencephalograph (EEG), 358
Electroglottograph (EGG), 102, 296
Emotionality, 115
  levels of in adults who stutter, 284–285
Empathy, 130
  problem-specific, 131–133
Employment, the teenager who stutters and, 275–276
Enthusiasm for changing people and behavior, 55
Equatorial/interactionist apporach, 339–340
Error
  false negative, 10
  false positive, 10
Evaluation, as precedent to remediation, 329–331
Expressive/receptive language, 96–99
  syntax, 96–97
  vocabulary, 97–99
Expressive Vocabulary Test (EVT), 97, 128

Family physician, maintaining contact with, 278
Fault line hypothesis, 34
Flexibility, 130
Fluency, assessment of, 78–96
Fluency "stress test," 273–274
Fluharty Preschool Speech and Language Screening Test, 96
Forward movement, 198–202, 207–208
Frequency of disfluency, 9–10
Functional magnetic resonance imaging (fMRI), 358
Fundamental frequency, 100
Future directions, 344–374
  general considerations, 344–348
    advancing by small increments, 346–347
    change, the one constant, 344–345
    importance of replication, 347–348
    information, effects of, 345–346
  opportunities, 348–374
    Attention Deficit Hyperactivity Disorder (ADHD), 351–352
    children, 348–350
    concomitant speech and language problems, 356–357
    cortical activity and structure, 357–360
    linguistic activities and syntactic, semantic, and phonological encoding, 354–356

naturalness, suitability, and utility of speech, 371–372

self-help organizations, 372–374

subgroups, 350–351

temperament, 352–354

temporal coordination of tongue and jaw movements during speech, 360–364

transitions, 364–366

treatment efficacy, 366–371

Gamma phase, 87

Garden hose analogy, 193–198

Generalizations about stuttering, 17–22

Genuineness, 130

Goldman-Fristoe Test of Articulation (GFTA), 94, 159, 160

Group therapy, adult, 289–292

Habituated speech, 257

Hard and easy speech, 178–180, 227

Hearing, 102–103

Homework, adult, 316–317

Identification, 237–239, 331–334

analogies, use of, 237–238

child's desire for "passive" cure, 239

clinician's ability to identify, 332–333

doing it "to" clients *vs.* clients doing "for" themselves, 333–334

identifying doesn't take place of modification, 333

imitation *vs.* mocking, 238

importance of physically feeling behavior, 331–332

problem sounds, 237

unnecessary emphasis on nonspeech behavior, 238–239

Inattentive listeners, as fluency inhibitor, 231–232

Individual differences in ability to communicate, 53

Individual therapy, adult, 292–322

Information, effects of, 345–346

Informed consent; client's right-to-know, 64

Ingredient-specific (I-S) models of stuttering, 30–33

table, 31

Insurance reimbursement, 375

Interaction of psyche and soma, 339–340

Interiorizing of stuttering, 256

Interview procedure, issues and concerns, 75–78

common listening problems, 75–76

deductive reasoning, 77

following up on questions, 76–77

inductive reasoning, 77–78

listening to and following up on answers, 76

Interview questions for parent(s) of disfluent child, 379–382

Iowa Scale for Rating the Severity of Stuttering, 15, 79, 91, 92

Jumping into swimming pool analogy, 191–192

Larynx, 99

as articulator, 99

as phonatory vibrator, 99

Learning disability (LD), 277–278

Lemma, or syntactic word, 29

Leyton Obsessional Inventory-Child Version, 107

Lidcombe program, 334, 343

Lily pad analogy, 198–200

Listener judgments, role of, 7

Listening, 130

Log jam analogy, 196–198

Maintenance/followup therapy, adults, 320–322

Mean length of utterance (MLU), 96

Measuring stuttering, 8–15

change as a constant, 14–15

"effortless-avoidance" continuum, 12–13

frequency of disfluency, 9–10

norms, 13–14

type of speech disfluency, 10–12

Mechanism-specific (M-S) models, 33–38

table, 31

Mental health professionals, referral to, 113–114

Mental whiteout, 132–133

Minimal brain dysfunction (MBD), 108

Mismatches

nature-nurture interaction, 46–48

people who stutter and environments, 45–46

time, 37–38, 38–48

Mistakes observed during diagnostic, ten common, 401–403

Modification, 240–253, 334–340

appropriate use of placebo effect, 253

behavior modification, 334

changes in time and tension, 243–244

changing speech postures, 246–247

collaborative efforts between public schools and clinics, 250–251

counting behavior, 240

(dis)continuing therapy, 252–253

Modification (*continued*)
  engaged parents, 251
  getting "unstuck," 244
  I forgot to practice, 249
  inability to make change, 245–246
  modeling change, 246
  need to speak, 247–248
  parental observation, 251–252
  parents' role, 250
  physical tension levels, 241–242
  practice, 248–249
  present modification doesn't guarantee future suc-
      cess, 334–336
  psyche, soma, and interaction, 339–340
  spoken *vs.* orthographic behavior, 338–339
  stuttered speech production, some facts, 337–338
  tension during speech production, 242
  typical improvements, 240–241
  whiteout, 245
  working from simple to complex, 338
Motivation, 112, 236
Multifactorial model, 32–33

Naturalness, suitability, and utility of speech, 371–372
Nature-nurture interaction, 376
Nature *vs.* nurture, 136–138
Nonspeech behaviors, 15–16, 91–92
Nonverbal behavior
  interacting with peers, older children and teenagers,
      233–234
Norms to establish whether a person stutters, 13–14
Note to beginning speech-language pathologist,
      383–389
Number of units of repetition per sound/syllable repe-
      tition, 88

Objective behavioral descriptions, 50
Obsessive-compulsive behavior (OCB), 107
Off-line analysis, 298
On-line analysis, 298
Oppositional-defiant behavior, 114–115
Oral Motor Assessment Scale, 109
Orthographic behavior, spoken behavior *vs.*, 338–339
Out of sight, out of mind analogy, 189–190

Parallel process, 15
Parental guilt, 151
Parent-child communication behavior, relationships,
      49

Parent/child fluency group, 167–177
  changing speech-prodcution behavior, 170–171
  child's group, 169–170
  grouping by age, 168
  logistics, 168
  maintenance therapy, 173
  means of changing pragmatic skills, 171–172
  parents' group, 172–173
  pragmatic difficulties, typical, 171
  preliminary treatment outcome data, 173–177
  reason for changing pragmatic behaviors, 171
Parents of older child and teenager, understanding,
      219–220
Parents' reading to children, 182–185
Patterned Elicitation Syntax Test (PEST), 128
Peabody Picture Vocabulary Test (PPVT-III), 97, 207
People who stutter, characteristics of, 23–26
  frequency, 25
  intelligence, 24
  personality, 24–25
  predictability, 25
  psychosocial adjustment, 24
  speech and language abilities, 25–26
Performance-ability (P/A) gap, 42
Persistent, predictable, consistent (PPC), 120
Phonologically disordered, 93
Physical effort, tension, avoidance, 12–13
Positron emission tomography (PET), 358
Practice and/or carryover of change, 271–273
  conducting and evaluating outside assignments, 272
  road trips, 271
  use of phone, 272
Preschool Language Scale, 96
Psyche, 339–340
Psycholinguistic factor, 34
Psychosocial adjustment, 111–115, 164–165
Psychosocial issues
  older children and teenagers, 270–271, 276

Questions (in interview procedure), 66–75
  area and style of, 66–67
  general issues, 68–69
    answered by inference and guesstimation, 68
    directly asked of client and associates, 68
    leading to testing, 68
  specific, 69–75
    academic information, 71
    anxiety/situational hierarchy, 72–73
    family history, 70

family interaction, 73–74
general development, 70
history/description of associated behavior, 72
history/description of problem, past and present, 71
introduction, 70
kind of "help" received, 73
social/behavioral, 74–75
speech/language abilities, 71–72
speech/language development and history, 70–71
wrap up, 75
specific types, 67–68
direct, 67
leading, 67
loaded, 67
mirror, 67
nondirective, 67
open-ended, 67
verbal probes, 67
yes-response, 67
Quick, accurate behavioral observations, 131
Quick Neurological Screening Test (QNST), 110

Rate and rhythmicity of repetition, 88
Rationales vs. recipes, 56–57
Reactivity, 115
Reading, 103–104
for content vs. for development of oral reading skills, 184–185
Recipe or cookbook approach, 57
Referrals to other professionals, 212–213
Referrals to therapy, 118–125
children, 122
general, 120
at low to no risk for continuing stuttering, 121
at moderate risk for continuing stuttering, 120–121
older clients for whom treatment is uncertain, 124
older clients who need therapy, 123
older clients with problems other than stuttering, 125
parents and relatives of children, 122–123
those who appear to stutter in their heads not their mouths, 124–125
Reinforcement, 312–313
Reiterative disfluencies, 222
Reluctance to deal with stuttering, 133–134
Remediation: adults who stutter, 283–325
ABCs of stuttering, 287–289
group therapy, 289–292

adult fluency groups, 289
client reluctance, 289–290
composition, 290
by itself, 291
logistics, 290
mechanics vs. feelings about speech, 291–292
SLP as group leader, 291
habitual inappropriate behavior as normal, 283–285
cautious optimism, 285
emotionality, levels of, 284–285
individual therapy, 292–322
bridging to modification, 304–306
if identification doesn't develop, 305–306
spontaneous modification, 305
identification, 295–306
adults' reactions, 296–297
bridge between off-line and on-line, 301
continuation of, 298–299
devices used, 296
early signs of improvement, 297–298
further reactions to, 303–304
identifying and physically feeling behavior, 295–296
off-line, 299–300
on-line, 301–303
time spent on per session, 297
maintenance/followup therapy, 320–322
modification, 306–320
after and then during instance of stuttering, 309–311
changing speech in conversation, 315–316
client reactions to change, 317–318
homework, 316–317
knowing when to dismiss, 318–320
movement between sounds, 306
nature of speech behavior as problem, 307
within therapy carryover, 313–315
when client fails to change, 311–312
when client produces real change, 312–313
where and what to modify, 307–309
starting up, 292–295
first impressions, 292–293
number of times per week, 294
trial therapy, 294–295
influence of the past, 283
problem dictates procedure, 285–289
late onset, 285–286
referrals from employers, 286–289
similarities to other problems, 286

Remediation: children who stutter, 129–216

children with some stuttering whose parents are also concerned, 177–186

child's "pragmatic" or usage abilities, 181–182

choosing more direct approach, 185–186

concept of hard and easy speech, 178–180

nature of communicative interaction between clinical and client, 180–181

parents' reading to children, 182–185

starting therapy, 177–178

children with some stuttering whose parents are unconcerned, 153–177

children who stutter who are almost or completely unintelligible, 161–162

child who begins to stutter after therapy for articulation problems, 160

child who stutters and exhibits speech sound problems, 161

concomitant speech and/or language problems, 155–156

dealing with articulation concerns, 158–160

dealing with language delays, 157–158

modifying stuttering, 166–167

other problems, 163–166

parent/child fluency group, 167–177

using concomitant problem to initiate therapy, 156–157

voice problems, 162–163

who knows who will become fluent and who will continue to stutter?, 154–155

children with some to great deal of stuttering whose parents are reasonably concerned, 187–215

cursive writing analogy, 208–210

don't bug children, 188

garden hose analogy, 193–198

helping child accept more active role in change, 188–189

helping child see, hear, feel stuttering, 205–207

helping child understand "forward movement," 207–208

helping parents understand unseen aspects of speaking, 189–190

helping parents understand what stuttering feels like, 190–193

not turning off child and parents to therapy, 210–212

other analogies, 199–205

referrals to other professionals, 212–214

clinician, role of, 129–138

clinician/client reluctance to deal with childhood stuttering, 133–134

parental involvement, 135–136

parents want to do the right thing, 138

pertinent literature, 134–135

problem-specific empathy, 131–133

six characteristics, 130–131

talking to parents about causes of stuttering, 136–138

stuttering as disorder of childhood, 129

therapy, 138–145

age grouping for, 144–145

child's age in relation to, 143

describing child's speech— the "s" word, 141

direct vs. indirect approaches, 143–144

suggested guidelines, 139–140

talking about talking, 141–142

when to start, how long, how often, 138–139

young children with no communicative problems whose parents are reasonably to quite concerned, 145–153

counseling parents and keeping in touch, 150–152

parents' concerns, 147–150

reevaluation of child and keeping in touch with parents, 153

Remediation: older children and teenagers who stutter, 217–281

desensitization, 228–235

"barbs" or fluency inhibitors, 230–231

encouraging child to (non)verbally interact with peers, 233–234

evaluating successfulness, 232–233

how to begin, 228–230

inattentive listeners, 231–232

learning or learning about learning, 234–235

differences in older children, 217–219, 220–221

differences in stuttering problems, 222–223

age as guide only, 223

variations among older children and teenagers, 223–224

older children with definite (cognitive/emotional) awareness of stuttering, 235–253

identification, 237–239
  modification, 240–253
  motivation, 236
older children with minimal or little awareness of
    stuttering, 224–228
  description of awareness, 224–226
  "everybody makes mistakes" approach, 227–228
  use of matter-of-fact, objective approach,
    226–227
teenagers with definite awareness of stuttering,
    254–278
  academics, social life, employment, 274–279
  assessing changes outside of therapy, 273–274
  demographics about teenagers who stutter,
    257–260
  differences between young teenagers and
    younger children who stutter, 257
  interest in and cooperation with therapy, 255–256
  motivating client to make speech changes,
    270–271
  objectively changing speech behavior, 264–269
  planning therapy: factors to consider, 260–263
  practice and carryover of change, 271–273
  12- to 14-year-olds, 254
  using other people to assist with therapy program,
    256–257
  when to begin and not begin therapy, 263–264
  understanding parents of, 219–220
Replication, importance of, 347–348
Report writing concerns, 397–400

School personnel, maintaining contact with, 278–279
Secondary or associated behaviors, 90; see also Non-
    speech behaviors
Selected Neuromotor Task Battery (SNTB), 110
Self-help organizations, 373–375
Skier vs. pogo stick analogy, 267–268
Slow-to-activate speech movement model, 34
Sociability, 115
Soma, 339–340
Sound activation vs.45 sound selection, 42–
Sound prolongations ("blocks"), 87
Sound-syllable repetition, 87
Special needs, children with, 163
Speech behavior, changing, 263–269
  distinguishing between categorical and continuous
    forms of speech production, 266–269
  learning easier onsets, 266

  learning how to change, 265
  making speech "visible," 263–264
  phasing out use of instrumentation, 266
  use of VU meter, 264
Speech disfluency, type of, 10–12
Speech Viewer, 296
Spontaneous modification, 305
Stocker Probe Technique, 79, 91
Stuttering, as childhood disorder, 129
Stuttering, awareness of, 224–226
  difference vs. disorder, 225
  type, not mere presence, 225–226
Stuttering, basic assumptions, facts, and generaliza-
    tions about, 16–23, 327–329
  table, 18
Stuttering, causes of, 26–38
  discussing with parents, 136–138
  lay opinion, 26
  professional opinions, 26
  theories of, 27–38
Stuttering, descriptions of, 3–8
  definition, 4–8
  differences between speakers and listeners, 7–8
  listener judgments, role of, 7
  relative vs. absolute, 3–4
  vs. people who stutter, 4–7
Stuttering, how to talk about with clients and families,
    50–51
Stuttering, measuring, 8–15
  change as a constant, 14–15
  frequency of disfluency, 9–10
  norms, 13–14
  physical effort, tension, avoidance, 12–13
  type of speech disfluency, 10–12
Stuttering, treatment of, general orientation, 48
Stuttering Foundation of America, 374
Stuttering-like disfluencies, 5
Stuttering-Like Disfluencies (SLD) measure, 81
Stuttering Prediction Instrument, 13, 79, 91, 92, 122,
    222
  for Young Children, 86
Stuttering Severity Instrument, 13, 15, 79, 91, 122
Subjective labels, 50
Suggestions for classroom teacher for children who
    stutter, 405–406
Syntactic, semantic, and phonological encoding,
    354–356
Syntactic encoding, 29

Talking about talking, 141–142

Teasing/mocking, 276–277

Temperament, 115–118, 352–354

Temperament Characteristics Scale (TCS), 117

Temporal coordination of tongue and jaw movements during speech, 360–364

Temporal misalignment, 38–48
  assembly-line analogy, 40–45
  mismatches between people and environment, 45–46
  mismatches due to nature interacting with nurture, 46–48

Tension *vs.* feelings of fear, 197–199

Test of Early Language Development, 96
  Primary 2, 96

Test of Word Finding, 111
  in Discourse, 111

Theories of stuttering, 27–38
  ingredient-specific (I-S) models, 30–33
    demands and capacities model, 32
    multifactorial model, 32–33
    three-factor model, 31–32
  mechanism-specific (M-S) models, 33–38
    covert repair hypothesis, 35–37
    dyssynchronous syllable frames and segment content model, 34–35
    fault line hypothesis, 34
    slow-to-activate speech movement model, 34
  nature, nurture, or interaction, 27–28

Therapy, benefit of, 123

Three-factor model, 31–32

Threshold of acceptability, 11

Thumb and opposing fingers analogy, 201, 203

Touching hot stove burner analogy, 192–193

Tourette's syndrome, 107–108

Transfer, 340–344
  carryover problems, 341–342
  maintaining modification, 340–341
  need for pre- *vs.* post-therapy research, 342–344

Transitions, 364–366

Treatment efficacy, 367–371

Trial therapy, adult, 294–295

Vanderbilt University
  Disfluency Frequency Count Sheet, 82–83
  Fluency Diagnostic Summary Sheet, 80–81

Verbal expression, 181

Video recordings, 63–64
  child's reaction to, 205–206

Visi-Pitch, 264, 296

Voice, 99–102

Voice onset time (VOT), 347

Voice problems, 162–163
  hoarseness, 163
  low-pitched monotone (Johnny-one-note), 162–163

Warmth, 130

What has to be changed analogy, 268–269

Whole-word repetition, 87

Within-word disfluencies, 5, 9, 79

Woodstock reading test, 110

Word finding, 110–111